CONSUMERS' GUIDE TO

Hospitals

BY THE EDITORS OF CONSUMERS' CHECKBOOK MAGAZINE

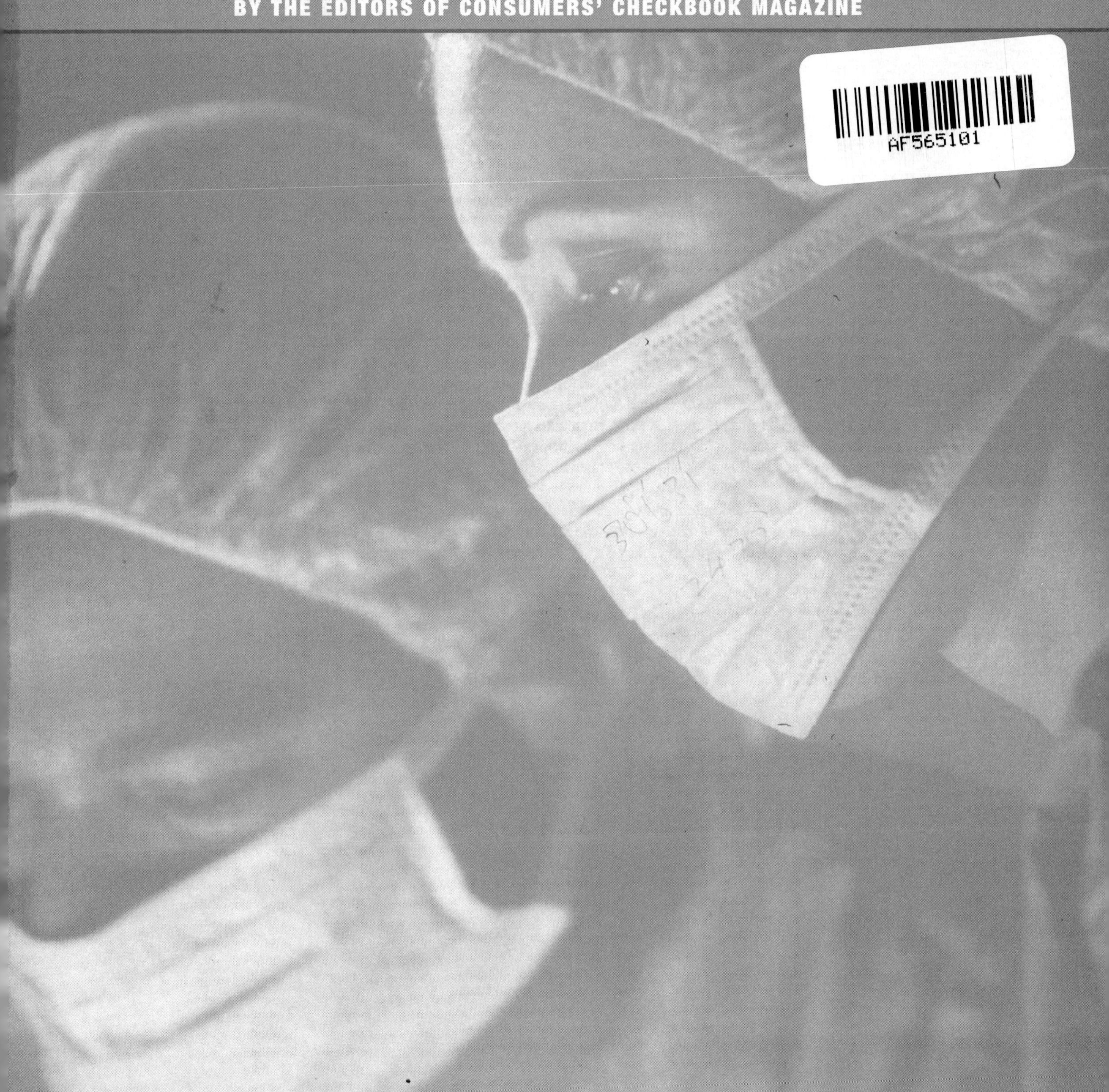

Consumers' CHECKBOOK is a program of the Center for the Study of Services, a nonprofit organization dedicated to helping consumers get the most for their money when they buy services. Founded in 1974, the Center is supported by subscribers to the two magazines it publishes in the Washington, DC, and San Francisco Bay areas, by sales of special books and reports in print and on the Web, by sales of other consumer information services, and by sales of survey, research, and analysis services. Its magazines, entitled *Washington Consumers' CHECKBOOK* and *Bay Area Consumers' CHECKBOOK*, rate the quality and prices of local service firms of various kinds, ranging from auto repair shops to banks to physicians. The Center plans to begin publishing additional versions of *Consumers' CHECKBOOK* magazine in other metropolitan areas in the near future. This book is a special *Consumers' CHECKBOOK* publication.

ISBN 1-888124-12-1 Library of Congress Control Number 2002104079

Consumers' CHECKBOOK
733 15th Street NW, Suite 820
Washington, DC 20005
202-347-7283
www.checkbook.org

Contents

Preface

Few of us look forward enthusiastically to a stay in a hospital. That's as it should be. Hospital stays are not fun, and stays at even the very best hospitals pose significant risks of infections and other mishaps.

But you'll be more comfortable entering a hospital if you know that the hospital stay is really necessary, that the hospital was selected carefully, and that you know how to deal effectively with the hospital's staff. This book is intended to help you find that peace of mind.

For each of 4,500 acute care hospitals nationwide, this book gives you important information on what has actually happened to each hospital's patients: estimates of the percent of patients with various types of cases who have died or experienced adverse outcomes, including complications. It also gives you scores from on-site inspections and reviews conducted by the Joint Commission on the Accreditation of Healthcare Organizations. In addition, the book gives you other key facts that relate to quality: information on hospital size and information on programs at each hospital for ongoing training of physicians. For hospitals in major metropolitan areas, we give you results from a major survey we conducted, in which we gathered ratings from more than 16,000 physicians in those areas: we tell you how each hospital was judged by those physicians.

Whatever hospital you choose, you'll want to get the best care the hospital has to offer. What you get depends in part on how well you are informed about what to expect during your stay—why you are there, what drugs and procedures you're to be exposed to, how much attention you should get from the nursing staff, etc. It also depends on how carefully you and your family and friends keep an eye on what the staff is doing. This book will help you prepare for your stay and play a useful role in your care.

Finally, you'll find advice on ways to help keep down the cost of your hospital stay. That's good for you and good for the community.

Hospitals in Major Metropolitan Areas That Received Our Top Rating (✓)

The hospitals listed here are those that received *Consumers' CHECKBOOK*'s checkmark (✓), indicating a top rating for quality. These hospitals were selected based on having met or exceeded thresholds we set for ratings by physicians, adjusted mortality rates, and overall evaluation scores from the Joint Commission on the Accreditation of Healthcare Organizations. The scoring is based entirely on data presented in the table beginning on page 32, so you are free to make different selections based on the same data. Please see an explanation, beginning on page 14, of all of the types of data used in this book.

In cases where some types of data were not available for a hospital, the hospital may have suffered a disadvantage in *CHECKBOOK*'s scoring. For example, specialty children's hospitals could not score high enough to receive our checkmark because we did not have mortality rate information for them or sufficient ratings information from surveyed physicians. Also, the hospitals listed here were selected only from the hospitals in the major metropolitan areas listed on the "Metro Areas" table beginning on page 32. This geographic limitation excluded some excellent hospitals located in less populous areas. (The clearest example of an exclusion of this kind is the Mayo Clinic hospitals—Saint Marys and Rochester Methodist—in Rochester, Minnesota. These hospitals have low adjusted mortality rates and were widely praised by doctors we surveyed in other areas.)

For more information on hospitals, please see the tables beginning on page 32 and on page 74. You will also find information on nationally recognized centers for difficult cases on page 352 and on cancer specialty centers on page 353.

Arizona

Arizona Heart, Phoenix
Desert Samaritan, Mesa
Good Samaritan Regional, Phoenix
Mayo Clinic, Phoenix
St Joseph's, Phoenix
Scottsdale Healthcare - Osborn, Scottsdale
Scottsdale Healthcare - Shea, Scottsdale

California

California Pacific - California Campus, San Francisco
Cedars - Sinai, Los Angeles
Eisenhower, Rancho Mirage
El Camino, Mountain View
Good Samaritan, Los Angeles
Hoag Presbyterian, Newport Beach
Huntington, Pasadena
John Muir, Walnut Creek
LAC - Harbor - UCLA, Torrance
Long Beach Memorial, Long Beach
Mercy General, Sacramento
Methodist Hospital of Southern California, Arcadia
Mission Regional, Mission Viejo
Providence Holy Cross, Mission Hills
Providence St Joseph, Burbank
St Johns, Santa Monica
San Francisco General, San Francisco
Scripps Green, La Jolla
Stanford Hospital, Stanford
UCLA, Los Angeles
University of California - Irvine, Orange
USC University, Los Angeles

Colorado

Denver Health, Denver
Rose, Denver
Swedish, Englewood
University of Colorado, Denver

Connecticut

Hartford Hospital, Hartford
Hospital of St Raphael, New Haven
St Francis, Hartford
St Vincent's, Bridgeport
University of Connecticut - John Dempsey, Farmington
Yale - New Haven, New Haven

Delaware

Christiana Care, Newark

District of Columbia

George Washington University, Washington
Georgetown University, Washington
Sibley, Washington
Washington Hospital Center, Washington

Florida

Baptist, Miami
Bayfront, St Petersburg
Boca Raton Community, Boca Raton
Broward General, Fort Lauderdale
Cedars, Miami
Holy Cross, Fort Lauderdale
Jackson Memorial, Miami
JFK, Atlantis
Morton Plant Mease, Clearwater
Mt Sinai, Miami Beach
Mt Sinai & Miami Heart Institute, Miami Beach
Orlando Regional, Orlando
St Joseph's, Tampa
Sarasota Memorial, Sarasota
South Miami, Miami
Tampa General, Tampa
University of Miami - Sylvester Cancer Center, Miami

Georgia

Crawford Long - Emory University, Atlanta
Emory University, Atlanta
Northside, Atlanta
Piedmont, Atlanta
St Joseph's, Atlanta

Illinois

Advocate Good Samaritan, Downers Grove
Advocate Lutheran/Lutheran Children's, Park Ridge
Evanston Northwestern, Evanston
Loyola University, Maywood
Northwestern, Chicago
Rush - Presbyterian - St Lukes, Chicago
University of Illinois, Chicago

Indiana

Clarian Health Partners, Indianapolis
St Vincent, Indianapolis
Wishard, Indianapolis

Kansas

Shawnee Mission Medical Center, Shawnee Mission

Louisiana

Memorial - Baptist Campus, New Orleans
Touro Infirmary, New Orleans
Tulane University, New Orleans

Maryland

Greater Baltimore, Baltimore
Johns Hopkins, Baltimore
Johns Hopkins Bayview, Baltimore
Sinai, Baltimore
Suburban, Bethesda
Union, Baltimore
University of Maryland, Baltimore

Massachusetts

Beth Israel Deaconess, Boston
Boston Medical Center, Boston
Brigham and Women's, Boston
Massachusetts General, Boston
Mt Auburn, Cambridge
New England Baptist, Boston
New England Medical Center, Boston
St Elizabeth's, Brighton

Michigan

Detroit Receiving, Detroit
Harper University, Detroit
Henry Ford, Detroit
St John, Detroit
William Beaumont, Royal Oak
William Beaumont, Troy

Minnesota

Methodist, St Louis Park
Regions, St Paul

Missouri

Barnes - Jewish, St Louis
Research, Kansas City
St John's Mercy, Creve Coeur
St Louis University, St Louis
St Luke's, Chesterfield
St Luke's, Kansas City

Nevada

University, Las Vegas

New Jersey

Deborah Heart and Lung, Browns Mills
Englewood Hospital, Englewood
Hackensack University, Hackensack
Newark Beth Israel, Newark
Overlook, Summit
Robert Wood Johnson University, New Brunswick
St Barnabas, Livingston
St Peter's University, New Brunswick
University, Newark
Valley, Ridgewood

New York

Bellevue, New York
Genesee, Rochester
Hospital for Special Surgery, New York
Lenox Hill, New York
Long Island Jewish, New Hyde Park
Memorial Sloan - Kettering Cancer, New York
Montefiore, Bronx
Mt Sinai, New York
New York Presbyterian, New York
New York Weill Cornell of NY Presbyterian, New York
North Shore University, Manhasset
NYU Hospital Center, New York
Rochester General, Rochester
St Francis, Roslyn
Strong, Rochester
University, Stony Brook
Winthrop - University, Mineola

North Carolina

Carolinas, Charlotte
North Carolina Baptist, Winston-Salem
Presbyterian, Charlotte
Rex, Raleigh
University of North Carolina, Chapel Hill
Wakemed, Raleigh

Ohio

Arthur G James Cancer/Richard J Solove, Columbus
Christ, Cincinnati
Cleveland Clinic Foundation, Cleveland
Hillcrest, Mayfield Heights
Metrohealth, Cleveland
Ohio State University Medical Center, Columbus
University, Cincinnati
University, Cleveland

Pennsylvania

Abington Memorial, Abington
Allegheny General, Pittsburgh
Bryn Mawr Hospital, Bryn Mawr
Hahnemann University, Philadelphia
Lankenau, Wynnewood
Magee - Womens, Pittsburgh
Mercy, Pittsburgh
Pennsylvania, Philadelphia
Presbyterian, Philadelphia
Temple University, Philadelphia
Thomas Jefferson University, Philadelphia
University of Pennsylvania, Philadelphia
UPMC Presbyterian, Pittsburgh
UPMC Shadyside, Pittsburgh

Rhode Island

Miriam, Providence
Rhode Island, Providence

Tennessee

Baptist, Nashville
Centennial, Nashville
St Thomas, Nashville
Vanderbilt University, Nashville

Texas

Harris Methodist Fort Worth, Fort Worth
Medical City Dallas Hospital, Dallas
Methodist, Houston
Parkland, Dallas
St David's, Austin
St Lukes Episcopal, Houston
Zale Lipshy University, Dallas

Utah

LDS, Salt Lake City
St Mark's, Salt Lake City
University of Utah, Salt Lake City

Virginia

Inova Fairfax, Falls Church
Sentara Leigh, Norfolk
Sentara Norfolk General, Norfolk

Washington

Swedish, Seattle
Swedish - Providence Campus, Seattle
University of Washington, Seattle

Wisconsin

Froedtert Memorial Lutheran, Milwaukee
St Luke's, Milwaukee

Chapter 1:

Learning About Your Case

To make the best possible choice of hospital, you must learn as much as time allows about your case. This education is also essential for you to answer two other critical questions: what is really wrong with you and what is the best approach to treatment? In addition, whatever you learn will help you play an active role later on in monitoring your care.

If a doctor recommends hospitalization, here are a few questions for you to ask (often in this book when we refer to "you," we assume it is relatives or friends who will take responsibility for a sick patient):

- What is the basis for the diagnosis? Are there other possible explanations for your symptoms? Might it make sense to do further tests or simply to wait awhile to get a surer diagnosis?
- What are the alternative ways of treating your problem? What are the pros and cons of each—the chances of various outcomes in terms of your lifestyle and ability to function?
- Why are the particular hospital, and the particular doctor who would care for you, good choices for your care?
- How complicated is the treatment you will get? Does it require sophisticated medical staff or advanced equipment?
- What are the risks of complications? Will it be important to have close monitoring and quick access to sophisticated medical staff and equipment at all times?
- Is your required treatment one for which special training or frequent experience is important? Are there certain hospitals or specialists who have more skill, more experience, and higher success rates than others with this treatment?

Up-to-date physicians will encourage you to ask such questions, will offer answers, and will steer you to sources for further research. Don't be concerned about insulting your physician by asking questions. It helps to write out your questions as a reminder. If your doctor is hard to talk with, take along a friend to help you press for answers.

A good physician will also encourage you to seek a second opinion. Get one.

Get your second opinion from an entirely independent doctor. If a surgeon who has recommended surgery refers you to another surgeon for a second opinion, it will be difficult for the second doctor to recommend against the advice (and the economic interests) of the first. To find a doctor to use for a second opinion, you can ask friends and co-workers for recommendations, contact a medical school, or ask for a referral from a well-regarded hospital. *Consumers' CHECKBOOK*'s book, *Consumers' Guide to Top Doctors*, identifies more than 15,000 top physician specialists who can give second opinions in 34 specialty fields. (That book can be ordered by calling 1-800-213-7283 or the information can be accessed directly on the Web at *www.checkbook.org*. The price is $19.95 either for the book or for two years of online access to the information.) If you read up on your type of case—especially if it is of a type that is being actively researched at certain medical centers—you may come upon names of leading specialists who might be available for advice. When two doctors from whom you get opinions disagree or are uncertain, you may want to seek additional opinions.

To keep down the cost and time required for a second opinion, have your first doctor send copies of your medical records, x-rays, and lab results to the second opinion doctor. This is standard procedure.

Medicare and most insurance plans will pay for second opinions, and in some circumstances plans may pay for third opinions. In some types of cases, insurance plans *require* second opinions.

Don't assume that because yours is a straightforward, uncomplicated case there is nothing to learn and there are no decisions to be made. In most cases, there are choices.

This point is brought home by studies done by Dartmouth Medical School researchers and others, looking at variations in medical practice in common types of cases across similar geographic areas. These studies have found, for example, that about 75 percent of the elderly men in one Maine town had undergone prostate surgery, compared with fewer than 25 percent of men the same age in an adjacent town. Similar variations have been found in rates of hysterectomies, caesarean sections, and other common procedures. Significantly, studies generally find no evidence that such medical practice differences result in differences in the health status of the affected populations.

The implication is that big differences in the ways patients are treated result from differences in the beliefs and customs of different physicians in different communities—possibly influenced by financial considerations—the need to generate fees—and not necessarily based on sound evidence of likely benefits to the patient. Even in a common type of case, you can't assume that a physician's recommendation is the best option for you.

To learn about your case, you can start with one of the family health books available in most bookstores and public libraries. Examples are the *Harvard Medical School Family Health Guide*, the *Mayo Clinic Family Health Book*, and the *American College of Physicians Complete Home Medical Guide*. To learn more about your case, you can take advantage of much more extensive information available in libraries. At public libraries, you can look at consumer-oriented newsletters and at medical textbooks. For more in-depth information, you can use a medical school library. These libraries will have both general textbooks and texts in specialty fields. They will also have peer-reviewed medical journals, which will have articles on new developments not yet reflected in textbooks. Contact the most conveniently located medical school and ask what the rules are for public access. Medical school libraries may also be able to help you find support groups and organizations that regularly provide information on your type of medical problem.

You can also find an enormous amount of information online. You can use any major search engine to find information on a disease, test, or treatment. But be careful about the information you use. Inaccurate information can find its way to the Web just as easily as reliable information. And much of what you find on the Web is paid for by drug companies and other commercial interests, with resulting biases. A Federal government website with basic information is *www.healthfinder.gov*. A valuable resource for a wide variety of information is the website of the National Library of Medicine of the Federal government's National Institutes of Health at *www.nlm.nih.gov*. In addition to other information available at this website, you can use the site to locate the most authoritative articles on any medical subject. You can read summaries of many articles online and then order copies, for a fee, from a participating medical library.

As you learn more about your treatment choices, you'll also learn about hospital choices. If yours is a case that requires a high degree of specialization that is currently available only at a few medical centers, you will want to use one of these centers for treatment. If yours is a complicated, high-risk case, you will want to use a hospital with sophisticated capabilities to deal with complications. If the case is low-risk, you might choose to give substantial consideration to the pleasantness of the staff and facility and its convenience to your home, family, and friends.

Chapter 2:
Why Your Choice of Hospital Matters

Today's hospitals can shatter kidney stones with sound waves; can look at tissues deep inside a patient's body without ever making a cut; have machines to take over when organs fail; in short, can do what only a few decades ago was beyond belief.

But hospitals remain today, as they always have been, dangerous places. Where else do you allow someone to cut deep into your body, inject potent chemicals into your veins, feed you strong drugs, and intervene in your life in so many other ways? In the operation of such powerful forces, at a time when you are sick and vulnerable, a single mistake can have catastrophic consequences.

And mistakes do occur: missed diagnoses as a result of inaccurate lab or x-ray results, administration of unprescribed medication, too slow response in emergencies, infections passed among patients, heart attacks caused by feeding the wrong solution into an IV hookup, operations on the wrong patient or the wrong organ, unintended lacerations of healthy organs, patients falling down or falling out of bed while under sedation, chokings from vomiting of meals improperly given before surgery, and many more.

In 2000, the Institute of Medicine of the National Academy of Sciences released an estimate of the extent of the problem in a shocking report, "To Err Is Human." Extrapolating from the results of two large studies of hospital cases, in 1984 and 1992, the Institute concluded that "at least 44,000 and perhaps as many as 98,000 Americans die in hospitals each year as a result of medical errors"—preventable adverse events. That is more than the number of deaths attributable to motor vehicle accidents, breast cancer, or AIDS.

There are also many other cases where hospital or doctor negligence, while not causing death, slows recovery or leads to short-term or long-term disability.

And those are the cases of negligence. There are countless cases where doctors and hospitals are not negligent but do fail to provide the best possible care—the kind of innovative, skilled, responsive care that might give you better than average chances of a successful and speedy cure or recovery.

In a 1999 speech, Donald M. Berwick, a well-known physician, Harvard Medical School professor, and chief executive of the Institute for Healthcare Improvement, put a human face on the problem. He described—with his wife, Ann's, permission—the experience he and Ann had endured during the previous year, in which Ann had six hospitalizations for a total of over 60 inpatient days in three institutions:

> "Let me first say that this painful summer and fall has left me more impressed than I have ever been before with the good will, kindness, generosity, commitment, and dignity of the people who work in health care—almost all of them...
>
> "Which makes it hard to tell the other side of the story. Put very, very simply: the people work well by and large, but the system often does not...
>
> "[Medication errors] were not rare, they were the norm. The neurologist in one admission told us in the morning, 'by no means should you be getting anticholinergic agents,' and a medication with profound anticholinergic side effects was given that afternoon. The attending neurologist in another admission told us by phone that a crucial and potentially toxic drug should be begun immediately. He said, 'time is of the essence.' That was on Thursday morning at 10:00 a.m. The first dose was given 60 hours later... Colace was discontinued by a physician's order on Day 1, and was nonetheless brought by the nurse every single evening throughout a 14-day admission...
>
> "A spinal tap was done for a crucial test for Lyme disease, but the doctor collected too little fluid for the test, and the tap had to be repeated. During a crucial phase of diagnosis, one doctor told us to hope that the diagnosis would be of a certain disease, because that disease has a benign course. The same evening, another doctor told us to hope for the opposite, because that same disease is relentless—sometimes fatal... [Information was] collected in disorganized, narrative formats, embedded in nursing notes and daily forms... As a result, physicians often reached erroneous conclusions about the past...
>
> "On at least three occasions, Ann waited alone for over an hour, cold, and frightened on a Gurney in the waiting area outside an MRI unit in a sub-basement in the middle of the night... Ann's bedtime was 10:00 p.m., but her sleeping medication was often brought at 8:00 p.m. to accommodate changes in nursing shifts... One place gave a sleeping pill at 3:00 a.m., and then routinely woke Ann at 4:00 a.m. to take her blood pressure, which never varied from normal."

These were just some of the examples Berwick reported. Fortunately, by the time he delivered the speech, he could report that Ann's condition had clearly begun to improve. But he and Ann, among the most sophisticated of all possible patients, much more able than most to recognize problems, had seen both the best and the worst of hospital care. Berwick used his and his wife's personal story as part of his life's work—to exhort his professional colleagues to make the system work better. The rest of us can take from it a warning that we must be vigilant in the selection of hospitals for care, and we must be vigilant and actively involved in our care in whatever hospital we use.

What you want for your care is a hospital that will keep mistakes to a minimum and that will help you quickly improve your medical condition and your ability to function; limit your discomfort; improve, or at least maintain, your morale; and make your stay reasonably pleasant.

One of Berwick's conclusions about the hospitals in which his wife received care was that "some were, in fact, much better than others."

That is a conclusion supported by the data in this book and by much other research. There are differences in how astute medical staffs are at spotting changes in a patient's condition, how adept nursing staffs are at instilling optimism in their patients, how good a facility's entire staff is at maintaining sanitary conditions, and myriad other aspects of hospital performance.

In addition to the inherent difficulty of delivering and coordinating complex care simultaneously to hundreds of patients in large institutions, hospitals face the stress of having to deliver this care under financial pressures. In many cases today, hospitals are paid a fixed amount per patient based on what Medicare or another private or public insurance program has determined is the average cost for patients with similar diagnoses. As a result, a hospital can achieve surplus income by cutting the cost of serving each patient or can take a loss if it keeps its patients too long or gives them care that is too intensive.

Since giving high-quality care—and avoiding complications—is often the best way to get patients out of the hospital quickly, and since early release appears to be good for the health of many patients, this payment system, with its incentives to reduce unnecessary care, is not necessarily bad for quality. But it definitely creates incentives that may cause hospitals in some circumstances to give less, or lower quality, care than would be in your best interest. This possibility reinforces the need for effective hospital-to-hospital quality comparison.

Certainly, if you are among the roughly one out of ten Americans who will be admitted to a hospital this year, you will want to be sure it's the best. But judging hospital quality is complex. Differences in hospitals' death rates among heart attack patients, for example, might simply mean that some hospitals get sicker, more frail patients; or that some send their patients prematurely to nursing homes, where they die; or that some are used by a few incompetent physicians who lose their patients despite the best possible care from the hospitals' own staffs.

In this book, we advise you on some facts to look for in selecting a hospital and we suggest ways you can enhance the quality of care you receive at whichever hospital you choose. The book includes extensive information on individual hospitals to help you choose a good one. We report data on death rates and rates of other adverse outcomes, results of surveys in which thousands of physicians rated hospitals, results of inspections by experts who visited the hospitals as part of the accreditation process, information on training programs in the hospitals, and other facts.

Unfortunately, these data do not give a clearcut way to sort the best hospitals from the worst. All of the measures have some methodological shortcomings, which are discussed at some length in Chapter 4. Some hospitals look good on some measures and not on others. But this information will enable you to find a few hospitals that look good across the board, and will add to what you know about almost any hospital you might consider. The information will help you have informed discussions about hospital choice with your physician.

By making the data in this book accessible to consumers, we hope we have strengthened incentives for government, the hospital industry, and health care researchers to continue to make improvements in methods for comparing hospitals.

Chapter 3:

The Need to Choose

Much of the responsibility for choosing the right hospital for you rests with your doctor. But you too must play an important role.

Your choice of hospital will generally be rather narrow if your primary care doctor proposes admitting you to a hospital under his or her own care. Most doctors have arranged privileges for themselves to admit patients only at a few hospitals, or a single hospital. In surveys we have conducted of physicians in the Washington, DC, and San Francisco Bay areas, we have found that, among those who admit at least 25 patients per year, about half use only a single hospital for almost all (at least 95 percent) of their cases. An additional 30 percent or so use only two hospitals almost all the time, and fewer than 10 percent put any significant number of their patients in four or more different hospitals.

But there's a good chance your primary care doctor will refer you to a specialist who will be the one who arranges for your admission to a hospital. You can consider hospital affiliation as one basis for selecting the specialist you will use.

Your primary care doctor will probably favor a specialist who practices at one of his or her own hospitals. These are usually the specialists your doctor knows best. Also, your doctor may want to see you in the hospital and work with the specialist. But the choices need not be limited to your doctor's hospitals. You will want your primary care doctor to remain involved in your case, to advise you and assure that all aspects of your care are coordinated, but the doctor might not have to have privileges at the hospital where you will be admitted in order to play this role. Discuss this issue with your primary care doctor. Ask your doctor if he or she can arrange to keep up-to-date on your care by communicating with the doctor or doctors who will be responsible for you in the hospital.

All this presumes that you have a doctor. But there is another point at which comparison of hospitals is important: when you are first choosing a doctor or health plan. There are two reasons to look for a doctor or health plan that uses high-quality hospitals. First, this will enhance your chances of being admitted to such a hospital in the future if the need arises. Second, it enhances your chances that your doctor will be a top-quality professional: good hospitals can be expected to attract good physicians.

A comparison of hospitals is especially important if you are considering a health maintenance organization (HMO) or a preferred provider organization (PPO). If an HMO or PPO uses high-quality hospitals, that suggests that its overall medical care standards are high.

Chapter 4:

Choosing the Best Hospital

Given the importance of choosing a high-quality hospital, much of this book is devoted to helping you make a good selection. There will be no clear-cut answers, but we can give you key information to help you judge most of the hospitals in the U.S., and we can advise on additional information you can collect on your own.

This chapter is divided into two main sections. The first is an overview, with a brief description of the information this book provides you on individual hospitals, additional information you can gather on your own, and how you can use the information to make a hospital choice. The second—for those who are interested—is a more detailed description of our data on individual hospitals and the strengths and weaknesses of these data.

Overview

This book contains two large tables, the Key Ratings for Metro Areas table (which we will refer to as the "Metro Areas" table), beginning on page 32, and the Detailed Ratings for All Areas table (which we will refer to as the "All Areas" table), beginning on page 74. The Metro Areas table includes hospitals in the central portions of the 50 largest Metropolitan Statistical Areas (MSAs) or Primary Metropolitan Statistical Areas (PMSAs) in the U.S., and an additional 21 MSAs or PMSAs that are, for the most part, adjacent to the 50 largest ones. The All Areas table includes all the hospitals listed on the Metro Areas table and also hospitals throughout the remainder of the U.S.

The tables in this book include nearly every short-term hospital for acute inpatient care in the U.S. except Veterans and military hospitals. (A few other hospitals are left out because of difficulties in matching data from multiple sources.) There are more than 1,300 hospitals on the Metro Areas table and more than 4,500 hospitals on the All Areas table. (See Notes on Identifying and Naming Hospitals on page 350.)

The Metro Areas Table

The Metro Areas table includes the following data—

- **Doctors' ratings.** These are the percentages of physicians who, in a large survey we conducted, rated each hospital "very good" or "excellent" for "surgery on an adult in cases where the risk of complications is high." We also show the number of doctors who rated each hospital on this question.
- **Desirability scores from doctors.** These are the results when we asked each surveyed physician to name the two hospitals, from a list in the physician's metropolitan area, that he or she would consider "most desirable" and the two he or she would consider "least desirable" for several different types of health care needs, from "uncomplicated delivery of a baby" to "medical care for an adult in complex cases." We report for each hospital for each type of case the percentage of its mentions that were favorable: that is, the number of times physicians mentioned it as desirable as a percentage of the total times physicians mentioned it as either desirable or undesirable.
- **Adjusted death rates.** These are the percentages of each hospital's patients, for a three-year period, who died within 30 days of the time they were admitted to the hospital. These rates are adjusted—to the extent we were able—for differences in how sick and frail each hospital's patients were. Rates are reported for selected, relatively high-risk cases in three categories: medical cases, surgical cases, and a combination of medical and surgical cases.
- **Adjusted adverse outcome rates.** These are similar to the death rates except that adverse outcomes include both deaths and complications (estimated by us) that resulted in extended stays in the hospital.
- **Overall scores on accreditation review.** These are scores the hospitals received on their most recent full review by the Joint Commission on the Accreditation of Healthcare Organizations (JCAHO), which sends on-site inspectors to hospitals no less often than once every three years.
- **Major medical school affiliations.** This is simply one indicator of the extent of each hospital's teaching programs for doctors.

For each of these measures, we indicate with blue type the most favorable scores and with ***bold-italic*** type the least favorable scores. In addition, we give our checkmark (✓) to hospitals that rated high on an overall score we calculated across a range of measures.

The All Areas Table

The All Areas table includes the following data—

- **Adjusted death rates for all selected cases.** This measure is the same as the figure reported on the Metro Areas table for the combination of medical and surgical cases. In addition, we report the number of cases each hospital had of the types included in the analysis. In addition, we include actual death rates—the rates found for each hospital before our adjustment for how sick and frail each hospital's patients were.

- **Whether death rates were better or worse than average.** For each hospital, for various categories of cases, we indicate with a star (★) if the hospital's death rate was better than would be expected, given how sick and frail its patients were. We indicate with an × if the hospital's death rate was worse than would be expected. To get a star (or an ×), a hospital had to do enough better (or worse) than expected that we could be quite confident that its better (or worse) performance was not just a matter of luck. We use a blue star (★) or a bold ✖ for the results we are most confident about. Many hospitals simply have blanks on the table for most or all categories of cases. That simply means that we could not be confident that their outcomes were different from what would be expected, given how sick and frail their patients were. There are also many hospitals that have a "—" on the table for many categories of cases. That means these hospitals had a relatively small number of cases in these categories—so small that we could not make a judgment on their outcomes.
- **Whether adverse outcome rates were better or worse than average.** This is like the death rate information except it takes into account both deaths and complications (our estimate) that resulted in extended lengths of stay in the hospital. Adverse outcome rates are reported only for surgical cases.
- **Accreditation status.** This is the status the hospital received on its last full review by JCAHO. All listed hospitals received (in order of desirability) accreditation with full standards compliance, accreditation with requirements for improvement, or conditional accreditation.
- **Overall JCAHO evaluation score.** This measure is the same as the figure shown on the Metro Areas table.
- **Number of beds.** This gives you a sense of a hospital's size. There is some evidence that larger hospitals have better outcomes.
- **Major medical school affiliations.** This information is the same as what is shown on the Metro Areas table.
- **Number of residents.** This is the number of doctors who work at each hospital as part of programs for advanced post-medical school training. It is an indicator of the extent of a hospital's teaching programs.
- **Computerized drug order entry system.** This measure, which is meaningful only for a limited number of hospitals in areas where the information on these systems was actively solicited, indicates whether hospitals have computerized systems that can be expected to reduce the risk of drug errors, a common type of complication. In coming months, many other hospitals in other parts of the country can be expected to report having such systems.

As with the Metro Areas table, we indicate with **blue** type the most favorable scores and with ***bold-italic*** type the least favorable scores. Note that on the All Areas table we have no information from our survey of physicians. That's because we did that survey only in 71 major metropolitan areas.

Other Hospital Listings

In addition to our two main tables, we have some other information on hospitals. On our survey of doctors, we asked each doctor: "If there are any major types of cases in which you would want your loved one to get care at a medical center in some other part of the country, please tell us below the type(s) of cases and the name(s) and location(s) of the facility or facilities you would recommend." This is a very unstructured approach, but gave the doctors an opportunity to share their expertise in an informal way. We share some of the information from this part of the survey in the listing on page 352. We also have included a special list of distinguished cancer treatment centers, on page 353, and a list of hospitals that have gained recognition for the quality of their nursing care, on page 355.

You might reasonably be interested in knowing how well patients rate hospitals. We are collecting such information in a number of metropolitan areas for our local consumer magazine, *Consumers' CHECKBOOK*. As we go to press, *Consumers' CHECKBOOK* magazine is published only in the Washington, DC, and San Francisco Bay areas, where it includes ratings of various types of local service firms, from auto repair shops to plumbers to hospitals. Soon additional versions will be launched in the Boston, Chicago, Philadelphia, Seattle, and Twin Cities areas. All of those magazines will include consumer ratings of hospitals.

Other Information You Can Gather On Your Own

In addition to the information on our tables, there is additional information you can gather on your own.

The Hospitals' Doctors

If you have a strong relationship with a physician who would care for you during a hospital stay, you will want to be wary of making a hospital selection that will force you to give up, or strain, that relationship. This is especially true if your case is one—knee ligament surgery, for instance—in which there is low risk of hospital-caused death or serious complications, but surgeon-to-surgeon differences in outcome in terms of your ability to function as you would like are substantial.

Before letting a physician relationship dictate choice of hospital, check whether the physician you prefer can be flexible. If it is your primary care physician whom you want involved in your case but you are going to have surgery or some other treatment that will be managed by a specialist while you are in the hospital, you might want to choose a specialist affiliated with the hospital you would prefer. You can ask your primary care physician to arrange to communicate regularly with that specialist.

Also, before choosing a hospital based on a physician relationship, be sure the physician or physicians you are counting on will actually be caring for you. Find out which doctor will be in charge of your care in the hospital. Will it be your primary care doctor, a surgeon, or some other doctor? Find out how often each doctor will be visiting you. If you have arranged for surgery from a well-known surgeon, make sure that this is the surgeon who will actually do the hands-on surgery. Some big name surgeons set up and supervise surgery but leave it to their assistants to do most of the work; if that is the plan, you might want to change surgeons.

Regardless of whether you currently have a strong relationship with a physician, one way to judge hospitals is by checking whether they have high-quality physicians affiliated with them. The best physicians are not likely to send their patients to low-quality hospitals. If there are physicians you know to be excellent, find out which hospitals they use. *Consumers' CHECKBOOK*'s book, *Consumers' Guide to Top Doctors* (which can be ordered by calling 1-800-213-7283), is a source of names of top-quality doctors whose hospital affiliations you can check out.

Special Services

You might want to consider whether a hospital has special services, programs, and strengths of kinds that are not addressed on our data tables. For example, if you are likely to need rehabilitation services, you might want a hospital that has strong capabilities in that field. You can ask your physician which hospitals have such special capabilities. You can also check with your state or local hospital association. The list on page 353 includes hospitals that specialize in one type of care, cancer care.

Consumer Reviews

You can learn a lot of important information about hospitals by making your own visits or talking with other consumers who have been patients in, or regularly visited, available facilities. The best way to learn about a facility is to observe when visiting friends of loved ones (or being a patient, of course), but you can also learn by calling the administrator's office at any hospital you are considering and arranging a tour. There's much to look for—

- Check the rooms. Are they roomy enough? How noisy are they? Is there privacy in patient beds and in bathrooms—from the hall and from the other patient in semi-private rooms? Are private rooms available and at what cost? Are the rooms clean and attractive? Are there windows with a pleasant view, and can they be opened for fresh air? Is there good lighting? Is there an easily accessible call button at bedside and in the bathroom? Are TV sets placed where they can be easily viewed? Can headphones be arranged so that you and your roommate, if you have one, can avoid disturbing one another? Is there air conditioning? Can temperatures be controlled on a room-by-room basis?
- Check the halls. Are they clean? Are they free of foul smells? Are they free of heavy smells of deodorizers that might be masking cleanliness problems?
- Check the other patient areas. Are there pleasant sitting areas and places where patients can walk close to their rooms? Can patients walk or sit outside in a safe and convenient place on pleasant days? Are there a cafeteria, newsstand, lobby and other facilities that will make the facility pleasant for visitors?
- Ask for a list of hospital policies. Are the visiting hours reasonable? What are the hours for receiving phone calls? Can children visit? How much flexibility is there on mealtimes and bedtimes? Can arrangements be made for a relative or close friend to sleep-in near the patient? In general, do policies seem reasonable?
- Check the staff. Do nurses and other staff members seem responsive to patient needs? Do they respond promptly when called? Do they take the time to listen and answer questions? Are they gentle? Are they respectful? Do they seem competent?
- Check the food. Does it seem fresh and attractive? Are fresh fruits served, and are fresh vegetables not overcooked? Do hot meals arrive hot and cold meals cold? Do patients who are not on physician-ordered diets have any choice of meals? Can arrangements be made for vegetarian, kosher, or other special diets?
- Check the social work services. What are the staff's capabilities for arranging needed services after discharge? Do they follow through?

The data on the tables in this book relate to serious, high-risk cases. Even in such cases, having pleasant surroundings, good meals, and other comforts will be important to you, but these features deserve special weight in low-risk cases. In all cases, it is very important that family and friends can conveniently visit you. Visitors can bolster your morale and thus speed your recovery. The presence of visitors puts the hospital staff on notice that someone cares about you; that might make the hospital staff more attentive also. In addition, having family or friends to observe the care you are getting is critical. They can help you look out for medication errors, gaps in staff followup, inattention to your pain, hospital routines like middle of the night wakeups that are unnecessarily disruptive, and many other care and service problems. And they can speak up on your behalf.

Talking with Your Doctor

The information on individual hospitals reported in this book and gathered on your own will help you in selecting a hospital. We strongly recommend that you discuss the data with a physician or physicians you trust. This discussion should be a two-way street; your opinions, information, and preferences matter. If your physician recommends a facility that you would not have chosen, ask why. Keep in mind that physicians may have reasons for hospital choice that are unrelated to your well-being. Your doctor might find it more convenient to have all his or her patients in the same facility. Within a managed care plan, there may be financial penalties for the doctor if the doctor doesn't use specific hospitals. You at least deserve to have an explanation of the reasons your doctor thinks a specific hospital is best for you.

More About Our Data

The following is a more detailed discussion of our data and how they should be interpreted.

Physician Ratings

To collect physicians' ratings of hospitals, we mailed questionnaires to more than 260,000 physicians in the summer and fall of 2001 and received more than 16,000 responses.

We gave each physician a list of hospitals in his or her metropolitan area and asked the physician to rate each **"for surgery on an adult in cases where the risk of complications is high."** The physicians were asked to use a five-point scale: "excellent," "very good," "good," "fair," or "poor," and simply to leave the form blank for hospitals for which they couldn't answer.

The Metro Areas table shows for each hospital the percentage, among the physicians who rated it, who said it was either "very good" or "excellent." The table also shows the number of raters for each hospital. We have not reported data on any hospital rated by fewer than 25 physicians. Some hospitals were rated "very good" or "excellent" by more than 90 percent of the physicians who rated them, while some got such favorable ratings from fewer than 20 percent.

We believe these ratings are a useful indicator of hospital quality, but you should keep several caveats in mind—

- In some cases, physicians may not have had a good basis for judging hospitals. A physician who regularly visits a hospital can get a good perspective on how responsive and thorough the nurses and other staff are, how clean and organized the facility is, and other aspects of quality. But most physicians don't see all parts of a hospital or see how it performs with all types of cases. And many of the ratings were likely based on reputations among the physicians' peers rather than direct experience.
- Physicians may have had biases—and possibly financial and professional interests based on their hospital affiliations—that influenced their ratings of specific hospitals.
- The types of physicians who responded to our survey might have had different opinions of the hospitals than the types who chose not to respond.
- Even if there was no consistent difference between the types of physicians who responded and the types who did not, we know that for each hospital there is a mix of opinions among physicians, and it is

possible that some hospitals got relatively low (or high) scores simply because they had bad (or good) luck in who happened to respond. For example, for one hospital, our survey may have reached a few physicians with the most negative opinions on a day when these physicians had time to respond while physicians who would have given negative ratings of another hospital were too busy to respond on the day the survey reached them. Naturally, such bad or good luck is less likely to be the explanation for one hospital's being rated higher than another if the number of raters was large or the two hospitals' scores are very different. On the Metro Areas table, we have used **blue** type for a physician ratings score if the score is substantially above average and if it is sufficiently high and the number of respondents was sufficiently large that the above-average score is very unlikely (less than one chance in 40) to have resulted simply from luck. We have marked in ***bold-italic*** type any below-average score that is sufficiently low and very unlikely (less than one chance in 40) to have resulted simply from luck.

It is interesting to note that doctors' ratings of hospitals are significantly (although not strongly) correlated to patients' ratings of the same hospitals. We surveyed consumers for their ratings of hospitals in 11 major metropolitan areas. We have 25 or more consumer ratings for 231 hospitals for which we also have 25 or more doctors' ratings. The figure below shows how the ratings compared when we grouped hospitals into three groups, based on doctors' ratings. The hospitals that were rated "very good" or "excellent" by fewer than 20 percent of the doctors who rated them were rated "very good" or "excellent" on average by 64 percent of the patients who rated them. Those that were rated "very good" or "excellent" by more than 40 percent of the doctors who rated them were rated "very good" or "excellent" on average by 70 percent of the patients who rated them.

Physicians and consumers tend to favor the same hospitals.

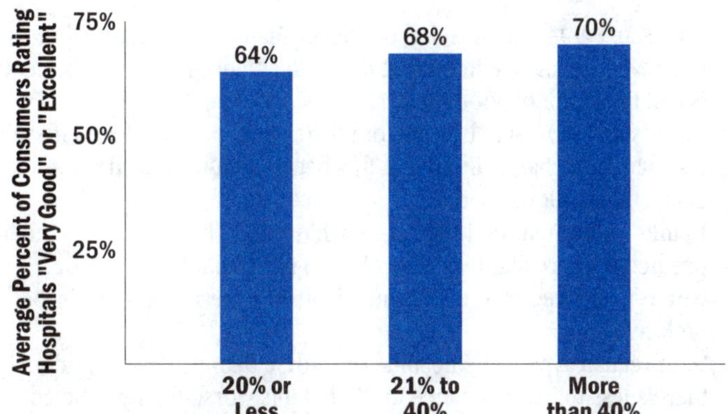

We also asked the physicians to tell us which two hospitals in their metropolitan areas were most desirable and which were least desirable for various types of cases—

- Uncomplicated delivery of a baby
- High-risk delivery of a baby
- Surgery on a child in cases where the risk of complications is high
- Surgery on an adult in cases where the risk of complications is high
- Surgery on an adult in cases where the risk of complications is low
- Medical care for an adult in complex cases

For each type of case, we counted the total number of times each hospital was mentioned favorably and compared that number to the total number of times it was mentioned at all (either favorably or unfavorably). The Metro Areas table shows, for each hospital for each type of case, the percentage of mentions that were favorable. For example, if a hospital was mentioned for a given type of case as most desirable in its local area by eight doctors and as least desirable by two doctors, that would give it a score of 80 percent (eight favorable mentions divided by 10 total mentions). On the table, we have not reported scores for a type of case for any hospital that was mentioned fewer than five times, and we have marked with an asterisk (*) any score that is based on fewer than 10 mentions.

This most desirable/least desirable approach to scoring doesn't allow formal assessments of the statistical significance of hospital-to-hospital differences. But hospitals that look good based on the most desirable/least desirable approach tend also to look good when rated on the five-point poor-to-excellent scale. Since we used both types of questions to ask about "adult surgery in cases where the risk of complications is high," we can compare the results. Consider, for instance, hospitals with at least 10 most desirable/least desirable mentions and at least 25 ratings on the poor-to-excellent scale. Of those that scored in the top half based on most desirable/least desirable mentions, 91 percent were also in the top half based on their score on the poor-to-excellent scale.

You can, on a smaller scale, collect the same kind of information that we collected from physicians. You can ask physicians you know for their recommendations, and you can ask your friends to get the thoughts of physicians they know.

Death Rates

In choosing a hospital, you will want to know how successful the facilities you are considering have been in delivering good results for other patients. The most important result is keeping you alive.

On the Metro Areas table beginning on page 32, we report risk-adjusted death rates. These rates were adjusted in an effort to take into account the fact that some hospitals treat sicker and frailer patients who are at greater risk of dying than patients at other hospitals.

The adjusted death rates are based on analysis of records of hospital stays of Medicare patients 65 or older admitted to hospitals in three Federal Fiscal Years, from October 1, 1996, through September 30, 1999—about 30 million hospital admissions nationwide. This is the only available uniform, nationwide data file of hospital cases.

The hospitals submit records to Medicare in order to be reimbursed for services rendered. Medicare adds one fact to the records submitted by the hospitals—whether the patient died within a specified number of days after hospital admission. Medicare gets this information on deaths, even on deaths that occurred after a patient's discharge from the hospital, by using Social Security records.

Our mortality rate analysis was conducted by **Michael Pine and Associates, Inc.**, a Chicago-based firm that is expert in evaluating the clinical quality of hospitals.

The analysis began with the selection of a subset of cases. We selected types of cases that are relatively common and that have substantial death rates which might be affected by the quality of a hospital's care. The cases included acute myocardial infarction (heart attack), obstructive pulmonary disease, cerebrovascular accident (stroke), and seven other types of cases in which patients were treated medically. They also included 11 types of surgical cases, such as coronary artery bypass graft surgery, large bowel surgery, and total hip replacement. The cases were selected from the Medicare records based on detailed definitions using standard diagnosis and procedure codes.

On the table, you will see, for example, a column showing "adjusted death rate for all [selected] case types." You will see that for some hospitals, the rate is below eight percent; for others, it is above 14 percent. This difference suggests that, among similar patients with serious medical problems or surgical procedures, those going into one of the high-death-rate hospitals have a six percentage point higher chance of dying than those going into one of the low-death-rate hospitals. A six percentage point difference in chance of dying in a few days is something that most people will be intently interested in avoiding.

It is important to note that we did not look at *all* cases. The average death rate across all hospitals for all the types of *Medicare* cases we *selected* is higher than the death rate would be if we reported on all cases the hospitals treated. So hospitals are not as dangerous overall as the death rates our selected cases might suggest, but the adjusted death rates we present are useful in comparing the hospitals for a broad group of serious types of cases.

Adjusted death rates were calculated in several steps.

First, for each type of case, we calculated the actual death rate for each hospital. We counted all deaths that occurred within 30 days of admission, even if they occurred after the patient was discharged from the hospital. Checking for this 30-day period eliminates the possibility that a hospital might have relatively low death rates only because it discharges patients to home, hospice care, or a nursing home when they are on the verge of death.

We then calculated a "predicted" death rate for each type of case for each hospital. The predicted death rate tells what percent of the hospital's patients would have died if the hospital were just as successful as the average of all U.S. hospitals in keeping similar patients alive. The patient characteristics that were taken into account in determining whether patients were similar were age, gender, the presence or absence of selected principal and secondary diagnoses, and whether certain surgical procedures were performed. For example, a hospital that had heart attack patients who were mostly over age 85 with secondary diagnoses like congestive heart failure, diabetes, and malnutrition, might have a considerably higher predicted death rate for heart attack cases than a hospital whose heart attack patients were mostly age 65 to 70 and had few other medical problems.

Next, we used each hospital's predicted death rate and actual death rate along with the national average death rate to calculate an "adjusted" death rate for the hospital. The simplest way to calculate an adjusted rate is in two steps. First, we can calculate the ratio of the actual rate to the predicted rate. If, for example, Hospital A has an actual death rate of five percent but would be predicted to have a death rate of 10 percent based on how sick and frail its patients are, then the ratio is 0.5 (five percent divided by 10 percent). Second, we can multiply this ratio by the national average death rate to get the adjusted death rate. If the national average death rate were 12 percent, then the adjusted death rate for Hospital A would be six percent (12 percent multiplied by the 0.5 ratio). In fact, we used a more complicated formula (using odds ratios) for calculating adjusted rates, but the result is very nearly the same.

For each hospital for each category of cases, we also checked whether the difference between the actual death rate and the predicted death rate was "statistically significant." For example, if the actual rate was nine percent and the predicted death rate was 10 percent, what are the chances that the one percentage point difference was the result of the hospital's simply having had unusually good luck with its patients during the three-year period we analyzed?

We know that some patients survive when the average patient in a similar condition who experienced the same treatment would be expected to die, and some die when the average similar patient given the same treatment would be expected to survive. Since the difference in result can't be explained, we call it good luck or bad luck. And any given hospital might have a string of good luck or bad luck with its patients. But big differences between actual and predicted death rates for large numbers of cases are not likely to be the result of luck alone. For each hospital for each category of cases on the Metro Areas table, we have used different type faces for the adjusted death rate to indicate whether the difference between the hospital's actual death rate and its predicted death rate was "statistically significant":

- **Blue** type—the hospital did better than predicted, and there's less than one chance in 40 that this better-than-predicted experience is just the result of good luck.
- Regular type—although the hospital may have done better or worse than predicted, there's at least one chance in 20 that its better- or worse-than-predicted experience is just the result of good or bad luck.
- ***Bold-italic*** type—the hospital did worse than predicted, and there's less than one chance in 40 that this worse-than-predicted experience is just the result of bad luck.

On the Metro Areas table, we show adjusted death rates and statistical significance for three categories of cases: all selected case types (medical and surgical combined), all selected medical cases, and all selected surgical cases.

On the All Areas table, which begins on page 74, we present death analysis results on those three categories of cases and also on more specific categories of cases, such as heart attack, stroke, pneumonia, and large bowel surgery. The All Areas table presents the data different from how they are presented on the Metro Areas table. Instead of reporting adjusted death rates, we simply indicate whether the hospital's actual death rate for each category of cases was statistically significantly better or worse than predicted, given the hospital's mix of patients. We score the hospitals as follows:

- Blue star (★)—the hospital did better than predicted, and there's less than one chance in 40 that this better-than-predicted experience is just the result of good luck.
- Black star (★)—the hospital did better than predicted, and there's less than one chance in 20 that this better-than-predicted experience is just the result of good luck.
- Blank—although the hospital may have done better or worse than predicted, there's at least one chance in 10 that its better- or worse-than-predicted experience is just the result of good or bad luck.
- × in regular type—the hospital did worse than predicted, and there's less than one chance in 20 that this worse-than-predicted experience is just the result of bad luck.
- **✖** in bold type—the hospital did worse than predicted, and there's less than one chance in 40 that this worse-than-predicted experience is just the result of bad luck.

If a hospital's number of cases or predicted number of deaths was too small, we did not report adjusted death rates nor the significance of the difference between actual and predicted death rates. For such hospitals, the tables show a "—" for "insufficient data."

On both the Metro Areas table and the All Areas table, the national average death rate for each category of cases appears at the top of each page. This is the average of the death rates for each hospital that had a sufficient number of cases for data to be reported.

Interpreting the Death Rate Data

Let's look a little more fully at the strengths and weaknesses of the death rate data. How valuable are they in choosing a hospital for your care?

The data are helpful in predicting a hospital's outcomes—especially among hospitals with a reasonably large number of cases. For example, consider hospitals for which we could calculate death rates for both 1997 and 1999. If you knew nothing more about these hospitals, your chances of picking one with a statistically significantly better-than-predicted death rate in the "all selected cases" category in 1999 would be about 11 percent. But, as the figure below shows, by choosing a hospital with a 1997 death rate that was significantly better than predicted, you would increase to 41 percent your chances that its 1999 death rate would also be statistically significantly better than predicted.

Hospitals with better mortality rates tend to stay that way from year to year.

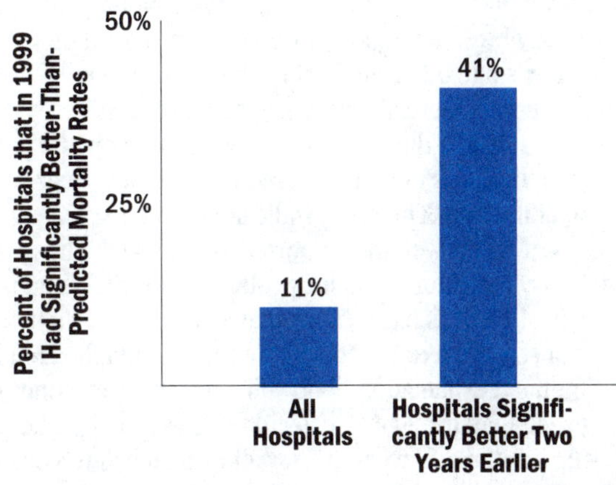

While the data have predictive power, there is much debate about the usefulness of such data for comparing hospitals. The following are some limitations that are important to keep in mind when considering the data on different hospitals—

- From the billing records submitted to Medicare by the hospitals and used for our analysis, it is impossible to know for sure whether secondary diagnoses existed when the patient entered the hospital or whether they occurred during the hospital stay. In many cases, one can confidently make an assumption about where a secondary condition started. Consider heart attack cases. If the patient's record says the patient also had diabetes, we can be confident that the diabetes was there on admission. In contrast, if the record says the patient had pneumonia, we can't tell whether the patient came into the hospital with the pneumonia or acquired it in the hospital. Medicare should, but doesn't, require hospitals to indicate on each patient record for each secondary diagnosis whether the problem was present at the time of admission. Without knowing this, we can't know whether to give the hospital credit for having more difficult cases if it has an unusually large number of heart attack cases with pneumonia. We wouldn't want to give the hospital such credit in our analysis if the hospital is *causing* the pneumonia. Some states require hospitals to indicate for each secondary diagnosis whether it was present upon admission to the hospital, and in our analysis, Michael Pine and Associates used data from state records to determine which secondary diagnoses were likely to have been present at the time of admission.

  This is an innovative approach. But using this approach or any other available approach, it is inevitable that some secondary diagnoses will be miscoded as having been present at admission when in fact they occurred in the hospital and others will be miscoded as complications that occurred in the hospital, when in fact they were present at admission.
- Because of data limitations, various underlying characteristics of patients could not be considered. Suppose, for example, you are looking at a public hospital that caters to low-income, uninsured patients. There's a good chance that the hospital's patients might have social problems—such as the absence of emotionally supportive family members—that are not reported in the data available for analysis but that might affect death rates within 30 days of hospital admission.
- Within any one of the types of cases we looked at, patients may have diseases at different stages of progression, with very different risks of death. Some hospitals' pneumonia cases, for example, might include a disproportionately large number of cases in which the disease was at an advanced stage by the time the patient was admitted. The data we were working with did not include information on laboratory or x-ray results, which would make it possible to distinguish among patients on the basis of these findings. Undetected differences in patient mix are especially likely when comparing hospitals if one hospital is a regional referral center to which other hospitals send their difficult cases.
- Cases were followed for only up to 30 days after admission. Problems caused by some hospitals may not result in death until later than that. (Longer follow-up periods, of course, have their own set of problems since more time increases the chances of death from causes unrelated to the hospital stay.)
- Some differences in death rates may result from differences in community practices or in the availability of non-hospital facilities to care for patients. In some communities, for example, patients in final stages of emphysema (obstructive pulmonary disease) may be allowed to die in their homes or in nursing facilities, while in other communities these patients may be admitted to hospitals for their final few days.
- Some of the data for some hospitals may not be accurate. There are, no doubt, many innocent errors when so many records are processed by hospital coding staff. In addition, it is likely that some hospitals follow different coding guidelines in describing diagnoses in the records they report to Medicare in their efforts to get the highest allowable reimbursements for the cost of care.
- Some of the data are incomplete. For example, the billing record that is the source of the data has space for hospitals to list only eight other diagnoses in addition to the principal diagnosis. If a patient had nine or more secondary diagnoses, the adjustment process was not able to allow for the secondary diagnoses in excess of eight.
- Time has elapsed since the period to which the data apply. The Medicare records of hospital cases don't become immediately available to the public or to researchers, and it took time for us to do our analyses.
- The data are for patients 65 or older. It is possible that hospitals that perform well with that age group don't do so well with younger patients.
- High or low hospital death rates may result from the quality of treatment provided by specific doctors, not from the quality of the hospital's performance. If a hospital does well because of specific doctors, that may do you no good if you use a different doctor.

What to Look For

To use our data on death rates, first look for categories of cases like yours on the All Areas table. If you are looking for a hospital to use for major bowel surgery, for example, look for hospitals with death rates that were significantly better than predicted in that category. Their results are shown as a star (★) (as a **blue** star in cases where we can be most confident that the difference between actual and predicted death rates is not a matter of luck).

If your case doesn't fit any of the categories on our table, or if you are selecting a hospital in advance of the need (for example, as a consideration in choosing a physician or HMO), look for a hospital with results marked with a star (★) in the "all selected cases" category and possibly in several other categories of cases of interest to you.

It is interesting to note that hospitals that had significantly better than predicted mortality rates in the "all selected cases" category—marked in **blue**—also tended to get higher ratings than other hospitals from surveyed physicians, as reported on the Metro Areas table beginning on page 32. As the figure below shows, the hospitals that had significantly better than predicted mortality rates were rated "very good" or "excellent" on average for "surgery on an adult in cases where the risk of complications is high" by 37 percent of surveyed physicians. Hospitals that had significantly worse than predicted mortality rates—marked in ***bold italic***—got such favorable ratings from significantly fewer (only 27 percent) of surveyed physicians. (For the hospitals for which we had consumer ratings, we found no significant relationship between mortality rates and consumer ratings.)

Physicians gave higher ratings to hospitals with better mortality rates.

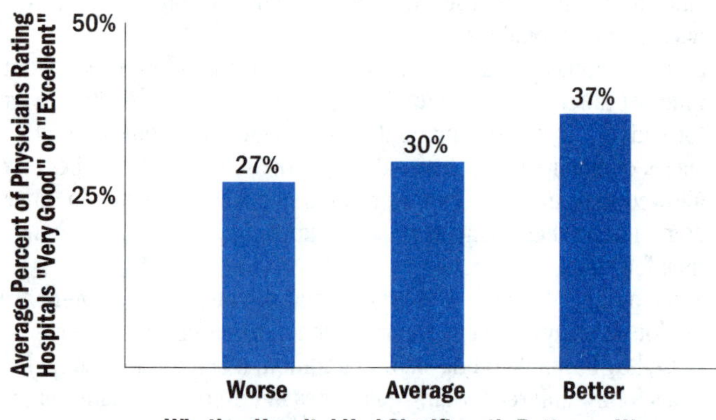

Be sure to discuss the death rate data with your doctor. Ask for any information he or she has that might explain an especially high or low adjusted rate. In addition, we recommend asking hospitals for their comments on their death rates. Call the hospitals' public relations departments.

In a few states, state agencies publish data on hospital outcomes. For example, New York state has for many years published data on death rates for hospitals, and for individual surgeons, for heart bypass surgery. You can ask your state health department if any such data are available for hospitals you are considering.

Rates of Adverse Outcomes

The death rate information we have presented focuses only on that one bad outcome: death. But there are other bad outcomes. You don't want to contract an infection in the hospital, have a bad reaction to a drug, fall out of bed, or have any of many other types of complications even if you ultimately survive. Some complications cause permanent disability or disfigurement; others just make your hospital stay longer and more unpleasant. You want neither.

We would have liked to be able simply to report risk-adjusted complication rates for the hospitals alongside the risk-adjusted death rates. Because of the nature of the Medicare records, however, it's not so straightforward. As mentioned above, the records Medicare gets from the hospitals list secondary diagnoses but don't indicate whether these problems started in the hospital or were present at the time of admission. It's obvious that diabetes was not caused by the hospital, and it's very likely that an infection in a surgical wound is a complication that occurred in the hospital. But a secondary diagnosis of pneumonia might reflect a condition that occurred in the hospital or one that existed at the time of admission. Clearly Medicare should fix this data problem by requiring the data to be reported differently. But with the current system, we can't tell for many secondary diagnoses whether they are complications or conditions that existed at the time of hospital admission, called "comorbidities." In addition, there is evidence that not all complications are reported on the records that are submitted.

To give you information that might alert you to high complication rates, we took a roundabout approach.

We looked for complications only in surgical cases. Our assumption was that for most of the surgeries, timing was discretionary, and patients would not generally be admitted to a hospital for surgery if they currently had an infection or some other medical problem that might be expected to go away if the surgery were simply delayed. Using these cases, Michael Pine and Associates, which did the analysis for us, developed a proxy indicator for complications in cases where death did not occur within 30 days of hospital admission. The proxy indicator is intended to highlight complications even if they were not reported as such in the hospital records. This proxy indicator looks for prolonged hospital lengths of stay. Analyses of medical records have shown that a large proportion of prolonged lengths of stay are associated with important complications.

Here is a simplified explanation of how that analysis was done. The analysis recognized that, for a given category of cases, a given hospital will have varying lengths of stay, even after allowing for differences in patients' characteristics. But after allowing for differences in patient characteristics, most of this variation will be clustered around the hospital's average length of stay for that category of cases. Cases in which the length of stay is not within a hospital's predicted cluster are likely to involve complications. For each category of cases for each hospital, the analysis identified cases that had lengths of stay outside the predicted cluster of lengths of stay. These were deemed to have prolonged lengths of stay. Such prolonged lengths of stay, like deaths, might occur more often in hospitals with especially sick or frail patients, so the analysis calculated a predicted percentage of prolonged lengths of stay for each hospital based on the mix of characteristics of the hospital's patients.

The predicted percentage of prolonged lengths of stay was then combined with the predicted percentage of deaths to come up with a predicted percentage of "adverse outcomes" for each hospital. At the same time, the actual percentage of prolonged lengths of stay was combined with the actual percentage of deaths to come up with an actual percentage of "adverse outcomes" for each hospital. The predicted adverse outcome rate was compared to the hospital's actual adverse outcome rate to calculate a ratio that was in turn used to calculate a risk-adjusted adverse outcome rate. This was done by following the same steps, described above, that were used in calculating a risk-adjusted death rate from the actual, predicted, and all-hospital death rates. The risk-adjusted adverse outcome rates for each hospital, which take into account both deaths and prolonged lengths of stay, are shown on our Metro Areas ratings table for surgical cases.

On the All Areas table, we also report for each hospital whether its actual adverse outcomes rate is significantly different from the predicted adverse outcomes rate in various specific categories of cases.

It is important to keep in mind that most of the caveats set out above with regard to adjusted death rates also apply to adjusted adverse outcome rates. In addition, while the death rates measure directly something we care about—death—the adverse outcome rates use a proxy—length of stay—as an indicator of the thing we care about—complications.

Surprisingly, we found no substantial relationship between adjusted death rates and adjusted adverse outcome rates (once we eliminated deaths from the adverse outcome rates). While these two rates are measures of different types of outcomes, one might expect that hospitals that are relatively good at preventing complications would also be relatively good at preventing deaths. But similar analyses done by others, also looking at complications and deaths, have had similar findings. When we ranked hospitals, we put more weight on death rates than on adverse outcome rates, but both types of rates appear on the hospital ratings tables.

Information from Accreditation Reviews

Our ratings tables show information from reviews conducted by the principal hospital accrediting agency in the U.S., the Joint Commission on the Accreditation of Healthcare Organizations (JCAHO). Accreditation by JCAHO is voluntary, but fulfills hospital licensure requirements in many states, is required by many health plans before they will contract with a hospital, and can be used as a substitute for surveys by federal inspectors by hospitals that wish to qualify to participate in Medicare or Medicaid. According to JCAHO, about 80 percent of U.S. hospitals—accounting for 90 percent of all inpatient admissions—seek JCAHO accreditation.

To maintain accreditation, a hospital must undergo an on-site survey by a JCAHO survey team at least every three years. JCAHO survey teams review a hospital's medical and nursing care, physical condition, life safety program, special care units, pharmaceutical services, infection control procedures, and a number of other areas affecting patient care. Based on the review, JCAHO assigns an accreditation status to each hospital and also gives scores for various areas of performance and an overall evaluation score.

On the All Areas table beginning on page 32, we report the level of accreditation each hospital had achieved on its last full accreditation review according to data supplied to us by JCAHO in September 2001. On both the All Areas and Metro Areas tables, we also report the overall evaluation score each hospital achieved at the time of its last full review. After a full review, hospitals can improve their accreditation status and overall evaluation score by making changes and having followup reviews; our tables do not show the status or scores that resulted from such followup reviews.

Hospitals with better JCAHO overall evaluation scores did not have better or worse adjusted death rates.

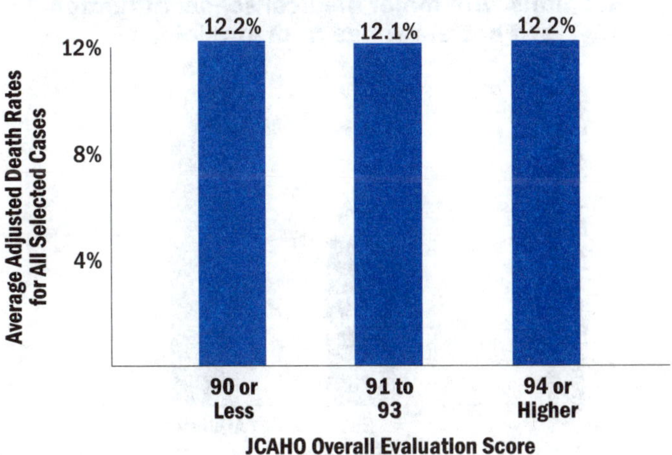

Hospitals with better JCAHO overall evaluation scores received better ratings from physicians.

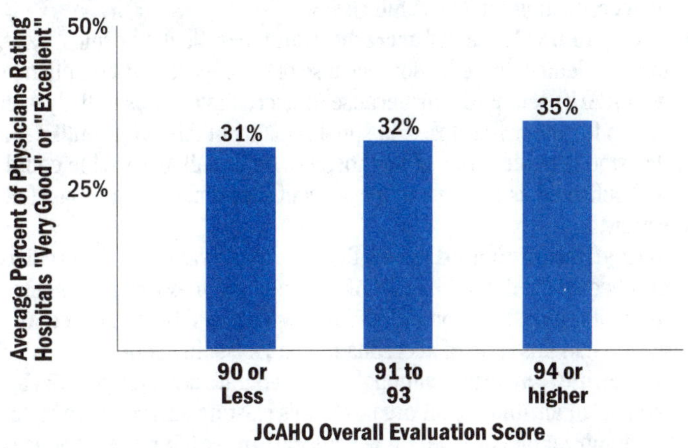

There are the following possible levels of accreditation status:

- **Accreditation with full standards compliance** means that the hospital met JCAHO standards in all performance areas on its most recent full review (in all cases, when we refer to the last review, we mean the last review shown on the records JCAHO supplied to us). Some hospitals, for which the last full accreditation review was before 2000, were given the status **accreditation with commendation** if they met standards in all performance areas and they can still use that language to refer to their accreditation status. But since the start of 2000, **accreditation with full standards compliance** has been the description of the highest accreditation level. About six percent of all the hospitals on the All Areas table beginning on page 74 could be confirmed as having had the highest level of accreditation on their last full review.
- **Accreditation with requirements for improvement** means that a hospital generally met JCAHO standards but did not meet important JCAHO standards in at least one category on its most recent full review. Hospitals with this result after a full review are required to make the required improvements within a specified time period. About 67 percent of all the hospitals on the All Areas table could be confirmed as having had this level of accreditation on their last full review.
- **Conditional accreditation** means that a hospital did not meet standards in some important ways and was performing only marginally at the time of its most recent full review. It might also indicate that one or more serious events had occurred for which the organization could be held accountable and which required followup improvement efforts. Hospitals with this result after a full review are required to make the required improvements within a specified time period, as confirmed by an additional on-site survey by JCAHO. About one percent of all the hospitals on the All Areas table could be confirmed as having had this level of accreditation on their last full review.
- **Provisional accreditation** is the result of an early partial survey, which is used for hospitals that are new to the accreditation process. It reflects general compliance with selected standards. Once the hospital has implemented its new systems, policies, and procedures, a full accreditation survey is conducted. The second survey is performed approximately six months after the first, allowing the hospital

to demonstrate a "track record" of performance. None of the hospitals on the All Areas table could be confirmed as having had this level of accreditation on its last full review.

- **Preliminary denial of accreditation** means that a hospital was initially denied accreditation because of significant non-compliance with JCAHO standards, or because its accreditation was initially withdrawn for other reasons. A hospital remains in this status until a final decision is made. None of the hospitals on the All Areas table could be confirmed as having had this level of accreditation on its last full review.
- **Accreditation denied** means that a hospital was denied accreditation because it did not meet JCAHO standards or key requirements. None of the hospitals on the All Areas table could be confirmed as having had this level of accreditation on its last full review.
- **Accreditation watch**, although not a separate accreditation decision, is an attribute of an organization's existing accreditation status. An organization is placed on **accreditation watch** if it experiences a sentinel event—an unexpected occurrence involving death or serious physical or psychological injury, or the risk thereof—and JCAHO determines that there is a reasonable potential for reducing the likelihood of such events in the future.

For 26 percent of hospitals on the All Areas table, we have indicated that the accreditation status could not be confirmed. This may mean that the hospital is not accredited by JCAHO, and thus is missing an important indicator of quality. But because of difficulties matching the names and ID numbers of hospitals listed on the data file JCAHO provided us with names and ID numbers of hospitals for which we have mortality and physician survey data, it may be that some hospitals are not given credit for an accreditation status they had achieved. It is also important to note that hospitals go through full reviews at least every three years and, in many cases, go through followup reviews as well. So we advise checking the most current accreditation information on JCAHO's excellent website at *www.jcaho.org*.

On our tables, we report each hospital's overall evaluation score if we could confirm it with the information we received from JCAHO. The scores range from 72 to 100, with an average a little above 91. These scores are calculated by JCAHO based on scores on individual "grid elements" relating to specific areas of performance—such as operating room procedures, drug dispensing procedures, anesthesia procedures, and infection control programs. We have reported the scores achieved by the hospitals at the time of the most recent full review, according to the file we received from JCAHO in September 2001. Hospitals can improve their scores with followup reviews.

As the figures on the previous page show, JCAHO's overall evaluation scores are not strongly related to death rates or physician ratings. We divided the hospitals into three groups of roughly equal numbers of hospitals based on JCAHO overall evaluation scores—a group with scores of 90 or below, a group with scores of 91 to 93, and a group with scores 94 or higher. The average adjusted mortality rates for all selected cases for hospitals with at least 1,000 cases were very nearly the same for all three groups of hospitals. The average percentage of physicians who rated the hospitals very good or excellent for hospitals with at least 25 physician ratings ranged from 31 percent for the group with the lowest JCAHO scores to 32 percent for the middle group to 35 percent for the group with the highest JCAHO scores. Although the hospitals with the best JCAHO scores averaged slightly better percentages of physicians rating them very good or excellent than the hospitals with the worst JCAHO scores, the difference was not statistically significant. (We also found no significant relationship between JCAHO overall evaluation scores and consumer ratings of hospitals for the hospitals for which we have at least 25 consumer ratings.)

These are surprising results. One would expect hospitals with better JCAHO scores to do considerably better on mortality rates and physician ratings than hospitals with worse JCAHO scores. The fact that such a relationship is not present may reasonably give you some concern about the meaningfulness of any of the scores. We can't relieve that concern. In our own evaluation of the hospitals, we have put more weight on the adjusted mortality rates and physician ratings than on the JCAHO overall evaluation scores. But that is not necessarily the correct balance. You may be safest with a hospital that scores at least above average on all three types of measures.

Teaching Programs

Our tables also show which hospitals had major affiliations with medical schools according to April 2001 Medicare records. An affiliation with a medical school generally means that various doctors and medical students check patients' records and interview the patients. That can result in your getting a variety of perspectives brought to bear on your case. Also, doctors who are at the cutting edge of research and practice tend to have at least some of their practice at hospitals affiliated with medical schools. This means that the doctors practicing at these hospitals tend to be exposed to the newest developments and to have their ideas challenged by sophisticated colleagues. In addition, hospitals affiliated with medical schools are likely to have advanced diagnostic and treatment equipment.

On the other hand, hospitals affiliated with medical schools are generally larger than average. The care may be relatively impersonal. And it can be annoying to be bothered by a continuing stream of students and trainees, all with an academic—but often not very personal—interest in your case.

The figure below shows the relationship between major medical school affiliation and physician ratings. As you can see, the hospitals with major medical school affiliations were rated much higher than other hospitals by surveyed physicians. As the figure on the facing page shows, hospitals with major medical school affiliation also had slightly (but statistically significantly) better adjusted mortality rates than other hospitals. Both the figures are for hospitals rated by at least 25 physicians and for which we were able to analyze at least 1,000 cases in calculating adjusted mortality rates for the "all selected cases" category. (Among the hospitals for which we had consumer ratings, those with major medical school affiliations rated almost exactly the same with consumers as those that did not have such affiliations.)

Hospitals with major medical school affiliation get better ratings from physicians.

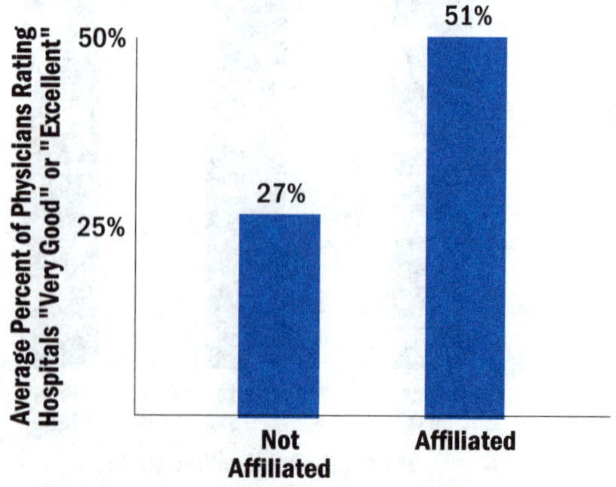

Hospitals with major medical school affiliation had slightly better adjusted death rates.

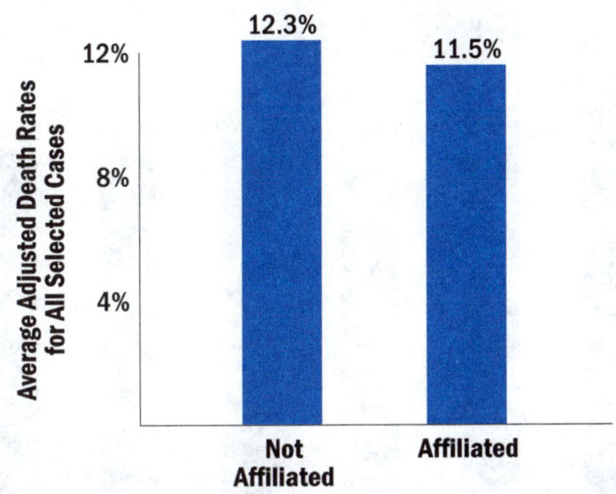

The All Areas table beginning on page 74 reports on a second measure of the extent of teaching programs—the number of residents who were working at each hospital according to 2001 industry or government sources. Residents are doctors who have graduated from medical school and who are getting more advanced training and experience in a specialty field. The residents get their training from more experienced physicians. The exchange of dialogue may result in useful perspectives and expertise being brought to your case. In addition, hospitals with residency programs are more likely than other hospitals to have doctors in the hospital 24 hours per day. But these advantages may also come with a degree of impersonality and with frequent intrusions upon your peace and privacy. In addition, you may find that some decisions affecting your care are made by the residents rather than by your personal physician.

As with medical school affiliation, the existence of residency programs at a hospital is associated with slightly (but significantly) better than average adjusted all-selected-cases death rates. But hospitals with residency programs were rated neither higher nor lower than other hospitals by surveyed physicians.

Computerized Drug Ordering and Control Systems

Our All Areas table, beginning on page 74, shows data on whether hospitals have computerized systems for doctors to use when ordering prescription medicine for their patients, referred to as Computerized Physician Order Entry (CPOE) systems.

Thousands of patients die each year as a result of drug errors in hospitals. Substantial numbers of these deaths could be avoided if hospitals used computerized systems for physicians to order prescriptions. With CPOE systems, doctors enter orders into a computer rather than writing them down on paper, and the prescription can be automatically checked against the patient's current information for potential mistakes or problems. For example, before the doctor can complete the prescription order, the computer checks to see if the new prescription might interact badly with another drug the patient is taking, or if the patient has a known allergy to it. This type of system also reduces mistakes that occur from misreading a doctor's handwriting. Studies show a computerized prescription system can reduce serious medication mistakes by up to 86 percent.

Unfortunately, for most hospitals, we don't have good documentation as to whether they have well-implemented computerized prescription order entry systems. But there is a group that is beginning to track hospitals' implementation of these systems. It is called The Leapfrog Group.

Founded by The Business Roundtable, a national association of chief executives of Fortune 500 companies, The Leapfrog Group was created to "help save lives and reduce preventable medical mistakes by mobilizing employer purchasing power to initiate breakthrough improvements in the safety of health care and by giving consumers information to make more informed hospital choices." Since the summer of 2001, the group has allowed hospitals to fill out a detailed online questionnaire about their programs in several different areas that relate to patient safety: implementation of CPOE, volume of cases in certain types of procedures for which there is known to be a relationship between volume and outcomes, and physician staffing of intensive care units. While all hospitals have been allowed to submit data, hospitals in just six urban area regions of Atlanta, Georgia; California; East Tennessee; Minnesota; Seattle/Tacoma/Everett, Washington; and St. Louis, Missouri were the focus of Leapfrog's data-solicitation efforts prior to March 2002. To be accepted by The Leapfrog Group, the information on a hospital's questionnaire must be affirmed in writing by the hospital's chief executive or his or her designated agent.

On the All Areas table, we indicate what level hospitals had achieved as of February 28, 2002, on Leapfrog's CPOE measure, with number designations as shown below, or a symbol for "no data." We used numbers to indicate five levels—

5—Fully implemented Leapfrog's recommended safety practice.

4—Good progress in implementing Leapfrog's recommended safety practice. (The hospital has already begun to implement the practice, has a clear action plan, and has committed the resources to achieve full implementation of the patient safety practice within the next few years.)

3—Good early stage effort in implementing Leapfrog's recommended safety practice. (The hospital has developed an action plan and is committed to implementing the practice in the next few years.)

2—Willing to report publicly: does not yet meet Leapfrog's criteria for a good early stage effort. (The hospital, while willing to report its implementation status, does not meet Leapfrog's criteria for a good early stage effort at implementing Leapfrog's recommended patient safety practice.)

1—Did not submit this information. (The hospital was invited to fill out the survey but did not. Currently, this status applies only to the hospitals in the six initial urban regions of Atlanta, Georgia; California; East Tennessee; Minnesota; Seattle/Tacoma/Everett, Washington; and St. Louis, Missouri where

Hospitals that met Leapfrog standards for computerized prescription drug order entry (CPOE) systems had relatively good adjusted death rates.

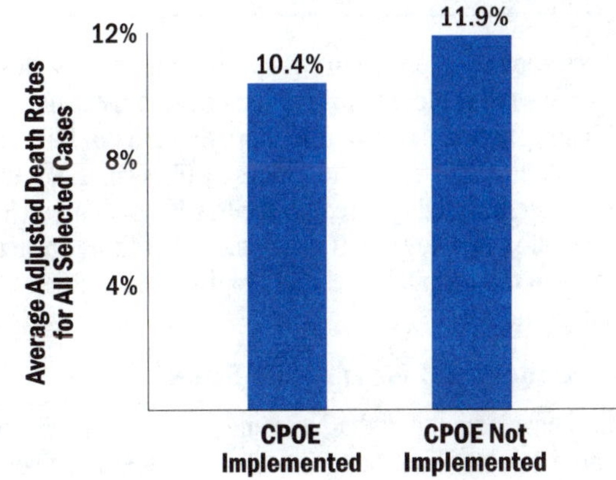

Leapfrog focused its efforts to get hospitals to fill out the survey. Hospitals in other parts of the country were welcome to participate but not actively recruited by Leapfrog or by the employers and health plans that are supporting Leapfrog.)

No data—indicated by a "—". (The hospital was not in a part of the country where Leapfrog focused its efforts to get hospital participation. Nonparticipation by these hospitals is not regarded as a negative sign.)

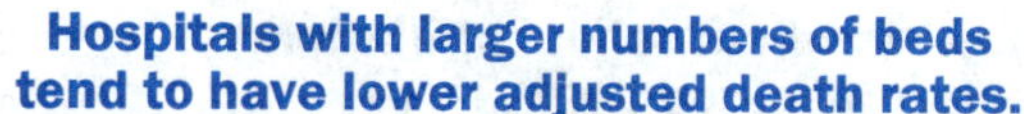

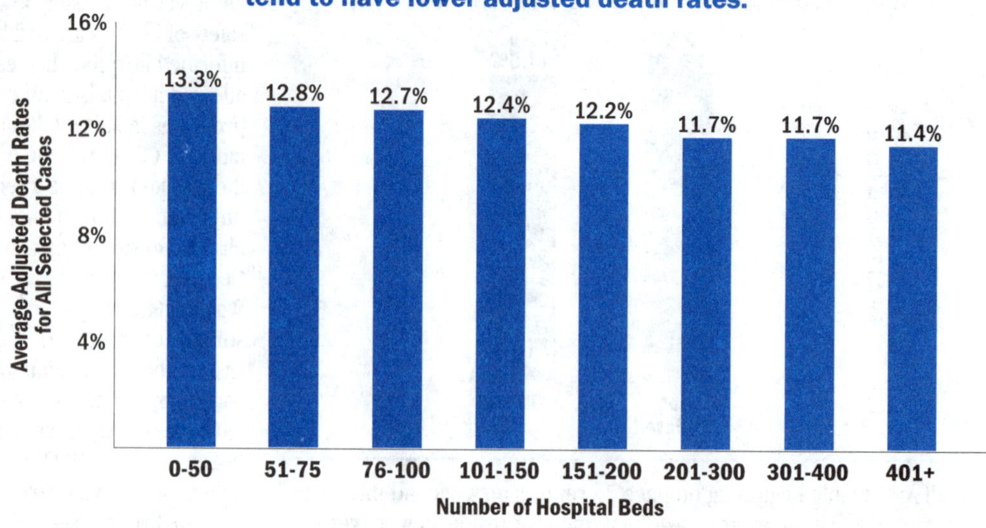

You will note that only 15 hospitals are reported as having had full CPOE implementation as measured by Leapfrog by February 28, 2002. That is the only status that indicates that you can currently expect that you will get the actual patient safety benefits from CPOE. The other levels on the Leapfrog scale can be achieved by planning and progress without full implementation.

We have not reported on Leapfrog's measures other than on CPOE. You can check on these other measures and get updates on hospitals' performance on the CPOE measure at Leapfrog's website, *www.leapfroggroup.org*. You will want to check this website, because many more hospitals are expected to meet Leapfrog's standards over coming months and years.

Hospitals that met Leapfrog standards for computerized prescription drug order entry (CPOE) systems were rated relatively high by physicians.

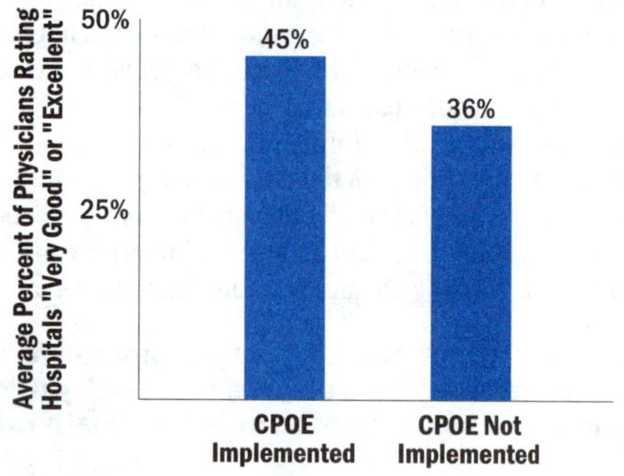

As the figures above and on the previous page indicate, the hospitals that met Leapfrog's full standards for computerized prescription systems scored significantly better, compared to those that did not fully meet the standard, on both mortality rates and ratings by physicians. We also looked at how these hospitals scored on the JCAHO evaluation element related to medication use; for that JCAHO score, there was no significant difference between the hospitals that met Leapfrog's full CPOE standard and those that did not.

How Many Cases and How Many Beds

Many studies have concluded that, in some types of cases, hospitals that handle large volumes have better results than other hospitals—that, in effect, practice makes perfect. Our tables don't report on hospitals' volumes for specific types of cases, but you can ask your doctor or the public information staffs of hospitals you are considering how many cases like yours they handle each year. Your doctor may have to help you define your case type in a precise enough way for the information to be meaningful. The following are types of cases for which The Leapfrog Group has concluded that there is substantial evidence of the benefits of volume (and the desired volume cutoffs for each type of case)—

- Coronary artery bypass surgery (volume of at least 500 cases per year)
- Coronary angioplasty (volume of at least 400 cases per year)
- Abdominal aortic aneurysm repair (volume of at least 30 cases per year)
- Carotid endarterectomy (volume of at least 100 cases per year)
- Esophageal cancer surgery (volume of at least seven cases per year)
- Delivery with pre-natal diagnosis of major congenital abnormalities, or delivery with expected birthweight less than 1,500 grams or gestational age less than 32 weeks (in states that identify regional neonatal intensive care units, volume of such a unit should be an average daily census of at least 15)

On the All Areas table, we have reported on number of beds. That may be a rough indicator of volume except for types of cases where hospitals tend to specialize. On that table, there is also another overall volume indicator for relatively difficult cases: the "number of cases" for "all selected case types." Keep in mind that the number of cases count is only selected Medicare cases and is for a three-year period (except for a few hospitals for which data were available for only one or two years of cases).

The figure above shows that hospitals with more beds tend to have lower adjusted death rates for "all selected [medical and surgical] cases" than hospitals with lower numbers of beds.

Our Checkmark (✓) for Quality

Using the measures on the Metro Areas table, we calculated an overall hospital score for each hospital on that table. Those that got our top scores got checkmarks (✓) on the table. Our overall scores reflect the specific weighting and cutoffs we applied to the measures. You might weight the measures differently and single out different hospitals.

Chapter 5:
How to Get Good Care Wherever You Go

Regardless of which hospital you are admitted to, you and your family or friends can do a lot to influence the quality of care you receive. What matters most is your attitude. It is important that you feel involved in, and responsible for, your own care—that you view the hospital and staff only as the setting and the means to help you get well. Two excellent books that will prepare you for the hospital experience are *Take This Book to the Hospital*, by Charles B. Inlander and Ed Weiner, and *How to Get Out of the Hospital Alive*, by Sheldon P. Blau and Elaine Fantle Shimberg. The following advice also should help you.

Before You Arrive

If there is time, a little care in getting ready for your hospital stay will serve you well later on.

If you will be getting care from a surgeon or other specialist, meet with this doctor. Get a full explanation of exactly what will be done. Get an understanding of who will be doing your surgery and what role assistants might play. Find out who will be caring for you as you recover after surgery and after you leave the hospital. If you are not happy with the answers, this would be the time to change doctors.

If you will be having surgery, try to meet also with the anesthesiologist. It is better to have this meeting in the more relaxed atmosphere of an office visit than to meet with the anesthesiologist, in the typical way, for a few hurried minutes right before the operation. Arranging an appointment in advance is not easy to do (and be sure to confirm that your insurance will cover it), but it is worthwhile, given the importance to your safety of his or her work. You can ask your surgeon to give you the name of the anesthesiologist and to help you make an appointment. When the anesthesiologist asks questions, be sure to give thorough answers—about high blood pressure, heart problems, allergies, or other conditions that might put you at risk when under anesthesia. Also, confirm that the anesthesiologist will actually be present with you in the operating room, not a subordinate.

If you might need blood transfusions in connection with surgery, ask your surgeon whether autologous transfusion makes sense for you—giving your own blood and having it stored for your own later use. You might be able to give a unit a week for several weeks before surgery.

Decide whether you will want a private or semi-private room. With a private room, you avoid any problems with roommates who might be noisy or have annoying visitors. But sharing a room with someone else gives you a little company, is likely to increase the frequency of nurse visits to your room since there are two patients to visit, and gives you someone who might be able to call for help for you in a crisis.

Think carefully about packing for the hospital. Be sure to take a toilet kit with toothbrush, shampoo, deodorant, and other items just as you would if you were going on a vacation. Also, bring along a clock, things to read, and things to write with. And bring pajamas, a robe, and non-skid slippers.

Don't bring a valuable watch or expensive jewelry. They might get stolen. You will not be able to keep an eye on it all the time—certainly not when you are in surgery or recovery. Don't bring more than a few dollars in cash. Bringing a credit card, and a phone card if you will want to make call out-of-area calls, is a good idea. You might want to bring a few pictures to keep you company and possibly a few other items of sentimental value, but label anything you bring with your full name and realize that you might lose it.

Check in advance with your doctor which of your regular medications, including vitamin supplements, you will be continuing to take while in the hospital. Bring a list of these medications, noting the dosage and frequency. If you bring the actual medications, have your doctor mark in your medical record that you are to take these medications and that the nurses are to find a place to store them; be sure to label them clearly as yours. Bring them in their original bottles with labels.

Monitor Your Own Care

Learn as much about your condition as possible before going to the hospital by talking to your doctor and doing research in libraries and on the Web. Ask your doctor to tell you what treatment is recommended, what alternatives are available, and the consequences of each. Find out what medications, if any, you will be taking, what they look like, and any possible side effects. If you and your doctor go over these things before you are in the hospital, you will be better prepared to deal with each treatment step and less likely to be surprised or feel pressured about making decisions.

During treatment, keep notes on the results of tests. Also keep track of changes in medications or diet and their effects.

Write down questions you want to ask the doctor or the unit's head nurse during his or her visit and record the answers.

By keeping track of these things, you will know more about your condition and what to expect. You will also know enough to question the arrival of the wrong meal or a new pill. It may not be yours.

Be Yourself

Simply as a part of being in the hospital, many people become more passive and dependent than usual. Inactivity and concern about your condition contribute to this; so does the typical hospital routine of frequent interruptions and continual waiting—for meals, tests, visits from the doctor and friends, and medication. To help you be yourself, try to personalize your day and your surroundings by putting out a few personal (not valuable) items from home, by wearing your own clothes where possible, by calling friends and asking them to bring you snacks (provided you are not on a restricted diet), or by doing some work or reading. If not disruptive to others or harmful to your condition, these kinds of activities might help you resist becoming excessively reliant on the hospital and staff—and will help to assure that staff members regard you as a person, not just a case. We know one patient who purposely wore bright red pajamas and did aerobic exercises every day just so she would not be typed simply as "thyroid tumor in 302."

In general, do all you can for yourself. No one expects you to jump out of bed hours after you come out of the operating room. But as you and your doctor feel you are able, try to feed yourself, get out of bed by yourself, and generally take on as much as you can of your own care. This is therapeutic for you and will gain you the respect of the staff.

Be sure to express your appreciation for the good care you receive. Nurses have a demanding job and, like everyone else, need a little feedback. If one of your visitors can bring a gift or some flowers for the nurses, rather than for you, that will be appreciated. Also, learn your nurses' names and call them by name.

Protect Yourself

Given the high risks of infections, drug errors, and other hospital mishaps, it is essential that you take steps to protect yourself. If this means you are not the most agreeable patient, so be it. This is a matter of life and death. The information that follows is drawn from various sources, including an excellent report issued by the U.S. Agency for Healthcare Research and Quality (AHRQ), entitled *Making Health Care Safer*.

Protect Yourself Against Infections

Hospital-caused infections are a major killer—and a major cause of suffering, anxiety, and extended hospital stays. AHRQ's *Making Health Care Safer* report states that such infections "occur in seven to 10 percent of hospitalized patients and account for approximately 80,000 deaths per year in the United States."

Most infections are the result of the spreading of "germs" from patient to patient on the hands of physicians, nurses, and other hospital workers. The best way to reduce this problem is very low-tech: the people who touch you in the hospital just need to wash their hands. Numerous studies have demonstrated that handwashing sharply reduces rates of patient infections. Although this has been known for 150 years, hospital workers simply don't always follow the basic rules of hygiene. In 11 studies cited in the AHRQ report, nine noted that compliance with basic handwashing practices was below 50 percent. Most healthcare workers understand the importance of handwashing but simply don't do it consistently—and aren't even aware of how poorly they are doing.

The solution for you? **Ask every healthcare worker—including your doctor—who will be having direct contact with you to wash his or her hands** before touching you, your food, your medications, or equipment that will come into contact with you. Studies have found that one of the most effective ways—better than training programs or rewards and punishments—to get health care workers to wash their hands is for patients to ask them to do so.

Washing hands with disinfectant soap and water is one effective technique. But it takes 15 to 30 seconds to do it right; it takes time for the hands to dry; and washing hands many times per day can be irritating to the skin. A faster, less irritating, and equally effective alternative is hygienic hand-wipes.

Take to the hospital with you a supply of sanitizing hand-wipes, which you can buy in the drug store, and keep them in a prominent place at your bedside. These alcohol-based hand-wipes generally have emollients that make them easy on the skin.

You may feel awkward interfering in the health care workers' routines. Overcome it. Be polite, but not passive. The stakes are too high. Some hospitals have found that instructing patients at admission that the patients should ask every healthcare worker to wash his or her hands is an effective way to increase handwashing compliance. But hospitals don't typically take this approach. You need to do it on your own. You can simply explain that you are doing as you were told by a book you read.

Ask also about equipment that will come into contact with you. That stethoscope should also be cleaned with a sanitizing wipe. Contaminated catheters, infusion pumps, endoscopes, and bronchoscopes can also be a problem, though one you will have a harder time monitoring.

If your roommate or the roommate's visitors show signs of contagious illness, like sneezing or coughing, ask your doctor about changing rooms.

Protect Yourself Against Drug Errors

The Institute of Medicine report, *To Err Is Human*, highlighted the shocking frequency of medication errors in hospitals. The Institute cited numerous studies to document the problem. For example, one study of a 37-day period in a sophisticated urban hospital found 27 cases of "injury resulting from a medical intervention related to a drug."

Hospitals could do, and long since should have done, much to reduce this problem, including the introduction of Computerized Physician Order Entry (CPOE) systems discussed in Chapter 4. But there is also a lot you can do to protect yourself.

The key is to have a written list of the medications—including medications taken via IV hookup—you will be receiving, why, how often, and what the proper dosage is. If a medication looks different from what you have been getting, stop and ask the nurse about it. Maybe it is just a generic-equivalent substitute, but maybe it is the wrong drug. Be sure the hospital staff knows about all the medications you and your doctors have agreed you will be taking.

Make notes of when you get medications. If you don't get one on schedule, ask the nurse why not. You and the nurse can confirm the missed dose by checking your chart.

If you have an unexpected reaction to a drug, bring it to the attention of the nurse immediately. Some, but not all, of the types of reactions to look out for are tightness in your chest, shortness of breath or trouble breathing, pain, burning sensations, dizziness, confusion, numbness, or itching.

Avoid Falling

Hospital patients are at substantial risk of falling, even patients who are young and strong and would not normally be considered to be at risk. You may be weak from illness or injury or from too much time in bed, or you may be dizzy or confused from medications. Falls can cause hip fractures, other types of fractures, concussions, or other injuries.

There are various precautions you can take to avoid falling—

- Before getting out of bed sit still on the edge of the bed with your feet dangling until you are sure you have your balance. If you still feel at all unsteady, call a nurse or aide to help—and wait for the help.
- If you have been instructed not to get up without help, follow that instruction.
- Keep your eyeglasses by the side of your bed. Be sure you can see normally, that your vision is not suffering from side effects of treatment, before trying to walk.
- Wear slippers that have non-skid soles and that will stay on your feet. If there are wet spots on floors, ask someone to dry them before proceeding.
- Make sure that furniture is not in your way. Before going to bed at night, check that furniture is arranged so that it won't interfere with you if you have to go to the bathroom.
- Take your time. Even a few days in the hospital can sap your strength. Use a walker if that will help.
- Don't get out of bed until your bed is cranked down and never try to climb over raised side rails. Ask a nurse or aide to fix your bed so that you can get out.

Be Able to Get Help When You Need It

When you first arrive in your room, locate the call buttons at bedside and in the bathroom. Tell the nurses that you want to test them, and do so.

When you use a call button, you should expect an immediate response—at least by intercom—to find out how urgent your need is.

If you don't get a quick enough response, call again. If you feel desperate, use your outside phone line to call the hospital and ask to be connected to the nursing station that serves your room number. If that, too, fails to get a response, call your doctor.

Insist on Attentive Nursing Care

Expect at least the following from the nursing staff—

- Nurses should observe you every few hours if you are not seriously ill—every few minutes if you are critically ill.
- They should spend time with you to ask about any changes in your condition, any pain, any new complaints.
- They should call your doctor if an unexpected change occurs—or if you are concerned enough that you think the doctor should know.
- There should be some continuity of the nursing staff—not a constant daily turnover of new faces.

Don't Get Cut in the Wrong Place

Wrong-site surgery—operating on the wrong body part—is the kind of mishap that gets dramatic attention in the press. Fortunately, it is not very common. Unfortunately, it is still too common. The Joint Commission on the Accreditation of Healthcare Organizations identified 114 such cases, based mainly on voluntary reports by hospitals, for a roughly six-year period ending in early 2001. There is some evidence, from jurisdictions where reporting is mandatory, that the actual incidence of wrong-site surgery may be as much as 20 times that high.

A key measure to avoid such catastrophes is to mark the surgery site with a permanent marker, during a preoperative visit, before the day of the operation. In 1998, the American Academy of Orthopaedic Surgeons endorsed a surgical site identification program called "Sign Your Site," modeled on the "Operate through your initials" campaign instituted by the Canadian Orthopaedic Association from 1994 to 1996. Ask your surgeon what site-marking procedure he or she uses, and then mark the site together while you are at the doctor's office.

Take Charge of Communication

Be sure the nursing staff knows about your conditions—what you are in the hospital for and other conditions that might affect the care you should receive. Hospitals are big places. Hospital workers care for dozens of patients every day. One worker takes over when another worker goes home. A lot of information can get lost in the shuffle; confusion can ensue. Computerized medical records, if properly used, would help. But most hospitals are shamefully backward in implementation of such systems, relying instead on the same types of patient records they have used for many years. It is, unfortunately, important for you, if you are able, to keep track of what is going on and make sure the right information gets from one caregiver to another.

First, make sure they know who you are. Make sure your wristband is accurate. To help everyone keep things straight, use a piece of posterboard to make a sign with your name, serious allergies, and chronic medical conditions and post it at the head of your bed. Some hospitals actually supply posters for this purpose.

Be particularly vigilant at shift changes—to be sure the new folks know what went on, or didn't go on, on the previous shift. The sign-out procedures used in most hospitals when a physician goes off duty to pass information to the "cross-covering" physician who will take care of patients in the interim is often informal and unstructured. Errors are more likely to occur during the coverage period of the cross-covering physician than when the regular physician is on duty.

Keep a log of what happens to you each day. If something seems to have been missed, or if there is an attempt to repeat some test or treatment that you think is unnecessary because it has already been done, ask about it. Refer to your log and your medical record.

Eat Right

Eating right is important for you to feel right when you are at home, so it's not surprising that it is also important when you are in a hospital. Unfortunately, that is not always easy. The food often leaves a lot to be desired. If the food is not as hot or as cold as it should be, ask the staff if that can be improved. If you find it just too unpleasant to eat, ask your doctor to authorize you to get food from the outside and ask friends to bring meals to you. Ask to have a small space arranged for you to store your food in a hospital refrigerator. Be sure to label it.

If you routinely take vitamin supplements, get your doctor's permission to take them in the hospital. Even if you don't take such supplements regularly, they might make sense for you in the hospital since your other nutritional intake may be deficient. Ask your doctor to arrange for your vitamins to be properly labeled, stored, and dispensed by the nursing staff.

Ask to see a hospital dietician if you have problems with food. Eat well, but be sure to follow orders about not eating before surgery.

Demand the Basic Comforts

It is important to your recovery that you be as comfortable and happy as possible. If your roommate or the roommate's visitors are too noisy, discuss it with your roommate. If that doesn't work, or if something your roommate can't control like incessant coughing is making it very difficult for you to relax or sleep, ask to have your room changed. If there is too much noise in the hall, ask what can be done about that. Another possible solution to noise problems is a radio, or a tape or CD player, with headphones.

Negotiate about schedule. If the staff routinely wakes you up three times in the middle of the night, ask whether all those disturbances are needed. See if you can take the medication or have the readings taken right before bedtime or right after you wake up. If you are normally a late sleeper, see if your normal schedule can be accommodated. If you don't want sleeping pills, ask not to be given them.

If you want someone to sleep-in with you, ask for that to be arranged. A comfortable chair should be arranged, and many hospitals will provide cots.

Don't Accept Treatment Without Your Consent

You have a right—based on law and on medical ethics—to be treated only after giving your informed consent. Before surgery, you will be asked to sign a consent form. In the absence of consent, a surgeon's cutting you open with a knife would be deemed negligence in some states, battery in others. Yet studies have found that substantial percentages of patients do not fully understand what their physicians have described about a procedure, and many would like more explanation.

If you don't understand the risks, the benefits, the alternatives, and other important aspects of a procedure, ask for more information. Do this even if you have already signed a consent form. It is not too late to change your mind right up until the procedure begins. This applies not only to surgery, but also to radiology procedures, drug treatments, blood transfusions, and other procedures that may pose risks to you.

Consider Carefully Participation in Clinical Trials

You may be offered a chance to participate in a clinical trial. A clinical trial is research in which the use of new drugs or medical devices is tested in humans. The purpose of such trials is to learn whether new treatments will benefit future patients.

Although the new treatment being tested might be better than alternative treatments, it might be worse. Also, if you participate in a trial, you might be assigned to the "control" group that gets a standard treatment rather than the new treatment. (In cases of life-threatening disease, control groups virtually always get a treatment that has been judged to have some value, not just no treatment at all.) There is some evidence that patients who have participated in trials have survived longer than patients who chose to get treatment outside a trial. An explanation for such a difference might be that patients in a trial may receive closer medical attention and more follow-up visits than patients who are not in a trial.

A very valuable resource to help you make a decision about participation in a clinical trial is *Should I Enter a Clinical Trial?*, a guide prepared by ECRI, a nonprofit health services research organization. The guide is available at *www.ecri.org*. Drawing on the guide, we list below several types of information you will want to get to help you decide whether to participate in a clinical trial—

- A summary of results from previous trials that led to this trial.
- The purpose of the new research—what it is trying to achieve.
- How long the trial will last for you if you remain in it to the end.
- A detailed description of each test and treatment that will be given according to the trial plan.
- The timing and the location of those tests and treatments and how they are scheduled for you.
- Identification of any procedures that are experimental.
- A description of any reasonably foreseeable risks or discomforts to you (for example, pain or minor and major side effects) from any test or treatment that will be given.
- A description of any possible benefits to you or to others.
- A description of any alternative procedures or courses of treatment that might be advantageous to you.
- A statement that participation is voluntary and that you may refuse or discontinue participation at any time without penalty or loss of benefits.
- A statement that significant new findings that may relate to your willingness to participate.
- An itemization of any costs to you as a result of participation.
- A description of anticipated circumstances under which the investigator may terminate your participation without regard to your consent.
- A description of the consequences of your decision to withdraw, if you decide to do so, and the procedures for withdrawal.
- The approximate number of participants involved in the study.
- A full disclosure of any financial interests the participating researchers and institutions have in the research.
- Travel and lodging information for you and loved ones accompanying you.
- A description of support that you might require from family and friends for daily activities or daily needs while in the trial.
- A statement describing the extent to which confidentiality of your records will be maintained.
- An explanation of whether any compensation and/or medical treatments are available if injury occurs from treatment in the trial and, if so, what they are and who will provide them.
- Information on whom to contact with questions about the trial and your rights.
- Information on whom to contact in the event of a research-related injury.

Don't Suffer Pain Silently

Nearly half of all surgery patients do not receive adequate pain relief. The practice of delaying or withholding pain relief medications due to fear of masking symptoms is widespread. Many patients mistakenly worry that taking pain medication will lead to addiction. Inappropriate treatment of pain results from poor understanding and skills of providers and inadequate patient education. The American Pain Foundation (APF), an organization devoted to educating consumers about pain, wants consumers to have the following facts about pain, whether in-hospital or elsewhere—

- **Pain is not something you "just have to live with."** Treatments are available to relieve or lessen most pain. If untreated, pain can make other health problems worse, slow recovery, and interfere with healing. Get help right away, and don't let anyone suggest that your pain is simply "in your head."
- **Not all doctors know how to treat pain.** Your doctor should give the same attention to your pain as to any other health problems. But many doctors have had little training in pain care. If your doctor is unable to deal with your pain effectively, ask the doctor to consult with a specialist, or consider switching doctors.
- **Pain medications rarely cause addiction.** Morphine and similar pain medications, called opioids, can be highly effective for certain conditions. Unless you have a history of substance abuse, there is little risk of addiction when these medications are properly prescribed by a doctor and taken as directed. Physical dependence—which is not to be confused with addiction—occurs in the form of withdrawal symptoms if you stop taking these medications suddenly. This usually is not a problem if you go off your medications gradually.
- **Most side effects from opioid pain medications can be managed.** Nausea, drowsiness, itching, and most other side effects caused by morphine and similar opioid medications usually last only a few days. Constipation from these medications can usually be managed with laxatives, adequate fluid intake, and attention to diet. Ask your doctor to suggest ways that are best for you.
- **If you act quickly when pain starts, you can often prevent it from getting worse.** Take your medications when you first begin to experience pain. If your pain does get worse, talk with your doctor. Your doctor may safely prescribe higher doses or change the prescription. Non-drug therapies such as relaxation training and others can also help give you relief.

The APF (*www.painfoundation.org*) has issued a pain care bill of rights. Although these are not legal rights, they are standards that you should expect to have observed. According to the APF, you have—

- The right to have your report of pain taken seriously and to be treated with dignity and respect by doctors, nurses, pharmacists and other healthcare professionals.
- The right to have your pain thoroughly assessed and promptly treated.
- The right to be informed by your doctor about what may be causing your pain, possible treatments, and the benefits, risks, and costs of each.
- The right to participate actively in decisions about how to manage your pain.

- The right to have your pain reassessed regularly and your treatment adjusted if your pain has not been eased.
- The right to be referred to a pain specialist if your pain persists.
- The right to get clear and prompt answers to your questions, take time to make decisions, and refuse a particular type of treatment if you choose.

You should be aware that in 1999 the Joint Commission on the Accreditation of Healthcare Organizations approved pain management standards as part of its overall accreditation standards. The first standard states that "every patient has a right to have pain assessed and managed appropriately."

Remember, you have a role here. You must communicate about your pain to your doctors and nurses.

Have Your End-of-Life Wishes Prevail

At some point, patients, their families, and friends may have to decide whether to extend life-sustaining treatment with measures such as resuscitation, endotracheal intubation, feeding tubes, and administration of IV fluids. If you want your end-of-life wishes honored, you will need to have discussions with your family or other representatives and your physician in advance. Good communication at the end of life can also help patients achieve closure and meaning in the final days of their life.

In 1990, the Federal Patient Self-Determination Act was passed by Congress to encourage competent adults to complete advance directives. The act requires hospitals, nursing homes, health maintenance organizations, and hospices that participate in Medicare and Medicaid to ask if patients have advance directives, to provide information about advance directives, and to incorporate advance directives into the medical record.

Advance directives are any expression by a patient intended to guide care, should they lose their medical decision-making capacity. Although both oral and written statements are valid, the added effort required to complete written statements gives them greater weight. In addition to their use when patients lose competence, advance directives also help patients consider the type of care they would want in the future, even if they retain decision-making capacity. Advance directives have legal validity in almost every state.

There are two principal forms of written advance directives: living wills and durable powers of attorney for healthcare. A *living will* is a document that allows you to indicate the interventions you would want if you were terminally ill, comatose with no reasonable hope of regaining consciousness, or in a persistent vegetative state with no reasonable hope of regaining significant cognitive function. A *durable power of attorney for healthcare* is a more comprehensive document that allows you to appoint a person as a proxy to make healthcare decisions for you should you lose decision-making capacity.

Unfortunately, the potential for advance directives to guide patient care is often not realized. Many patients don't complete such directives, and often the directives are not available or adequately communicated at the time end-of-life decisions must be made. Even when a written advance directive document is prepared, it may not meet its objective. One study found that only 12 percent of patients with an advance directive had talked with a physician when completing the document and only 25 percent of physicians were aware of their patients' advance directives. One study that surveyed elders in community settings found that 81 percent desired to discuss their preferences with their physicians if they were terminally ill, but only 11 percent had done so. In one survey of 200 patients, only 18 percent had filled out an advance directive and of these, 50 percent had secured the only copy in a safety deposit box.

Copies of advance directives often are not transferred from nursing homes to hospitals on admission. One study found that physicians documented advance directives or discussions with appointed proxies about treatment decisions in only 11 percent of admission notes. While 90 percent of Americans say they want to die at home, four out of five die in a hospital or other healthcare facility.

If you wish to have control over your own end-of-life decisions, you will need to discuss your preferences with your family and physician, complete the documentation, and make sure, on your own or through a representative, that the documentation is included in your medical record at hospitals or other care facilities you enter.

Leave with a Map

Before it is time to leave the hospital, be sure you have a realistic plan for your care. Will you be able to care for yourself at home? Will you be able to get along with the help of an available family member? Will you need a visiting nurse or aide? Meals On Wheels? A nursing home? Make contact early, even before you enter a hospital if possible, with a hospital social worker and with other community social service agencies you are familiar with.

You will also need to make sure that there is a plan for your medical care and management by a physician after you leave the hospital. Will you turn to your primary care doctor or to a specialist who treated you in the hospital? If a doctor other than the doctor who managed your care in the hospital will be responsible, you will need to take steps to assure that the doctor who will be taking over has full information about you and your case right away.

That kind of information is supposed to be contained in a well-organized and thorough "discharge summary," which is supposed to be communicated promptly to the doctor who will be caring for you. Unfortunately, it doesn't always work that way.

Discharge summaries often are in a relatively unstructured, narrative format that invites inaccuracies. In addition, there can be significant delays transmitting discharge summaries to the doctors who need them.

In one study examining the effectiveness of inpatient follow-up care, nearly ten percent of discharged patients experienced worsening of symptoms or functional capacity as a result of an inadequately managed discharge process. Another study demonstrated that patients may be less likely to be readmitted to the hospital if their primary care provider receives a discharge summary. Yet one study found that only 34 percent of patients had a discharge summary sent to their outpatient care provider.

Be active in planning the care you will receive after discharge. Before leaving the hospital, ask your doctor when a discharge summary will be prepared, to whom it will be sent, and how it will be sent. Ask that a copy be sent to you. Then keep track of whether you get one and check with your outpatient care provider to be sure that provider's copy arrived.

Be Aware of Your Rights and Complain Where Necessary

If you feel you are not being treated with the proper respect or care, talk with the staff concerned. If that fails, talk with the nurse who works on the floor most regularly or with the head nurse on the floor. You can also check whether the hospital has a patient representative or ombudsman department. You can call a patient representative to talk about anything from cold food to rude staff. This person is charged with taking the problem to the responsible department and checking back with you to assure that the problem is corrected.

To help you insist on the care you deserve, it is useful to know your rights as a patient. Every hospital should have a statement of patient rights. You might ask for a copy of this statement at the time of admission or before. It should cover such matters as the right to informed consent and participation in your medical care, the right to privacy during physical examination, and the right to refuse to participate in any hospital research experiments. The American Hospital Association's standard Patient's Bill of Rights is reproduced in Appendix D.

If you consider a complaint serious enough—you believe your health is in jeopardy or the quality of care is simply very bad—talk with your doctor about having you transferred to another unit of the hospital or another hospital, or just sending you home. The doctor should recognize that your tension or unhappiness is not making you feel any better, and should be willing to try something else.

Don't Let Yourself Be Dumped

Because hospitals are paid by the case by Medicare and in a similar fashion by some other insurance plans, a hospital may come out better financially by discharging patients prematurely. Don't let this happen to you. First, tell your doctor that you don't feel well enough to go home. If he or she can't or won't stop the discharge process and if you are on Medicare, the hospital is required to give you a written description of an appeal procedure. During your appeal, which usually takes a day or two, you can stay in the hospital.

Chapter 6:

Keeping Costs Down

Most consumers care much more about a hospital's quality than about its prices. That's because under many insurance policies, your hospital bills will be paid in full even at the most expensive of hospitals.

But if your policy is less generous—for example, requiring you to pay 20 percent of hospital costs—your share of the differences in hospitals' charges can be significant. In our surveys, we have found that in the same community the daily rate for a semi-private room is sometimes twice as high at some hospitals as at others. And hospitals' average charges for specific types of cases also vary dramatically. In a survey of Utah hospitals, for example, average charges for an appendectomy ranged from less than $2,700 to nearly $7,500. In a survey of hospitals in Seattle, Washington, average charges for a normal childbirth ranged from less than $2,700 to more than $4,600. In a survey in the Chicago area, charges for a semi-private room ranged from less than $500 to more than $1,100.

You can call hospitals to inquire about charges for a semi-private room and other basic services, and you can ask about typical charges for your type of case. Also, check whether an agency in your state regularly publishes comparisons of charges.

Whatever hospital you choose, there are various ways to keep costs down. For example—

- Ask your doctor if you can have any needed tests—complete blood count, urinalysis, etc.—done by an outside lab or as a hospital outpatient before you are admitted to a hospital. You save by finding a less expensive lab and by avoiding a day or more in the hospital. Also, check whether every test the hospital wants to give you at entry is necessary and has been ordered by your doctor. Your health insurance may not reimburse for tests routinely done on admission unless specifically ordered.
- Ask your doctor if a hospital is the only place where your treatment can be done. Perhaps several visits to a hospital or a clinic as an outpatient will do just as well. If surgery is planned, check whether it is one of the many procedures now being performed on an outpatient basis.
- Check in late and check out early. Hospitals work like hotels; there is a time when the admission day begins and ends. Find out when it is. If you can come in the same day as your procedure, you will not have to pay to sit around. Short hospital stays are becoming more common. Ask your doctor if you can go home as soon as you feel like it. Many people feel better resting at home anyway.
- If your recuperation is likely to be long and you still require nursing assistance, find out about home health services. Care in your home is often much less expensive than prolonged hospital care, and may be more convenient for your family. Your doctor or the hospital's patient representative or social services department can help you get care at home. Medicare and most insurance plans will cover some portion of the costs of this kind of care if you have been in the hospital and the doctor recommends it.
- If you need blood transfusions, find out whether you can be your own donor. If surgery is planned several weeks away, you may be able to give a few units, which will replace themselves before the surgery. Find out if you can donate for yourself or have friends and family donate for you.
- If your health insurance plan requires that you get authorization from it before hospital admission in non-emergency cases and shortly after admission in emergency cases, be sure to get these authorizations so you won't be stuck with the bill. Also, be sure to find out whether a second opinion is required before admission.
- Check your bill. Be sure you aren't being charged by a hospital for more days than you were there. Also, check that you're only charged for medications you actually received and for tests and x-rays that actually took place. If a planned series of tests was canceled, be sure the charges didn't make it onto your bill.
- Don't pay twice. If a hospital's staff does a test or x-ray improperly or misplaces the results, be sure you are not billed for the retests.

Key Ratings for Metro Areas

See more information on "Detailed Ratings for All Areas" table beginning on page 74

✓ means hospital receives our top rating
Blue is most favorable
Bold Italic is least favorable
"–" means insufficient data

	Doctors' ratings of hospitals for high-risk adult surgery		Desirability scores from doctors (0 to 100, higher is better)					Measures of outcomes for selected cases (lower % is better)					
	Percent rating "very good" or "excellent"	Number of ratings	Low-risk adult surgery	Complex medical care for adults	High-risk child surgery	High-risk delivery of a baby	Uncomplicated delivery of a baby	Adjusted death rate for all case types (%)	Adjusted death rate for medical cases (%)	Adjusted death rate for surgical cases (%)	Adjusted adverse outcome rate for surgical cases (%)	Overall score on accreditation review (higher is better)	Major affiliation with a medical school?
National Average	32	–	59	50	40	46	58	12.1	14.8	2.3	7.7	91	–
Arizona													
Phoenix Area													
✓ Arizona Heart, Phoenix	**60**	107	57*	58	–[3]	–[4]	–[4]	11.9	13.3	2.8	8.3	–[6]	No
Arizona Surgical, Phoenix	–	–	***No data collected***					14.5	17.2	–	–	92	No
Arrowhead, Glendale	***8***	76	33	***8***	–[3]	***0***	44	12.5	15.1	–	9.2	92	No
Chandler Regional, Chandler	19	80	46	29	***0****	***0****	55	12.4	15.0	3.2	6.8	–[6]	No
Del E Webb, Sun City West	18	66	***0****	–	–[3]	–[4]	–[4]	12.1	14.7	2.3	8.9	**94**	No
✓ Desert Samaritan, Mesa	**68**	106	**100**	**97**	**86**	**100**	**100**	11.6	13.7	***3.0***	8.9	**95**	No
✓ Good Samaritan Regional, Phoenix	**89**	147	**100**	**100**	–[3]	**99**	**97**	11.7	14.1	2.5	9.5	93	**Yes**
John C Lincoln - Deer Valley, Phoenix	21	72	43*	14*	–	–	33*	11.3	13.3	3.5	7.4	–[6]	No
John C Lincoln - North Mountain, Phoenix	43	93	**92**	75*	–	–	69	***13.6***	***16.6***	2.7	8.2	–[6]	No
Maricopa, Phoenix	33	109	***0****	38	25	53	***18***	***14.2***	***17.0***	***7.8***	13.4	***88***	**Yes**
Maryvale, Phoenix	***3***	78	***0***	***0***	***0***	***0***	***5***	12.1	14.6	2.9	8.0	***88***	No
✓ Mayo Clinic, Phoenix	**73**	120	**91**	**99**	–[3]	–[4]	–[4]	**8.7**	**11.1**	1.2	7.7	**98**	**Yes**
Mesa General, Mesa	***6***	81	***7***	***0***	***0***	***0***	***3***	11.7	14.4	2.0	**5.3**	93	No
Mesa Lutheran, Mesa	17	84	70	33*	–	20*	67*	***13.8***	***16.6***	***3.2***	9.7	**97**	No
Paradise Valley, Phoenix	21	86	46	***8***	17*	***0****	52	***13.7***	***16.5***	3.6	7.6	**95**	No
Phoenix Baptist, Phoenix	25	88	55	44	–	–	69	12.0	14.6	2.3	8.7	91	No
Phoenix Children's, Phoenix	–[2]	–[2]	–[2]	–[2]	**100**	**96**	**90**	***No data collected***				**94**	–[6]
Phoenix Indian, Phoenix	–	–	***No data collected***					9.6	12.0	–	–	90	No
Phoenix Memorial, Phoenix[1]	***4***	81	***10***	***5***	7	7	***13***	10.4	12.8	1.6	8.0	93	No
✓ St Joseph's, Phoenix	**76**	139	**98**	**100**	**99**	**99**	**94**	11.9	14.5	2.3	8.4	–[6]	**Yes**
St Luke's, Phoenix	31	93	57*	–	–[3]	–[4]	–[4]	***14.6***	16.5	***4.8***	***15.2***	91	No
✓ Scottsdale Healthcare - Osborn, Scottsdale	**62**	107	88	**100**	33*	63*	86	11.2	**13.6**	2.3	9.7	93	No
✓ Scottsdale Healthcare - Shea, Scottsdale	**65**	113	**96**	**95**	33*	83	**98**	**10.6**	**13.0**	1.8	7.9	93	No
Tempe St Luke's, Tempe	***9***	77	***14***	19	7	6	***12***	13.3	16.1	–	9.5	**94**	No
Thunderbird Samaritan, Glendale[1]	**57**	86	88	64	–	80*	**97**	***13.2***	***16.0***	2.8	10.0	89	No
Valley Lutheran, Mesa	26	68	55	50*	–	20*	63*	12.3	15.0	2.1	8.2	**96**	No
Walter O Boswell, Sun City	33	67	63*	60*	–[3]	–[4]	–[4]	***12.7***	***15.8***	**1.8**	9.5	93	No
Wickenburg Regional, Wickenburg	***4***	50	***0***	***0***	***0***	–[4]	–[4]	**8.6**	10.6	–	–	91	No
California													
Los Angeles and Orange Counties													
Alhambra Hospital, Alhambra	***7***	56	–	***0****	–[3]	–[4]	–[4]	**8.4**	**10.2**	–	7.4	***86***	No
Anaheim General, Anaheim	***12***	52	–	–	–	–	38*	11.2	13.6	–	8.9	89	No
Anaheim Memorial, Anaheim	31	67	–	–	–[3]	–	–	11.7	14.2	2.4	8.2	93	No
Antelope Valley, Lancaster	***13***	60	–	–	–	–	–	12.2	14.6	3.4	8.2	93	No

Footnotes are on page 73. *Hospital's score based on relatively little data. See page 16.

Key Ratings for Metro Areas

See more information on "Detailed Ratings for All Areas" table beginning on page 74

✓ means hospital receives our top rating
Blue is most favorable
Bold Italic is least favorable
"–" means insufficient data

	Doctors' ratings of hospitals for high-risk adult surgery		Desirability scores from doctors (0 to 100, higher is better)					Measures of outcomes for selected cases (lower % is better)					
	Percent rating "very good" or "excellent"	Number of ratings	Low-risk adult surgery	Complex medical care for adults	High-risk child surgery	High-risk delivery of a baby	Uncomplicated delivery of a baby	Adjusted death rate for all case types (%)	Adjusted death rate for medical cases (%)	Adjusted death rate for surgical cases (%)	Adjusted adverse outcome rate for surgical cases (%)	Overall score on accreditation review (higher is better)	Major affiliation with a medical school?
National Average	32	–	59	50	40	46	58	12.1	14.8	2.3	7.7	91	–
California *(continued)*													
Los Angeles and Orange Counties *(continued)*													
Bellflower Medical Center, Bellflower	***13***	46	–	29*	–[3]	***0****	***20***	**9.3**	**11.4**	–	10.8	***84***	No
Bellwood General, Bellflower	***9***	34	–	***0****	–[3]	–	–	*No data collected*				90	–[6]
Beverly, Montebello	15	74	71*	–	–	–	60*	12.7	15.4	3.0	7.3	92	No
Brea Community, Brea	***7***	45	–	–	–	–[4]	–[4]	14.0	16.6	–	6.7	**98**	No
Brotman, Culver City	18	119	43*	27	–[3]	***0****	***0****	**9.0**	**10.9**	2.5	8.1	**95**	No
California, Los Angeles	***14***	93	–	–	33*	38*	50*	**9.2**	**11.2**	–	8.3	93	No
✓ Cedars - Sinai, Los Angeles	**83**	317	**96**	**96**	**92**	**96**	**92**	**9.4**	**11.5**	**1.6**	8.8	**97**	**Yes**
Centinela, Inglewood	40	127	75*	–	–	–	50*	**10.0**	**12.1**	2.3	7.7	**96**	No
Century City, Los Angeles	29	105	**89***	–	–[3]	–[4]	–[4]	**9.5**	**11.6**	2.0	9.1	***87***	No
Chapman, Orange	18	56	***25****	***0****	***0****	***0****	***0****	***14.9***	***18.3***	–	–	92	No
Children's, Orange	–[2]	–[2]	–[2]	–[2]	**98**	–[4]	–[4]	*No data collected*				–[6]	–[6]
Childrens, Los Angeles	–[2]	–[2]	–[2]	–[2]	**100**	–[4]	–[4]	*No data collected*				89	–[6]
Citrus Valley, West Covina	25	44	60*	57*	60*	75*	75*	10.9	13.2	2.3	7.3	90	No
Citrus Valley Intercommunity, Covina	24	41	71*	67*	–	–	–	12.5	15.0	3.0	8.7	–[6]	No
City of Angels, Los Angeles	–	–	*No data collected*					–	–	–	–	91	No
City of Hope National, Duarte	**83**	150	–	70	–	–[4]	–[4]	13.3	16.2	–	–	93	No
Coast Plaza Doctors, Norwalk	***9***	34	***0****	***0****	–[3]	***0****	***0****	13.8	16.7	–	–	***80***	**Yes**
Coastal Communities, Santa Ana	***7***	45	***20***	13*	20*	***0****	30	13.1	16.0	–	5.9	**96**	No
Community, Gardena	–	–	–	–	–[3]	–[4]	–[4]	9.8	11.6	–	–	***81***	No
Community, Huntington Park[1]	–	–	–	–	–	–	–	**6.6**	**8.0**	–	7.4	91	No
Daniel Freeman Marina, Marina Del Rey	23	105	38*	***0****	–[3]	–[4]	–[4]	**10.2**	**12.4**	–	6.3	***87***	No
Daniel Freeman Memorial, Inglewood	25	124	50	29*	–	14*	29*	**8.6**	**10.4**	2.4	8.7	***87***	No
Doctors, West Covina	***4***	26	–	–	–	–	–	**2.9**	**3.1**	–	–	**95**	No
Downey Regional, Downey	24	50	50*	50*	–	–	***20****	12.7	15.6	2.1	7.2	91	No
East Los Angeles Doctors, Los Angeles	***4***	48	***0****	–	–	***0****	***11****	**5.5**	**6.8**	–	–	92	No
Encino - Tarzana Regional, Encino	29	90	–	–	–[3]	–[4]	–[4]	12.4	15.2	2.1	5.8	–[6]	No
Encino - Tarzana Regional, Tarzana	46	95	**95**	**100**	**100***	86	87	**9.8**	**12.2**	**1.3**	7.2	92	No
Foothill Presbyterian, Glendora	18	33	–	–	–	–	–	***14.9***	***17.9***	–	10.1	**94**	No
Fountain Valley Regional, Fountain Valley	35	81	33*	46	43*	39	40	**9.7**	**11.7**	2.4	6.7	**100**	No
Garden Grove Hospital, Garden Grove	20	51	33*	***0****	***0****	***0****	31	12.0	14.5	2.5	5.7	93	No
Garfield, Monterey Park	***11***	72	60*	17*	–	–	33*	**6.7**	**8.1**	1.9	7.2	90	No
Glendale Adventist, Glendale	42	131	71*	71*	–	83*	62	12.1	14.7	2.3	7.0	**96**	**Yes**
Glendale Memorial, Glendale	35	80	86*	67*	–	57*	78*	**8.8**	**10.6**	2.4	8.9	90	No
✓ Good Samaritan, Los Angeles	**67**	148	**100**	**90**	–[3]	**100**	**100**	**9.5**	**11.0**	***3.2***	***10.0***	90	**Yes**

Footnotes are on page 73. *Hospital's score based on relatively little data. See page 16.

Key Ratings for Metro Areas

See more information on "Detailed Ratings for All Areas" table beginning on page 74

✓ means hospital receives our top rating
Blue is most favorable
Bold Italic is least favorable
"–" means insufficient data

	Doctors' ratings of hospitals for high-risk adult surgery		Desirability scores from doctors (0 to 100, higher is better)					Measures of outcomes for selected cases (lower % is better)					
	Percent rating "very good" or "excellent"	Number of ratings	Low-risk adult surgery	Complex medical care for adults	High-risk child surgery	High-risk delivery of a baby	Uncomplicated delivery of a baby	Adjusted death rate for all case types (%)	Adjusted death rate for medical cases (%)	Adjusted death rate for surgical cases (%)	Adjusted adverse outcome rate for surgical cases (%)	Overall score on accreditation review (higher is better)	Major affiliation with a medical school?
National Average	32	–	59	50	40	46	58	12.1	14.8	2.3	7.7	91	–
California *(continued)*													
Los Angeles and Orange Counties *(continued)*													
Granada Hills Community, Granada Hills	16	45	–	–	–[3]	***0****	***0****	8.1	9.7	2.4	6.7	–[6]	No
Greater El Monte, South El Monte	***5***	38	–	–	–	–	–	7.8	9.5	–	–	***83***	No
Henry Mayo Newhall, Valencia	***12***	75	***13****	***0***	–[3]	***0***	***8***	9.1	11.1	1.5	4.5	***79***	No
✓ Hoag Presbyterian, Newport Beach	78	174	95	94	67	88	91	10.6	12.9	1.7	8.9	95	No
Hollywood Community, Hollywood	***8***	37	***0****	–	–[3]	–[4]	–[4]	6.9	8.4	–	–	***86***	No
✓ Huntington, Pasadena	84	160	100	100	94	98	98	10.6	12.9	2.2	9.2	92	No
Huntington Beach Hospital, Huntington Beach	18	45	–	–	–[3]	–[4]	–[4]	11.8	14.2	–	8.5	92	No
Huntington East Valley, Glendora	–	–	–	20*	–[3]	–	–	9.0	10.7	–	–	***83***	No
Irvine Regional, Irvine	35	78	57	40	57*	50*	71	11.5	13.9	–	6.0	92	No
Kaiser Permanente, Anaheim	48	97	73	54	67*	75	78	12.6	15.8	0.9	5.3	***87***	No
Kaiser Permanente, Baldwin Park	49	104	85	60	–[3]	64	82	***40.0***	***50.9***	–	–	–[6]	No
Kaiser Permanente, Bellflower	42	126	60	71*	60	68	53	***14.2***	***17.5***	1.6	8.3	93	No
Kaiser Permanente, Harbor City	38	103	60*	60*	–	–	–	13.1	***16.5***	0.4	6.6	***87***	No
Kaiser Permanente, Panorama City	37	108	69	62	40*	67*	82	12.3	14.8	3.1	8.0	***85***	No
Kaiser Permanente, Woodland Hills	47	130	92	89*	83*	88	86	***13.5***	***16.4***	2.7	8.3	***87***	No
Kaiser Permanente Los Angeles, Los Angeles	63	188	88	85	81	92	86	***13.4***	***16.3***	2.5	9.4	89	Yes
Kaiser Permanente West Los Angeles, Los Angeles	43	135	63*	–	–	–	67*	13.0	***15.9***	2.4	9.7	90	No
La Palma Intercommunity, La Palma	***8***	48	***20****	–	–[3]	–	67*	8.7	10.6	–	–	***88***	No
LAC + USC, Los Angeles	46	223	***12***	44	–	81[5]	***27***[5]	10.1	12.3	–	–	***85***	No
✓ LAC - Harbor - UCLA, Torrance	65	232	55	83	67	75	***27***	11.1	13.6	–	–	91	Yes
LAC - High Desert, Lancaster	***10***	52	–	***0****	–	–[4]	–[4]	–	–	–	–	98	No
Lakewood Regional, Lakewood	23	56	–	–	–[3]	–	–	12.0	14.5	2.5	8.4	90	No
Lancaster Community, Lancaster	22	36	–	–	–[3]	–[4]	–[4]	10.3	12.6	2.0	6.7	***87***	No
Lincoln, Los Angeles	–	–	***0****	–	***0****	–	–	2.7	–	–	–	***83***	No
Little Company of Mary, Torrance[1]	46	112	85	67	29*	70	90	10.9	13.2	2.2	10.1	93	No
Long Beach Memorial, Long Beach	24	59	***20****	14*	14*	14*	–	12.9	15.5	***3.5***	10.2	–[6]	No
✓ Long Beach Memorial, Long Beach	73	178	100	100	100	100	100	11.7	14.3	2.0	7.7	96	Yes
Los Alamitos Medical Center, Los Alamitos	35	71	100	78*	–[3]	80*	90	11.8	14.3	2.5	8.0	91	No
Los Angeles Community, Los Angeles[1]	***7***	29	–	–	–	–	–	5.9	7.3	–	3.1	***86***	No
Los Angeles Metropolitan, Los Angeles	***8***	25	–	–	–	–	–	8.5	10.3	–	–	***83***	No
Los Angeles Metropolitan - Hawthorne, Hawthorne[1]	–	–	–	–	–[3]	–[4]	–[4]	*No data collected*				–[6]	–[6]
Martin Luther King - Drew, Los Angeles	***14***	154	***0***	***3***	***0***	6	***4***	8.9	10.8	–	–	***82***	No
Memorial, Gardena	***7***	27	–	–	–	–	–	12.6	14.9	***6.6***	***19.2***	90	No
✓ Methodist Hospital of Southern California, Arcadia	54	46	86*	–	–	–	90	9.8	12.1	1.2	6.6	92	No

Footnotes are on page 73. *Hospital's score based on relatively little data. See page 16.

Key Ratings for Metro Areas

See more information on "Detailed Ratings for All Areas" table beginning on page 74

✓ means hospital receives our top rating
Blue is most favorable
Bold Italic is least favorable
"–" means insufficient data

	Doctors' ratings of hospitals for high-risk adult surgery		Desirability scores from doctors (0 to 100, higher is better)					Measures of outcomes for selected cases (lower % is better)					
	Percent rating "very good" or "excellent"	Number of ratings	Low-risk adult surgery	Complex medical care for adults	High-risk child surgery	High-risk delivery of a baby	Uncomplicated delivery of a baby	Adjusted death rate for all case types (%)	Adjusted death rate for medical cases (%)	Adjusted death rate for surgical cases (%)	Adjusted adverse outcome rate for surgical cases (%)	Overall score on accreditation review (higher is better)	Major affiliation with a medical school?
National Average	32	–	59	50	40	46	58	12.1	14.8	2.3	7.7	91	–
California *(continued)*													
Los Angeles and Orange Counties *(continued)*													
Midway, Los Angeles	24	62	62	40*	***0****	–[4]	–[4]	9.8	11.8	3.1	7.4	***86***	No
Mission - Panorama, Panorama City	***4***	25	–	–	–[3]	–[4]	–[4]	7.6	9.3	–	–	96	No
✓ Mission Regional, Mission Viejo	56	71	90	89	100[5]	90	90	11.8	13.9	***3.6***	7.5	90	No
Monrovia Community, Monrovia	–	–	–	–	–[3]	–[4]	–[4]	11.6	14.1	–	–	92	No
Monterey Park Hospital, Monterey Park	***6***	47	–	–	–[3]	–	–	6.4	7.8	–	7.5	***88***	No
Motion Picture and Television Fund, Woodland Hills	–	–			***No data collected***			11.4	14.3	–	–	91	No
Northridge - Roscoe Blvd Campus, Northridge	22	67	–	–	–	***0****	***14****	9.1	11.0	1.8	8.3	93	No
Northridge - Sherman Way Campus, Van Nuys	41	83	100	100*	–[3]	90	92	8.9	11.0	–	6.4	93	No
Orange Coast, Fountain Valley	23	53	83*	–	–[3]	–	86*	12.1	14.4	***4.0***	7.6	94	No
Orthopaedic, Los Angeles	63	87	–	–	–	–[4]	–[4]	–	–	–	13.1	***87***	No
Pacific, Long Beach	***9***	45	***10***	***0***	–[3]	11*	***11****	10.1	12.3	–	–	***83***	No
Pacific Alliance, Los Angeles	17	30	–	–	–	–	–	6.9	8.4	1.8	3.8	91	No
Pacifica, Sun Valley	***8***	26	–	***0****	***0****	***0****	***0****	12.5	15.2	–	–	***82***	No
Placentia Linda, Placentia	***13***	39	100*	–	–[3]	–	–	***15.1***	***18.4***	–	3.9	96	No
Pomona Valley, Pomona	32	53	100*	–	–	100*	100*	9.6	11.3	3.0	8.1	94	No
Presbyterian Intercommunity, Whittier	60	53	88	86*	–	89*	94	12.1	14.9	1.7	7.3	91	No
✓ Providence Holy Cross, Mission Hills	51	43	100*	–	–	–	100*	9.0	10.9	2.1	8.4	90	No
✓ Providence St Joseph, Burbank	62	45	93	88*	–	67*	82	9.3	11.3	2.1	6.7	90	No
Queen of Angels - Hollywood Presbyterian, LA	25	95	56*	29*	50*	38*	42	7.5	9.0	2.9	8.2	***87***	No
Robert F Kennedy, Hawthorne	***11***	45	***11****	***0****	–[3]	–[4]	–[4]	9.3	11.2	–	–	91	No
Saddleback, Laguna Hills	55	91	94	100	–[3]	84	89	***13.3***	***16.4***	1.6	5.8	94	No
St Francis, Lynwood	22	60	–	40*	–	–	***17****	10.5	12.7	2.6	9.9	93	No
✓ St Johns, Santa Monica	78	130	100	97	90	88	100	8.0	9.8	1.0	7.0	92	No
St Joseph, Orange	75	119	97	97	–[3]	98	95	12.5	15.5	1.7	7.2	93	No
St Jude, Fullerton	71	87	83*	100*	–	100*	100	***13.5***	***16.6***	2.1	9.6	97	No
St Luke, Pasadena	16	49	–	–	–	–	–	7.7	9.2	3.0	10.3	–[6]	No
St Mary, Long Beach	36	67	75*	83*	60*	86*	92	9.5	11.4	2.6	7.4	92	No
St Vincent, Los Angeles	69	88	100	100*	–	–[4]	–[4]	8.3	9.9	2.2	8.4	***86***	No
San Clemente Hospital, San Clemente	***4***	46	***20****	***0****	–[3]	***0****	***0****	11.8	14.3	–	5.4	98	No
San Dimas Community, San Dimas	15	26	–	–	–	–	–	12.9	15.6	–	4.1	***88***	No
San Gabriel Valley, San Gabriel	29	48	–	–	–	–	83*	9.3	11.4	1.4	6.3	90	No
San Pedro Peninsula, San Pedro	***12***	33	–	–	–	–	–	12.1	14.9	1.5	7.1	92	No
Santa Ana Hospital, Santa Ana	***8***	36	***13****	***0****	17*	***0****	***11****	11.5	13.7	–	1.7	91	No
Santa Marta, Los Angeles	***12***	34	–	–	–[3]	–	–	6.0	7.3	–	4.9	95	No

Footnotes are on page 73. *Hospital's score based on relatively little data. See page 16.

Key Ratings for Metro Areas

See more information on "Detailed Ratings for All Areas" table beginning on page 74

✓ means hospital receives our top rating
Blue is most favorable
Bold Italic is least favorable
"–" means insufficient data

	Doctors' ratings of hospitals for high-risk adult surgery		Desirability scores from doctors (0 to 100, higher is better)					Measures of outcomes for selected cases (lower % is better)					
	Percent rating "very good" or "excellent"	Number of ratings	Low-risk adult surgery	Complex medical care for adults	High-risk child surgery	High-risk delivery of a baby	Uncomplicated delivery of a baby	Adjusted death rate for all case types (%)	Adjusted death rate for medical cases (%)	Adjusted death rate for surgical cases (%)	Adjusted adverse outcome rate for surgical cases (%)	Overall score on accreditation review (higher is better)	Major affiliation with a medical school?
National Average	32	–	59	50	40	46	58	12.1	14.8	2.3	7.7	91	–
California *(continued)*													
Los Angeles and Orange Counties *(continued)*													
Santa Monica UCLA, Santa Monica	**58**	169	86	79	75*	**92**	**96**	**10.1**	**12.5**	1.4	**4.9**	***84***	No
Santa Teresita, Duarte	***12***	33	***0****	–	–[3]	–	–	11.3	13.7	–	–	91	No
Sherman Oaks Hospital, Sherman Oaks	26	54	–	–	–	–[4]	–[4]	***15.2***	***18.5***	–	7.0	93	No
South Coast, Laguna Beach	***6***	52	–	***0****	***0****	–	–	12.1	15.2	0.5	**3.2**	**98**	No
Suburban, Paramount	–	–	–	–	–	–	–	11.9	14.2	–	–	**94**	No
Temple, Los Angeles	***7***	29	–	–	–[3]	–[4]	–[4]	**5.0**	**6.2**	0.5	6.4	93	No
Torrance Memorial, Torrance	**60**	101	**100**	**100**	**100***	**100**	**100**	11.6	14.0	2.5	8.9	***87***	No
Tri-City Regional, Hawaiian Gardens	–	–			*No data collected*			13.4	15.9	–	11.1	89	No
Tustin Hospital, Tustin	***7***	42	***0****	***0****	–[3]	–[4]	–[4]	2.5	3.1	–	–	***80***	No
✓ UCLA, Los Angeles[1]	**90**	328	88	**98**	**96**	**97**	82	**9.9**	**12.2**	**1.2**	7.7	–[6]	**Yes**
✓ University of California - Irvine, Orange	**70**	156	88	**97**	**90**	**92**	71	10.5	13.2	1.2	6.8	**96**	**Yes**
USC - Kenneth Norris Cancer, Los Angeles	**89**	179	67*	80	–[3]	–[4]	–[4]	12.8	16.7	–	5.3	–[6]	No
✓ USC University, Los Angeles	**80**	261	81	**88**	–[3]	–[4]	–[4]	**7.4**	**8.5**	1.6	**6.3**	91	**Yes**
Valley Care - Los Angeles County UCLA, Sylmar	29	147	–	–	–	67*	60*	14.6	17.4	–	–	93	No
Valley Presbyterian, Van Nuys	36	77	40*	–	17*	44	36	**10.7**	**12.9**	2.2	6.9	89	No
Verdugo Hills, Glendale	***14***	57	–	–	–[3]	–	80*	***13.8***	***16.8***	2.3	7.2	–[6]	No
West Anaheim Medical Center, Anaheim	16	49	–	–	–	–	–	13.0	15.6	3.6	7.2	92	No
West Hills, Canoga Park	35	52	**100**	**100***	44*	83	**94**	11.6	14.0	2.4	7.8	93	No
Western, Anaheim	31	81	70	67*	–[3]	63*	33*	12.8	15.1	3.5	12.5	92	No
Western, Santa Ana	18	50	–	–	–	–	57*	13.1	15.6	***4.4***	8.6	91	No
White, Los Angeles	33	129	83*	80*	–	**100***	83*	**7.9**	**9.5**	2.7	7.5	**97**	**Yes**
Whittier Hospital, Whittier	24	63	60*	20*	–	20*	60*	***14.0***	***16.8***	–	–	93	No
Riverside and San Bernardino Counties													
Arrowhead Regional, Colton	**52**	65	33*	67	67*	43*	***14****	11.3	13.6	–	–	***86***	No
Barstow Community, Barstow	***3***	33	–	–	***0****	–	***0****	12.2	15.0	–	8.7	***83***	No
Bear Valley, Big Bear Lake	***3***	32	***0****	***0****	–[3]	–[4]	–[4]	16.0	19.5	–	–	***84***	No
Chino Valley, Chino	20	30	63*	40*	–	***0****	–	**8.9**	**10.8**	–	**3.2**	**95**	No
Colorado River, Needles	–	–	–	–	–	–	–	12.6	15.3	–	–	***84***	No
Community, San Bernardino	***11***	45	–	–	–	–	***20****	12.0	14.4	3.3	10.3	93	No
Corona Regional, Corona	20	35	50*	–	–	–	33*	12.1	14.7	2.8	10.5	***84***	No
Desert Regional, Palm Springs	46	39	**100***	–	–	83*	71*	***13.1***	15.7	***3.5***	8.8	90	No
Desert Valley, Victorville	16	32	60*	–	–	–	50*	***15.2***	***18.5***	–	3.6	**94**	No
Doctors', Montclair	***8***	40	***13***	***8***	***0***	***0***	***7***	***16.2***	***19.4***	–	–	89	No
✓ Eisenhower, Rancho Mirage	**67**	55	**100**	**91**	–	75*	**92**	11.6	14.2	2.0	8.5	**97**	No

Footnotes are on page 73. *Hospital's score based on relatively little data. See page 16.

Key Ratings for Metro Areas

See more information on "Detailed Ratings for All Areas" table beginning on page 74

✓ means hospital receives our top rating
Blue is most favorable
Bold Italic is least favorable
"–" means insufficient data

	Doctors' ratings of hospitals for high-risk adult surgery		Desirability scores from doctors (0 to 100, higher is better)					Measures of outcomes for selected cases (lower % is better)					
	Percent rating "very good" or "excellent"	Number of ratings	Low-risk adult surgery	Complex medical care for adults	High-risk child surgery	High-risk delivery of a baby	Uncomplicated delivery of a baby	Adjusted death rate for all case types (%)	Adjusted death rate for medical cases (%)	Adjusted death rate for surgical cases (%)	Adjusted adverse outcome rate for surgical cases (%)	Overall score on accreditation review (higher is better)	Major affiliation with a medical school?
National Average	32	–	59	50	40	46	58	12.1	14.8	2.3	7.7	91	–
California *(continued)*													
Riverside and San Bernardino Counties *(continued)*													
Hemet Valley, Hemet	***11***	38	–	–	–	–	33*	***14.9***	***17.7***	***4.7***	11.0	89	No
Hi-Desert, Joshua Tree	***9***	34	***14****	17*	20*	–[4]	–[4]	***14.8***	***17.5***	***4.7***	10.1	91	No
Inland Valley Regional, Wildomar	23	30	–	–	–[3]	–	–	9.4	10.8	***4.7***	8.0	94	No
John F Kennedy, Indio	18	38	–	***0****	–	17*	40	10.8	13.0	2.5	6.3	93	No
Kaiser Permanente, Fontana	63	70	87	91	81	94	93	***15.3***	***18.7***	2.9	8.1	92	No
Kaiser Permanente, Riverside	49	57	83	63*	33*	43*	73	***15.1***	***18.1***	***3.9***	8.9	92	No
Loma Linda University (Anderson St), Loma Linda[1]	86	93	100	100	100	100	100	12.6	15.6	1.8	***11.4***	–[6]	Yes
Loma Linda University (Barton Rd), Loma Linda	52	69	80	94	96	–[4]	–[4]	***No data collected***				–[6]	–[6]
Menifee Valley, Sun City	***13***	32	***20****	–	–	–	–	11.2	13.1	***6.0***	9.2	91	No
Moreno Valley Community, Moreno Valley	***11***	35	–	–	–	–	–	10.1	12.4	–	4.1	92	No
Mountains, Lake Arrowhead	***10***	30	***0****	***0****	–	–	–	8.0	9.9	–	–	***81***	No
Palo Verde, Blythe	–	–	***29****	20*	–[3]	17*	***17****	***15.6***	***18.7***	–	–	–[6]	No
Parkview, Riverside	18	49	100*	–	–	100*	89*	***14.8***	***17.7***	***4.6***	10.6	89	No
Rancho Springs, Murrieta	–	–	–	–	–	–	–	10.5	12.7	2.2	3.6	95	No
Redlands Community, Redlands	50	56	94	80	–	60*	96	***15.2***	***18.8***	2.5	6.9	92	No
Riverside Community, Riverside	43	53	86	85	50*	75*	86	12.9	15.3	***3.6***	10.5	97	No
Riverside County Regional, Moreno Valley	54	57	–	75*	–	50*	40*	***16.7***	***20.3***	–	–	94	Yes
St Bernardine, San Bernardino	61	72	100	100*	60*	100*	100*	12.4	15.1	2.5	***11.0***	89	No
St Mary Regional, Apple Valley	25	40	–	–	–	–	83*	12.5	14.5	***4.5***	10.4	***88***	No
San Antonio, Upland	55	58	94	85	88*	89*	93	12.5	15.1	3.0	9.3	–[6]	No
San Gorgonio, Banning	***8***	37	***0****	***0****	***0****	***0****	***0****	***18.3***	***22.2***	–	8.6	93	No
Victor Valley, Victorville	***5***	38	***13****	***0****	***0****	***0****	***0****	***14.2***	***17.2***	–	7.6	–[6]	No
Sacramento Area													
Kaiser Permanente Sacramento, Sacramento	53	91	66	69	53	69	56	***14.5***	***17.7***	2.7	8.5	***88***	No
Kaiser Permanente South Sacramento, Sacramento	42	89	60	55	–[3]	34	74	***15.3***	***18.9***	1.7	8.1	94	Yes
Mercy, Folsom	16	73	***29***	13	–[3]	***0***	41	12.5	15.2	2.4	7.1	95	No
✓ Mercy General, Sacramento	65	93	90	93	36	47	82	10.7	13.3	1.5	5.6	94	Yes
Mercy San Juan, Carmichael	52	83	79	71	50	82	78	12.5	15.1	2.7	7.9	92	No
Methodist, Sacramento	***10***	77	***13***	***3***	***0***	8	***17***	13.0	15.8	2.8	7.5	97	No
Sutter General, Sacramento	73	89	94	95	–[3]	–[4]	–[4]	***13.4***	***16.8***	1.9	9.6	***84***	No
Sutter Memorial, Sacramento	64	90	85	81	97	97	94	***No data collected***				–[6]	–[6]
University of California - Davis, Sacramento	65	97	48	91	94	74	33	12.4	15.3	1.3	9.3	91	Yes
San Diego Area													
Alvarado, San Diego	30	101	75	72	–[3]	30	55	11.6	14.0	2.5	7.2	***87***	No

Footnotes are on page 73. *Hospital's score based on relatively little data. See page 16.

Key Ratings for Metro Areas

See more information on "Detailed Ratings for All Areas" table beginning on page 74

✓ means hospital receives our top rating
Blue is most favorable
Bold Italic is least favorable
"–" means insufficient data

	Doctors' ratings of hospitals for high-risk adult surgery		Desirability scores from doctors (0 to 100, higher is better)					Measures of outcomes for selected cases (lower % is better)					
	Percent rating "very good" or "excellent"	Number of ratings	Low-risk adult surgery	Complex medical care for adults	High-risk child surgery	High-risk delivery of a baby	Uncomplicated delivery of a baby	Adjusted death rate for all case types (%)	Adjusted death rate for medical cases (%)	Adjusted death rate for surgical cases (%)	Adjusted adverse outcome rate for surgical cases (%)	Overall score on accreditation review (higher is better)	Major affiliation with a medical school?
National Average	32	–	59	50	40	46	58	12.1	14.8	2.3	7.7	91	–
California *(continued)*													
San Diego Area *(continued)*													
Children's, San Diego	89	79	–	–	100	–[4]	–[4]	***No data collected***				91	–[6]
Fallbrook Hospital, Fallbrook[1]	***2***	65	***6***	***0***	***0***	***0***	***8***	12.2	15.1	–	3.7	***87***	No
Grossmont, La Mesa	35	100	88	93	–	50	91	12.6	***15.6***	1.5	7.3	92	No
Kaiser Permanente, San Diego[1]	39	102	75	62	59	68	59	***13.6***	***16.9***	1.7	7.1	94	No
Palomar, Escondido	31	87	30	14*	–	–	38*	***13.2***	***16.1***	2.3	8.0	***87***	Yes
Paradise Valley, National City	***1***	80	***0***	***0***	***0***	***0***	***8***	7.4	9.0	–	7.4	92	No
Pomerado, Poway	18	83	55	29*	–[3]	11*	57	***14.1***	***17.3***	2.3	5.2	–[6]	No
Scripps, Chula Vista	17	82	60*	–	–	–	–	11.5	14.1	1.9	8.7	–[6]	No
Scripps, Encinitas	32	91	89	75	–[3]	–	82	11.7	14.6	1.1	5.5	93	No
✓ Scripps Green, La Jolla	60	107	95	93	–[3]	–[4]	–[4]	11.0	14.1	1.2	6.3	90	No
Scripps Memorial, La Jolla	73	120	94	89	38*	78	89	10.5	13.0	1.6	7.5	***82***	No
Scripps Mercy, San Diego	70	118	88	89	63*	85	88	9.9	11.8	2.7	7.5	***88***	No
Sharp, Chula Vista	24	76	100*	67*	–	–	89*	10.7	12.9	2.1	8.7	93	No
Sharp, Coronado	***8***	75	***0****	–	–[3]	***0****	***17****	***14.3***	***17.4***	–	–	93	No
Sharp Mary Birch Hospital for Women, San Diego	81	80	80*	78*	–[3]	99	98	–	–	–	–	95	No
Sharp Memorial, San Diego	80	122	98	98	–[3]	100*	–	12.2	15.0	2.1	8.2	91	No
Tri-City, Oceanside	40	94	60	60	***0***	18	40	12.4	15.1	2.6	9.6	92	No
UCSD - La Jolla/Thornton, La Jolla	69	118	89	97	33*	75	78*	***No data collected***				–[6]	–[6]
University of California - San Diego, San Diego	73	129	74	95	94	96	59	12.8	15.7	2.2	7.6	93	Yes
Villaview, San Diego	***3***	73	***3***	***0***	–[3]	–[4]	–[4]	12.5	14.7	–	–	92	No
San Francisco Bay Area													
Alameda County, Oakland	30	131	***11***	35	***0***	10	***11***	10.2	12.5	–	–	–[6]	No
Alameda Hospital, Alameda	***8***	72	***13****	14*	–[3]	13	***0***	13.0	15.7	3.0	6.5	***87***	No
Alta Bates, Berkeley	65	194	98	94	–[3]	98	96	11.0	13.5	1.9	9.1	***83***	No
✓ California Pacific - California Campus, San Francisco[1]	74	174	98	96	95	99	99	10.3	12.8	1.4	6.3	90	Yes
California Pacific - Davies Campus, San Francisco[1]	48	106	83*	50*	–[3]	–[4]	–[4]	9.0	10.9	–	–	90	No
California Pacific - East Campus, San Francisco[1]	49	76	–	–	–	–	–	***No data collected***				90	–[6]
California Pacific - Pacific Campus, San Francisco[1]	77	137	96	94	83	88	82	***No data collected***				90	–[6]
Children's, Oakland	–[2]	–[2]	–[2]	–[2]	100	–[4]	–[4]	***No data collected***				***88***	–[6]
Chinese, San Francisco[1]	18	74	36	21	–[3]	***0****	***0****	9.1	11.0	2.0	5.8	97	No
Community, Los Gatos	24	108	71	40	***0***	17	68	11.4	13.8	2.6	6.9	–[6]	No
Contra Costa Regional, Martinez	16	81	***0***	***8***	***0***	***0***	***6***	11.2	13.7	–	–	91	No
Doctors, Pinole	***10***	77	–	–	–[3]	–[4]	–[4]	13.5	15.7	***6.2***	***14.9***	91	No
Doctors, San Pablo	***10***	72	54	47	–[3]	***0****	31	12.9	15.6	2.9	6.9	93	No

Footnotes are on page 73. *Hospital's score based on relatively little data. See page 16.

Key Ratings for Metro Areas

See more information on "Detailed Ratings for All Areas" table beginning on page 74

✓ means hospital receives our top rating
Blue is most favorable
Bold Italic is least favorable
"–" means insufficient data

	Doctors' ratings of hospitals for high-risk adult surgery		Desirability scores from doctors (0 to 100, higher is better)					Measures of outcomes for selected cases (lower % is better)					
	Percent rating "very good" or "excellent"	Number of ratings	Low-risk adult surgery	Complex medical care for adults	High-risk child surgery	High-risk delivery of a baby	Uncomplicated delivery of a baby	Adjusted death rate for all case types (%)	Adjusted death rate for medical cases (%)	Adjusted death rate for surgical cases (%)	Adjusted adverse outcome rate for surgical cases (%)	Overall score on accreditation review (higher is better)	Major affiliation with a medical school?
National Average	32	–	59	50	40	46	58	12.1	14.8	2.3	7.7	91	–
California *(continued)*													
San Francisco Bay Area *(continued)*													
Eden, Castro Valley	36	106	**90**	**89***	–	75*	83	***13.3***	***16.2***	2.5	**6.1**	93	No
✓ El Camino, Mountain View	**66**	177	**95**	84	50*	78	**97**	11.6	14.3	1.7	**5.9**	**94**	No
Good Samaritan, San Jose	47	150	88	86	**83**	87	**91**	11.6	14.1	2.3	7.4	***86***	No
Healdsburg General, Healdsburg	***11***	37	–	***0****	–	–	***0****	14.0	17.2	2.4	7.1	89	No
✓ John Muir, Walnut Creek[1]	**75**	178	**90**	87	64	**90**	**90**	11.8	14.5	2.0	7.7	**96**	No
Kaiser Permanente, Hayward[1]	**54**	153	79	70	–	72	**89**	12.4	15.2	2.0	7.2	***86***	No
Kaiser Permanente, Oakland	**61**	195	**90**	86	81	77	76	***13.1***	***16.0***	2.0	8.5	***86***	No
Kaiser Permanente, Redwood City	**65**	135	**89***	–	–	–	**88***	12.6	15.5	2.1	**5.6**	***85***	No
Kaiser Permanente, Richmond	32	119	40	25*	–[3]	–[4]	–[4]	***No data collected***				–[6]	–[6]
Kaiser Permanente, San Francisco	**69**	219	86	**91**	**83**	82	84	12.3	15.3	1.9	7.3	–[6]	No
Kaiser Permanente, San Rafael	**69**	128	**91**	78	–	–[4]	–[4]	***13.8***	***17.1***	1.7	8.1	–[6]	No
Kaiser Permanente, Santa Clara	**70**	223	**94**	**94**	**89**	**94**	**93**	***13.5***	***16.5***	2.0	7.7	89	**Yes**
Kaiser Permanente, Santa Rosa	**66**	105	**100**	75*	–	86*	**100**	13.3	16.2	2.5	**6.0**	90	No
Kaiser Permanente, South San Francisco	**59**	113	**100***	–	–	–	–	***13.4***	***16.4***	1.6	6.5	–[6]	No
Kaiser Permanente, Vallejo[1]	**65**	98	80	71	–	–	**89***	***13.1***	***16.3***	**1.1**	7.9	***88***	No
Kaiser Permanente, Walnut Creek	**68**	176	84	78	22*	**88**	85	***13.7***	***16.7***	2.4	7.3	***85***	No
Kaiser Permanente Santa Teresa, San Jose	**53**	124	87	81	50	56*	87	12.7	15.4	2.6	7.0	93	No
Lucile Packard Children's, Palo Alto	–[2]	–[2]	–[2]	–[2]	**99**	**98**	**91**	***No data collected***				90	–[6]
Marin General, Greenbrae	43	122	77	44*	29*	22*	73	***14.1***	***17.4***	2.1	**6.9**	**96**	No
Menlo Park Surgical, Menlo Park	15	26	–	–	–[3]	–[4]	–[4]	–	–	–	–	**99**	No
Mills - Peninsula, Burlingame[1]	49	72	–	–	–	–	**100***	12.8	***15.9***	1.6	**5.7**	92	No
Mt Diablo, Concord	**59**	136	**91**	**89**	–	18	70	***14.2***	***17.7***	1.8	7.2	**97**	No
Nelson Holderman, Yountville[1]	–	–	***No data collected***					***15.0***	***18.2***	–	–	–[6]	No
Northbay, Fairfield[1]	21	42	–	–	–	–	–	***18.9***	***22.9***	–	10.7	**96**	No
Novato Community, Novato	***14***	63	–	–	–	***0****	***14****	***14.0***	***17.2***	–	9.0	**95**	No
O'Connor, San Jose	38	135	76	50	14*	15	73	**10.6**	**13.0**	1.8	7.9	***88***	No
Palm Drive, Sebastopol	***6***	33	–	***0****	–[3]	–[4]	–[4]	10.7	13.3	–	9.5	91	No
Petaluma Valley, Petaluma	***8***	39	–	–	–	***0****	40*	11.9	14.4	3.3	7.8	***83***	No
Queen of the Valley, Napa	42	78	71*	67*	–	–	60*	11.7	14.3	1.8	7.2	89	No
Regional, San Jose	15	98	***29***	17	20	13	***25***	**9.8**	**12.0**	1.3	5.2	93	No
St Francis, San Francisco	34	104	86	80	–[3]	–[4]	–[4]	11.0	13.5	1.5	**5.1**	***87***	No
St Helena, Deer Park	25	52	–	–	–	–	–	**9.9**	**11.8**	2.0	8.2	–[6]	No
St Louise Regional, Gilroy	***5***	86	***0***	***0***	***0***	***0***	***5***	13.5	16.4	–	8.0	***88***	No
St Luke's, San Francisco	***10***	104	***7***	***0***	***0***	***0***	***18***	**10.2**	**12.4**	2.2	8.5	***78***	No

Footnotes are on page 73. *Hospital's score based on relatively little data. See page 16.

Key Ratings for Metro Areas

See more information on "Detailed Ratings for All Areas" table beginning on page 74

✓ means hospital receives our top rating
Blue is most favorable
Bold Italic is least favorable
"–" means insufficient data

	Doctors' ratings of hospitals for high-risk adult surgery		Desirability scores from doctors (0 to 100, higher is better)					Measures of outcomes for selected cases (lower % is better)					
	Percent rating "very good" or "excellent"	Number of ratings	Low-risk adult surgery	Complex medical care for adults	High-risk child surgery	High-risk delivery of a baby	Uncomplicated delivery of a baby	Adjusted death rate for all case types (%)	Adjusted death rate for medical cases (%)	Adjusted death rate for surgical cases (%)	Adjusted adverse outcome rate for surgical cases (%)	Overall score on accreditation review (higher is better)	Major affiliation with a medical school?
National Average	32	–	59	50	40	46	58	12.1	14.8	2.3	7.7	91	–
California *(continued)*													
San Francisco Bay Area *(continued)*													
St Mary's, San Francisco	49	130	80	55	–[3]	–[4]	–[4]	**10.2**	**12.5**	1.6	***10.4***	***88***	No
St Rose, Hayward	***8***	88	***21***	20	–[3]	14	***18***	**9.7**	**11.9**	1.3	6.7	93	No
✓ San Francisco General, San Francisco	**71**	222	***23***	83	39	38	***14***	11.4	14.0	–	5.9	***88***	**Yes**
San Jose Medical Center, San Jose	23	131	***25***	28	14	5	***5***	11.4	13.9	2.1	8.5	**97**	No
San Leandro Hospital, San Leandro	***12***	69	60*	40*	–[3]	–[4]	–[4]	**10.7**	**13.1**	1.5	**5.8**	**98**	No
San Mateo County General, San Mateo	16	45	–	–	–[3]	–[4]	–[4]	11.8	14.6	–	–	**96**	No
San Ramon Regional, San Ramon	46	103	87	50	–[3]	38*	80	**9.5**	**11.4**	2.4	5.4	92	No
Santa Clara Valley, San Jose	**60**	178	31	74	64	71	32	***13.4***	***16.3***	–	**2.4**	***84***	**Yes**
Santa Rosa Memorial, Santa Rosa	48	61	**89***	**90**	–	86*	**89***	12.8	15.6	2.4	7.7	***86***	No
Sequoia, Redwood City	**62**	79	**100***	–	–	–	83*	**10.6**	13.4	**1.3**	**6.2**	***88***	No
Seton, Daly City	47	90	–	–	–	***0****	–	**9.8**	**12.0**	1.7	7.9	90	No
Sonoma Developmental Center, Eldridge	–	–	***No data collected***					8.3	10.2	–	–	–[6]	No
Sonoma Valley, Sonoma[1]	17	30	–	–	–[3]	–	–	10.8	13.3	–	7.3	–[6]	No
✓ Stanford Hospital, Stanford[1]	**89**	283	79	**98**	–[3]	–[4]	–[4]	11.9	14.2	2.8	***10.3***	92	**Yes**
Summit, Oakland	**50**	147	**92**	**92**	–[3]	**96**	**92**	**8.8**	**10.8**	**1.6**	7.3	***77***	No
Sutter, Santa Rosa	37	52	86*	**88***	**89***	**93**	83	***15.2***	***18.6***	–	–	**94**	No
Sutter Delta, Antioch	***6***	94	***8***	***0***	***0***	***0***	***8***	11.8	14.2	3.2	8.5	93	No
Sutter Solano, Vallejo	21	53	–	–	20*	–	***17****	***16.3***	***19.8***	–	8.3	**94**	No
UCSF, San Francisco	**91**	296	85	**98**	**98**	**96**	83	12.2	15.0	1.7	8.1	89	**Yes**
VacaValley, Vacaville[1]	***14***	29	–	–	–[3]	–[4]	–[4]	***20.1***	***23.7***	–	–	**96**	No
Valley Care, Pleasanton	31	77	63*	63*	–	–	67	***No data collected***				–[6]	–[6]
Valley Care - Valley Memorial, Livermore[1]	–	–	***No data collected***					11.1	13.1	***4.5***	7.2	***86***	No
Washington, Fremont[1]	30	98	53	54	20*	40	47	**10.1**	**12.4**	1.7	9.4	***83***	**Yes**
Colorado													
Denver Area													
Centura St Anthony Central, Denver	**60**	110	64	86	9	29	31	***13.6***	***16.6***	2.5	7.5	***82***	No
Centura St Anthony North, Westminster	25	85	50	24	***0****	***0***	33	13.4	16.1	3.3	7.0	–[6]	No
Children's, Denver	–[2]	–[2]	–[2]	–[2]	**99**	–[4]	–[4]	***No data collected***				**94**	–[6]
✓ Denver Health, Denver[1]	**63**	117	***15***	50	48	39	***7***	10.6	12.8	–	–	90	**Yes**
Exempla Lutheran, Wheat Ridge	**67**	99	**90**	76	–	67	**90**	***13.2***	***16.0***	2.8	7.2	91	No
Exempla St Joseph, Denver	**58**	113	83	84	33	**90**	87	***13.5***	***16.7***	1.6	**6.9**	92	No
Littleton Adventist, Littleton[1]	31	95	84	17	20	25	77	***No data collected***				***86***	–[6]
Medical Center of Aurora, Aurora	17	81	***22***	21	5	4	***13***	11.8	14.3	2.6	7.0	93	No
National Jewish, Denver	–	–	***No data collected***					7.9	9.7	–	–	**98**	No

Footnotes are on page 73. *Hospital's score based on relatively little data. See page 16.

Key Ratings for Metro Areas

See more information on "Detailed Ratings for All Areas" table beginning on page 74

✓ means hospital receives our top rating
Blue is most favorable
Bold Italic is least favorable
"–" means insufficient data

	Doctors' ratings of hospitals for high-risk adult surgery		Desirability scores from doctors (0 to 100, higher is better)					Measures of outcomes for selected cases (lower % is better)					
	Percent rating "very good" or "excellent"	Number of ratings	Low-risk adult surgery	Complex medical care for adults	High-risk child surgery	High-risk delivery of a baby	Uncomplicated delivery of a baby	Adjusted death rate for all case types (%)	Adjusted death rate for medical cases (%)	Adjusted death rate for surgical cases (%)	Adjusted adverse outcome rate for surgical cases (%)	Overall score on accreditation review (higher is better)	Major affiliation with a medical school?
National Average	32	–	59	50	40	46	58	12.1	14.8	2.3	7.7	91	–
Colorado *(continued)*													
Denver Area *(continued)*													
North Suburban, Thornton	***8***	80	***8***	***3***	***0***	***0***	***17***	***14.7***	***17.5***	***4.6***	6.6	**94**	No
Platte Valley, Brighton	***0***	57	***0***	***0***	***0***	***0***	***0***	11.2	13.3	–	–	92	No
Porter Adventist, Denver[1]	43	98	82	75	***0****	13	***27***	12.1	14.6	2.7	8.7	***86***	No
Presbyterian - St Luke's, Denver	**57**	117	70	67	81	**90**	62	11.7	14.1	2.5	7.5	***88***	No
✓ Rose, Denver	**73**	117	**91**	85	46	**93**	**95**	11.8	14.3	2.7	8.3	92	No
✓ Swedish, Englewood	**78**	113	**98**	**94**	69	**95**	**98**	11.7	14.6	**0.9**	**5.0**	**94**	No
✓ University of Colorado, Denver	**73**	121	65	**98**	**83**	**90**	47	10.8	13.0	3.0	9.2	–[6]	**Yes**
Connecticut													
Fairfield and New Haven Counties													
Bridgeport Hospital, Bridgeport	**60**	133	65	81	**89**	87	56	***13.1***	***16.0***	2.2	***10.6***	**96**	**Yes**
Danbury Hospital, Danbury	40	117	**95**	79	75*	63*	74	**10.0**	**12.2**	**1.4**	9.2	93	**Yes**
Greenwich Hospital, Greenwich[1]	40	110	**96**	63	32	58	**95**	**10.6**	**12.8**	2.1	8.2	**96**	No
Griffin, Derby	***7***	108	***17***	***5***	***0***	***0***	***25***	***13.8***	***16.9***	2.1	***12.4***	92	**Yes**
✓ Hospital of St Raphael, New Haven	**78**	129	**93**	**92**	**86**	**93**	**92**	**9.8**	**11.9**	**1.9**	***11.3***	92	**Yes**
Masonic Geriatric, Wallingford	–	–	***No data collected***					14.7	17.7	–	–	**97**	No
Midstate, Meriden	***13***	78	***11***	***0***	***0***	***0***	***17***	***15.3***	***18.8***	2.2	7.0	***87***	No
Milford Hospital, Milford	***10***	99	***24***	***7***	***0***	***0***	***26***	12.1	14.8	1.8	6.8	89	No
Norwalk Hospital, Norwalk[1]	36	118	**92**	80	54	68	79	12.3	15.0	2.4	10.2	***83***	**Yes**
St Mary's, Waterbury[1]	20	94	32	***8***	***0***	***0***	33	12.0	14.8	1.7	7.7	93	**Yes**
✓ St Vincent's, Bridgeport	**52**	122	85	74	28	42	69	11.5	14.1	1.8	***10.1***	92	**Yes**
Stamford Hospital, Stamford[1]	**54**	114	**90**	81	46	81	**88**	12.9	15.5	3.1	***10.6***	**94**	**Yes**
Waterbury Hospital, Waterbury	22	93	57	42	8	25	55	***13.0***	***15.8***	2.8	***11.4***	***86***	**Yes**
✓ Yale - New Haven, New Haven	**92**	171	87	**99**	**100**	**100**	81	11.6	14.4	**1.6**	9.2	**94**	**Yes**
Hartford Area													
Bradley, Southington	***4***	55	***7***	***4***	–[3]	–[4]	–[4]	***13.7***	***16.9***	1.1	6.2	91	No
Bristol Hospital, Bristol	***7***	61	***27***	23	4	4	***23***	11.6	14.1	2.3	9.3	–[6]	**Yes**
Connecticut Children's, Hartford	–[2]	–[2]	–[2]	–[2]	**99**	–[4]	–[4]	***No data collected***				–[6]	–[6]
✓ Hartford Hospital, Hartford	**96**	83	**92**	**97**	–[3]	**95**	87	**11.0**	**13.5**	**1.8**	8.1	93	**Yes**
Manchester Memorial, Manchester	17	59	71	25*	9	***0****	**90**	***13.9***	***17.1***	2.0	8.8	**94**	No
New Britain General, New Britain	45	65	85	80	–	**88***	**89**	**11.1**	**13.6**	1.8	9.3	90	No
Rockville General, Rockville	***7***	55	***10***	***0***	***0***	***0***	***19***	***13.8***	***16.9***	1.8	9.0	**94**	No
✓ St Francis, Hartford	**71**	77	**90**	**93**	71	**93**	**89**	**11.3**	14.0	**1.7**	8.1	92	No
✓ University of Connecticut - John Dempsey, Farmington	**55**	82	84	**91**	–[3]	**96**	70	10.7	**12.9**	2.2	10.7	92	**Yes**

Footnotes are on page 73. *Hospital's score based on relatively little data. See page 16.

Key Ratings for Metro Areas

See more information on "Detailed Ratings for All Areas" table beginning on page 74

✓ means hospital receives our top rating
Blue is most favorable
Bold Italic is least favorable
"–" means insufficient data

	Doctors' ratings of hospitals for high-risk adult surgery		Desirability scores from doctors (0 to 100, higher is better)					Measures of outcomes for selected cases (lower % is better)					
	Percent rating "very good" or "excellent"	Number of ratings	Low-risk adult surgery	Complex medical care for adults	High-risk child surgery	High-risk delivery of a baby	Uncomplicated delivery of a baby	Adjusted death rate for all case types (%)	Adjusted death rate for medical cases (%)	Adjusted death rate for surgical cases (%)	Adjusted adverse outcome rate for surgical cases (%)	Overall score on accreditation review (higher is better)	Major affiliation with a medical school?
National Average	32	–	59	50	40	46	58	12.1	14.8	2.3	7.7	91	–
Delaware													
Delaware Valley Area													
Alfred I Dupont Hospital for Children, Wilmington	–[2]	–[2]	–[2]	–[2]	**93**	–[4]	–[4]	***No data collected***				***88***	–[6]
Christiana, Wilmington	21	77	–	–	–	–	–	***No data collected***				–[6]	–[6]
✓ Christiana Care, Newark[1]	**74**	121	**90**	**100**	–	**100**	**100**	**10.8**	**13.1**	2.0	9.4	**95**	**Yes**
St Francis, Wilmington[1]	***13***	77	–	–	–	20*	43*	12.0	14.7	2.0	6.8	***87***	**Yes**
District of Columbia													
Children's National, Washington	–[2]	–[2]	–[2]	–[2]	**99**	–[4]	–[4]	***No data collected***				92	–[6]
Columbia Hospital for Women, Washington	34	235	60*	–	67*	**89**	83	–	–	–	10.8	91	No
District of Columbia General, Washington	***4***	231	***0***	***2***	2	1	***1***	12.2	14.8	–	–	–[6]	**Yes**
✓ George Washington University, Washington	**66**	382	**90**	**98**	–[3]	**92**	83	**10.2**	**12.3**	2.5	9.0	91	**Yes**
✓ Georgetown University, Washington	**66**	395	88	**97**	**94**	**97**	**92**	**9.5**	**11.7**	1.4	8.4	***86***	**Yes**
Greater Southeast, Washington	***3***	233	***0***	***2***	***0***	***0***	***3***	**8.6**	**10.4**	2.5	7.9	***84***	No
Hadley, Washington	***1***	159	***0***	***0***	–[3]	–[4]	–[4]	**9.2**	**11.0**	–	–	**96**	No
Howard University, Washington	***14***	256	***22***	26	10	13	***18***	**7.6**	**9.0**	***4.5***	***12.9***	93	**Yes**
Providence, Washington	***13***	228	33	***0***	–[3]	14	33	**9.2**	**11.2**	2.0	***11.9***	**94**	**Yes**
✓ Sibley, Washington	**52**	332	**98**	70	25	52	**97**	**9.8**	**12.1**	**1.4**	***10.8***	92	**Yes**
✓ Washington Hospital Center, Washington	**87**	396	**90**	**98**	–[3]	**89**	71	**9.0**	**10.3**	2.6	***11.0***	**95**	No
Florida													
Brevard, Orange, Seminole, and Volusia Counties													
Atlantic, Daytona Beach	–	–	–	–	–	–[4]	–[4]	11.5	13.7	–	–	89	No
Bert Fish, New Smyrna Beach	***10***	30	***22****	13*	–[3]	–[4]	–[4]	**10.7**	**12.9**	2.3	7.3	92	No
Cape Canaveral, Cocoa Beach	***8***	36	78*	40*	–	–	80	**10.5**	**12.7**	2.4	8.8	90	No
Central Florida Regional, Sanford	24	46	50	39	25	30	53	**8.8**	**10.6**	1.8	8.5	–[6]	No
Florida, Altamonte Springs	**54**	57	85	75*	–	40*	71	***No data collected***				–[6]	–[6]
Florida, Apopka	***6***	52	***0****	***0***	***0****	***0****	***0****	***No data collected***				–[6]	–[6]
Florida, Deland	***3***	30	33*	–	–	***0****	***20****	**10.6**	**12.9**	2.0	7.8	91	No
Florida, Orlando	**84**	86	**89**	**97**	**98**	**98**	**92**	**10.6**	**13.0**	**1.9**	**7.6**	***88***	No
Florida - East Orlando, Orlando	15	61	36	27	***0****	18	***17***	***No data collected***				–[6]	–[6]
Florida - Fish Memorial, Orange City	21	33	67*	–	–[3]	–[4]	–[4]	10.9	**13.2**	2.5	8.8	**95**	No
Halifax, Daytona Beach	**67**	42	**100**	**100**	**100**	**90**	86	12.3	14.9	2.6	8.8	**94**	**Yes**
Health Central, Ocoee	***12***	51	33	***0***	10	8	***25***	12.1	14.7	–	11.7	**95**	No
Holmes Regional, Melbourne	43	37	79	**88**	**83***	82	85	**11.0**	**13.5**	**1.7**	8.7	93	No
Memorial - Ormond Beach, Ormond Beach	44	34	78	**100**	–[3]	–	**100**	**10.4**	**12.4**	2.4	**7.0**	–[6]	No
Memorial - Peninsula, Ormond Beach	***0***	27	***0****	***0***	–[3]	–[4]	–[4]	***13.5***	***16.4***	–	8.2	–[6]	No
✓ Orlando Regional, Orlando[1]	**87**	87	**96**	**98**	**100**[5]	**100**[5]	**99**[5]	**10.8**	**12.9**	2.7	8.5	91	**Yes**

Footnotes are on page 73. *Hospital's score based on relatively little data. See page 16.

Key Ratings for Metro Areas

See more information on "Detailed Ratings for All Areas" table beginning on page 74

✓ means hospital receives our top rating
Blue is most favorable
Bold Italic is least favorable
"–" means insufficient data

	Doctors' ratings of hospitals for high-risk adult surgery		Desirability scores from doctors (0 to 100, higher is better)					Measures of outcomes for selected cases (lower % is better)					
	Percent rating "very good" or "excellent"	Number of ratings	Low-risk adult surgery	Complex medical care for adults	High-risk child surgery	High-risk delivery of a baby	Uncomplicated delivery of a baby	Adjusted death rate for all case types (%)	Adjusted death rate for medical cases (%)	Adjusted death rate for surgical cases (%)	Adjusted adverse outcome rate for surgical cases (%)	Overall score on accreditation review (higher is better)	Major affiliation with a medical school?
National Average	32	–	59	50	40	46	58	12.1	14.8	2.3	7.7	91	–
Florida *(continued)*													
Brevard, Orange, Seminole, and Volusia Counties *(continued)*													
Orlando Regional Lucerne, Orlando	28	57	50*	–	–[3]	***0****	***17****	***No data collected***				–[6]	–[6]
Parrish, Titusville	***5***	37	***0****	***0****	***0****	***0****	***20***	10.8	13.2	1.9	6.9	96	No
Sand Lake (Orlando Regional), Orlando	52	60	91	60*	–	***0****	43*	***No data collected***				–[6]	–[6]
Wuesthoff, Rockledge[1]	***13***	38	73	57*	–	71*	56*	11.2	13.4	2.7	8.3	93	No
Charlotte, Collier, and Lee Counties													
Bon Secours St Joseph, Port Charlotte	–	–	88*	56*	36	36	79	9.9	11.9	2.4	6.4	89	No
Cape Coral Hospital, Cape Coral	46	28	91	80*	60*	100	94	***12.8***	***15.6***	2.4	6.4	–[6]	No
Charlotte Regional, Punta Gorda	–	–	54	60	–[3]	–[4]	–[4]	10.3	12.1	2.7	8.1	***86***	No
East Pointe, Lehigh Acres	***7***	28	***0***	***0***	***0****	***0****	***8***	11.9	14.2	3.6	***13.0***	92	No
Fawcett, Port Charlotte	36	25	71	71*	–	–[4]	–[4]	12.1	14.7	2.4	7.1	97	No
Gulf Coast, Fort Myers	***14***	29	31	14	–[3]	25	44	13.1	15.8	2.9	6.4	96	No
Healthpark, Fort Myers	68	31	91	91	100[5]	97	97	***No data collected***				–[6]	–[6]
Lee, Fort Myers[1]	70	33	81	87	86	84	67	11.4	14.0	1.8	6.0	***88***	No
Naples Community, Naples	–	–	92	91	57*	63*	85	10.9	13.2	2.1	8.2	94	No
Southwest Florida Regional, Fort Myers	53	32	86	90	–	–[4]	–[4]	***13.4***	***16.1***	***3.2***	7.9	92	No
Hillsborough, Manatee, Pinellas, Polk, and Sarasota Counties													
All Children's, St Petersburg	–[2]	–[2]	–[2]	–[2]	100	–[4]	–[4]	***No data collected***				97	–[6]
Bartow Memorial, Bartow	***5***	41	***0****	***0****	***0****	***0****	***0****	***14.6***	***17.7***	–	4.8	***82***	No
✓ Bayfront, St Petersburg	79	107	84	97	90	92	68	11.7	14.0	2.8	9.7	96	Yes
Blake, Bradenton	45	47	73	64	33*	29*	75	***12.7***	15.4	2.7	8.5	97	No
Bon Secours - Venice, Venice[1]	18	39	67*	40	–[3]	–[4]	–[4]	12.5	15.4	1.7	9.1	***86***	No
Brandon Regional, Brandon	22	82	55	50*	11*	29	46	10.0	12.1	2.6	9.3	***87***	No
Doctors, Sarasota	35	51	77	43*	–[3]	30	77	10.9	13.2	2.2	7.8	***88***	No
Edward White, St Petersburg	***12***	59	46	***0****	–[3]	–[4]	–[4]	10.7	12.9	2.6	5.5	92	No
Englewood Community, Englewood	***3***	35	***0****	***0****	–[3]	–[4]	–[4]	10.3	12.4	2.3	7.8	93	No
H Lee Moffitt Cancer Center, Tampa[1]	78	125	63*	79	20*	–[4]	–[4]	14.3	***18.4***	1.6	5.0	94	No
Heart of Florida Regional, Davenport	***5***	38	***17****	–	***0****	–[4]	–[4]	12.2	14.7	3.7	9.9	98	No
Helen Ellis, Tarpon Springs	22	64	33*	***0****	–	***0****	38*	10.2	12.4	2.1	7.9	96	No
Lake Wales Medical Center, Lake Wales[1]	***3***	38	–	–	–	–	–	***13.9***	***17.1***	1.2	4.2	–[6]	No
Lakeland Regional, Lakeland	56	59	100	100	–	94	100	12.0	14.8	1.9	8.7	95	No
Largo Medical Center, Largo	45	77	100	92	–[3]	43*	83	10.7	13.2	1.5	5.5	96	No
Manatee, Bradenton	36	55	73	60*	–	56*	62	***12.7***	15.2	***3.5***	9.6	95	No
Mease, Dunedin	44	66	100*	83*	–	71*	69	11.9	14.5	2.2	7.4	91	No
Mease Countryside, Safety Harbor	52	71	100*	100*	–[3]	–[4]	–[4]	12.0	14.4	3.1	7.8	–[6]	No

Footnotes are on page 73. *Hospital's score based on relatively little data. See page 16.

Key Ratings for Metro Areas

See more information on "Detailed Ratings for All Areas" table beginning on page 74

✓ means hospital receives our top rating
Blue is most favorable
Bold Italic is least favorable
"–" means insufficient data

	Doctors' ratings of hospitals for high-risk adult surgery		Desirability scores from doctors (0 to 100, higher is better)					Measures of outcomes for selected cases (lower % is better)					
	Percent rating "very good" or "excellent"	Number of ratings	Low-risk adult surgery	Complex medical care for adults	High-risk child surgery	High-risk delivery of a baby	Uncomplicated delivery of a baby	Adjusted death rate for all case types (%)	Adjusted death rate for medical cases (%)	Adjusted death rate for surgical cases (%)	Adjusted adverse outcome rate for surgical cases (%)	Overall score on accreditation review (higher is better)	Major affiliation with a medical school?
National Average	32	–	59	50	40	46	58	12.1	14.8	2.3	7.7	91	–
Florida *(continued)*													
Hillsborough, Manatee, Pinellas, Polk, and Sarasota Counties *(continued)*													
Memorial, Tampa	17	83	68	46	–[3]	–[4]	–[4]	11.6	14.3	1.8	**5.5**	90	No
✓ Morton Plant Mease, Clearwater	**69**	94	**100**	**95**	67*	84	**92**	**10.2**	**12.3**	2.1	8.1	93	No
Northside, St Petersburg[1]	30	60	40*	31	–[3]	–[4]	–[4]	11.3	**13.4**	***3.3***	8.7	**97**	No
Palms of Pasadena, St Petersburg	30	56	57*	56*	–[3]	–[4]	–[4]	**10.0**	**12.3**	1.6	**7.1**	**94**	No
Regency, Winter Haven	16	31	–	–	–	–	**100***	***No data collected***				–[6]	–[6]
St Anthony's, St Petersburg	42	71	80	77	–[3]	–	–	**10.1**	**12.2**	2.2	8.1	**96**	No
✓ St Joseph's, Tampa	**79**	121	**94**	87	**97**[5]	60*	44*	**10.0**	**11.8**	***3.4***	9.6	**95**	No
St Joseph's Women's, Tampa	**58**	90	88*	**100***	–[3]	**97**	**96**	***No data collected***				–[6]	–[6]
St Petersburg Medical Center, St Petersburg	***13***	63	***15***	***8***	***0****	27	53	11.3	13.4	***3.6***	8.2	**94**	No
✓ Sarasota Memorial, Sarasota	**69**	65	**100**	**100**	70	**100**	**97**	11.7	14.5	**1.9**	**7.6**	**97**	No
South Bay, Sun City Center	***8***	52	***10***	***9***	–[3]	–[4]	–[4]	11.4	13.8	2.3	6.8	***86***	No
South Florida Baptist, Plant City	***13***	56	***9***	***9***	***0***	***0****	***25****	10.8	**12.6**	***3.8***	8.9	93	No
Sun Coast, Largo	18	65	***23***	25	***0***	***0****	***8***	***No data collected***				–[6]	–[6]
✓ Tampa General, Tampa	**82**	137	**95**	**99**	**98**	**92**	73	11.9	14.5	2.4	9.6	***88***	**Yes**
Town and Country, Tampa	***9***	79	40	20	–[3]	–[4]	–[4]	12.3	14.8	3.1	**4.2**	92	No
University, Tampa	44	106	85	79	50	85	**91**	11.4	13.7	2.5	8.3	**98**	No
University - Carrollwood, Tampa	22	89	53	57*	–[3]	–[4]	–[4]	11.0	13.4	–	6.2	–[6]	No
Winter Haven Hospital, Winter Haven	33	43	86*	71*	–	–	–	12.1	14.6	3.0	9.6	89	No
South Florida													
Aventura Hospital, Aventura	21	151	65	50	33	29	50	12.0	14.6	2.8	9.8	**94**	No
✓ Baptist, Miami	**79**	236	**92**	**96**	74	**89**	**93**	**9.4**	**11.3**	2.2	10.0	**98**	No
Bethesda, Boynton Beach	29	131	81	79	40	67	79	11.4	13.9	2.1	8.7	**97**	No
✓ Boca Raton Community, Boca Raton	**59**	152	**93**	**90**	59	76	**91**	**10.4**	**12.5**	2.4	9.6	92	No
✓ Broward General, Fort Lauderdale	**63**	205	53	84	**90**	**89**	58	10.8	13.2	2.1	10.4	**94**	No
✓ Cedars, Miami	**53**	182	68	71	–[3]	–[4]	–[4]	**9.9**	**11.7**	3.1	***11.5***	**94**	No
Cleveland Clinic, Fort Lauderdale	41	184	45	67	–[3]	–[4]	–[4]	11.0	13.8	**1.3**	**5.1**	**97**	No
Columbia, West Palm Beach	***11***	94	***29***	19	–[3]	18	50	12.3	15.0	2.3	7.4	**96**	No
Coral Gables Hospital, Coral Gables	***10***	139	44	14*	–[3]	–[4]	–[4]	**10.0**	**12.0**	3.1	8.3	90	No
Coral Springs Medical Center, Coral Springs	18	152	77	22*	31	47	87	10.9	12.8	***4.4***	9.2	**95**	No
Delray Medical Center, Delray Beach	37	131	63	52	–[3]	–[4]	–[4]	**10.0**	**12.1**	2.0	**7.0**	**98**	No
Fishermen's, Marathon	***7***	81	43*	***0****	–[3]	–[4]	–[4]	***14.5***	***17.8***	–	5.2	***81***	No
Florida, Fort Lauderdale	23	158	63	57	–[3]	–[4]	–[4]	**11.1**	**13.5**	2.3	8.8	**97**	No
Glades General, Belle Glade	***4***	82	***0***	***0***	***0***	***0***	***6***	14.7	17.8	–	–	***86***	No
Good Samaritan, West Palm Beach	47	119	74	82	67*	57	50	**10.8**	**13.1**	2.4	9.9	–[6]	No

Footnotes are on page 73. *Hospital's score based on relatively little data. See page 16.

Key Ratings for Metro Areas

See more information on "Detailed Ratings for All Areas" table beginning on page 74

✓ means hospital receives our top rating
Blue is most favorable
Bold Italic is least favorable
"–" means insufficient data

	Doctors' ratings of hospitals for high-risk adult surgery		Desirability scores from doctors (0 to 100, higher is better)					Measures of outcomes for selected cases (lower % is better)					
	Percent rating "very good" or "excellent"	Number of ratings	Low-risk adult surgery	Complex medical care for adults	High-risk child surgery	High-risk delivery of a baby	Uncomplicated delivery of a baby	Adjusted death rate for all case types (%)	Adjusted death rate for medical cases (%)	Adjusted death rate for surgical cases (%)	Adjusted adverse outcome rate for surgical cases (%)	Overall score on accreditation review (higher is better)	Major affiliation with a medical school?
National Average	32	–	59	50	40	46	58	12.1	14.8	2.3	7.7	91	–
Florida *(continued)*													
South Florida *(continued)*													
Healthsouth Doctors', Coral Gables	33	152	95	100*	–	–	40*	9.8	12.2	0.7	7.8	95	No
Hialeah Hospital, Hialeah	***7***	137	***12***	***0***	***0***	14	***25***	9.6	11.7	1.8	6.4	93	No
Hollywood Medical Center, Hollywood	29	153	54	33	–[3]	–[4]	–[4]	12.8	15.1	***4.8***	9.2	97	No
✓ Holy Cross, Fort Lauderdale	54	177	84	91	47	60	82	10.7	13.1	1.8	7.8	90	No
Homestead Hospital, Homestead	***2***	118	***0****	***0***	***0****	***0****	***11****	12.5	15.3	–	0.0	93	No
Imperial Point, Fort Lauderdale	19	139	81	67*	–[3]	–[4]	–[4]	11.6	14.3	–	7.6	96	No
✓ Jackson Memorial, Miami	86	282	81	97	98	98	49	10.4	12.2	***3.7***	8.8	90	Yes
Jackson South, Miami	***5***	135	***27***	***0****	***0****	***0***	***20***	***16.0***	***19.2***	–	–	96	No
✓ JFK, Atlantis	50	135	82	86	–[3]	–[4]	–[4]	11.9	14.4	2.4	7.9	96	No
Jupiter Medical Center, Jupiter	33	89	100	100*	–	–[4]	–[4]	9.0	10.7	2.5	9.1	***88***	No
Kendall, Miami	15	138	40	36	14*	25	47	9.5	11.5	2.5	9.0	97	No
Larkin, South Miami	***4***	130	***27***	***0***	–[3]	–[4]	–[4]	8.8	10.6	–	–	98	No
Lower Keys, Key West	***4***	72	***0****	***0****	***0****	***0****	43*	13.6	16.4	3.2	9.6	93	No
Mariners, Tavernier	***8***	84	–	–	–[3]	–[4]	–[4]	11.8	14.8	–	–	91	No
Memorial - Pembroke, Pembroke Pines	22	124	–	–	–	–	–	13.0	16.0	–	13.5	99	No
Memorial Regional, Hollywood	69	160	96	100	98	99	96	12.5	15.2	2.5	9.9	94	No
Memorial West, Pembroke Pines	43	142	100	100	71	100	100	9.5	11.6	1.9	6.6	97	No
Mercy, Miami	48	184	86	78	–[3]	67	91	8.5	10.2	2.5	7.9	90	No
Miami Children's, Miami	–[2]	–[2]	–[2]	–[2]	98	–[4]	–[4]	***No data collected***				93	–[6]
Miami Jewish Home for the Aged, Miami	–	–	***No data collected***					***16.0***	***19.3***	–	–	96	No
✓ Mt Sinai, Miami Beach	73	232	82	84	44*	71	79	10.1	12.3	2.1	8.2	***82***	Yes
✓ Mt Sinai & Miami Heart Institute, Miami Beach	61	182	70	86	–[3]	–	–	8.5	10.1	2.2	9.1	–[6]	No
North Broward, Pompano Beach	38	149	67	57*	20*	–[4]	–[4]	***14.9***	***18.0***	3.7	7.6	94	No
North Ridge, Fort Lauderdale	48	155	83	80	–	***0****	***20****	9.3	11.4	1.6	9.3	92	No
North Shore, Miami	***9***	131	67*	–	–	–	67*	12.0	14.5	–	6.9	94	No
Northwest, Margate	***12***	109	40	25*	***0****	20	63	10.7	12.9	3.0	6.9	92	No
Palm Beach Gardens Med Ctr, Palm Beach Gardens	33	99	80	79	–	43*	69	10.7	12.9	2.2	***9.9***	91	No
Palm Springs General, Hialeah	***3***	103	30	17	–[3]	–[4]	–[4]	9.9	12.0	3.1	6.3	89	No
Palmetto General, Hialeah	16	148	46	43*	–[3]	44*	58	9.2	11.1	2.6	6.6	93	No
Palms West, Loxahatchee	23	92	82	75	73	67	76	9.9	12.0	2.4	10.2	93	No
Pan American, Miami	***6***	136	***5***	***5***	–[3]	–[4]	–[4]	7.9	9.6	2.2	6.3	90	No
Parkway Regional, North Miami Beach	***9***	156	***29***	17*	***0****	20	33	***15.0***	***18.0***	***4.4***	***14.0***	92	No
Plantation General, Plantation	17	144	41	29	44	76	77	10.9	13.1	–	***14.6***	96	No
St Mary's, West Palm Beach	45	120	65	75	92	87	64	12.8	15.5	2.6	10.3	–[6]	No

Footnotes are on page 73. *Hospital's score based on relatively little data. See page 16.

Key Ratings for Metro Areas

See more information on "Detailed Ratings for All Areas" table beginning on page 74

✓ means hospital receives our top rating
Blue is most favorable
Bold Italic is least favorable
"–" means insufficient data

	Doctors' ratings of hospitals for high-risk adult surgery		Desirability scores from doctors (0 to 100, higher is better)					Measures of outcomes for selected cases (lower % is better)					
	Percent rating "very good" or "excellent"	Number of ratings	Low-risk adult surgery	Complex medical care for adults	High-risk child surgery	High-risk delivery of a baby	Uncomplicated delivery of a baby	Adjusted death rate for all case types (%)	Adjusted death rate for medical cases (%)	Adjusted death rate for surgical cases (%)	Adjusted adverse outcome rate for surgical cases (%)	Overall score on accreditation review (higher is better)	Major affiliation with a medical school?
National Average	32	–	59	50	40	46	58	12.1	14.8	2.3	7.7	91	–
Florida (continued)													
South Florida (continued)													
✓ South Miami, Miami	59	172	98	93	90	98	99	8.5	10.3	1.7	7.8	94	No
South Shore, Miami Beach	6	111	0*	0*	–	–[4]	–[4]	11.7	14.2	–	12.9	87	Yes
University, Tamarac	14	132	44*	10	0*	–[4]	–[4]	12.4	15.0	3.1	9.7	96	No
✓ University of Miami - Sylvester Cancer Center, Miami[1]	73	181	100	100	93	–[4]	–[4]	10.9	13.1	–	–	96	Yes
Wellington Regional, West Palm Beach	14	96	58	29	38*	57	70	11.9	14.2	–	8.2	92	Yes
West Boca, Boca Raton	26	129	29	16	–[3]	67	71	11.1	13.3	3.4	8.7	97	No
Westchester General, Miami	2	117	0	0	0	–[4]	–[4]	9.9	11.3	–	–	–[6]	No
Westside Regional, Plantation	20	131	80	39	14*	0*	13*	11.1	13.6	1.8	7.9	97	No
Georgia													
Atlanta Area													
Atlanta Medical Center, Atlanta	19	115	39	46	20*	33	29	12.5	14.9	3.7	8.6	89	No
Children's Healthcare at Egleston, Atlanta	–[2]	–[2]	–[2]	–[2]	99	–	–	No data collected				–[6]	–[6]
Children's Healthcare at Scottish Rite, Atlanta	–[2]	–[2]	–[2]	–[2]	99	–[4]	–[4]	No data collected				–[6]	–[6]
✓ Crawford Long - Emory University, Atlanta	68	149	89	94	–[3]	94	77	10.2	12.3	2.2	9.9	96	Yes
Decatur Hospital, Decatur	12	75	–	17*	–	–[4]	–[4]	No data collected				93	–[6]
Dekalb, Decatur	48	140	80	75	–	81	73	14.0	17.0	3.1	9.2	90	No
Emory - Adventist, Smyrna	6	82	11*	0*	–[3]	–[4]	–[4]	12.1	14.9	–	–	96	No
Emory Dunwoody, Atlanta	10	91	67	40	–[3]	30	42	10.2	12.4	–	4.5	93	No
Emory Eastside, Snellville	19	85	57	33*	–[3]	20	73	12.5	15.1	3.1	7.8	87	No
Emory Northlake Regional, Tucker	10	97	22*	0*	–[3]	0*	0*	10.9	13.3	–	8.7	93	No
Emory Parkway, Lithia Springs	5	78	–	0*	–	–	14*	12.9	15.7	2.4	4.8	83	No
✓ Emory University, Atlanta	83	166	89	95	–[3]	–[4]	–[4]	11.0	13.2	2.4	9.9	96	Yes
Fayette Community, Fayetteville	–	–	No data collected					14.9	18.3	–	6.6	92	No
Grady, Atlanta[1]	57	157	7	50	44*	73	0	12.8	15.4	4.8	12.6	83	Yes
Gwinnett, Lawrenceville	36	109	92	57*	–	80	78	11.5	13.8	3.5	8.8	97	No
Henry, Stockbridge	7	87	14	0	0*	0	23	14.2	17.0	4.0	9.7	92	No
Hughes Spalding Children's, Atlanta	23	70	–	–	53	–	–	No data collected				–[6]	–[6]
Joan Glancy, Duluth	8	77	0*	0*	0*	–	–	No data collected				–[6]	–[6]
North Fulton Regional, Roswell	18	104	63*	43*	–[3]	17*	67	13.3	16.3	1.5	5.0	98	No
✓ Northside, Atlanta	84	183	95	96	88*	99	95	11.6	13.7	3.8	8.1	97	No
Northside - Cherokee, Canton	15	78	50*	–	–	87	81	15.6	18.8	–	9.4	–[6]	No
✓ Piedmont, Atlanta	84	188	99	98	–	99	99	11.7	14.1	2.5	8.4	91	No
Rockdale, Conyers[1]	11	85	56	15	0*	0	33	14.1	17.3	1.8	5.4	95	No
✓ St Joseph's, Atlanta	94	172	98	100	–[3]	–[4]	–[4]	11.3	13.7	2.3	9.5	94	No

Footnotes are on page 73. *Hospital's score based on relatively little data. See page 16.

Key Ratings for Metro Areas

See more information on "Detailed Ratings for All Areas" table beginning on page 74

✓ means hospital receives our top rating
Blue is most favorable
Bold Italic is least favorable
"–" means insufficient data

	Doctors' ratings of hospitals for high-risk adult surgery		Desirability scores from doctors (0 to 100, higher is better)					Measures of outcomes for selected cases (lower % is better)					
	Percent rating "very good" or "excellent"	Number of ratings	Low-risk adult surgery	Complex medical care for adults	High-risk child surgery	High-risk delivery of a baby	Uncomplicated delivery of a baby	Adjusted death rate for all case types (%)	Adjusted death rate for medical cases (%)	Adjusted death rate for surgical cases (%)	Adjusted adverse outcome rate for surgical cases (%)	Overall score on accreditation review (higher is better)	Major affiliation with a medical school?
National Average	32	–	59	50	40	46	58	12.1	14.8	2.3	7.7	91	–
Georgia *(continued)*													
Atlanta Area *(continued)*													
Shepherd Center, Atlanta	**75**	89	–	–	–	–	–	***No data collected***				93	–[6]
South Fulton, East Point	***4***	99	***15***	***11***	–[3]	***0***	***13***	**10.3**	**12.4**	3.0	7.6	–[6]	No
Southern Regional, Riverdale	***11***	120	***12***	***0***	***0***	14	***18***	***13.1***	***15.8***	3.3	**6.4**	92	No
Southwest, Atlanta	***2***	66	***0****	***0***	***0****	***0****	***0****	11.0	13.4	–	–	89	No
Wellstar Cobb, Austell	23	97	69	71*	***0****	33*	67*	***12.9***	15.6	3.2	9.7	**94**	No
Wellstar Douglas, Douglasville	***9***	65	40*	–	–[3]	–	–	***14.2***	***17.4***	–	4.1	92	No
Wellstar Kennestone, Marietta	46	112	**90**	75	14*	78	86	11.7	14.4	**1.5**	8.0	93	No
Wesley Woods Center of Emory University, Atlanta	–	–	***No data collected***					12.5	15.2	–	–	91	No
Illinois													
Chicago Area													
Advocate Bethany, Chicago	***3***	106	–	***0****	***0***	***0****	***0****	**7.5**	**9.2**	–	–	90	No
Advocate Christ and Hope Children's, Oak Lawn	**70**	184	**90**	86	**83**[5]	**93**	**91**	12.1	14.7	2.4	9.4	93	**Yes**
✓ Advocate Good Samaritan, Downers Grove	**64**	129	87	**100**	–	–	**94**	**10.6**	**12.7**	2.5	9.6	–[6]	No
Advocate Good Shepherd, Barrington	21	80	–	–	–	–	80*	12.1	14.8	1.6	7.1	93	No
Advocate Illinois Masonic, Chicago[1]	45	177	**94**	**93**	–	85	**94**	**10.2**	**12.4**	2.3	6.5	90	**Yes**
✓ Advocate Lutheran/Lutheran Children's, Park Ridge[1]	**82**	222	**94**	87	**100**	**98**	**89**	**9.6**	**11.8**	**1.2**	9.0	92	**Yes**
Advocate Ravenswood, Chicago	***7***	121	***29****	17*	–	***0****	33*	10.9	**13.0**	3.6	9.1	–[6]	No
Advocate South Suburban, Hazel Crest	15	80	60*	–	–	–	83*	**9.7**	**11.6**	2.6	7.7	–[6]	No
Advocate Trinity, Chicago	***8***	74	***15***	***0****	***0****	***0****	***17****	**7.7**	**9.5**	1.4	4.9	92	No
Alexian Brothers, Elk Grove Village	40	159	86	83*	–	–	83	11.5	14.1	1.8	8.4	**95**	No
Catholic Health Partners Columbus, Chicago	16	133	–	–	–	20*	***20****	**8.1**	**9.9**	–	8.3	89	**Yes**
Central DuPage, Winfield	48	112	**94**	80	–	**100***	**100**	***13.4***	***16.4***	2.6	8.8	91	No
Children's, Chicago	–[2]	–[2]	–[2]	–[2]	**100**	**93**	80*	***No data collected***				91	–[6]
Condell, Libertyville	16	102	50*	–	–	–	–	***13.5***	***16.5***	2.4	6.7	**98**	No
Cook County, Chicago	38	218	***18***	20	15	28	***3***	**7.5**	**8.9**	–	12.8	***86***	**Yes**
Delnor, Geneva	16	63	55	25*	–	–	60*	13.2	***16.2***	1.9	9.7	**95**	No
Edgewater, Chicago	***2***	119	***0***	***0***	–[3]	–[4]	–[4]	**5.8**	**7.1**	2.2	6.3	92	No
Edward, Naperville[1]	41	111	**100***	80*	–	40*	**90**	12.5	15.2	2.5	9.8	91	No
Elmhurst Memorial, Elmhurst	27	112	88*	80*	–	–	**90**	**10.6**	**12.9**	1.7	8.0	***88***	No
✓ Evanston Northwestern, Evanston	**75**	213	**98**	**96**	**86***	**97**	**97**	11.9	14.5	2.2	***10.5***	**95**	**Yes**
Glenbrook, Glenview	44	151	**100***	–	–	–	–	***No data collected***				–[6]	–[6]
Glenoaks, Glendale Heights	***13***	69	***29****	***0****	***0****	***0****	***25****	***16.7***	***20.1***	–	–	89	No
Gottlieb, Melrose Park	***10***	119	50*	–	–	–	–	**9.2**	**11.3**	1.7	6.6	**98**	No
Grant, Chicago	***4***	136	***25****	20*	–[3]	–[4]	–[4]	**9.7**	**11.9**	1.3	7.1	***84***	No

Footnotes are on page 73. *Hospital's score based on relatively little data. See page 16.

Key Ratings for Metro Areas

See more information on "Detailed Ratings for All Areas" table beginning on page 74

✓ means hospital receives our top rating
Blue is most favorable
Bold Italic is least favorable
"–" means insufficient data

	Doctors' ratings of hospitals for high-risk adult surgery		Desirability scores from doctors (0 to 100, higher is better)					Measures of outcomes for selected cases (lower % is better)					
	Percent rating "very good" or "excellent"	Number of ratings	Low-risk adult surgery	Complex medical care for adults	High-risk child surgery	High-risk delivery of a baby	Uncomplicated delivery of a baby	Adjusted death rate for all case types (%)	Adjusted death rate for medical cases (%)	Adjusted death rate for surgical cases (%)	Adjusted adverse outcome rate for surgical cases (%)	Overall score on accreditation review (higher is better)	Major affiliation with a medical school?
National Average	32	–	59	50	40	46	58	12.1	14.8	2.3	7.7	91	–
Illinois *(continued)*													
Chicago Area *(continued)*													
Harvard Memorial, Harvard	***8***	36	–	–	–	–	–	13.3	16.2	–	–	89	No
Highland Park Hospital, Highland Park	34	122	**100**	–	–	–	**100**	12.4	15.1	2.5	**6.0**	–[6]	No
Hinsdale Hospital, Hinsdale	**56**	139	**100**	**100**	60*	**88**	**97**	11.5	13.8	2.8	***10.1***	***88***	No
Holy Cross, Chicago	***3***	101	–	–	–	17*	***0****	11.5	14.0	2.5	8.5	***86***	**Yes**
Holy Family, Des Plaines	***5***	103	40*	14*	–	–	40*	12.4	14.7	***4.4***	***11.6***	92	No
Ingalls, Harvey	16	111	33*	–	–	17*	50*	**10.6**	**12.9**	2.1	9.1	90	No
Jackson Park, Chicago[1]	***2***	111	***0***	***10***	***0****	***0***	***7***	**9.2**	**11.1**	–	–	92	No
La Grange Memorial, La Grange	29	112	**89***	80*	–	–	67*	**10.0**	**12.1**	2.0	9.1	***87***	No
La Rabida Children's, Chicago	**57**	77	–	–	**83***	–	–	***No data collected***				**96**	–[6]
Lake Forest Hospital, Lake Forest	31	101	83	–	–	–	**94**	11.6	14.4	1.5	10.9	91	No
Little Company of Mary, Evergreen Park[1]	***11***	120	–	–	–	***0****	40*	12.0	14.7	2.2	8.9	90	No
Loretto, Chicago	***6***	109	***6***	***0***	6	–[4]	–[4]	**7.9**	**9.4**	–	–	***86***	No
Louis A Weiss, Chicago	18	137	–	–	–[3]	–	–	**10.2**	**12.4**	2.0	***12.0***	***88***	**Yes**
✓ Loyola University, Maywood	**85**	234	**96**	**97**	**88**	**99**	**89**	11.3	13.5	2.4	9.5	**95**	**Yes**
MacNeal, Berwyn	21	153	46	27	9	20	30	12.1	14.9	1.6	7.8	***86***	**Yes**
Memorial, Woodstock	19	37	60*	–	–	–	–	***13.6***	***16.4***	3.1	**5.9**	***87***	No
Mercy, Chicago	17	130	–	–	–	–	***20****	11.9	14.5	2.4	9.9	91	No
Methodist, Chicago	***3***	59	–	–	–[3]	–[4]	–[4]	**8.7**	**10.5**	2.7	9.0	92	No
Michael Reese, Chicago	17	151	–	22*	–[3]	–	71*	**10.4**	**12.6**	2.7	8.9	***79***	No
Midwestern Regional, Zion	–[2]	–[2]	–[2]	–[2]	–	–[4]	–[4]	***16.2***	***19.5***	–	–	**97**	No
Mt Sinai, Chicago	16	125	–	–	–	17*	***0****	**8.6**	**10.4**	–	8.2	93	**Yes**
Northern Illinois, McHenry	22	54	–	–	–	–	–	***13.9***	***16.9***	2.4	8.4	***88***	No
Northwest, Arlington Heights	35	145	80	60	–	–	**93**	12.5	15.3	2.2	8.1	91	No
✓ Northwestern, Chicago	**89**	248	**95**	**98**	–[3]	**97**	**94**	**9.7**	**12.1**	**1.2**	9.4	**97**	**Yes**
Norwegian - American, Chicago	***1***	87	***22****	***0****	–	33*	56*	11.3	13.7	–	11.6	**97**	No
Oak Park Hospital, Oak Park	***13***	116	–	20*	17*	–[4]	–[4]	**9.9**	**11.8**	3.0	6.8	92	No
Our Lady of the Resurrection, Chicago	***11***	97	–	–	–[3]	–[4]	–[4]	***12.9***	***15.6***	2.8	**5.6**	**98**	No
Palos Community, Palos Heights	***14***	104	86*	–	–	–	**100***	11.9	14.6	1.6	8.0	93	No
Provena Mercy, Aurora	***12***	42	–	–	–	–	–	***13.9***	***17.1***	2.3	7.6	90	No
Provena St Joseph, Elgin	***14***	44	–	–	–	–	–	12.8	15.7	2.1	9.5	***88***	No
Provena St Joseph, Joliet	34	58	88*	–	–	–	–	11.8	14.5	2.0	8.4	–[6]	No
Provident of Cook County, Chicago	***3***	87	–	20*	***0****	***0****	40*	10.0	12.1	–	–	89	No
Resurrection, Chicago	32	130	69	55	***0****	–	79	***13.4***	***16.1***	***2.9***	8.9	**96**	**Yes**
Roseland, Chicago	***1***	68	***0****	***0***	***0****	***0***	***0***	12.8	15.7	–	–	93	No

Footnotes are on page 73. *Hospital's score based on relatively little data. See page 16.

Key Ratings for Metro Areas

See more information on "Detailed Ratings for All Areas" table beginning on page 74

✓ means hospital receives our top rating
Blue is most favorable
Bold Italic is least favorable
"–" means insufficient data

	Doctors' ratings of hospitals for high-risk adult surgery		Desirability scores from doctors (0 to 100, higher is better)					Measures of outcomes for selected cases (lower % is better)					
	Percent rating "very good" or "excellent"	Number of ratings	Low-risk adult surgery	Complex medical care for adults	High-risk child surgery	High-risk delivery of a baby	Uncomplicated delivery of a baby	Adjusted death rate for all case types (%)	Adjusted death rate for medical cases (%)	Adjusted death rate for surgical cases (%)	Adjusted adverse outcome rate for surgical cases (%)	Overall score on accreditation review (higher is better)	Major affiliation with a medical school?
National Average	32	–	59	50	40	46	58	12.1	14.8	2.3	7.7	91	–
Illinois *(continued)*													
Chicago Area *(continued)*													
Rush - Copley, Aurora[1]	23	78	–	–	–	–	–	12.6	15.6	1.8	7.4	93	Yes
✓ Rush - Presbyterian - St Lukes, Chicago	83	226	95	99	90	93	90	8.3	10.0	1.6	7.9	***87***	Yes
Rush North Shore, Skokie	33	153	71	55	33*	30	36	9.6	11.8	1.2	8.7	91	Yes
Sacred Heart, Chicago	***4***	50	–	–	–[3]	–[4]	–[4]	5.7	7.1	–	3.6	***88***	No
St Alexius, Hoffman Estates	29	87	100	–	–	–	100*	11.6	14.0	2.9	9.3	90	No
St Anthony, Chicago	***4***	74	–	–	***0****	–	–	8.9	10.9	–	3.4	***87***	No
St Bernard, Chicago	***2***	88	***0***	***0***	***0****	***0***	***0***	11.3	13.8	–	–	89	No
St Elizabeth, Chicago	***9***	92	–	–	–	–	–	8.6	10.3	3.8	***12.9***	98	No
St Francis, Blue Island	22	95	80*	–	–	–	–	9.7	11.7	2.2	7.6	91	No
St Francis, Evanston	36	144	83*	80*	–	–	60*	11.0	13.3	2.5	9.0	***82***	No
St James, Chicago Heights	***13***	72	–	–	–	–	–	11.0	13.4	2.2	8.5	93	No
St James, Olympia Fields[1]	***13***	72	–	–	–	–	–	11.8	14.0	***3.9***	9.2	–[6]	No
St Joseph, Chicago	20	113	–	–	–	–	80*	10.2	12.2	2.7	10.0	***84***	Yes
St Mary of Nazareth, Chicago	***7***	85	40*	–	–	–	–	7.3	8.7	1.9	6.1	90	No
Sherman, Elgin	20	66	–	–	–	–	–	11.8	14.5	2.1	8.8	92	No
Silver Cross, Joliet	28	69	–	17*	–	–	–	11.3	13.8	1.8	9.3	89	No
South Shore, Chicago	***3***	65	***0****	***0****	–	–[4]	–[4]	8.4	10.4	–	2.3	***86***	No
Swedish Covenant, Chicago	***11***	120	33*	33*	–	–	60*	11.6	14.0	2.8	8.4	90	No
Thorek, Chicago	***3***	113	***4***	***4***	–[3]	–[4]	–[4]	8.8	10.8	–	4.9	89	No
University of Chicago, Chicago	81	207	91	98	97[5]	100[5]	83[5]	12.0	14.2	***3.5***	***12.0***	95	Yes
✓ University of Illinois, Chicago	59	199	89*	96	83	93	80*	7.8	9.0	3.4	7.3	90	Yes
Victory, Waukegan[1]	***5***	61	–	–	–	–	–	10.6	12.5	***4.0***	9.3	91	No
Vista Health Provena St Therese, Waukegan	***6***	54	–	–	–	–	–	***13.7***	***16.4***	4.1	10.2	95	No
West Suburban, Oak Park	27	122	71*	60*	–	20*	77	9.9	11.9	2.4	6.2	***80***	No
Westlake, Melrose Park	***12***	98	***14****	***0****	–	–	***0****	7.6	9.2	1.8	5.9	***88***	Yes
Indiana													
Indianapolis Area													
✓ Clarian Health Partners, Indianapolis	95	66	95	96	92	94	76	10.2	12.0	***2.9***	9.2	91	Yes
Community East, Indianapolis[1]	38	52	80	67	–	–	60	9.8	11.8	2.3	***9.8***	***87***	No
Community North, Indianapolis	40	53	95	64	–	63*	91	*No data collected*				***87***	–[6]
Community South, Indianapolis	***12***	51	44*	14*	–	13*	50	13.0	15.5	3.5	8.9	***88***	No
Indiana University, Indianapolis	83	64	72	100	100[5]	100	70	*No data collected*				–[6]	–[6]
St Francis, Beech Grove[1]	49	53	75	71*	–	***0****	63*	12.1	14.7	2.4	8.5	89	No
✓ St Vincent, Indianapolis[1]	77	64	98	94	83	94	90	11.3	13.4	***2.8***	8.9	***88***	Yes

Footnotes are on page 73. *Hospital's score based on relatively little data. See page 16.

Key Ratings for Metro Areas

See more information on "Detailed Ratings for All Areas" table beginning on page 74

✓ means hospital receives our top rating
Blue is most favorable
Bold Italic is least favorable
"–" means insufficient data

	Doctors' ratings of hospitals for high-risk adult surgery		Desirability scores from doctors (0 to 100, higher is better)					Measures of outcomes for selected cases (lower % is better)					
	Percent rating "very good" or "excellent"	Number of ratings	Low-risk adult surgery	Complex medical care for adults	High-risk child surgery	High-risk delivery of a baby	Uncomplicated delivery of a baby	Adjusted death rate for all case types (%)	Adjusted death rate for medical cases (%)	Adjusted death rate for surgical cases (%)	Adjusted adverse outcome rate for surgical cases (%)	Overall score on accreditation review (higher is better)	Major affiliation with a medical school?
National Average	32	–	59	50	40	46	58	12.1	14.8	2.3	7.7	91	–
Indiana *(continued)*													
Indianapolis Area *(continued)*													
Westview, Indianapolis	***2***	51	***2***	***0***	–[3]	–[4]	–[4]	10.5	12.7	–	6.0	–[6]	No
Winona, Indianapolis	***2***	52	***0***	***0***	***0***	–[4]	–[4]	11.4	13.9	–	5.4	–[6]	No
✓ Wishard, Indianapolis	**59**	58	32	65	23	33	***20***	**10.7**	**12.8**	4.5	7.4	***86***	**Yes**
Women's, Indianapolis	21	43	–	***0****	–[3]	**88**	**91**	–	–	–	–	***87***	No
Kansas													
Kansas City Area													
Bethany, Kansas City	***1***	68	***0***	***0***	***0***	***0***	***0***	11.3	13.6	2.9	8.6	93	**Yes**
Children's Mercy South, Overland Park	48	67	–	–	**93**	–	–	***No data collected***				–[6]	–[6]
Menorah, Overland Park	45	136	83	67	9	33	84	11.5	14.6	1.0	8.1	**99**	No
Olathe Medical Center, Olathe	47	116	**94**	**93**	–	60*	86	11.3	14.0	1.4	**5.9**	91	**Yes**
Overland Park Regional, Overland Park	41	125	85	60	40	**88**	**89**	**9.9**	**12.3**	**1.0**	**6.3**	**97**	No
Providence, Kansas City	***14***	93	***22****	13*	***0****	***0****	***25****	**10.4**	**12.6**	2.3	9.9	**94**	No
St Luke's South, Overland Park	25	108	47	27	10	8	60	6.8	7.1	–	–	**95**	No
✓ Shawnee Mission Medical Center, Shawnee Mission	**82**	128	**96**	**92**	**88***	**91**	**97**	**10.9**	**13.4**	1.9	8.1	91	No
University of Kansas, Kansas City[1]	**61**	137	72	**94**	**90**	**93**	45	13.3	16.1	2.8	8.4	–[6]	**Yes**
Louisiana													
New Orleans Area													
Lakeland, New Orleans	27	30	80*	–	–	22*	71*	11.4	13.4	***4.0***	9.2	**95**	No
Med Ctr of LA - University Campus, New Orleans	49	43	30	82	33*	68	32	***No data collected***				–[6]	–[6]
Med Ctr of LA at New Orleans, New Orleans	45	44	***17***	46	30	14*	***0***	12.5	14.9	4.1	9.3	–[6]	**Yes**
✓ Memorial - Baptist Campus, New Orleans	**79**	42	**97**	**100**	**100***	**100**	**100**	**10.0**	**12.0**	2.9	9.1	90	No
Memorial - Mercy Campus, New Orleans[1]	**51**	35	**89***	–	–	–[4]	–[4]	***No data collected***				–[6]	–[6]
Ochsner Foundation, New Orleans	**85**	46	86	**94**	**83**	**93**	77	12.6	15.3	2.7	**6.8**	92	No
Pendleton Methodist, New Orleans	43	30	71*	60*	–	***0****	67*	11.1	13.6	1.9	9.3	**94**	No
St Charles General, New Orleans	***6***	33	***21***	***0***	–[3]	–[4]	–[4]	**6.4**	**7.6**	–	–	**96**	No
St Claude, New Orleans	***0***	32	***0***	***0***	***0***	***0***	***0***	10.3	12.6	–	–	***83***	No
✓ Touro Infirmary, New Orleans	**59**	46	**96**	**100**	–[3]	80	**93**	11.9	14.4	2.6	7.5	93	**Yes**
✓ Tulane University, New Orleans	**58**	43	64	**91**	**83**	87	82	10.7	13.2	1.5	7.2	92	**Yes**
Maryland													
Baltimore Area													
Bon Secours, Baltimore[1]	***0***	94	***0***	***0***	–[3]	–[4]	–[4]	**9.5**	**11.6**	1.7	7.6	92	No
Franklin Square, Baltimore[1]	20	102	53	18	11*	44	68	**11.2**	**13.6**	2.4	9.0	**96**	No
Good Samaritan, Baltimore	17	99	54	30	–[3]	–[4]	–[4]	**9.2**	**11.1**	2.3	10.1	93	No

Footnotes are on page 73. *Hospital's score based on relatively little data. See page 16.

Key Ratings for Metro Areas

See more information on "Detailed Ratings for All Areas" table beginning on page 74

✓ means hospital receives our top rating
Blue is most favorable
Bold Italic is least favorable
"–" means insufficient data

	Doctors' ratings of hospitals for high-risk adult surgery		Desirability scores from doctors (0 to 100, higher is better)					Measures of outcomes for selected cases (lower % is better)					
	Percent rating "very good" or "excellent"	Number of ratings	Low-risk adult surgery	Complex medical care for adults	High-risk child surgery	High-risk delivery of a baby	Uncomplicated delivery of a baby	Adjusted death rate for all case types (%)	Adjusted death rate for medical cases (%)	Adjusted death rate for surgical cases (%)	Adjusted adverse outcome rate for surgical cases (%)	Overall score on accreditation review (higher is better)	Major affiliation with a medical school?
National Average	32	–	59	50	40	46	58	12.1	14.8	2.3	7.7	91	–
Maryland *(continued)*													
Baltimore Area *(continued)*													
✓ Greater Baltimore, Baltimore	**68**	116	**99**	**96**	**88**	**96**	**98**	**10.3**	**12.6**	1.7	8.5	90	No
Harbor, Baltimore	***2***	95	***0***	***0***	3	***0***	***0***	**9.4**	**11.4**	2.3	8.1	***88***	No
James Lawrence Kernan, Baltimore	–	–			*No data collected*			**2.3**	3.2	–	4.6	91	No
✓ Johns Hopkins, Baltimore	**93**	125	78	**99**	**99**	**97**	50	**9.9**	**11.6**	2.4	***11.8***	91	**Yes**
✓ Johns Hopkins Bayview, Baltimore	**52**	107	47	81	62	71	29*	11.4	13.9	1.9	7.8	92	**Yes**
Maryland General, Baltimore	***6***	98	***7***	***0***	***0***	***0***	***9***	**10.1**	**12.1**	3.4	10.0	91	**Yes**
Mercy, Baltimore	42	106	**92**	78*	33*	71	85	**8.8**	**10.3**	3.1	8.5	90	**Yes**
Northwest, Randallstown	***7***	98	48	***5***	–[3]	–[4]	–[4]	11.4	13.8	2.9	8.2	**98**	No
St Agnes, Baltimore[1]	31	98	76	69	–[3]	29	78	11.8	14.3	2.5	9.6	92	No
St Joseph, Towson	**54**	114	**100**	**94**	–	**89**	**100**	12.5	***15.6***	2.0	9.1	***81***	No
✓ Sinai, Baltimore	**55**	113	**100**	84	**90**	**96**	87	**10.6**	**12.9**	2.0	8.9	93	No
✓ Union, Baltimore	**50**	109	78	64	***0***	9	56	11.1	13.7	**1.6**	8.5	**94**	No
✓ University of Maryland, Baltimore[1]	**83**	122	72	**99**	**100**	**97**	45	**10.7**	**12.9**	2.3	7.1	91	**Yes**
Washington, DC, Area													
Anne Arundel, Annapolis	29	106	70	40*	–	60*	80	11.5	14.1	1.6	7.2	93	No
Doctors, Lanham	***13***	144	39	13	–[3]	–[4]	–[4]	**9.8**	**12.0**	2.1	8.8	***88***	No
Fort Washington Medical Center, Fort Washington	***3***	104	***0****	***0****	–[3]	–[4]	–[4]	**10.1**	**12.2**	–	6.8	***88***	No
Holy Cross, Silver Spring	49	290	**94**	**88**	78*	**97**	**98**	11.8	14.5	1.7	8.5	**96**	**Yes**
Howard County General, Columbia	15	123	–	–	–	17*	50	11.5	13.8	3.2	9.1	**97**	No
Laurel Regional, Laurel	***7***	120	50*	13*	–[3]	***0****	***20***	12.3	14.9	2.7	7.5	91	No
Montgomery General, Olney	17	222	50	20	***0***	***0***	39	11.8	14.4	2.0	10.0	**95**	No
North Arundel, Glen Burnie	***12***	97	–	–	–	–[4]	–[4]	11.7	14.1	2.8	***11.1***	89	No
Prince George's, Cheverly[1]	***13***	149	***18***	***7***	***0***	13	***12***	**10.6**	**12.6**	***3.8***	***12.6***	**94**	No
Shady Grove Adventist, Rockville	30	277	75	24	44	67	84	***13.7***	***16.7***	2.9	***11.7***	**99**	No
Southern Maryland, Clinton[1]	***8***	138	***24***	***0***	***0***	***0***	***7***	**11.0**	**13.5**	1.4	8.8	90	No
✓ Suburban, Bethesda[1]	**60**	306	**96**	83	33	–[4]	–[4]	**10.2**	**12.5**	1.7	***10.5***	92	No
Washington Adventist, Takoma Park	44	214	79	77	–[3]	–	63	**9.4**	**11.4**	1.7	9.7	**98**	No
Massachusetts													
Boston Area													
Addison Gilbert, Gloucester	***3***	74	–	–	–	–	–		*No data collected*			–[6]	–[6]
Anna Jaques, Newburyport	***6***	96	33*	***0****	–	–	33*	11.1	13.5	1.9	**5.1**	***84***	No
✓ Beth Israel Deaconess, Boston	**76**	286	**90**	**94**	–[3]	**96**	**95**	**11.1**	**13.6**	**1.7**	9.0	92	**Yes**
Beverly Hospital, Beverly[1]	***14***	115	60*	–	–	–	85	12.5	15.1	3.2	9.9	90	**Yes**
✓ Boston Medical Center, Boston[1]	**66**	254	87	**96**	64	71	63	**9.4**	**11.3**	2.0	8.6	90	**Yes**

Footnotes are on page 73. *Hospital's score based on relatively little data. See page 16.

Key Ratings for Metro Areas

See more information on "Detailed Ratings for All Areas" table beginning on page 74

✓ means hospital receives our top rating
Blue is most favorable
Bold Italic is least favorable
"–" means insufficient data

	Doctors' ratings of hospitals for high-risk adult surgery		Desirability scores from doctors (0 to 100, higher is better)					Measures of outcomes for selected cases (lower % is better)					
	Percent rating "very good" or "excellent"	Number of ratings	Low-risk adult surgery	Complex medical care for adults	High-risk child surgery	High-risk delivery of a baby	Uncomplicated delivery of a baby	Adjusted death rate for all case types (%)	Adjusted death rate for medical cases (%)	Adjusted death rate for surgical cases (%)	Adjusted adverse outcome rate for surgical cases (%)	Overall score on accreditation review (higher is better)	Major affiliation with a medical school?
National Average	32	–	59	50	40	46	58	12.1	14.8	2.3	7.7	91	–
Massachusetts *(continued)*													
Boston Area *(continued)*													
✓ Brigham and Women's, Boston	**91**	312	**95**	**98**	–[3]	**99**	**96**	**10.1**	**12.8**	**1.4**	8.5	***88***	**Yes**
Brockton Hospital, Brockton	***12***	140	80*	–	–	20*	31	12.0	14.6	2.3	8.5	**95**	**Yes**
Cambridge Hospital, Cambridge[1]	18	154	64	–	–	20*	46	12.0	14.7	1.8	7.2	90	**Yes**
Caritas, Norwood	***11***	119	67	20*	***0****	–	62	12.6	15.5	1.5	**5.4**	***82***	**Yes**
Caritas Good Samaritan, Brockton	16	104	67*	–	–	–	55	12.4	15.0	2.4	9.3	–[6]	No
Caritas Southwood, Norfolk	–	–	*No data collected*					11.5	14.0	–	5.5	–[6]	No
Carney, Boston	***11***	140	64	25	13*	–[4]	–[4]	**7.9**	**9.6**	1.6	9.1	–[6]	**Yes**
Charlton - Fall River Site of Southcoast, Fall River[1]	***10***	83	50*	–	–	–	**88***	**10.3**	**12.5**	2.0	***11.6***	93	No
Children's, Boston	–[2]	–[2]	–[2]	–[2]	**100**	**100***	–	*No data collected*				**94**	–[6]
Dana-Farber Cancer Institute, Boston	**85**	169	–	–	–	–[4]	–[4]	***21.0***	***23.8***	–	–	**95**	**Yes**
Deaconess, Waltham	***8***	109	***11****	***0****	–	–	***0****	**9.2**	**11.3**	1.4	6.8	***86***	No
Deaconess - Glover, Needham	16	110	50*	–	–	–[4]	–[4]	12.8	15.7	0.9	4.4	93	No
Deaconess - Nashoba, Ayer	***10***	81	–	–	–	–[4]	–[4]	11.1	13.6	–	6.5	93	No
Emerson, West Concord	23	129	75*	–	–	–	**91**	**10.6**	13.1	**0.9**	6.9	91	No
Faulkner, Boston	34	172	**90**	80*	–[3]	–[4]	–[4]	**9.8**	**12.0**	1.5	6.0	92	No
Franciscan Children's, Boston	31	65	–	–	60*	–	–	*No data collected*				91	–[6]
Hale, Haverhill	***4***	85	***0***	***0***	***0****	***0****	***0***	***14.9***	***18.1***	2.7	8.3	93	No
Hallmark Health - Lawrence, Medford[1]	***7***	83	67*	–	–	–	–	*No data collected*				90	–[6]
Hallmark Hlth - Melrose-Wakefield Campus, Melrose	***7***	86	46	13*	–	***0****	46	**9.6**	**11.7**	1.7	9.1	**97**	No
Holy Family, Methuen	24	89	62	–	–	–	70	12.8	15.7	1.6	9.4	93	No
Jordan, Plymouth	***13***	107	56*	***0****	–	***0****	39	***13.9***	***17.0***	2.5	10.4	**94**	No
Lahey Clinic, Burlington	**73**	222	**94**	84	17*	–[4]	–[4]	**10.5**	**12.9**	1.8	9.5	***88***	No
Lahey Clinic Northshore, Peabody	28	99	–	–	–	–	–	*No data collected*				–[6]	–[6]
Lawrence F Quigley, Chelsea[1]	–	–	*No data collected*					9.7	11.8	–	–	–[6]	No
Lawrence General, Lawrence	18	107	69	38*	–	***0****	60	12.5	15.3	1.3	8.1	***83***	**Yes**
Lemuel Shattuck, Jamaica Plain	***6***	93	***0****	***0****	***0****	–[4]	–[4]	*No data collected*				***88***	–[6]
Lowell General, Lowell	18	107	63*	40*	–	13*	50*	***13.6***	***16.5***	3.0	9.1	**94**	No
Marlborough Hospital, Marlborough	25	71	–	–	–	–[4]	–[4]	11.7	14.1	3.4	8.0	89	No
✓ Massachusetts General, Boston	**93**	309	**94**	**99**	**98**	**94**	84	**10.1**	**12.6**	**1.5**	9.1	92	**Yes**
Metrowest, Natick[1]	***10***	97	–	–	–	–	–	*No data collected*				–[6]	–[6]
Metrowest, Framingham	25	119	33*	–	–	33*	83*	12.3	15.0	2.4	8.8	92	No
Milton Hospital, Milton	***8***	109	63*	33*	–	–[4]	–[4]	13.0	15.8	2.4	9.8	**96**	No
Morton, Taunton	***6***	69	–	–	–	–	60*	***14.1***	***17.1***	2.8	10.3	**97**	No
✓ Mt Auburn, Cambridge	**54**	175	**97**	83	–	50*	**100**	11.8	14.5	1.4	9.5	**94**	**Yes**

Footnotes are on page 73. *Hospital's score based on relatively little data. See page 16.

Key Ratings for Metro Areas

See more information on "Detailed Ratings for All Areas" table beginning on page 74

✓ means hospital receives our top rating
Blue is most favorable
Bold Italic is least favorable
"–" means insufficient data

	Doctors' ratings of hospitals for high-risk adult surgery		Desirability scores from doctors (0 to 100, higher is better)					Measures of outcomes for selected cases (lower % is better)					
	Percent rating "very good" or "excellent"	Number of ratings	Low-risk adult surgery	Complex medical care for adults	High-risk child surgery	High-risk delivery of a baby	Uncomplicated delivery of a baby	Adjusted death rate for all case types (%)	Adjusted death rate for medical cases (%)	Adjusted death rate for surgical cases (%)	Adjusted adverse outcome rate for surgical cases (%)	Overall score on accreditation review (higher is better)	Major affiliation with a medical school?
National Average	32	–	59	50	40	46	58	12.1	14.8	2.3	7.7	91	–
Massachusetts *(continued)*													
Boston Area *(continued)*													
✓ New England Baptist, Boston	**64**	163	**100**	–	–[3]	–[4]	–[4]	**8.6**	**10.8**	**0.7**	9.9	**94**	No
✓ New England Medical Center, Boston[1]	**79**	228	**96**	**98**	**94**	**96**	**100**	**9.5**	**11.4**	2.0	9.7	**96**	**Yes**
Newton - Wellesley, Newton Lower Falls	45	212	**94**	75*	29*	35	83	**9.2**	**11.2**	1.5	8.1	93	**Yes**
Quincy Medical Center, Quincy	***9***	108	***29***	13*	–	–	***0****	***13.3***	***16.2***	2.3	6.9	**96**	No
St Anne's, Fall River[1]	***11***	72	–	–	–	–[4]	–[4]	**10.5**	**13.0**	1.1	7.4	–[6]	No
✓ St Elizabeth's, Brighton	**50**	189	**100**	**100**	–[3]	83	**89**	**9.8**	**12.2**	**1.1**	8.9	–[6]	**Yes**
St Luke's, New Bedford	18	78	–	20*	–	–	–	***No data collected***				90	–[6]
Saints, Lowell	***12***	73	–	–	–	–	71*	***14.3***	***17.4***	2.6	10.0	92	No
Salem Hospital, Salem[1]	32	103	**100***	67*	–	–	79	12.5	15.2	2.1	8.5	89	No
Somerville Hospital, Somerville	***3***	89	–	–	–	–[4]	–[4]	***No data collected***				–[6]	–[6]
South Shore, South Weymouth	35	119	88	–	–	–	**91**	12.1	14.8	**1.4**	**6.6**	**97**	No
Sturdy, Attleboro	***4***	82	–	–	***0****	–	–	***14.3***	***17.6***	1.8	**5.9**	**94**	No
Tobey - Southcoast, Wareham	***3***	75	***20****	***0****	***0****	–	–	***No data collected***				**95**	–[6]
Union, Lynn	***12***	73	80*	50*	–[3]	–[4]	–[4]	***13.1***	***16.1***	1.8	8.3	***85***	No
Whidden, Everett	***8***	86	33*	13*	–[3]	–[4]	–[4]	***No data collected***				93	–[6]
Winchester Hospital, Winchester	24	118	**100**	60*	–	33*	87	**10.8**	13.4	1.4	8.9	90	No
Michigan													
Greater Detroit Area													
Bi-County, Warren	***5***	184	***10***	***4***	***0***	***0***	***15***	12.1	14.7	2.3	9.5	–[6]	**Yes**
Bon Secours, Grosse Pointe[1]	19	195	72	50	***0****	***0****	83	**10.9**	**13.4**	1.6	8.4	***84***	No
Botsford General, Farmington	22	225	46	19	***0***	***0***	32	12.3	14.9	2.7	8.8	–[6]	**Yes**
Chelsea Community, Chelsea	17	157	73	13*	***0****	–[4]	–[4]	***14.4***	***17.4***	–	6.0	**97**	No
Children's, Detroit	–[2]	–[2]	–[2]	–[2]	**98**	–[4]	–[4]	***No data collected***				**96**	–[6]
Cottage, Grosse Pointe Farms[1]	***8***	167	–	14*	–[3]	–[4]	–[4]	12.1	14.7	–	5.1	–[6]	No
Crittenton, Columbus	***11***	202	73	–	–	22*	71	**10.0**	**12.3**	1.4	**6.6**	–[6]	No
✓ Detroit Receiving, Detroit	**68**	247	63	87	–[3]	–[4]	–[4]	**10.6**	**12.7**	***4.7***	***17.8***	**98**	**Yes**
Garden City Osteopathic, Garden City	***6***	189	***7***	***4***	4	***0***	***9***	11.6	14.1	2.1	8.1	–[6]	**Yes**
✓ Harper University, Detroit	**66**	234	**94**	**94**	–[3]	**89***	–	**9.9**	**11.7**	2.6	***11.1***	92	**Yes**
✓ Henry Ford, Detroit[1]	**76**	280	**90**	**93**	63	79	76	**9.4**	**11.3**	2.5	***11.1***	–[6]	**Yes**
Henry Ford, Wyandotte	***11***	160	–	–	–	–	–	11.4	13.8	2.6	8.8	***87***	No
Huron Valley - Sinai, Commerce	27	203	77	44*	20	43	81	12.4	15.3	1.6	9.6	**98**	No
Hutzel, Detroit	**58**	196	–	–	–	**97**	79	***No data collected***				–[6]	–[6]
Madison Community, Madison Heights	***1***	142	***0***	***5***	–[3]	–[4]	–[4]	**8.5**	**10.4**	–	–	***79***	No
Mt Clemens General, Mt Clemens	18	189	61	30	9	31	55	***14.8***	***18.0***	2.8	9.3	–[6]	**Yes**

Footnotes are on page 73. *Hospital's score based on relatively little data. See page 16.

Key Ratings for Metro Areas

See more information on "Detailed Ratings for All Areas" table beginning on page 74

✓ means hospital receives our top rating
Blue is most favorable
Bold Italic is least favorable
"–" means insufficient data

	Doctors' ratings of hospitals for high-risk adult surgery		Desirability scores from doctors (0 to 100, higher is better)					Measures of outcomes for selected cases (lower % is better)					
	Percent rating "very good" or "excellent"	Number of ratings	Low-risk adult surgery	Complex medical care for adults	High-risk child surgery	High-risk delivery of a baby	Uncomplicated delivery of a baby	Adjusted death rate for all case types (%)	Adjusted death rate for medical cases (%)	Adjusted death rate for surgical cases (%)	Adjusted adverse outcome rate for surgical cases (%)	Overall score on accreditation review (higher is better)	Major affiliation with a medical school?
National Average	32	–	59	50	40	46	58	12.1	14.8	2.3	7.7	91	–
Michigan *(continued)*													
Greater Detroit Area *(continued)*													
North Oakland, Pontiac	***6***	170	50*	29	20*	50*	46	11.2	13.5	2.7	8.7	***86***	No
Oakwood, Dearborn	32	205	79	50*	–	71	78	**10.7**	**13.2**	**1.7**	***12.3***	91	**Yes**
Oakwood Annapolis, Wayne	***6***	172	***18***	***5***	***0***	5	***25***	11.7	14.1	3.4	8.4	***88***	No
Oakwood Heritage, Taylor	***5***	151	***13****	***0****	–	–[4]	–[4]	***15.0***	***18.3***	1.7	10.1	***81***	No
Oakwood Seaway, Trenton	***4***	152	***15***	***6***	***0***	***0***	***6***	***13.6***	***16.8***	1.5	7.5	92	No
POH, Pontiac	***9***	182	***20***	16	***0***	***0***	***0***	11.3	13.8	1.8	7.0	–[6]	**Yes**
Providence, Southfield	47	262	**93**	86	56*	**90**	**96**	**11.1**	**13.6**	**1.6**	**6.9**	***86***	No
Riverside Osteopathic, Trenton	***4***	167	***22***	***10***	***0***	***0***	33	13.2	16.0	2.7	6.8	–[6]	No
✓ St John, Detroit	**63**	218	**93**	**89**	77	**95**	**97**	**11.0**	**13.4**	2.1	***10.4***	**95**	**Yes**
St John Detroit Riverview, Detroit	***9***	149	***25****	–	–	14*	43*	**9.1**	**11.1**	2.8	10.4	***87***	No
St John Macomb, Warren	23	171	79	56*	***0****	20*	69	**10.8**	**13.2**	2.0	8.9	***87***	No
St John Northeast, Detroit	***8***	131	***29****	20*	–	–[4]	–[4]	11.6	14.0	3.4	***13.9***	89	No
St John Oakland, Madison Heights[1]	21	162	73	33*	–	–[4]	–[4]	11.6	13.9	3.6	9.0	***88***	**Yes**
St Joseph Mercy, Ann Arbor[1]	**72**	229	**97**	**97**	78*	**97**	**99**	***13.1***	***16.0***	2.6	9.3	**97**	**Yes**
St Joseph Mercy Oakland, Pontiac	29	184	**100**	**90**	63*	80	87	11.9	14.5	2.3	***11.3***	**95**	No
St Joseph's Mercy - East, Mt Clemens	***8***	139	–	–	–	–	–	*No data collected*				–[6]	–[6]
St Joseph's Mercy of Macomb, Clinton Township[1]	***13***	148	67	20*	***0****	***0****	55	**11.2**	**13.5**	2.8	8.1	***83***	No
St Mary Mercy, Livonia	***7***	166	33	18	***0****	8	55	12.1	14.8	1.7	8.5	**96**	No
Saline Community, Saline	***11***	152	63*	13*	–	–[4]	–[4]	12.1	14.6	–	–	**97**	No
Sinai - Grace, Detroit	30	199	33	38	13*	42	42	**10.1**	**12.1**	***4.0***	***11.9***	92	**Yes**
University of Michigan, Ann Arbor	**91**	299	**89**	**99**	**99**[5]	**98**[5]	**92**[5]	12.2	14.7	2.5	***10.3***	**95**	**Yes**
✓ William Beaumont, Royal Oak	**81**	314	**96**	**95**	**87**	**95**	**93**	**10.1**	**12.3**	**1.7**	9.2	**96**	**Yes**
✓ William Beaumont, Troy	**55**	253	88	74	57	61	**88**	**10.5**	**12.6**	2.8	***10.8***	92	No
Minnesota													
Twin Cities Area													
Abbott Northwestern, Minneapolis	**90**	292	**97**	**97**	–[3]	**99**	**96**	**9.8**	**11.9**	**1.8**	**7.2**	***88***	No
Buffalo Hospital, Buffalo	***6***	114	***9***	***0***	***0***	***0***	***6***	12.6	15.3	–	5.1	***85***	No
Children's, Minneapolis	–[2]	–[2]	–[2]	–[2]	**100**	–[4]	–[4]	*No data collected*				–[6]	–[6]
Children's, St Paul	–[2]	–[2]	–[2]	–[2]	**99**	–[4]	–[4]	*No data collected*				–[6]	–[6]
Fairview - Riverside Campus, Minneapolis	44	232	51	44	32	81	64	12.2	15.1	1.9	9.0	***84***	No
Fairview - University Campus, Minneapolis[1]	**68**	260	50	**92**	**84**	69	***17***	*No data collected*				–[6]	–[6]
Fairview Ridges, Burnsville	22	186	68	13	***0***	***0***	75	11.5	14.1	1.4	**5.6**	***85***	No
Fairview Southdale, Edina	43	257	72	47	5	33	66	**10.2**	**12.3**	2.0	7.5	***85***	No
Hennepin County, Minneapolis	**83**	278	60	**90**	71	79	***24***	**9.4**	**11.4**	2.1	6.2	***83***	No

Footnotes are on page 73. *Hospital's score based on relatively little data. See page 16.

Key Ratings for Metro Areas

See more information on "Detailed Ratings for All Areas" table beginning on page 74

✓ means hospital receives our top rating
Blue is most favorable
Bold Italic is least favorable
"–" means insufficient data

	Doctors' ratings of hospitals for high-risk adult surgery		Desirability scores from doctors (0 to 100, higher is better)					Measures of outcomes for selected cases (lower % is better)					
	Percent rating "very good" or "excellent"	Number of ratings	Low-risk adult surgery	Complex medical care for adults	High-risk child surgery	High-risk delivery of a baby	Uncomplicated delivery of a baby	Adjusted death rate for all case types (%)	Adjusted death rate for medical cases (%)	Adjusted death rate for surgical cases (%)	Adjusted adverse outcome rate for surgical cases (%)	Overall score on accreditation review (higher is better)	Major affiliation with a medical school?
National Average	32	–	59	50	40	46	58	12.1	14.8	2.3	7.7	91	–
Minnesota *(continued)*													
Twin Cities Area *(continued)*													
Lakeview, Stillwater	12	102	42	20	10	0*	78*	15.3	19.1	–	4.5	98	No
Mercy, Coon Rapids[1]	33	176	82	48	0	0	57	10.3	12.9	1.2	7.0	88	No
✓ Methodist, St Louis Park[1]	62	250	88	75	17	44	77	10.8	13.3	1.7	7.0	89	No
Monticello Big Lake, Monticello[1]	4	100	0	0	0	0	0*	16.5	20.3	–	–	94	No
North Memorial, Robbinsdale[1]	82	261	94	94	50	79	87	13.2	16.3	1.8	8.6	91	Yes
Regina, Hastings[1]	8	100	33*	0*	0*	0*	30	15.5	19.2	–	4.3	96	No
✓ Regions, St Paul	62	230	60	78	39	59	45	10.3	12.4	2.4	7.5	86	Yes
Ridgeview, Waconia	15	123	64	–	0	0*	100	12.5	15.2	2.2	6.1	92	No
St Francis Regional, Shakopee	7	135	17	0	0	0	19	13.3	15.5	5.2	9.1	88	No
St John's, Maplewood	31	175	87	36	17*	36	90	12.4	15.3	1.5	6.5	96	No
St Joseph's, St Paul	36	162	83	63	0	27	83	11.7	14.2	2.5	8.0	97	Yes
United, St Paul[1]	68	201	91	96	–[3]	98	97	8.9	10.8	1.9	7.5	84	No
Unity, Fridley[1]	22	174	70	19	0	11	48	11.2	13.8	1.5	7.7	88	No
Woodwinds, Woodbury	10	122	33	3	5	3	68	–	–	–	–	–[6]	No
Missouri													
Kansas City Area													
Baptist, Kansas City	19	118	46	25	7	24	36	12.5	15.4	1.9	6.9	92	No
Children's Mercy, Kansas City	–[2]	–[2]	–[2]	–[2]	100	85	–	*No data collected*				92	–[6]
Independence Regional, Independence	17	88	20	18	0*	–[4]	–[4]	12.9	15.7	2.4	6.2	–[6]	No
Lee's Summit Hospital, Lee's Summit	4	94	21	7	0	–[4]	–[4]	16.4	20.0	2.6	7.2	91	No
Medical Center, Independence	7	90	20*	0	0*	10	27	14.1	17.1	2.4	6.7	88	Yes
✓ Research, Kansas City	63	125	88	98	60*	89	68	11.6	14.2	2.0	10.1	89	No
St Joseph, Kansas City[1]	72	127	93	88	50*	79	87	11.1	13.5	2.4	6.6	86	No
✓ St Luke's, Kansas City	86	136	94	97	83	99	90	10.7	13.1	1.8	7.6	92	Yes
St Luke's Northland, Kansas City	27	81	–	–	–	–	–	*No data collected*				92	–[6]
St Mary's, Blue Springs	12	81	50	17*	0*	0*	78*	14.5	17.5	3.3	7.8	94	No
Trinity Lutheran, Kansas City	11	98	6	7	–[3]	–[4]	–[4]	10.7	12.9	2.3	8.8	87	No
Truman, Kansas City	33	107	29	43	–[3]	61	19	8.7	10.7	–	5.8	–[6]	Yes
Truman - Lakewood, Kansas City	6	86	0	0	0*	0*	27	16.9	20.4	–	–	–[6]	Yes
St. Louis Area													
✓ Barnes - Jewish, St Louis	90	78	86	98	–[3]	98	76	10.2	12.2	2.4	10.7	89	Yes
Barnes - Jewish West County, St Louis	33	58	69	50*	–[3]	–[4]	–[4]	9.7	12.4	0.7	12.3	90	No
Cardinal Glennon Children's, St Louis	–[2]	–[2]	–[2]	–[2]	99	–[4]	–[4]	*No data collected*				91	–[6]
Christian Northeast, St Louis[1]	13	56	63*	–	40*	14*	13*	11.2	13.5	2.9	8.3	95	No

Footnotes are on page 73. *Hospital's score based on relatively little data. See page 16.

Key Ratings for Metro Areas

See more information on "Detailed Ratings for All Areas" table beginning on page 74

✓ means hospital receives our top rating
Blue is most favorable
Bold Italic is least favorable
"–" means insufficient data

	Doctors' ratings of hospitals for high-risk adult surgery		Desirability scores from doctors (0 to 100, higher is better)					Measures of outcomes for selected cases (lower % is better)					
	Percent rating "very good" or "excellent"	Number of ratings	Low-risk adult surgery	Complex medical care for adults	High-risk child surgery	High-risk delivery of a baby	Uncomplicated delivery of a baby	Adjusted death rate for all case types (%)	Adjusted death rate for medical cases (%)	Adjusted death rate for surgical cases (%)	Adjusted adverse outcome rate for surgical cases (%)	Overall score on accreditation review (higher is better)	Major affiliation with a medical school?
National Average	32	–	59	50	40	46	58	12.1	14.8	2.3	7.7	91	–
Missouri *(continued)*													
St. Louis Area *(continued)*													
Christian Northwest, Florissant[1]	***7***	54	–	–	–	***0****	29*	12.6	15.4	–	–	**95**	No
DePaul, Bridgeton	18	51	–	–	–	***0****	***21***	11.5	13.8	***3.1***	9.3	91	No
Des Peres, St Louis	17	48	33	13*	–[3]	–[4]	–[4]	13.5	16.4	2.7	8.9	–[6]	**Yes**
Forest Park, St Louis	***9***	55	***18***	***6***	–[3]	11	***16***	12.8	15.4	3.2	8.8	93	No
Missouri Baptist, St Louis	**70**	71	**97**	**94**	–	**94**	**98**	11.6	14.3	1.9	7.9	***87***	No
St Alexius, St Louis	***8***	53	***0***	***3***	–[3]	–[4]	–[4]	11.3	13.9	1.6	7.9	**94**	No
St Anthony's, St Louis	24	62	55	14*	***0****	***0****	53	11.8	14.2	2.9	***11.5***	91	No
✓ St John's Mercy, Creve Coeur	**67**	66	**100**	**96**	58	**99**	**98**	11.9	14.5	2.3	8.4	92	No
St Louis Children's, St Louis	–[2]	–[2]	–[2]	–[2]	**98**	–[4]	–[4]	***No data collected***				**94**	–[6]
St Louis ConnectCare, St Louis	–	–	***No data collected***					**6.2**	**7.7**	–	–	–[6]	No
✓ St Louis University, St Louis	**74**	69	88	**94**	–[3]	–[4]	–[4]	**10.0**	**12.2**	1.6	8.7	**95**	**Yes**
✓ St Luke's, Chesterfield	**63**	64	**97**	**100**	–	**92**	**100**	**9.4**	**11.3**	2.0	9.1	**95**	No
St Mary's, Richmond Heights	43	61	**89***	60*	–[3]	**88**	**93**	**10.2**	**12.1**	2.9	8.4	–[6]	**Yes**
Southpointe, St Louis	***5***	41	***4***	***4***	–[3]	***0***	***0***	11.5	13.8	–	9.7	***86***	No
SSM St Joseph, Kirkwood	26	53	83*	–	–	20*	56*	11.1	13.5	2.3	10.2	**94**	No
Nevada													
Las Vegas Area													
Boulder City Hospital, Boulder City	***6***	50	***0***	***0***	***0***	–[4]	–[4]	13.2	15.8	–	–	–[6]	No
Desert Springs, Las Vegas	23	84	44	30	7	10	40	12.6	15.2	2.9	9.0	***85***	No
Lake Mead, North Las Vegas	***9***	78	***4***	***2***	***0***	***0***	***7***	13.0	15.4	***4.7***	10.0	–[6]	No
Mountainview, Las Vegas	35	84	86	69	31	33	74	***13.3***	***16.2***	2.7	9.6	**96**	No
St Rose Dominican, Henderson	–	–	***No data collected***					***15.5***	***18.7***	3.7	***11.1***	**96**	No
Summerlin, Las Vegas	19	85	62	39	13	10	62	12.1	14.5	–	8.9	**96**	No
Sunrise, Las Vegas	**73**	94	**94**	**96**	**97**	**96**	86	12.4	15.0	2.6	8.7	**94**	No
✓ University, Las Vegas	**65**	96	83	**96**	**96**	**93**	65	**9.2**	**11.1**	2.5	8.4	***86***	**Yes**
Valley, Las Vegas	36	91	53	53	30	63	69	***14.7***	***17.6***	***3.4***	9.4	**94**	No
New Jersey													
Delaware Valley Area													
Cooper, Camden[1]	**63**	145	73	81	68	**88**	61	12.6	15.4	2.4	9.8	92	**Yes**
✓ Deborah Heart and Lung, Browns Mills	**70**	112	–	–	–	–[4]	–[4]	**9.4**	**11.1**	1.9	***10.2***	93	No
Kennedy - University Medical Center, Cherry Hill	***12***	108	***10***	***0***	***0****	***0***	***11****	***No data collected***				–[6]	–[6]
Kennedy - University Medical Center, Stratford	***12***	107	43*	36	***0****	14*	29*	12.3	14.9	2.8	***11.2***	–[6]	**Yes**
Kennedy - University Medical Center, Turnersville	***11***	99	38*	14*	***0****	11*	33*	***No data collected***				–[6]	–[6]
Our Lady of Lourdes, Camden	33	120	**100***	**88***	–	**100***	**100***	12.4	14.7	***3.0***	***11.7***	**96**	**Yes**

Footnotes are on page 73. *Hospital's score based on relatively little data. See page 16.

Key Ratings for Metro Areas

See more information on "Detailed Ratings for All Areas" table beginning on page 74

✓ means hospital receives our top rating
Blue is most favorable
Bold Italic is least favorable
"–" means insufficient data

Hospital	Doctors' ratings of hospitals for high-risk adult surgery		Desirability scores from doctors (0 to 100, higher is better)					Measures of outcomes for selected cases (lower % is better)					
	Percent rating "very good" or "excellent"	Number of ratings	Low-risk adult surgery	Complex medical care for adults	High-risk child surgery	High-risk delivery of a baby	Uncomplicated delivery of a baby	Adjusted death rate for all case types (%)	Adjusted death rate for medical cases (%)	Adjusted death rate for surgical cases (%)	Adjusted adverse outcome rate for surgical cases (%)	Overall score on accreditation review (higher is better)	Major affiliation with a medical school?
National Average	32	–	59	50	40	46	58	12.1	14.8	2.3	7.7	91	–
New Jersey *(continued)*													
Delaware Valley Area *(continued)*													
Rancocas, Willingboro	3	96	0*	–	–	–	0*	13.5	16.3	3.2	10.3	93	No
Underwood - Memorial, Woodbury	14	90	30	17	0*	0	18	11.6	14.0	2.9	12.3	94	No
Virtua, Marlton[1]	22	103	100	–	–[3]	–[4]	–[4]	No data collected				–[6]	–[6]
Virtua, Mt Holly	24	93	92	–	–	–	92	12.5	15.3	2.2	9.2	–[6]	Yes
Virtua, Voorhees	21	102	94	82	40*	87	100	No data collected				–[6]	–[6]
Virtua West Jersey, Berlin	6	90	–	–	–[3]	–[4]	–[4]	No data collected				–[6]	–[6]
Northern and Central New Jersey													
Barnert, Paterson	5	82	11*	0*	0*	0*	8	9.2	11.0	–	10.8	96	No
Bayonne Hospital, Bayonne	10	84	–	–	–	–	–	9.5	11.7	1.5	7.0	88	No
Bayshore, Holmdel	8	72	22*	38*	0	–[4]	–[4]	11.0	13.5	1.5	10.5	86	No
Centrastate, Freehold[1]	8	74	39	20	0*	0*	46	10.4	12.4	3.8	10.0	93	No
Chilton, Pompton Plains	23	99	71	40	13*	17	68	12.4	15.2	1.7	9.8	96	No
Christ, Jersey City	13	93	78*	50*	40*	–	50*	10.2	12.4	2.2	10.4	86	No
Christian, Wyckoff	6	71	0	0	0	0	0	No data collected				94	–[6]
Clara Maass, Belleville[1]	18	113	60	44*	–	–	82	10.1	12.3	2.0	10.6	91	No
Columbus, Newark	12	92	57*	–	20*	43*	43	8.8	10.6	2.6	8.7	–[6]	No
East Orange General, East Orange	3	100	10	6	–[3]	–[4]	–[4]	8.5	10.3	4.4	10.5	91	No
✓ Englewood Hospital, Englewood	52	187	90	90	80	86	87	9.7	11.9	1.7	10.8	93	Yes
General, Passaic	21	82	100*	80	–	–	63*	11.1	13.5	2.1	10.5	94	No
Greenville, Jersey City	2	62	–	17*	–[3]	–[4]	–[4]	9.0	10.9	–	7.7	94	No
✓ Hackensack University, Hackensack	88	244	97	99	98	96	93	10.7	13.0	2.0	12.8	96	Yes
Hackettstown Community, Hackettstown	10	67	38*	17*	20*	20*	63*	11.3	13.6	3.2	8.2	94	No
Holy Name, Teaneck	38	170	96	85	30	55	93	10.4	12.6	2.1	9.5	97	No
Hospital Center, Orange	4	93	39	9	0	0*	–	8.1	9.6	3.2	9.9	91	No
Hunterdon, Flemington[1]	19	80	63*	–	–	–	69	11.5	14.1	1.4	7.7	94	No
Irvington General, Irvington	6	97	8	0*	–[3]	–[4]	–[4]	7.7	9.5	0.4	4.6	92	No
Jersey City Medical Center, Jersey City	11	116	8	18	22*	33	9	9.7	11.8	–	7.6	91	Yes
Jersey Shore, Neptune[1]	37	107	54	63	50	67	69	13.0	16.1	2.0	8.5	91	Yes
JFK, Edison	33	136	84	83	50*	60*	86	9.7	11.9	1.5	11.7	97	No
Meadowlands, Secaucus	2	97	22*	8	20	7	25	11.7	13.8	4.9	12.0	96	No
Monmouth, Long Branch	48	91	78	83	79	91	86	10.8	13.2	1.8	11.0	94	Yes
Morristown Memorial, Morristown	89	207	99	99	99	98	99	12.7	15.7	2.0	10.1	99	Yes
Mountainside, Montclair	27	134	85	60*	–	–	71*	11.6	14.1	2.7	13.5	99	No
Muhlenberg Regional, Plainfield	15	92	55	33*	17*	11*	46	11.7	14.2	2.5	11.2	–[6]	No

Footnotes are on page 73. *Hospital's score based on relatively little data. See page 16.

Key Ratings for Metro Areas

See more information on "Detailed Ratings for All Areas" table beginning on page 74

✓ means hospital receives our top rating
Blue is most favorable
Bold Italic is least favorable
"–" means insufficient data

	Doctors' ratings of hospitals for high-risk adult surgery		Desirability scores from doctors (0 to 100, higher is better)					Measures of outcomes for selected cases (lower % is better)					
	Percent rating "very good" or "excellent"	Number of ratings	Low-risk adult surgery	Complex medical care for adults	High-risk child surgery	High-risk delivery of a baby	Uncomplicated delivery of a baby	Adjusted death rate for all case types (%)	Adjusted death rate for medical cases (%)	Adjusted death rate for surgical cases (%)	Adjusted adverse outcome rate for surgical cases (%)	Overall score on accreditation review (higher is better)	Major affiliation with a medical school?
National Average	32	–	59	50	40	46	58	12.1	14.8	2.3	7.7	91	–
New Jersey *(continued)*													
Northern and Central New Jersey *(continued)*													
✓ Newark Beth Israel, Newark	**51**	175	79	87	**92**	77	86	**8.8**	**10.6**	2.1	8.3	**94**	**Yes**
Newton Memorial, Newton	***13***	67	38*	29*	***0****	***0****	44*	11.2	13.6	2.1	9.0	90	No
✓ Overlook, Summit	**60**	155	**93**	**93**	**88**	**91**	**96**	**10.8**	**13.4**	**1.3**	9.4	**97**	**Yes**
Palisades of New York Presbyterian, North Bergen	***0***	84	40*	17*	***0****	14*	***25***	**10.8**	**13.1**	2.7	7.7	**94**	No
Pascack Valley, Westwood	23	142	50	25	9	8	50	12.1	14.7	2.2	***10.7***	**98**	No
Passaic Beth Israel, Passaic	17	77	–	–	–	–[4]	–[4]	12.1	14.9	1.5	8.8	**96**	No
Rahway Hospital, Rahway	***10***	87	***22****	14*	***0****	–	***0****	12.7	15.5	2.7	***11.0***	**94**	No
Raritan Bay, Perth Amboy	***9***	85	***13****	***0****	***0****	***0****	***10***	**10.5**	**12.9**	1.4	8.8	93	No
Raritan Bay - Old Bridge Division, Old Bridge	***11***	79	33	***10***	***0****	***0***	***9***	*No data collected*				–[6]	–[6]
Riverview, Red Bank	24	72	72	78*	50*	38*	74	11.8	14.4	1.9	9.2	**96**	No
✓ Robert Wood Johnson University, New Brunswick	**86**	205	**93**	**97**	**98**	**93**	**88**	11.4	14.1	1.8	***10.8***	**97**	**Yes**
✓ St Barnabas, Livingston	**80**	239	**96**	**97**	**96**	**97**	**95**	**10.1**	**12.3**	**1.6**	9.0	**94**	**Yes**
St Claire's, Sussex[1]	***5***	58	***29****	13*	***0****	–[4]	–[4]	13.5	16.8	–	**3.4**	–[6]	No
St Clare's, Dover	***10***	84	***0****	***0****	–[3]	–[4]	–[4]	12.1	14.6	2.8	9.9	**97**	No
St Clares, Denville	30	102	73	55	20	39	76	11.7	14.3	2.2	10.4	**97**	**Yes**
St Francis, Jersey City	***2***	62	–	***0****	–	–[4]	–[4]	12.6	15.3	2.4	10.7	**97**	No
St James, Newark	***8***	84	–	***0****	***0****	17*	***0****	11.7	14.3	–	4.9	93	No
St Joseph's, Wayne	***8***	86	57*	***0****	–	***0****	38*	12.8	15.6	2.4	9.8	**95**	No
St Joseph's Regional, Paterson	**64**	140	86	**96**	**96**	**97**	**91**	12.3	14.7	3.0	***10.7***	**95**	No
St Mary, Hoboken	***14***	76	75*	71*	–	–	80	**10.5**	**12.8**	2.0	8.5	93	No
St Mary's, Passaic	***8***	61	33*	33*	20*	***0****	***25****	11.3	13.9	1.7	9.1	93	No
St Michaels, Newark	29	129	***0****	80	–	17*	***9***	**9.9**	**11.9**	2.3	8.7	***88***	No
✓ St Peter's University, New Brunswick	**71**	150	**90**	**92**	**93**	**97**	**97**	**11.0**	**13.4**	1.9	***11.9***	**96**	**Yes**
Somerset, Somerville	32	96	**100**	**91**	–	–	**100**	12.3	15.0	2.2	8.8	92	No
Trinitas (East Jersey St), Elizabeth[1]	19	72	–	60*	–	–	–	11.3	13.6	3.1	11.2	93	No
Trinitas (Williamson St), Elizabeth	15	82	–	–	–	50*	–	**8.8**	**10.6**	2.7	9.5	***87***	No
Union Hospital, Union	18	88	71	60	–[3]	–[4]	–[4]	11.7	14.2	2.4	***12.3***	**99**	**Yes**
✓ University, Newark	**65**	186	63	**98**	**91**	69	***26***	**10.1**	**11.7**	***4.2***	10.9	**97**	**Yes**
✓ Valley, Ridgewood	**65**	181	**95**	**96**	**86**	**95**	**96**	**10.8**	**13.3**	**1.5**	***10.5***	93	No
Warren, Phillipsburg	***4***	46	–	–	–	–	–	12.0	14.7	1.9	8.6	91	No
West Hudson, Kearny	***8***	59	60*	–	–	–[4]	–[4]	**10.5**	**12.9**	1.4	6.7	93	No
New York													
Buffalo Area													
Bertrand Chaffee, Springville	***0***	27	***14****	***0***	–	***0****	***17****	10.7	13.0	–	–	–[6]	No

Footnotes are on page 73. *Hospital's score based on relatively little data. See page 16.

Key Ratings for Metro Areas

See more information on "Detailed Ratings for All Areas" table beginning on page 74

✓ means hospital receives our top rating
Blue is most favorable
Bold Italic is least favorable
"–" means insufficient data

	Doctors' ratings of hospitals for high-risk adult surgery		Desirability scores from doctors (0 to 100, higher is better)					Measures of outcomes for selected cases (lower % is better)					
	Percent rating "very good" or "excellent"	Number of ratings	Low-risk adult surgery	Complex medical care for adults	High-risk child surgery	High-risk delivery of a baby	Uncomplicated delivery of a baby	Adjusted death rate for all case types (%)	Adjusted death rate for medical cases (%)	Adjusted death rate for surgical cases (%)	Adjusted adverse outcome rate for surgical cases (%)	Overall score on accreditation review (higher is better)	Major affiliation with a medical school?
National Average	32	–	59	50	40	46	58	12.1	14.8	2.3	7.7	91	–
New York *(continued)*													
Buffalo Area *(continued)*													
Children's, Buffalo	**71**	41	–	–	**100**	**98**	**93**	***No data collected***				–[6]	–[6]
Erie County, Buffalo	**53**	40	88*	**90**	–[3]	–[4]	–[4]	***14.8***	***18.1***	2.1	7.5	***85***	**Yes**
Kaleida Health - Buffalo General, Buffalo[1]	**56**	43	74	**91**	60*	–	38*	***12.7***	***15.5***	2.4	***9.7***	89	**Yes**
Kaleida Hlth - Millard Filmore Suburban, Williamsville	**63**	43	**97**	**94**	56*	58	87	***No data collected***				–[6]	–[6]
Kalieda Hlth - Millard Filmore - Gates Circle, Buffalo[1]	45	40	**93**	**93**	–[3]	–	–	***No data collected***				–[6]	–[6]
Kenmore Mercy, Kenmore	24	37	67*	–	–[3]	–[4]	–[4]	***13.5***	***16.7***	1.9	***11.8***	91	No
Mercy, Buffalo	26	35	78*	–	–	15	63	***13.2***	***16.2***	2.1	***10.1***	91	No
Our Lady of Victory, Lackawanna	***4***	26	***12***	***0***	–[3]	–[4]	–[4]	12.6	15.3	2.7	***12.8***	–[6]	No
Roswell Park Cancer Institute, Buffalo	**76**	38	83*	**89***	–	–[4]	–[4]	14.9	18.6	–	10.4	**96**	No
St Joseph, Cheektowaga	***11***	35	36	***9***	–[3]	–[4]	–[4]	11.5	14.0	2.3	9.1	**96**	No
Sheehan, Buffalo	***0***	31	***0***	***0***	***0***	–[4]	–[4]	**8.2**	**9.7**	–	–	***84***	No
Sisters of Charity, Buffalo	48	42	**90**	**93**	–[3]	77	**91**	11.9	14.5	2.4	***12.0***	***87***	No
New York City, Long Island, and Westchester County													
Allen Pavilion (New York Presbyterian), New York	**61**	237	**89***	**91**	**89***	**89***	79	***No data collected***				–[6]	–[6]
✓ Bellevue, New York	**52**	317	43*	50	50*	22*	***20***	**9.7**	**11.7**	2.3	7.2	93	**Yes**
Beth Israel - Kings Highway Division, Brooklyn	***6***	177	44*	17*	–[3]	–[4]	–[4]	***No data collected***				–[6]	–[6]
Beth Israel - Petrie Division, New York	44	268	73	56	41	52	60	**8.9**	**10.8**	**1.7**	8.3	**94**	**Yes**
Beth Israel - Singer Division, New York[1]	44	263	88	57*	–[3]	–[4]	–[4]	***No data collected***				–[6]	–[6]
Bronx - Lebanon, Bronx	***5***	176	***0****	13*	***0****	***0***	***0***	**10.4**	**12.5**	3.2	***15.7***	93	**Yes**
Brookdale, Brooklyn	***10***	220	33*	***11****	14*	22*	***27***	**10.4**	**12.5**	3.6	***12.0***	**96**	**Yes**
Brookhaven, Patchogue	***4***	93	–	***0****	–	***0****	***13****	***13.5***	***16.4***	2.5	8.0	93	No
Brooklyn - Caledonian Campus, Brooklyn	***4***	157	–	–	–	***0****	***0****	***No data collected***				–[6]	–[6]
Brooklyn Hospital Center, Brooklyn[1]	***10***	160	67*	60*	–	71*	75*	**10.7**	**13.0**	2.2	10.6	**96**	**Yes**
Brunswick General, Amityville	***2***	91	***13****	14*	14*	–[4]	–[4]	11.4	13.9	2.6	***12.9***	***81***	No
Cabrini, New York	***7***	235	***29***	15	–[3]	–[4]	–[4]	**8.4**	**9.8**	2.9	***11.2***	90	**Yes**
Calvary, Bronx	22	117	–	–	–	–	–	***No data collected***				**99**	–[6]
Central Suffolk, Riverhead	***0***	89	–	–	–	–	–	12.9	15.7	2.9	***12.4***	–[6]	No
Community, Dobbs Ferry	***6***	108	40*	***0****	–[3]	–[4]	–[4]	13.2	16.0	–	6.3	**98**	No
Coney Island, Brooklyn	***2***	213	***0***	***0***	***0***	***0***	***0***	12.1	14.6	4.0	6.5	**96**	**Yes**
Doctors', Staten Island	***4***	116	–	17*	–[3]	–[4]	–[4]	11.0	13.9	–	6.0	***87***	No
Eastern Long Island, Greenport	***1***	73	–	–	–	–[4]	–[4]	11.8	14.1	–	8.6	90	No
Elmhurst Hospital, Elmhurst[1]	16	185	33*	40*	–	–	67*	13.2	15.9	–	14.0	–[6]	**Yes**
Flushing Hospital, Flushing	***10***	157	–	–	–	–	67*	***12.8***	***15.6***	2.2	11.2	–[6]	**Yes**
Franklin, Valley Stream[1]	***6***	155	***17****	20	***0****	***0***	***17***	***14.5***	***17.8***	1.8	9.5	**96**	No

Footnotes are on page 73. *Hospital's score based on relatively little data. See page 16.

Key Ratings for Metro Areas

See more information on "Detailed Ratings for All Areas" table beginning on page 74

✓ means hospital receives our top rating
Blue is most favorable
Bold Italic is least favorable
"–" means insufficient data

	Doctors' ratings of hospitals for high-risk adult surgery		Desirability scores from doctors (0 to 100, higher is better)					Measures of outcomes for selected cases (lower % is better)					
	Percent rating "very good" or "excellent"	Number of ratings	Low-risk adult surgery	Complex medical care for adults	High-risk child surgery	High-risk delivery of a baby	Uncomplicated delivery of a baby	Adjusted death rate for all case types (%)	Adjusted death rate for medical cases (%)	Adjusted death rate for surgical cases (%)	Adjusted adverse outcome rate for surgical cases (%)	Overall score on accreditation review (higher is better)	Major affiliation with a medical school?
National Average	32	–	59	50	40	46	58	12.1	14.8	2.3	7.7	91	–
New York *(continued)*													
New York City, Long Island, and Westchester County *(continued)*													
Good Samaritan, West Islip	22	121	89	91	86*	91	94	***13.2***	***16.1***	2.4	***11.4***	94	Yes
Harlem, New York	***8***	243	***0***	***0***	***0***	***0***	***0***	9.5	11.6	–	***16.6***	93	Yes
Hospital for Joint Diseases, New York	–	–	*No data collected*					7.2	11.8	–	7.7	97	No
✓ Hospital for Special Surgery, New York	88	338	100	80*	88*	–[4]	–[4]	4.0	–	0.7	8.1	98	Yes
Hudson Valley, Peekskill	***5***	105	50*	17*	–	13*	55	12.9	15.7	2.4	7.1	–[6]	No
Huntington Hospital, Huntington	25	125	100*	–	–	–	89*	10.8	13.2	2.0	10.4	–[6]	No
Interfaith, Brooklyn	***1***	148	***0****	***9***	***0****	13*	***10***	8.7	10.4	–	–	–[6]	No
Interfaith - Brooklyn Jewish Division, Brooklyn	***3***	163	***0***	***0***	***0***	***0***	***0***	*No data collected*				89	–[6]
Island, Hempstead	***2***	107	***0****	–	–[3]	–[4]	–[4]	***15.1***	***18.1***	–	–	***77***	No
Jacobi, Bronx	31	239	50*	64	33*	33*	50	11.3	13.7	–	10.5	93	Yes
Jamaica Hospital, Jamaica	***10***	175	***17****	–	10	25*	***25****	10.8	13.2	2.1	9.6	95	No
John T Mather, Port Jefferson	24	96	100	100*	–	–[4]	–[4]	12.5	15.3	1.5	9.0	92	No
Kings County, Brooklyn	23	243	***0***	***0***	8	6	***0***	12.4	15.1	–	–	93	No
Kingsbrook Jewish, Brooklyn	***3***	143	–	–	–	–[4]	–[4]	10.1	12.3	3.0	9.5	92	No
Lawrence, Bronxville	***14***	140	78*	–	–	60*	81	10.7	13.0	2.0	7.9	96	No
✓ Lenox Hill, New York	69	345	95	91	71	88	97	8.8	10.6	1.8	***11.7***	–[6]	Yes
Lincoln Medical and Mental Health, Bronx	***5***	176	***0***	***0***	***0***	***0***	***0***	9.7	11.9	–	5.3	95	Yes
Long Beach Medical Center, Long Beach	***2***	126	***0****	–	25*	–[4]	–[4]	12.7	15.5	1.8	7.1	92	No
Long Island College, Brooklyn	26	226	93	71*	60	82	95	9.1	11.1	1.7	***11.2***	96	Yes
✓ Long Island Jewish, New Hyde Park	72	274	96	100	99[5]	97	97	11.5	14.0	2.1	***9.9***	–[6]	Yes
Lutheran, Brooklyn	***12***	172	56*	22*	***0****	20*	50*	9.9	11.8	2.9	***11.1***	92	Yes
Maimonides, Brooklyn	34	257	56	69	57*	79	79	8.8	10.8	1.6	9.6	90	Yes
Mary Immaculate (St Vincent Catholic), Jamaica	***5***	127	***0****	–	***0****	–	***0****	*No data collected*				–[6]	–[6]
Massapequa General, Seaford	***3***	131	***9***	***0****	–[3]	–[4]	–[4]	12.3	15.2	1.4	6.4	–[6]	No
✓ Memorial Sloan - Kettering Cancer, New York	90	398	78*	94	71*	–[4]	–[4]	10.6	13.4	0.8	9.0	98	Yes
Mercy, Rockville Centre	***13***	155	100	71*	–	–	80	10.8	13.3	1.1	7.7	96	No
Metropolitan, New York	***5***	231	***11***	***7***	6	11	***6***	8.0	9.5	–	11.1	–[6]	Yes
✓ Montefiore, Bronx	67	269	94	92	95	–	–	11.6	14.2	2.0	8.5	94	Yes
Montefiore - Jackie Weiler, Bronx	72	282	91	92	93	93	90	*No data collected*				–[6]	–[6]
✓ Mt Sinai, New York[1]	86	415	99	99	100	99	97	11.2	14.0	1.3	9.3	***88***	Yes
Mt Sinai of Queens, Long Island City[1]	16	152	83*	100*	–[3]	–[4]	–[4]	*No data collected*				***88***	–[6]
Mt Vernon Hospital, Mt Vernon	***4***	117	***11****	13*	***0***	***0****	***0****	7.6	9.2	2.5	10.2	***88***	No
Nassau University, East Meadow[1]	19	208	***13***	16	17	18	***22***	***15.3***	***18.5***	–	15.9	96	Yes
New Island, Bethpage	***5***	118	43	33*	–	11*	38	11.0	13.3	2.3	8.5	90	No

Footnotes are on page 73. *Hospital's score based on relatively little data. See page 16.

Key Ratings for Metro Areas

See more information on "Detailed Ratings for All Areas" table beginning on page 74

✓ means hospital receives our top rating
Blue is most favorable
Bold Italic is least favorable
"–" means insufficient data

	Doctors' ratings of hospitals for high-risk adult surgery		Desirability scores from doctors (0 to 100, higher is better)					Measures of outcomes for selected cases (lower % is better)					
	Percent rating "very good" or "excellent"	Number of ratings	Low-risk adult surgery	Complex medical care for adults	High-risk child surgery	High-risk delivery of a baby	Uncomplicated delivery of a baby	Adjusted death rate for all case types (%)	Adjusted death rate for medical cases (%)	Adjusted death rate for surgical cases (%)	Adjusted adverse outcome rate for surgical cases (%)	Overall score on accreditation review (higher is better)	Major affiliation with a medical school?
National Average	32	–	59	50	40	46	58	12.1	14.8	2.3	7.7	91	–
New York *(continued)*													
New York City, Long Island, and Westchester County *(continued)*													
New York, Brooklyn	***2***	123	***13****	***0****	–[3]	–[4]	–[4]	11.4	13.9	1.9	6.4	***87***	No
New York Hospital of Queens, Flushing	27	155	75*	67*	60*	75*	71*	***14.6***	***17.9***	2.0	***12.0***	96	Yes
New York Methodist, Brooklyn	24	176	73	75	60*	64	81	9.6	11.6	2.4	***12.9***	95	No
✓ New York Presbyterian, New York	90	410	100	100	99	99	97	11.5	14.2	1.8	9.4	–[6]	Yes
New York United, Port Chester	***10***	122	–	–	–	–	–	10.2	12.4	1.7	6.3	***84***	No
✓ New York Weill Cornell of NY Presbyterian, New York[1]	86	376	98	98	97	98	98	10.4	12.9	1.5	***10.1***	91	Yes
New York Westchester Square, Bronx	***12***	145	***29****	22*	–[3]	–[4]	–[4]	11.9	14.6	1.9	8.3	94	No
North Central Bronx, Bronx	***6***	190	***11****	***0****	***0****	–	***14***	8.1	9.9	–	–	97	No
North General, New York	***5***	177	***11****	***0***	***0****	–[4]	–[4]	***14.9***	***17.5***	***7.8***	***16.8***	93	Yes
North Shore University, Forest Hills	28	177	***20****	40*	–	29*	50*	11.9	14.3	3.7	***14.1***	–[6]	No
North Shore University, Glen Cove	28	181	77	–	–	20*	89*	12.1	14.6	2.5	9.0	97	No
✓ North Shore University, Manhasset	79	299	96	97	95	100	99	10.3	12.8	1.3	8.3	98	Yes
North Shore University, Plainview	22	161	86*	–	–	–	80	12.6	15.4	2.2	9.2	99	No
North Shore University, Syosset	18	163	93	–	–[3]	–	–	***No data collected***				100	–[6]
Northern Westchester, Mt Kisco	30	142	95	100*	–	83*	100	10.1	12.5	1.1	9.2	93	No
NYU Downtown, New York	37	256	83	78*	56*	71*	73	9.5	11.6	1.7	11.5	91	Yes
✓ NYU Hospital Center, New York	87	388	98	99	97	98	98	7.3	8.8	1.5	***10.3***	92	Yes
Our Lady of Mercy, Bronx[1]	***5***	163	–	–	–	–	60*	9.5	11.6	2.0	10.4	***88***	Yes
Our Lady of Mercy - D'Urso Pavilion, Bronx	***2***	121	–	–	–[3]	–[4]	–[4]	***No data collected***				–[6]	–[6]
Parkway, Forest Hills	***3***	152	***6***	***0***	–[3]	–[4]	–[4]	11.3	13.8	2.3	***12.3***	***84***	No
Peninsula, Far Rockaway	***3***	147	***17****	***0****	***0****	–[4]	–[4]	***14.0***	***16.9***	2.7	9.7	91	No
Phelps, North Tarrytown	17	134	71	50*	20*	–	71	11.6	14.4	0.9	10.7	96	No
Queens, Jamaica	***5***	144	***25***	20	9	15	***19***	10.7	13.3	–	–	94	Yes
St Agnes, White Plains[1]	***6***	125	40*	–	20*	–	67*	9.6	11.5	–	8.2	91	Yes
St Barnabas, Bronx	***10***	165	–	***0****	***0****	***0****	***0****	9.2	11.1	–	10.5	92	No
St Catherine of Siena, Smithtown	***12***	82	88*	–	–	–	89*	10.0	11.8	–	–	–[6]	No
St Charles, Port Jefferson[1]	22	94	89*	–	–	–	88	***15.7***	***19.4***	2.2	***11.9***	92	No
St Clare's, New York	***3***	180	***9***	***7***	–[3]	–[4]	–[4]	8.6	10.2	–	–	***87***	No
✓ St Francis, Roslyn	78	244	100	88	–	–[4]	–[4]	8.3	11.1	0.9	8.3	97	No
St John's Episcopal - South Shore, Far Rockaway	***3***	115	–	–	–	–	–	***No data collected***				93	–[6]
St John's Queens (St Vincent Catholic), Flushing	***4***	118	–	–	–	17*	50*	***No data collected***				–[6]	–[6]
St John's Riverside, Yonkers	***10***	112	–	–	–	–	88*	9.0	11.0	1.5	8.2	93	No
St Joseph's, Flushing[1]	***2***	107	–	20*	–[3]	–	–	***No data collected***				–[6]	–[6]
St Joseph's, Yonkers	***12***	102	63*	29*	–	–[4]	–[4]	12.3	14.9	2.8	8.4	91	No

Footnotes are on page 73. *Hospital's score based on relatively little data. See page 16.

Key Ratings for Metro Areas

See more information on "Detailed Ratings for All Areas" table beginning on page 74

✓ means hospital receives our top rating
Blue is most favorable
Bold Italic is least favorable
"–" means insufficient data

	Doctors' ratings of hospitals for high-risk adult surgery		Desirability scores from doctors (0 to 100, higher is better)					Measures of outcomes for selected cases (lower % is better)					
	Percent rating "very good" or "excellent"	Number of ratings	Low-risk adult surgery	Complex medical care for adults	High-risk child surgery	High-risk delivery of a baby	Uncomplicated delivery of a baby	Adjusted death rate for all case types (%)	Adjusted death rate for medical cases (%)	Adjusted death rate for surgical cases (%)	Adjusted adverse outcome rate for surgical cases (%)	Overall score on accreditation review (higher is better)	Major affiliation with a medical school?
National Average	32	–	59	50	40	46	58	12.1	14.8	2.3	7.7	91	–
New York *(continued)*													
New York City, Long Island, and Westchester County *(continued)*													
St Luke's - Roosevelt - Roosevelt Division, New York	38	287	**91**	67*	67*	82	80	*No data collected*				–[6]	–[6]
St Luke's - Roosevelt - St Luke's Division, New York	33	275	–	–	–	–	40*	**9.7**	**11.8**	1.7	***10.1***	***87***	**Yes**
St Mary's (St Vincent Catholic), Brooklyn	***4***	122	–	–	–	–	–	*No data collected*				–[6]	–[6]
St Vincent Catholic, Jamaica[1]	***7***	137	–	–	***0****	***0****	33*	***13.1***	***15.9***	***3.5***	9.5	89	**Yes**
St Vincent Catholic of New York, Staten Island	21	135	**92**	86*	**89***	**94**	**90**	*No data collected*				93	–[6]
St Vincents, New York	39	293	**100**	83	**100***	86*	**100**	11.2	13.9	**1.4**	***13.3***	90	**Yes**
St Vincents of New York - Bayley Seton, Staten Island	***12***	124	–	–	–[3]	–[4]	–[4]	**10.0**	**12.1**	–	9.8	–[6]	**Yes**
Sound Shore of Westchester, New Rochelle	15	131	78*	57*	50*	57*	80	11.9	14.6	2.1	6.6	**95**	**Yes**
South Nassau, Oceanside	18	147	63*	60*	14*	40	62	12.5	15.2	2.3	***11.5***	**94**	No
Southampton Hospital, Southampton	***6***	102	63*	–	–	–	**100***	11.8	14.6	1.2	8.9	90	No
Southside, Bay Shore	***14***	100	50*	33*	–	***0****	67	***13.2***	***15.9***	3.3	10.8	**96**	No
Staten Island University - North, Staten Island	27	153	79	75	50*	67*	79	***13.8***	***16.8***	2.5	***10.4***	–[6]	**Yes**
Staten Island University - South, Staten Island	18	145	–	–	–[3]	–[4]	–[4]	***13.8***	***16.8***	2.5	***10.4***	–[6]	**Yes**
SUNY Downstate, Brooklyn	41	209	60*	50*	**88***	57*	–	10.8	12.8	3.2	11.5	**96**	**Yes**
Union, Bronx	***2***	111	***0****	***0****	***0****	***0****	***0***	*No data collected*				–[6]	–[6]
✓ University, Stony Brook	**58**	144	67	82	**84**	**93**	**88**	**10.9**	**13.2**	2.3	9.1	89	**Yes**
Victory, Brooklyn	***3***	155	***21***	***6***	***0***	***0***	***21***	***14.0***	***17.0***	2.8	10.2	–[6]	No
Westchester, Valhalla[1]	**67**	238	63	**90**	**91**	**92**	71	12.0	15.5	1.7	9.2	**94**	**Yes**
White Plains Hospital, White Plains	37	164	**97**	**91**	71*	**91**	**94**	**10.7**	**13.2**	**1.2**	10.1	91	No
✓ Winthrop - University, Mineola	**64**	247	**97**	**96**	**92**	**98**	**100**	**10.4**	**13.2**	**1.0**	8.9	**97**	**Yes**
Woodhull, Brooklyn	***2***	183	***0***	***0***	***0***	***0***	***0***	**8.9**	**10.8**	–	–	**94**	No
Wyckoff Heights, Brooklyn	***3***	157	***0****	***0***	***0****	***0***	***0***	**9.3**	**11.4**	1.7	7.7	**96**	No
Rochester Area													
✓ Genesee, Rochester	**54**	37	62	41	20	36	67	**10.8**	**13.1**	2.5	9.0	–[6]	**Yes**
Highland, Rochester	41	111	76	44	–[3]	54	**88**	***14.3***	***17.5***	2.2	8.6	–[6]	**Yes**
Lakeside, Brockport	***3***	88	***9***	***2***	1	***0***	***6***	12.5	14.9	4.0	10.5	90	No
Park Ridge, Rochester	30	102	55	23	–[3]	3	42	11.4	14.0	1.4	9.8	***84***	No
✓ Rochester General, Rochester	**83**	118	87	**97**	**94**	**91**	73	**11.0**	**13.3**	2.4	***11.2***	**95**	No
✓ Strong, Rochester	**83**	122	72	**97**	**99**	**98**	71	11.6	14.4	1.9	***9.9***	92	**Yes**
North Carolina													
Charlotte Area													
✓ Carolinas, Charlotte[1]	**84**	82	79	**96**	**98**	**97**	68	11.7	13.9	***3.0***	***9.7***	**95**	**Yes**
Mercy, Charlotte	24	63	***28***	***10***	4	3	***12***	**10.1**	**12.1**	2.7	8.1	**94**	No
Mercy South, Charlotte	16	62	54	***7***	***0***	17	77	*No data collected*				–[6]	–[6]

Footnotes are on page 73. *Hospital's score based on relatively little data. See page 16.

Key Ratings for Metro Areas

See more information on "Detailed Ratings for All Areas" table beginning on page 74

✓ means hospital receives our top rating
Blue is most favorable
Bold Italic is least favorable
"–" means insufficient data

Hospital	Doctors' ratings of hospitals for high-risk adult surgery		Desirability scores from doctors (0 to 100, higher is better)					Measures of outcomes for selected cases (lower % is better)					
	Percent rating "very good" or "excellent"	Number of ratings	Low-risk adult surgery	Complex medical care for adults	High-risk child surgery	High-risk delivery of a baby	Uncomplicated delivery of a baby	Adjusted death rate for all case types (%)	Adjusted death rate for medical cases (%)	Adjusted death rate for surgical cases (%)	Adjusted adverse outcome rate for surgical cases (%)	Overall score on accreditation review (higher is better)	Major affiliation with a medical school?
National Average	32	–	59	50	40	46	58	12.1	14.8	2.3	7.7	91	–
North Carolina *(continued)*													
Charlotte Area *(continued)*													
✓ Presbyterian, Charlotte	**81**	80	84	**94**	**97**	**90**	85	11.8	14.4	2.3	8.7	**97**	No
Presbyterian, Matthews	32	62	58	22	7	6	73	10.7	13.2	1.8	6.3	–[6]	No
Presbyterian - Orthopaedic, Charlotte	–	–	***No data collected***					8.3	–	1.6	**5.3**	–[6]	No
University, Charlotte	26	62	54	19	9	19	43	12.1	14.6	2.8	10.1	**95**	No
Forsyth and Guilford Counties													
Forsyth, Winston-Salem	**55**	69	69	63	–[3]	**96**	**93**	***12.8***	***15.6***	2.5	***10.0***	**95**	**Yes**
High Point Regional, High Point[1]	38	50	44	31	16	13	46	11.6	14.0	2.7	8.4	**97**	No
Medical Park, Winston-Salem	25	52	58	***7***	–[3]	–[4]	–[4]	**2.5**	–	**0.5**	**5.3**	**97**	No
Moses H Cone, Greensboro[1]	**74**	58	86	**92**	**83**	**97**[5]	**97**[5]	12.0	14.8	1.9	9.0	91	No
✓ North Carolina Baptist, Winston-Salem	**95**	74	**92**	**94**	**97**	70	55	**11.2**	**13.4**	2.8	***11.0***	***87***	**Yes**
Wesley Long, Greensboro	33	27	60	56*	–	14*	***11****	12.9	***16.3***	1.6	**5.7**	–[6]	No
Triangle Area													
Duke University, Durham	**93**	101	74	**96**	**98**	**98**	51	12.0	14.9	1.9	8.4	**95**	**Yes**
Durham Regional, Durham	26	84	61	27	6	8	71	***15.1***	***18.5***	2.5	9.7	***87***	No
Raleigh Community, Raleigh	20	84	44	20	–[3]	***0***	42	**10.4**	**12.4**	2.6	8.8	90	No
✓ Rex, Raleigh[1]	**51**	88	87	67	27	44	**91**	**10.2**	**12.5**	**1.6**	8.6	92	No
✓ University of North Carolina, Chapel Hill	**85**	104	70	**92**	**95**	**92**	55	**10.4**	**12.8**	1.7	9.7	**95**	**Yes**
✓ Wakemed, Raleigh	**65**	85	78	73	**84**	**90**	76	**10.5**	**12.8**	**1.7**	8.3	**98**	**Yes**
Western Wake, Cary	16	77	32	***7***	–[3]	–[4]	–[4]	**10.2**	**12.2**	–	10.5	**99**	No
Ohio													
Cincinnati Area													
Bethesda North, Cincinnati[1]	**53**	76	**92**	75	–[3]	57	87	***14.1***	***17.1***	***3.1***	9.0	**97**	No
Children's, Cincinnati	–[2]	–[2]	–[2]	–[2]	**100**	–[4]	–[4]	***No data collected***				92	–[6]
✓ Christ, Cincinnati	**72**	83	**90**	**90**	–[3]	73	**89**	**10.6**	**12.6**	2.5	7.9	92	No
Deaconess, Cincinnati	18	67	46	29	–[3]	–[4]	–[4]	11.9	14.6	2.2	**6.2**	90	No
Good Samaritan, Cincinnati	**80**	80	**95**	**98**	**88**	**99**	**99**	12.1	14.7	2.2	7.9	93	**Yes**
Jewish, Cincinnati	33	73	62	54	–[3]	6	29	11.3	**13.6**	2.5	8.1	89	No
Mercy - Anderson, Cincinnati	***13***	60	63	***11****	–[3]	***0***	46	12.3	14.9	2.6	9.1	**95**	**Yes**
Mercy Franciscan - Mt Airy, Cincinnati[1]	***12***	57	***25***	***4***	–[3]	***0***	***14***	11.9	14.5	1.8	7.4	**99**	No
Mercy Franciscan - Western Hills, Cincinnati[1]	***11***	55	***23***	***10***	–[3]	–[4]	–[4]	11.5	14.0	2.3	8.0	**99**	No
✓ University, Cincinnati	**77**	79	50	87	–[3]	87	***24***	**10.2**	**12.2**	3.1	9.5	92	**Yes**
Cleveland Area													
✓ Cleveland Clinic Foundation, Cleveland	**85**	183	**92**	**95**	**93**	77	68	**9.3**	**12.0**	**1.2**	8.7	–[6]	No

Footnotes are on page 73. *Hospital's score based on relatively little data. See page 16.

Key Ratings for Metro Areas

See more information on "Detailed Ratings for All Areas" table beginning on page 74

✓ means hospital receives our top rating
Blue is most favorable
Bold Italic is least favorable
"–" means insufficient data

	Doctors' ratings of hospitals for high-risk adult surgery		Desirability scores from doctors (0 to 100, higher is better)					Measures of outcomes for selected cases (lower % is better)					
	Percent rating "very good" or "excellent"	Number of ratings	Low-risk adult surgery	Complex medical care for adults	High-risk child surgery	High-risk delivery of a baby	Uncomplicated delivery of a baby	Adjusted death rate for all case types (%)	Adjusted death rate for medical cases (%)	Adjusted death rate for surgical cases (%)	Adjusted adverse outcome rate for surgical cases (%)	Overall score on accreditation review (higher is better)	Major affiliation with a medical school?
National Average	32	–	59	50	40	46	58	12.1	14.8	2.3	7.7	91	–
Ohio *(continued)*													
Cleveland Area *(continued)*													
Deaconess, Cleveland	***4***	102	***15***	***8***	***0***	***0***	***0***	12.0	14.6	2.1	**4.8**	90	No
Euclid Hospital, Euclid	***10***	108	86*	29*	–	***0****	62	11.6	14.2	2.1	6.9	**96**	No
Fairview, Cleveland	38	128	86	67*	80*	**94**	**98**	**10.8**	**13.1**	1.9	**6.9**	89	No
Grace, Cleveland	***1***	93	***0***	***3***	***0***	–[4]	–[4]	***No data collected***				92	–[6]
✓ Hillcrest, Mayfield Heights	**53**	127	**95**	83	–[3]	**91**	**95**	**9.2**	**11.3**	**1.6**	8.2	91	No
Huron - Cleveland Clinic, Cleveland	***11***	100	***27***	20	–[3]	–[4]	–[4]	**8.9**	**10.7**	–	8.4	**94**	No
Lakewood Hospital, Lakewood[1]	17	103	86	–	–	20*	75	**10.4**	**12.5**	2.5	10.0	***87***	No
Lutheran, Cleveland	***12***	103	33	–	–[3]	–[4]	–[4]	12.1	14.9	1.6	8.8	***81***	No
Marymount, Garfield Heights	***8***	103	40	17*	–[3]	13*	64	**9.8**	**11.8**	3.0	9.2	**94**	No
✓ Metrohealth, Cleveland	**84**	162	**98**	**97**	**94**	**100**	**93**	11.6	14.1	2.4	9.2	90	**Yes**
Parma Community General, Parma	24	110	55	24	8	8	33	12.7	15.4	2.5	10.0	91	No
St John West Shore, Cleveland	***11***	99	38	33	–[3]	13	50	***13.2***	***16.0***	2.8	7.5	**95**	**Yes**
St Vincent Charity, Cleveland[1]	26	108	67	60*	–	–[4]	–[4]	**9.5**	**11.1**	2.5	8.6	91	No
South Pointe - Cleveland Clinic, Warrensville Heights[1]	***7***	103	53	18	–[3]	–[4]	–[4]	**10.2**	**12.4**	2.2	7.4	***85***	**Yes**
Southwest General, Middleburg Heights	32	111	**92**	78*	–	–	**95**	**10.7**	**13.1**	2.1	7.4	92	No
UHHS, Richmond Heights	***4***	93	***8***	***0***	–[3]	–[4]	–[4]	**10.4**	**12.8**	1.6	7.3	–[6]	**Yes**
University, Bedford[1]	***8***	90	***13***	***0***	***0***	***0***	***17***	13.0	15.7	2.7	6.6	93	No
✓ University, Cleveland	**83**	178	**96**	**97**	**99**	**99**	**93**	**9.5**	**11.6**	**1.6**	8.7	89	**Yes**
University St Michael, Cleveland	***2***	88	***0***	***0***	***0***	–[4]	–[4]	**8.7**	**10.5**	2.5	5.5	***87***	No
Columbus Area													
✓ Arthur G James Cancer/Richard J Solove, Columbus	**79**	70	75*	80	–[3]	33*	***13****	11.6	15.1	1.3	7.0	***87***	**Yes**
Children's, Columbus	–[2]	–[2]	–[2]	–[2]	**99**	–[4]	–[4]	***No data collected***				93	–[6]
Columbus Community, Columbus	***0***	53	***0***	***0***	–[3]	–[4]	–[4]	**9.6**	**11.6**	–	7.7	**94**	No
Doctors - Ohio Health, Columbus	***8***	60	***0***	***0***	10	***0***	***0***	**10.4**	**12.7**	2.1	9.3	**99**	No
Doctors West, Columbus	***13***	63	***19***	17	***0***	5	***16***	***No data collected***				–[6]	–[6]
Grant, Columbus	**53**	70	87	**92**	–[3]	58	67	***13.1***	15.7	***3.0***	8.9	–[6]	No
Mount Carmel East, Columbus	40	68	70	50	20*	9	61	***No data collected***				–[6]	–[6]
Mount Carmel St Ann's, Westerville	25	69	82	38*	–[3]	61	**92**	***15.1***	***18.2***	3.4	8.7	**96**	No
Mount Carmel West, Columbus[1]	**51**	69	74	74	–[3]	54	56	***14.4***	***17.6***	2.4	8.3	–[6]	No
Ohio State University East Hospital, Columbus	18	67	***12***	14	–[3]	–[4]	–[4]	**10.3**	**12.2**	***3.9***	***14.1***	93	No
✓ Ohio State University Medical Center, Columbus[1]	**78**	72	**90**	**95**	–[3]	**94**	76	**9.8**	**11.7**	2.3	9.4	***83***	**Yes**
Riverside Methodist, Columbus	**74**	70	**93**	**93**	–[3]	**92**	**91**	12.6	***15.7***	**1.8**	9.1	91	**Yes**

Footnotes are on page 73. *Hospital's score based on relatively little data. See page 16.

Key Ratings for Metro Areas

See more information on "Detailed Ratings for All Areas" table beginning on page 74

✓ means hospital receives our top rating
Blue is most favorable
Bold Italic is least favorable
"–" means insufficient data

	Doctors' ratings of hospitals for high-risk adult surgery		Desirability scores from doctors (0 to 100, higher is better)					Measures of outcomes for selected cases (lower % is better)					
	Percent rating "very good" or "excellent"	Number of ratings	Low-risk adult surgery	Complex medical care for adults	High-risk child surgery	High-risk delivery of a baby	Uncomplicated delivery of a baby	Adjusted death rate for all case types (%)	Adjusted death rate for medical cases (%)	Adjusted death rate for surgical cases (%)	Adjusted adverse outcome rate for surgical cases (%)	Overall score on accreditation review (higher is better)	Major affiliation with a medical school?
National Average	32	–	59	50	40	46	58	12.1	14.8	2.3	7.7	91	–
Oregon													
Portland Area													
Adventist, Portland	29	108	67	39	13*	***0****	50	***14.2***	***17.4***	2.8	8.2	95	No
Eastmoreland, Portland	***4***	95	***5***	***0***	–[3]	–[4]	–[4]	14.0	16.9	–	1.8	–[6]	Yes
Kaiser Sunnyside, Clackamas	41	108	56	50	19	21	53	***15.7***	***18.9***	3.5	8.3	89	No
Legacy Emanuel, Portland[1]	84	147	93	98	100	100	91	13.5	15.9	***3.9***	7.9	–[6]	Yes
Legacy Good Samaritan, Portland	73	135	98	98	–[3]	89*	97	12.3	15.5	1.7	6.3	–[6]	Yes
Legacy Meridian Park, Tualatin	42	116	90	44*	–[3]	33*	92	***14.9***	***18.5***	2.1	6.1	93	No
Legacy Mount Hood, Gresham	21	100	–	–	***0****	***0****	***17****	***15.5***	***18.7***	3.7	8.1	95	No
OHSU, Portland[1]	75	151	75	96	100[5]	96	55	12.1	14.8	2.3	7.9	89	Yes
Providence, Milwaukie	***14***	104	***11***	***7***	***0***	***0***	***20***	***19.3***	***24.2***	1.5	3.9	90	No
Providence, Portland	80	140	97	94	29	69	92	***13.5***	***16.7***	2.2	5.8	93	No
Providence St Vincent, Portland	81	156	93	94	53	85	88	***13.9***	***17.5***	2.0	7.3	***83***	Yes
Tuality, Forest Grove	***0***	78	***6***	***0***	***0***	–[4]	–[4]	***No data collected***				–[6]	–[6]
Tuality, Hillsboro	***11***	97	***21***	***6***	***0***	5	***12***	***16.2***	***19.8***	2.9	6.7	93	No
Willamette Falls, Oregon City	***11***	95	***28***	***8***	***0***	4	31	***16.1***	***19.7***	2.3	7.0	***86***	No
Woodland Park, Portland	***5***	86	***3***	***0***	–[3]	***0***	***3***	***15.5***	***18.7***	–	–	***83***	No
Pennsylvania													
Delaware Valley Area													
✓ Abington Memorial, Abington	67	208	97	93	–	88	91	11.4	13.8	2.6	9.8	93	No
Albert Einstein, Philadelphia	49	199	85	83*	–	56*	67	11.6	13.9	***3.3***	***11.3***	90	Yes
Brandywine, Coatesville[1]	15	98	–	–	–	***0****	***0****	12.1	14.7	2.3	10.0	95	No
✓ Bryn Mawr Hospital, Bryn Mawr[1]	58	198	100	92	71*	86	98	10.0	12.0	2.2	8.2	96	No
Chester County, West Chester	21	112	88*	–	–	57*	89*	11.3	13.5	3.4	8.9	92	No
Chestnut Hill, Philadelphia	19	167	82	–	–	–	80	12.5	15.5	0.7	5.6	97	No
Children's, Philadelphia	–[2]	–[2]	–[2]	–[2]	100	–[4]	–[4]	***No data collected***				–[6]	–[6]
Crozer - Chester, Upland	47	169	85	63*	***0****	80*	77	12.0	14.7	2.0	6.8	90	Yes
Delaware County, Drexel Hill	***11***	123	–	50*	–	–	–	11.5	14.0	2.2	9.9	93	No
Doylestown Hospital, Doylestown	26	121	90	86*	–	–	92	11.3	13.9	1.9	7.4	94	No
Elkins Park Hospital, Elkins Park	***4***	139	***22****	17*	–[3]	***0****	***7***	8.4	10.6	–	–	97	No
Episcopal, Philadelphia	***4***	142	***7***	***6***	–[3]	6	***5***	9.7	11.2	4.1	11.2	–[6]	Yes
Fox Chase Cancer Center, Philadelphia	73	194	–	–	–[3]	–[4]	–[4]	***17.4***	***22.2***	–	8.2	94	No
Frankford - Bucks County Campus, Langhorne	***14***	118	–	***0****	–	–	–	***No data collected***				–[6]	–[6]
Frankford - Frankford Campus, Philadelphia	18	147	–	–	–	–	–	***No data collected***				–[6]	–[6]
Frankford - Torresdale, Philadelphia	27	153	80	67*	–	29*	58	12.5	15.3	2.3	7.9	***85***	Yes
Germantown, Philadelphia	***4***	119	***0****	–	–[3]	–	–	***No data collected***				92	–[6]

Footnotes are on page 73. *Hospital's score based on relatively little data. See page 16.

Key Ratings for Metro Areas

See more information on "Detailed Ratings for All Areas" table beginning on page 74

✓ means hospital receives our top rating
Blue is most favorable
Bold Italic is least favorable
"–" means insufficient data

	Doctors' ratings of hospitals for high-risk adult surgery		Desirability scores from doctors (0 to 100, higher is better)					Measures of outcomes for selected cases (lower % is better)					
	Percent rating "very good" or "excellent"	Number of ratings	Low-risk adult surgery	Complex medical care for adults	High-risk child surgery	High-risk delivery of a baby	Uncomplicated delivery of a baby	Adjusted death rate for all case types (%)	Adjusted death rate for medical cases (%)	Adjusted death rate for surgical cases (%)	Adjusted adverse outcome rate for surgical cases (%)	Overall score on accreditation review (higher is better)	Major affiliation with a medical school?
National Average	32	–	59	50	40	46	58	12.1	14.8	2.3	7.7	91	–
Pennsylvania *(continued)*													
Delaware Valley Area *(continued)*													
Graduate, Philadelphia	34	188	67*	71*	–[3]	–[4]	–[4]	7.2	8.8	–	5.5	93	No
Grand View, Sellersville	***14***	111	–	40*	–	–	–	12.2	15.0	1.8	6.6	–[6]	No
✓ Hahnemann University, Philadelphia	52	214	69	79	–[3]	63	54	9.1	10.4	3.5	10.8	92	Yes
Holy Redeemer, Meadowbrook[1]	24	147	83	60*	20*	50*	86	11.2	13.6	2.1	***10.8***	***88***	No
Jeanes, Philadelphia	21	152	58	***9***	***0****	–	36	10.9	13.3	2.0	8.5	94	No
✓ Lankenau, Wynnewood	70	216	100	100	–	92	97	8.6	10.5	1.6	9.5	–[6]	Yes
Medical College of Pennsylvania, Philadelphia	49	200	64	67	–[3]	–[4]	–[4]	8.8	10.9	–	–	90	Yes
Mercy, Havertown	***7***	111	***14****	***0****	–	–[4]	–[4]	***14.8***	***18.0***	–	6.0	94	No
Mercy, Philadelphia	***5***	119	–	–	–	–	–	*No data collected*				–[6]	–[6]
Mercy Fitzgerald, Darby[1]	***11***	130	–	–	–	–	50*	11.9	14.4	2.2	10.2	89	Yes
Mercy Suburban, Norristown	***3***	111	–	***0****	–	***0****	***17****	***16.0***	***19.2***	4.0	10.4	***87***	Yes
Methodist, Philadelphia	***6***	128	40*	***0****	–	20*	60*	–	–	–	–	–[6]	Yes
Montgomery, Norristown	***7***	122	–	–	–	–	–	***13.9***	***16.8***	3.1	***10.9***	91	No
Nazareth, Philadelphia	***5***	129	57*	–	–	–	33*	10.9	13.4	1.9	7.5	89	No
North Penn, Lansdale	***7***	121	83*	50*	–	–	63*	***13.9***	***16.7***	3.2	10.2	–[6]	No
Northeastern, Philadelphia	***5***	117	***0****	–	–	–	***0****	*No data collected*				–[6]	–[6]
Paoli Memorial, Paoli	30	133	93	–	–	–	91	12.8	15.6	2.3	7.7	–[6]	No
✓ Pennsylvania, Philadelphia	71	232	98	97	–	99	97	8.4	10.1	1.5	***10.4***	98	Yes
Phoenixville Hospital, Phoenixville[1]	18	111	–	–	–	–	–	13.0	15.9	1.8	6.5	***85***	No
Pottstown Memorial, Pottstown	***1***	104	–	–	–	–	–	***16.0***	***19.2***	3.8	***12.0***	–[6]	No
✓ Presbyterian, Philadelphia	52	170	100*	100*	–[3]	–[4]	–[4]	9.3	11.3	1.8	7.9	92	No
Riddle, Media	***13***	126	60	–	–	–	91	***12.9***	***15.8***	2.0	7.7	–[6]	No
Roxborough, Philadelphia	***2***	126	***11****	***0****	–	***0****	–	10.6	12.7	4.1	8.0	91	No
St Agnes, Philadelphia	17	127	***0****	***0****	–[3]	–[4]	–[4]	9.5	11.5	3.9	8.1	***87***	No
St Christophers for Children, Philadelphia	76	174	–	–	96	–[4]	–[4]	*No data collected*				97	–[6]
St Joseph's, Philadelphia[1]	***4***	109	***15***	***7***	–[3]	–[4]	–[4]	9.2	11.1	–	–	94	Yes
St Lukes, Quakertown	***8***	83	–	–	–	–[4]	–[4]	13.2	16.2	–	5.5	***86***	No
St Mary, Langhorne	***14***	127	88*	–	–	–	71*	***14.1***	***17.3***	2.4	6.6	92	No
Southern Chester County, West Grove	***2***	83	–	–	–	–	***0****	11.6	14.2	2.0	6.4	91	No
Springfield Hospital, Springfield	***3***	105	40*	–	–[3]	–[4]	–[4]	*No data collected*				–[6]	–[6]
Taylor, Ridley Park	***7***	111	–	–	–[3]	–[4]	–[4]	*No data collected*				–[6]	–[6]
Temple - Lower Bucks, Bristol	***8***	119	–	***0****	–	40*	50*	12.8	15.6	2.5	9.5	92	Yes
✓ Temple University, Philadelphia	72	234	67	94	29	84	44	9.8	11.7	2.9	8.9	91	Yes
✓ Thomas Jefferson University, Philadelphia	92	255	95	98	88	95	94	9.4	11.5	1.6	***12.0***	***81***	Yes

Footnotes are on page 73. *Hospital's score based on relatively little data. See page 16.

Key Ratings for Metro Areas

See more information on "Detailed Ratings for All Areas" table beginning on page 74

✓ means hospital receives our top rating
Blue is most favorable
Bold Italic is least favorable
"–" means insufficient data

	Doctors' ratings of hospitals for high-risk adult surgery		Desirability scores from doctors (0 to 100, higher is better)					Measures of outcomes for selected cases (lower % is better)					
	Percent rating "very good" or "excellent"	Number of ratings	Low-risk adult surgery	Complex medical care for adults	High-risk child surgery	High-risk delivery of a baby	Uncomplicated delivery of a baby	Adjusted death rate for all case types (%)	Adjusted death rate for medical cases (%)	Adjusted death rate for surgical cases (%)	Adjusted adverse outcome rate for surgical cases (%)	Overall score on accreditation review (higher is better)	Major affiliation with a medical school?
National Average	32	–	59	50	40	46	58	12.1	14.8	2.3	7.7	91	–
Pennsylvania *(continued)*													
Delaware Valley Area *(continued)*													
✓ University of Pennsylvania, Philadelphia	**90**	251	**91**	**99**	–[3]	**94**	80	**10.1**	**12.1**	2.3	9.1	**95**	**Yes**
Warminster Hospital, Warminster	***4***	117	***17****	***0****	–[3]	***0****	***0****	10.9	13.5	–	–	**96**	No
Wills Eye, Philadelphia	–	–		*No data collected*				7.9	9.8	–	**3.8**	93	**Yes**
Pittsburgh Area													
Alle-Kiski, Natrona Heights	***10***	49	–	***0****	–	***0****	–	***12.9***	***15.8***	2.2	**6.7**	**96**	No
✓ Allegheny General, Pittsburgh	**73**	74	82	**97**	81	68	69	**10.0**	**12.0**	2.1	8.2	**97**	**Yes**
Children's, Pittsburgh	**78**	46	–	–	**100**	–[4]	–[4]		*No data collected*			92	–[6]
Forbes Regional, Monroeville	21	53	**100***	–	–	–	83*	12.4	15.2	1.7	8.4	**97**	No
Jefferson, Pittsburgh[1]	18	44	–	–	–	–[4]	–[4]	12.4	15.1	2.5	7.7	***86***	No
✓ Magee - Womens, Pittsburgh[1]	**77**	66	–	–	–	**98**	**94**	10.2	–	–	**4.1**	***84***	**Yes**
✓ Mercy, Pittsburgh	**57**	65	**90**	**100**	62	75*	69	**11.0**	**13.2**	2.4	9.2	92	No
Mercy Providence, Pittsburgh	***6***	47	–	–	–[3]	–[4]	–[4]	10.7	12.9	2.7	5.8	89	No
Pittsburgh's Ohio Valley General, McKees Rocks	***2***	52	***0****	***0****	–[3]	***0****	***0****	12.9	15.7	2.3	**4.4**	**97**	No
St Clair, Pittsburgh	21	58	50*	–	–	***0***	36	***14.8***	***18.2***	2.3	8.7	–[6]	No
St Francis Central Hospital, Pittsburgh	***6***	32	–	–	–	–[4]	–[4]	11.8	14.3	2.3	8.2	–[6]	**Yes**
St Francis Medical Center, Pittsburgh	19	58	33*	29*	–	–	–	**9.9**	**12.0**	1.8	7.7	***84***	**Yes**
Sewickley Valley, Sewickley	16	45	–	–	–	–	60*	12.7	15.4	2.6	***11.0***	**95**	No
Suburban General, Pittsburgh	***10***	48	***0****	***0****	–	–[4]	–[4]	11.4	13.8	2.4	7.6	91	No
UPMC Braddock, Braddock	***5***	59	***11***	***0****	***0****	–[4]	–[4]	11.8	14.6	1.3	9.1	92	No
UPMC McKeesport, McKeesport	***5***	56	***23***	***11****	***0****	***0****	***14****	**9.9**	**12.2**	1.7	8.5	92	No
UPMC Passavant, Pittsburgh	35	60	88*	–	–	***0****	86*	12.6	15.2	2.7	***11.7***	**97**	No
✓ UPMC Presbyterian, Pittsburgh	**90**	79	**89**	**94**	–	–[4]	–[4]	**10.5**	**12.9**	1.9	9.0	–[6]	**Yes**
UPMC St Margaret, Pittsburgh	**57**	60	**100**	–	–	–	–	12.6	15.3	2.5	8.1	**96**	**Yes**
✓ UPMC Shadyside, Pittsburgh	**76**	71	**94**	**93**	–[3]	55	87	**10.7**	**13.1**	1.9	8.8	–[6]	No
UPMC South Side, Pittsburgh	15	55	33*	–	–[3]	–[4]	–[4]	11.5	13.6	***3.7***	***11.4***	**94**	No
Western Pennsylvania, Pittsburgh	**74**	66	**96**	**100**	–	**95**	**90**	11.2	13.7	2.0	***10.4***	***86***	No
Rhode Island													
Kent County, Warwick	20	95	66	58	35	66	80	**11.3**	13.7	2.0	**6.9**	91	No
Landmark, Woonsocket	***5***	85	***19***	***5***	***0***	4	***21***	***14.2***	***17.3***	2.8	7.9	93	No
Memorial of Rhode Island, Pawtucket	18	88	74	59	38*	33	69	**10.2**	**12.2**	3.1	9.3	**94**	**Yes**
✓ Miriam, Providence	**72**	109	**93**	**97**	–[3]	–[4]	–[4]	**10.3**	**12.5**	2.1	8.4	93	**Yes**
Newport Hospital, Newport	22	81	58	***9***	***0****	8	56	11.2	13.7	1.8	7.1	**96**	No
✓ Rhode Island, Providence	**78**	117	81	**94**	**100**[5]	–[4]	–[4]	**10.9**	**13.3**	1.8	9.3	92	**Yes**
Roger Williams, Providence	44	99	85	82	–[3]	***0****	***0****	***12.9***	***15.6***	2.9	8.2	92	**Yes**

Footnotes are on page 73. *Hospital's score based on relatively little data. See page 16.

Key Ratings for Metro Areas

See more information on "Detailed Ratings for All Areas" table beginning on page 74

✓ means hospital receives our top rating
Blue is most favorable
Bold Italic is least favorable
"–" means insufficient data

	Doctors' ratings of hospitals for high-risk adult surgery		Desirability scores from doctors (0 to 100, higher is better)					Measures of outcomes for selected cases (lower % is better)					
	Percent rating "very good" or "excellent"	Number of ratings	Low-risk adult surgery	Complex medical care for adults	High-risk child surgery	High-risk delivery of a baby	Uncomplicated delivery of a baby	Adjusted death rate for all case types (%)	Adjusted death rate for medical cases (%)	Adjusted death rate for surgical cases (%)	Adjusted adverse outcome rate for surgical cases (%)	Overall score on accreditation review (higher is better)	Major affiliation with a medical school?
National Average	32	–	59	50	40	46	58	12.1	14.8	2.3	7.7	91	–
Rhode Island *(continued)*													
St Joseph of Rhode Island, Providence	20	83	56	32	17	9	31	**9.6**	**11.6**	2.3	7.0	89	**Yes**
South County, Wakefield	23	80	56	31	7	11	74	11.3	13.9	1.4	6.7	**94**	No
Westerly Hospital, Westerly	***11***	70	***23***	14	***0***	8	42	11.5	14.2	1.6	6.7	93	No
Women and Infants of Rhode Island, Providence	**73**	89	–	80*	–[3]	**100**	**97**	16.5	–	–	10.6	**94**	**Yes**
Tennessee													
Nashville Area													
✓ Baptist, Nashville	**76**	79	**96**	**95**	**97**	**99**	**99**	**11.3**	13.9	1.9	8.7	**94**	No
✓ Centennial, Nashville	**75**	80	83	81	47	73	87	11.7	13.7	***3.2***	9.7	**95**	No
Metropolitan Nashville General, Nashville	***5***	66	***4***	***0***	2	2	***2***	***14.8***	***17.7***	–	–	**96**	**Yes**
✓ St Thomas, Nashville[1]	**92**	79	**98**	**98**	–[3]	9	***14***	**9.8**	**12.1**	**1.4**	8.7	**95**	No
Skyline, Nashville	15	61	***18***	***0***	***0***	***0***	***0***	12.1	14.7	2.5	9.5	***87***	No
Southern Hills, Nashville	***11***	64	***20***	***0***	***0***	***0***	***21***	***13.4***	***16.3***	2.6	9.4	**95**	No
Summit, Hermitage	21	61	71	43*	–	–	57	11.0	13.3	2.6	9.3	90	No
Tennessee Christian, Madison	***7***	60	***7***	***0***	***0***	***0***	***3***	11.3	13.7	–	11.5	***87***	No
✓ Vanderbilt University, Nashville[1]	**85**	78	78	**97**	**100**	**99**	76	**10.5**	**12.6**	2.5	8.7	89	**Yes**
Texas													
Austin Area													
Brackenridge, Austin	**78**	58	52	74	**99**[5]	72	36	**9.9**	**12.0**	2.4	**4.4**	***83***	No
Heart Hospital, Austin	**56**	45	33	39	–[3]	–[4]	–[4]	***No data collected***				***85***	–[6]
North Austin Medical Center, Austin	39	46	52	42	–[3]	13	41	11.4	13.9	2.1	7.4	93	No
✓ St David's, Austin	**79**	58	**96**	**96**	–[3]	**97**	**97**	11.4	13.6	3.0	9.1	92	No
Seton Medical Center, Austin	**81**	57	**92**	**96**	78	**94**	**90**	11.8	14.2	2.5	***10.4***	***88***	No
Seton Northwest, Austin	24	45	32	***5***	6	17	50	***No data collected***				–[6]	–[6]
South Austin Hospital, Austin	29	48	41	12	5	***0***	32	**10.6**	**12.7**	2.9	8.6	**94**	No
Dallas-Ft. Worth Area													
All Saints Episcopal, Fort Worth	42	93	**100**	**93**	–	**92**	**93**	***14.9***	***17.9***	***3.5***	9.0	93	No
Arlington Memorial, Arlington	37	92	83	77	–	64	80	***15.8***	***19.2***	3.3	9.9	**98**	No
Baylor, Garland	23	103	83*	–	–	–	83*	***14.4***	***17.6***	2.3	6.8	92	No
Baylor, Grapevine	32	78	55	–	–	–	80	***14.1***	***17.3***	2.5	5.5	**94**	No
Baylor, Irving	28	111	**100***	80*	–[3]	–	80*	12.4	14.9	3.3	***11.2***	91	No
Baylor - Richardson Medical Center, Richardson	**91**	174	**97**	**98**	**88**	**97**	**97**	13.0	15.7	3.6	6.9	90	No
Baylor All Saints of Cityview, Fort Worth	***8***	75	***29****	17*	–	17*	–	***No data collected***				–[6]	–[6]
Baylor University, Dallas	25	110	–	–	–	–	60*	**10.6**	**13.0**	**1.7**	8.5	89	No
Charlton Methodist, Dallas	16	105	56*	14*	–	–	60	11.3	13.8	2.0	7.3	***84***	No

Footnotes are on page 73. *Hospital's score based on relatively little data. See page 16.

Key Ratings for Metro Areas

See more information on "Detailed Ratings for All Areas" table beginning on page 74

✓ means hospital receives our top rating
Blue is most favorable
Bold Italic is least favorable
"–" means insufficient data

	Doctors' ratings of hospitals for high-risk adult surgery		Desirability scores from doctors (0 to 100, higher is better)					Measures of outcomes for selected cases (lower % is better)					
	Percent rating "very good" or "excellent"	Number of ratings	Low-risk adult surgery	Complex medical care for adults	High-risk child surgery	High-risk delivery of a baby	Uncomplicated delivery of a baby	Adjusted death rate for all case types (%)	Adjusted death rate for medical cases (%)	Adjusted death rate for surgical cases (%)	Adjusted adverse outcome rate for surgical cases (%)	Overall score on accreditation review (higher is better)	Major affiliation with a medical school?
National Average	32	–	59	50	40	46	58	12.1	14.8	2.3	7.7	91	–
Texas *(continued)*													
Dallas-Ft. Worth Area *(continued)*													
Children's, Dallas	–[2]	–[2]	–[2]	–[2]	**98**	–[4]	–[4]	***No data collected***				**96**	–[6]
Cook Children's, Fort Worth	–[2]	–[2]	–[2]	–[2]	**99**	–[4]	–[4]	***No data collected***				91	–[6]
Dallas - Fort Worth, Grand Prairie	***1***	73	***0****	***0***	***0****	***0***	***0***	***14.2***	***16.8***	***4.9***	9.9	–[6]	No
Dallas Southwest, Dallas	15	81	***22****	17*	***0****	17*	***0****	10.3	12.5	–	6.2	92	No
Doctors, Dallas	19	115	64	42	***0****	11*	47	11.9	14.6	1.6	9.7	**96**	No
✓ Harris Methodist Fort Worth, Fort Worth	**79**	110	**97**	**96**	78*	**96**	**93**	12.0	14.4	2.9	8.7	**97**	No
Harris Methodist H-E-B, Bedford	43	80	**100**	**100***	–	**100***	**100**	***14.3***	***16.5***	***5.7***	9.0	–[6]	No
Harris Methodist Northwest, Azle	***8***	61	–	–	–	–[4]	–[4]	10.2	12.6	–	–	**96**	No
Harris Methodist Southwest, Fort Worth	25	77	**100***	–	–	–	**100**	***13.8***	***16.8***	2.9	6.3	**96**	No
Huguley, Fort Worth[1]	***13***	77	43*	***0****	***0****	***0****	***17****	***14.1***	***16.9***	***4.0***	8.6	89	No
JPS, Fort Worth[1]	36	109	***20***	42	22*	38	***18***	***16.2***	***19.5***	–	11.4	***88***	No
Lake Pointe, Rowlett	***6***	83	***9***	***0****	***0****	***0***	***0***	11.9	14.3	***4.8***	6.3	**97**	No
Las Colinas, Irving	***4***	89	–	17*	–	40*	44*	6.3	8.0	–	–	**94**	No
Leland, Garland	***2***	84	***0****	***0***	–[3]	–[4]	–[4]	***16.2***	***19.9***	–	–	90	No
Medical Center, Arlington	20	71	60*	40*	–	29*	63*	**10.4**	**12.6**	2.7	**4.5**	**95**	No
Medical Center, Lancaster	***3***	73	***0****	***0***	–[3]	***0***	***0***	11.2	13.4	–	10.7	**97**	No
Medical Center, Mesquite	***2***	89	***0****	***7***	–[3]	***0***	***22****	12.4	14.9	3.4	5.9	91	No
✓ Medical City Dallas Hospital, Dallas	**66**	144	87	**88**	80[5]	84	84	**10.9**	**13.3**	2.2	8.5	**97**	No
Mesquite Community, Mesquite	***5***	97	***18***	***6***	–[3]	***0***	***11***	***14.4***	***17.3***	***4.7***	7.8	92	No
Methodist, Dallas	**55**	124	80	73	–	83	79	11.2	13.5	2.6	8.6	***82***	No
North Hills, North Richland Hills	***12***	67	30	***8***	***0****	9	***17***	12.5	14.8	***4.5***	8.1	**98**	No
Osteopathic of Texas, Fort Worth	18	82	***12***	***10***	***0***	***0***	***18***	***14.0***	***16.8***	3.3	8.6	93	**Yes**
✓ Parkland, Dallas[1]	**81**	177	57	**96**	–[3]	**99**	47	11.0	13.2	3.2	8.6	**94**	**Yes**
Plaza, Fort Worth	31	87	46	39	–[3]	***0****	***0****	12.5	15.0	2.9	8.1	**97**	No
Presbyterian, Dallas	**82**	171	**95**	**98**	78*	**99**	**99**	12.2	14.5	***2.9***	9.5	**96**	No
RHD, Dallas	***13***	110	***27***	***0***	–[3]	***0***	***18***	12.5	15.0	3.7	***13.9***	**96**	No
St Paul University, Dallas	**60**	144	88	82	–[3]	**94**	**92**	12.4	14.9	2.9	10.2	**94**	No
Texas Scottish Rite for Children, Dallas	–[2]	–[2]	–[2]	–[2]	**100**	–[4]	–[4]	***No data collected***				**97**	–[6]
✓ Zale Lipshy University, Dallas	**84**	155	**100**	**100**	–[3]	–[4]	–[4]	10.5	13.1	1.5	8.0	**98**	**Yes**
Houston Area													
Baycoast, Baytown	***2***	57	***0****	–	***0****	***0****	***0****	10.2	12.5	–	–	***82***	No
Bayou City (Belleaire Blvd), Houston	***0***	69	***0****	–	–[3]	***0****[5]	***0****[5]	11.3	13.5	–	–	–[6]	No
Bayou City (Portsmouth St), Houston	***1***	67	–	***0****	–	***0****	***0****	***No data collected***				***83***	–[6]
Bayshore, Pasadena	***11***	79	33*	***0****	***0****	***0***	***10***	12.0	14.3	***3.6***	8.8	92	No

Footnotes are on page 73. *Hospital's score based on relatively little data. See page 16.

Key Ratings for Metro Areas

See more information on "Detailed Ratings for All Areas" table beginning on page 74

✓ means hospital receives our top rating
Blue is most favorable
Bold Italic is least favorable
"–" means insufficient data

Hospital	Doctors' ratings of hospitals for high-risk adult surgery		Desirability scores from doctors (0 to 100, higher is better)					Measures of outcomes for selected cases (lower % is better)				Overall score on accreditation review (higher is better)	Major affiliation with a medical school?
	Percent rating "very good" or "excellent"	Number of ratings	Low-risk adult surgery	Complex medical care for adults	High-risk child surgery	High-risk delivery of a baby	Uncomplicated delivery of a baby	Adjusted death rate for all case types (%)	Adjusted death rate for medical cases (%)	Adjusted death rate for surgical cases (%)	Adjusted adverse outcome rate for surgical cases (%)		
National Average	32	–	59	50	40	46	58	12.1	14.8	2.3	7.7	91	–
Texas *(continued)*													
Houston Area *(continued)*													
Bellaire, Houston	***2***	91	***0***	***0***	–[3]	***0***	***7***	9.2	11.3	–	–	89	No
Ben Taub General, Houston[1]	68	157	***29****	71*	62	41	***8***	***13.8***	***16.7***	–	7.6	***86***	Yes
Christus St John, Nassau Bay	***10***	78	100*	–	–	–	83*	***14.2***	16.9	–	***13.9***	95	No
Christus St Joseph, Houston	47	116	100*	100*	–	100*	100	12.3	15.0	2.0	7.2	93	No
Clear Lake Regional, Webster	26	91	–	–	–	–	88*	12.8	15.4	3.1	7.2	97	No
Columbia Spring Branch, Houston	18	78	–	–	–	–	–	11.7	14.3	1.9	7.0	96	No
Cypress Fairbanks, Houston	***11***	75	–	–	–	–	100*	11.7	14.2	–	9.2	***87***	No
Doctors - Parkway, Houston	***3***	71	***0***	***0***	***0***	***0***	***0***	9.5	11.4	–	9.0	–[6]	No
Doctors - Tidwell, Houston	***3***	67	***0***	***4***	***0***	***0***	***0***	6.8	8.0	–	–	89	No
East Houston Regional, Houston	***11***	66	***10***	***9***	***0****	***0****	***25***	11.9	14.5	–	5.2	91	No
Houston Northwest, Houston	38	89	85	86*	–	–	100	12.1	14.7	2.6	8.8	94	No
Kingwood Medical Center, Kingwood	***5***	77	***20****	–	***0****	***0****	***17****	10.7	12.9	–	7.2	98	No
Lyndon B Johnson General, Houston[1]	33	120	***18***	14*	***0****	27	***13***	***No data collected***				***86***	–[6]
Memorial Hermann, Houston	84	182	96	98	97	95	90	***13.4***	15.6	***5.1***	9.7	98	Yes
Memorial Hermann Memorial City, Houston	47	109	100	75*	–	–	100	12.3	15.0	2.3	9.4	96	No
Memorial Hermann Northwest, Houston	25	85	–	–	–	–	–	***No data collected***				98	–[6]
Memorial Hermann Southeast, Houston	23	92	67*	–	–	–	–	***No data collected***				–[6]	–[6]
Memorial Hermann Southwest, Houston[1]	59	140	96	100	–	80*	92	***No data collected***				97	–[6]
✓ Methodist, Houston	91	205	98	98	–[3]	90	85	11.6	13.7	2.7	9.0	96	Yes
Methodist Diagnostic, Houston	36	100	90	91	–[3]	–[4]	–[4]	9.5	11.8	1.1	5.0	93	No
Northeast, Humble	***13***	68	60	–	–	–	83*	11.4	13.8	2.7	7.8	***88***	No
Northside General, Houston	***0***	48	***0****	–	–	–[4]	–[4]	6.8	8.4	–	–	–[6]	No
Park Plaza, Houston	29	124	93	75	–	20*	78*	10.9	13.1	2.6	7.7	92	No
Riverside General, Houston	***0***	55	***0****	***0***	***0****	***0***	***0***	–	–	–	–	***88***	No
✓ St Lukes Episcopal, Houston[1]	92	194	99	99	–[3]	99	98	10.8	12.1	***3.3***	***9.9***	96	Yes
San Jacinto Methodist, Baytown	***12***	69	–	–	–	–	–	***13.1***	***15.9***	2.6	5.4	89	Yes
Texas Children's, Houston	–[2]	–[2]	–[2]	–[2]	100	–[4]	–[4]	***No data collected***				96	–[6]
Texas Orthopedic, Houston	–	–	***No data collected***					–	–	–	***13.9***	96	No
Tomball Regional, Tomball	***14***	70	60*	33*	–	–	–	10.5	12.7	2.3	7.2	94	No
University of Texas M D Anderson Cancer Ctr, Houston	94	171	100*	100	100*	–[4]	–[4]	***14.7***	***18.4***	1.5	11.4	97	No
West Houston Medical Center, Houston	15	74	67*	67*	–	–	56*	12.0	14.3	***4.1***	10.9	97	No
Woman's of Texas, Houston	62	122	–	–	–[3]	98	100	–	–	–	6.7	99	No
San Antonio Area													
Baptist, San Antonio[1]	22	85	46	48	19	6	***24***	11.4	13.8	2.5	***11.0***	***79***	No

Footnotes are on page 73. *Hospital's score based on relatively little data. See page 16.

Key Ratings for Metro Areas

See more information on "Detailed Ratings for All Areas" table beginning on page 74

✓ means hospital receives our top rating
Blue is most favorable
Bold Italic is least favorable
"–" means insufficient data

	Doctors' ratings of hospitals for high-risk adult surgery		Desirability scores from doctors (0 to 100, higher is better)					Measures of outcomes for selected cases (lower % is better)					
	Percent rating "very good" or "excellent"	Number of ratings	Low-risk adult surgery	Complex medical care for adults	High-risk child surgery	High-risk delivery of a baby	Uncomplicated delivery of a baby	Adjusted death rate for all case types (%)	Adjusted death rate for medical cases (%)	Adjusted death rate for surgical cases (%)	Adjusted adverse outcome rate for surgical cases (%)	Overall score on accreditation review (higher is better)	Major affiliation with a medical school?
National Average	32	–	59	50	40	46	58	12.1	14.8	2.3	7.7	91	–
Texas *(continued)*													
San Antonio Area *(continued)*													
Christus Santa Rosa (Babcock Rd), San Antonio	32	81	78*	58	–	63*	80	***No data collected***				–[6]	–[6]
Christus Santa Rosa (N Santa Rosa St), San Antonio[1]	27	79	57	55	**91**[5]	78	62	**9.6**	**11.6**	2.2	8.2	***88***	**Yes**
Methodist Ambulatory Surgery NW, San Antonio	–	–	***No data collected***					–	–	–	–	**96**	No
Methodist Specialty and Transplant, San Antonio[1]	**60**	82	**91**	**88**	–[3]	–[4]	–[4]	13.4	16.1	3.0	6.7	93	No
Metropolitan Methodist, San Antonio	33	83	50	47	–[3]	29	64	***No data collected***				–[6]	–[6]
Nix, San Antonio[1]	***12***	77	***17***	***6***	***0***	***0***	***14***	10.7	13.4	0.9	6.8	***87***	No
North Central Baptist, San Antonio	26	88	84	36	44	33	80	***No data collected***				–[6]	–[6]
Northeast Baptist, San Antonio	33	80	77	87	–	56*	85	***No data collected***				–[6]	–[6]
Northeast Methodist, San Antonio	***11***	76	44*	17*	–[3]	***0****	***17***	12.9	15.9	1.7	**3.4**	**98**	No
Southeast Baptist, San Antonio	***7***	67	33	***6***	–[3]	***0***	***20***	***No data collected***				–[6]	–[6]
Southwest General, San Antonio	***5***	73	***2***	***0***	***0***	***0***	***5***	**8.5**	**10.4**	–	7.9	92	No
Southwest Texas Methodist, San Antonio[1]	**87**	91	**99**	**99**	**100**[5]	**97**	**97**	11.8	14.3	2.3	8.9	***83***	No
University, San Antonio	**59**	93	50	85	74	86	49	12.5	14.9	3.1	9.1	***79***	**Yes**
Utah													
Salt Lake City Area													
Alta View, Sandy	16	64	50	***0***	–[3]	***0****	**94**	13.2	16.0	–	6.9	**95**	No
Cottonwood, Murray	35	72	88	55	43*	71*	**93**	**10.0**	**11.8**	3.5	9.5	90	No
Jordan Valley, West Jordan	***5***	64	***14***	***4***	***0***	***0***	31	***18.6***	***22.2***	–	–	91	No
✓ LDS, Salt Lake City	**96**	77	**98**	**99**	–[3]	**99**	**98**	**10.3**	**12.4**	1.9	8.9	90	No
Pioneer Valley, West Valley	***3***	61	***10***	***0***	4	***0***	***7***	12.4	15.0	–	***17.8***	**96**	No
Primary Children's, Salt Lake City	–[2]	–[2]	–[2]	–[2]	**100**	–[4]	–[4]	***No data collected***				**94**	–[6]
✓ St Mark's, Salt Lake City	**72**	71	**98**	**96**	–[3]	85	**97**	11.5	14.1	2.1	8.2	92	No
Salt Lake Regional, Salt Lake City	31	67	67	54	–[3]	11*	81	11.5	14.1	1.9	7.0	–[6]	No
✓ University of Utah, Salt Lake City[1]	**92**	78	80	**99**	**100**	**100**	55	10.8	13.1	2.0	7.2	***88***	**Yes**
Virginia													
Norfolk Area													
Bon Secours DePaul, Norfolk	31	32	71	61	17	30	67	12.4	14.9	3.0	8.9	91	**Yes**
✓ Sentara Leigh, Norfolk	**55**	33	**91**	80	10	48	**94**	**9.5**	**11.4**	2.1	8.4	–[6]	**Yes**
✓ Sentara Norfolk General, Norfolk	**85**	33	85	**93**	–[3]	**96**	70	**10.0**	**12.0**	2.1	8.0	**94**	No
Washington, DC, Area													
Inova Alexandria Hospital, Alexandria	37	223	**91**	87	38*	73	85	**10.6**	**12.8**	2.4	9.1	**96**	No
Inova Fair Oaks, Fairfax	36	228	**90**	72	57	74	**92**	11.1	13.6	1.6	8.3	**96**	No
✓ Inova Fairfax, Falls Church	**92**	355	**98**	**98**	**98**	**99**	**95**	**10.3**	**12.6**	**1.8**	8.5	93	No

Footnotes are on page 73. *Hospital's score based on relatively little data. See page 16.

Key Ratings for Metro Areas

See more information on "Detailed Ratings for All Areas" table beginning on page 74

✓ means hospital receives our top rating
Blue is most favorable
Bold Italic is least favorable
"–" means insufficient data

	Doctors' ratings of hospitals for high-risk adult surgery		Desirability scores from doctors (0 to 100, higher is better)					Measures of outcomes for selected cases (lower % is better)					
	Percent rating "very good" or "excellent"	Number of ratings	Low-risk adult surgery	Complex medical care for adults	High-risk child surgery	High-risk delivery of a baby	Uncomplicated delivery of a baby	Adjusted death rate for all case types (%)	Adjusted death rate for medical cases (%)	Adjusted death rate for surgical cases (%)	Adjusted adverse outcome rate for surgical cases (%)	Overall score on accreditation review (higher is better)	Major affiliation with a medical school?
National Average	32	–	59	50	40	46	58	12.1	14.8	2.3	7.7	91	–
Virginia *(continued)*													
Washington, DC, Area *(continued)*													
Inova Mount Vernon, Alexandria	21	183	69	40	0*	–[4]	–[4]	9.8	12.0	1.5	12.6	94	No
Loudoun, Leesburg	12	147	50	11*	0	20	38	12.4	14.8	3.5	8.9	97	No
Northern Virginia, Arlington	3	176	17	0	0	–[4]	–[4]	11.9	14.6	1.8	6.3	83	No
Potomac, Woodbridge	9	140	33	21	0	6	27	11.2	13.7	2.0	7.8	98	No
Prince William, Manassas	10	145	67	47	0	27	68	17.3	20.8	3.9	8.4	97	No
Reston Hospital, Reston	33	208	86	59	17*	50	83	10.9	13.4	1.2	9.6	86	No
Virginia, Arlington	41	239	93	84	33	67	90	10.2	12.4	2.1	9.8	90	No
Washington													
Seattle Area													
Allenmore, Tacoma	16	58	–	–	–[3]	–[4]	–[4]	*No data collected*				–[6]	–[6]
Auburn Regional, Auburn	5	96	8	0	0	0	13	12.7	15.5	2.4	7.1	88	No
Cascade Valley, Arlington	6	53	13*	0*	0*	0	18	12.1	15.3	–	1.1	90	No
Children's, Seattle	–[2]	–[2]	–[2]	–[2]	100	–[4]	–[4]	*No data collected*				96	–[6]
Enumclaw Community, Enumclaw	1	81	0	0	0	0	14*	15.6	18.3	–	12.9	–[6]	No
Evergreen, Kirkland	34	132	95	60	–	72	100	13.9	16.9	2.4	6.9	87	No
Good Samaritan, Puyallup	19	62	–	20*	–	–	–	13.8	16.8	2.5	7.1	94	No
Harborview, Seattle	86	200	55	86	90	44*	6	13.3	16.1	2.9	7.0	96	Yes
Harrison, Bremerton	8	74	33*	13*	–	0*	43*	12.0	14.6	2.2	6.4	81	No
Highline, Burien	5	115	23	0	0	0	29	13.6	16.6	2.3	7.0	94	No
Northwest, Seattle	33	146	72	20	–[3]	27	74	12.2	14.9	2.0	7.2	84	No
Overlake, Bellevue	60	148	93	84	–[3]	86	95	13.2	16.1	2.5	9.3	86	No
Providence, Everett	43	74	86*	67*	20*	–	56*	13.0	16.0	1.9	7.7	87	No
St Clare, Lakewood	9	54	57*	17*	–	–	40	11.7	14.3	2.2	4.4	–[6]	No
St Francis, Federal Way	16	95	50	–	0*	0*	50	11.5	13.9	2.6	6.7	–[6]	No
St Joseph, Tacoma	51	77	83*	91	–	90	91	11.8	14.4	2.2	7.7	80	No
Stevens, Edmonds	14	84	44*	27	0*	0*	64	12.9	15.7	2.6	9.0	94	No
✓ Swedish, Seattle	83	192	94	93	83	97	95	11.6	14.0	2.4	7.9	94	Yes
Swedish - Ballard, Seattle	26	124	93	25*	–	25*	89	*No data collected*				–[6]	–[6]
✓ Swedish - Providence Campus, Seattle	65	146	96	92	–[3]	92	85	11.8	14.2	2.6	8.4	–[6]	Yes
Tacoma General, Tacoma[1]	51	90	78*	85	40*	80	58	13.4	16.5	2.3	8.1	84	No
✓ University of Washington, Seattle	83	206	72	97	–[3]	97	51	11.3	13.7	2.3	7.4	91	Yes
Valley, Renton	38	134	31	0	11*	11*	47	12.6	15.5	1.5	6.0	92	No
Valley General, Monroe	14	58	17*	0*	0*	0*	14*	16.5	20.1	–	–	90	No
Virginia Mason, Seattle	73	172	94	93	–[3]	–[4]	–[4]	10.2	12.8	1.5	5.9	83	No

Footnotes are on page 73. *Hospital's score based on relatively little data. See page 16.

Key Ratings for Metro Areas

See more information on "Detailed Ratings for All Areas" table beginning on page 74

✓ means hospital receives our top rating
Blue is most favorable
Bold Italic is least favorable
"–" means insufficient data

	Doctors' ratings of hospitals for high-risk adult surgery		Desirability scores from doctors (0 to 100, higher is better)					Measures of outcomes for selected cases (lower % is better)					
	Percent rating "very good" or "excellent"	Number of ratings	Low-risk adult surgery	Complex medical care for adults	High-risk child surgery	High-risk delivery of a baby	Uncomplicated delivery of a baby	Adjusted death rate for all case types (%)	Adjusted death rate for medical cases (%)	Adjusted death rate for surgical cases (%)	Adjusted adverse outcome rate for surgical cases (%)	Overall score on accreditation review (higher is better)	Major affiliation with a medical school?
National Average	32	–	59	50	40	46	58	12.1	14.8	2.3	7.7	91	–
Wisconsin													
Milwaukee Area													
Children's of Wisconsin, Wauwatosa	–[2]	–[2]	–[2]	–[2]	**99**	–[4]	–[4]	***No data collected***				**94**	–[6]
Columbia, Milwaukee	44	84	**91**	86	13*	36	**90**	11.9	14.9	1.6	**6.9**	***86***	**Yes**
✓ Froedtert Memorial Lutheran, Milwaukee	**88**	97	**98**	**100**	–[3]	**95**	83	11.2	13.3	3.1	7.8	**98**	**Yes**
Northwest General, Milwaukee	–	–	***No data collected***					10.7	11.8	–	–	–[6]	No
St Francis, Milwaukee	***12***	77	***9***	14	***0***	***0***	***20***	12.1	14.3	***3.0***	***10.9***	91	No
St Joseph's, Milwaukee	42	74	75	86	**90**	**97**	**92**	12.6	15.3	2.3	8.4	90	No
St Joseph's Bluemound, Wauwatosa	***6***	52	***8***	***5***	***0***	–[4]	–[4]	***No data collected***				–[6]	–[6]
✓ St Luke's, Milwaukee	**84**	94	**96**	**95**	**100**	36	67	**10.9**	**13.3**	**1.9**	8.3	93	No
St Luke's South Shore, Cudahy	***8***	62	***0***	***8***	–[3]	***0***	***6***	***No data collected***				–[6]	–[6]
St Mary's, Milwaukee	39	74	86	75	40*	**89**	**89**	12.3	15.4	1.6	9.9	***83***	**Yes**
St Michael, Milwaukee	***10***	68	***10***	***0***	***0***	***0***	***12***	13.0	15.6	3.3	9.2	92	**Yes**
Sinai Samaritan, Milwaukee	32	75	45	55	***0***	69	42	11.1	13.3	2.9	8.6	92	No
West Allis Memorial, West Allis	24	74	81	25	–	50*	**93**	12.8	15.6	2.3	9.2	**96**	No

*Hospital's score based on relatively little data. See page 16.

Footnotes:

1 Some data for this hospital may reflect information from a larger entity or multiple hospitals.
2 Hospital provides primarily pediatric care.
3 Hospital does not generally provide pediatric care.
4 Hospital does not generally provide childbirth services.
5 Score is from an associated hospital.
6 Researchers could not determine information for this item from the data sources that were used.

Detailed Ratings for All Areas

See more information on "Key Ratings for Metro Areas" table beginning on page 32

Blue is most favorable
Bold Italic is least favorable
Blank means neither better nor worse than average
"–" means insufficient data

	Death rates for all selected case types			Hospital outcomes: better (★) or worse (×) than average — Adjusted Death rates											
					Medical Cases										
	Number of cases	Actual death rate (%)	Adjusted death rate (%) (lower is better)	All selected cases	All selected medical cases	Heart attack	Congestive heart failure	Obstructive pulmonary disease	Pneumonia	Respiratory failure and arrest	Septicemia	Stroke	Gastrointestinal hemorrhage	Fluid, electrolyte, & acid-base disorders	Kidney failure
National Average	–	–	12.1	12.1	14.8	21.2	10.6	6.5	16.9	34.4	25.1	18.4	6.7	11.0	20.9
Alabama															
Andalusia Regional, Andalusia	2,037	9.5	10.6	★	★				★	–					
Athens - Limestone, Athens	2,196	10.5	10.7	★	★					★					
Atmore Community, Atmore	1,190	12.5	11.0					★	★					★	–
Baptist East, Montgomery	2,228	10.5	11.0				★								
Baptist Montclair, Birmingham[1]	6,261	10.7	11.3		★					★		★			
Baptist Princeton, Birmingham	6,156	14.0	11.4		★			★					★	×	
Baptist South, Montgomery	7,719	11.7	12.3					✖							
Bessemer Carraway, Bessemer	3,096	16.4	12.2								✖				
Bibb, Centreville	305	17.0	***16.7***	✖	✖	–	–	–		–	–	–	–	–	–
Brookwood, Birmingham	5,741	11.5	***13.0***	✖	✖							★	✖		
Bryan W Whitfield, Demopolis	1,375	11.3	10.4	★	★				★						
Bullock County, Union Springs	469	8.5	8.7	★	★	–	★	–		–		–	–	★	–
Carraway Burdick West, Haleyville	1,722	12.7	12.2					★		–			★		
Carraway Methodist, Birmingham	4,496	13.2	***13.5***	✖	✖	✖			✖					×	
Carraway Northwest, Winfield	1,248	10.9	11.8										–		–
Cherokee Baptist, Centre	941	12.1	13.2					★		×		✖			
Chilton, Clanton	691	10.4	8.5	★	★	–			★		★		–		–
Citizens Baptist, Talladega	1,593	15.2	***16.2***	✖	✖	×	×		✖				✖		–
Clay County, Ashland	1,031	10.8	13.5			–			★	–		✖	–	–	–
Community, Tallassee	1,290	16.0	13.4	×	×				✖			✖			✖
Cooper Green, Birmingham	308	16.9	13.6			–	–			–		–	–	–	✖
Coosa Valley Baptist, Sylacauga	2,364	10.5	12.5			✖		×	✖		★	★			
Crenshaw Baptist, Luverne	628	16.1	13.9		×	–		✖		–			–		
Crestwood, Huntsville	1,911	12.0	12.9			×					✖				
Cullman Regional, Cullman	3,444	13.0	13.0	×		✖									
D W McMillan, Brewton	1,279	11.0	11.0			✖			★	★					
Dale, Ozark	1,507	12.5	12.2				×			–					
DCH Regional, Tuscaloosa	8,521	10.6	10.2	★	★		★	★	★		✖	★	★	★	
Decatur General, Decatur	3,131	11.6	11.9			✖									
DeKalb Baptist, Fort Payne	1,767	16.6	***14.7***	✖	✖				✖					×	
East Alabama, Opelika[1]	5,979	9.9	12.0										✖		
Edge Regional, Troy	1,377	11.8	12.1												
Elba General, Elba	364	11.5	14.6			–		–		–	–	–	–	–	–
Eliza Coffee, Florence	5,162	9.0	9.9	★	★	★	★	★				★	★	★	
Elmore, Wetumpka	650	13.2	13.6			–				–	✖		–		–

Footnotes are on page 350.

Hospital outcomes: better (★) or worse (×) than average											Results of accreditation review on full survey		Other facts			
Adjusted Death rates			Adjusted Adverse outcome rates													
Surgical cases			Surgical cases													
All selected surgical cases	Coronary artery bypass surgery	Large bowel surgery	All selected surgical cases	Coronary artery bypass surgery	Large bowel surgery	Gall bladder removal	Total knee replacement	Total hip replacement	Simple prostatectomy	Carotid endarterectomy	Accreditation status*	Overall evaluation score (higher is better)	Number of beds	Major medical school affiliation?	Number of residents	Computerized drug order system (1 to 5 scale, higher is preferred; see page 23 for details)
2.3	3.8	6.5	7.7	10.3	11.9	7.5	6.7	6.4	5.4	8.2	–	91	161	–	–	–
–	–	–		–			★	–	–	–	4	**88**	87	No	0	–
	–	–		–	✖		–	–	–	–	4	92	101	No	0	–
–	–	–	–	–	–	–	–	–	–	–	4	92	51	No	0	–
	–	–		–			–	–	–		4	**97**	130	No	0	–
		★	✖	✖							4	**88**	423	**Yes**	0	–
			✖	✖		✖		–			4	91	289	**Yes**	0	–
	✖			✖						★	4	**94**	343	No	0	–
	–			–			–	–	–		4	**87**	210	No	0	–
–	–	–	–	–	–	–	–	–	–	–	–[2]	–[2]	25	No	0	–
	✖			✖							4	93	497	No	6	–
–	–	–		–	–	–	–		–	–	4	**88**	99	No	0	–
–	–	–	–	–	–	–	–	–	–	–	–[2]	–[2]	30	No	0	–
–	–	–	–	–	–	–	–	–	–	–	4	**86**	43	No	1	–
✖	×		✖	✖				–			4	**95**	383	No	61	–
–	–	–		–		–	–	–	–	–	4	**95**	63	No	0	–
–	–	–	–	–	–	–	–	–	–	–	4	89	45	No	0	–
–	–	–	–	–	–	–	–	–	–	–	4	**85**	45	No	0	–
✖	–	–	×	–	–	–	–	–	–	–	4	**87**	97	No	0	–
–	–	–	–	–	–	–	–	–	–	–	–[2]	–[2]	43	No	0	–
–	–	–		–	–	–	–	–	–	–	–[2]	–[2]	69	No	0	–
–	–	–	–	–	–	–	–	–	–	–	4	**86**	141	No	0	–
×	–	–		–			–	–	–	–	4	**86**	176	No	4	–
–	–	–	–	–	–	–	–	–	–	–	–[2]	–[2]	52	No	0	–
	–			–				–	–	–	4	90	92	No	0	–
✖	–	✖		–				–			4	92	115	No	0	–
	–	–		–		–	–	–	–	–	–[2]	–[2]	67	No	0	–
–	–	–		–		–	–	–	–	–	4	**94**	59	No	0	–
✖			✖	×	✖		★			✖	–[2]	–[2]	383	**Yes**	0	–
	–			–	✖			–	–		4	**94**	256	No	0	–
	–	–		–			–	–	–	–	4	93	91	No	0	–
	★						★			✖	4	89	245	No	0	–
–	–	–		–	–	✖	–	–	–	–	4	89	87	No	0	–
–	–	–	–	–	–	–	–	–	–	–	–[2]	–[2]	20	No	2	–
✖	✖		✖	✖					✖	–	4	**98**	253	No	0	–
–	–	–	–	–	–	–	–	–	–	–	–[2]	–[2]	45	No	0	–

***Accreditation Status:** 5=Accredited with commendation or with full standards compliance; 4=Accredited with requirements for improvement; 3=Conditional accreditation.

Detailed Ratings for All Areas

See more information on "Key Ratings for Metro Areas" table beginning on page 32

Blue is most favorable
Bold Italic is least favorable
Blank means neither better nor worse than average
"–" means insufficient data

	Death rates for all selected case types			Hospital outcomes: better (★) or worse (×) than average — Adjusted Death rates											
					Medical Cases										
	Number of cases	Actual death rate (%)	Adjusted death rate (%) (lower is better)	All selected cases	All selected medical cases	Heart attack	Congestive heart failure	Obstructive pulmonary disease	Pneumonia	Respiratory failure and arrest	Septicemia	Stroke	Gastrointestinal hemorrhage	Fluid, electrolyte, & acid-base disorders	Kidney failure
National Average	–	–	12.1	12.1	14.8	21.2	10.6	6.5	16.9	34.4	25.1	18.4	6.7	11.0	20.9
Alabama *(continued)*															
Evergreen Medical Center, Evergreen	1,157	6.4	8.5	★	★	–	★	★		–			–	★	–
Fayette Medical Center, Fayette[1]	1,302	14.6	12.7			×				–			–		
Florala Memorial, Florala	391	5.6	7.6	★	★	–		–		–	–	–	–	–	–
Flowers, Dothan	6,393	9.5	10.0	★	★			★	★			★		★	
Gadsden Regional, Gadsden	5,857	13.3	12.7	×	×				✖						
George H Lanier, Valley	2,302	11.3	9.8	★	★				★	★				★	
Georgiana Hospital, Georgiana	732	10.7	10.8			–	★			–	–		×		–
Greene County, Eutaw[1]	155	11.6	12.5			–	–	–		–	–	–	–	–	–
Grove Hill Memorial, Grove Hill	492	12.4	12.8			–				–	✖	–	–		–
Hale County, Greensboro	326	8.6	10.2			–		–		–	–	–	–	–	–
Hartselle Medical Center, Hartselle	1,547	13.2	11.4							–					–
Healthsouth, Birmingham	2,828	8.1	***13.6***	✖	✖		✖			✖					
Healthsouth Metro West, Fairfield	2,506	15.6	12.3			×					✖				
Helen Keller, Sheffield	2,886	11.8	11.2								✖	★			★
Hill Hospital of Sumter County, York	203	5.9	6.1	★	★	–	–	–		–	–	–	–	–	–
Huntsville Hospital, Huntsville[1]	12,802	11.7	***12.7***	✖	×						✖		✖		
J Paul Jones, Camden	288	15.6	15.1			–		–			–	–	–		–
Jackson, Montgomery	5,861	14.4	***13.4***	✖	✖			✖	✖		✖				★
Jackson County, Scottsboro[1]	2,095	11.1	11.7											★	✖
Jackson Medical Center, Jackson	357	15.1	***16.2***	✖	✖	✖		–		–	–	✖	–	–	–
Jacksonville Hospital, Jacksonville	1,023	14.7	***15.1***	✖	✖	✖		–	×					–	–
L V Stabler, Greenville	1,142	13.4	13.4		×						✖		★		✖
Lakeshore, Dadeville	964	13.4	9.4	★	★	–			★	–			★		–
Lakeview, Eufaula	1,287	12.1	10.8			–	★			★					
Lawrence Baptist, Moulton	1,107	12.3	9.4	★	★			★	★	–				★	✖
Marion Regional, Hamilton	997	11.1	***14.8***	✖	✖	–	✖	–		✖			–		–
Marshall North, Guntersville	1,879	11.7	12.9			✖									
Marshall South, Boaz	2,590	15.9	***14.1***	✖	✖		×			✖		✖			✖
Medical Center, Enterprise	2,170	9.6	8.6	★	★		★	★	★	×	★		★	★	
Medical Center Blount, Oneonta	1,332	16.4	***14.4***	✖	✖	✖	✖			×					
Medical Center East, Birmingham	6,432	11.6	***13.9***	✖	✖	✖			×		✖	✖			
Mizell, Opp	1,121	12.5	12.4					★					–		
Mobile Infirmary, Mobile	11,839	10.6	11.0	★	★			★	★						
Monroe County, Monroeville	1,274	9.9	10.4	★								★		★	
North Baldwin, Bay Minette	738	17.3	***16.2***	✖	✖	✖				–	×	–	–		–

Footnotes are on page 350.

Hospital outcomes: better (★) or worse (×) than average											Results of accreditation review on full survey		Other facts			
Adjusted Death rates			Adjusted Adverse outcome rates													
Surgical cases			Surgical cases													
All selected surgical cases	Coronary artery bypass surgery	Large bowel surgery	All selected surgical cases	Coronary artery bypass surgery	Large bowel surgery	Gall bladder removal	Total knee replacement	Total hip replacement	Simple prostatectomy	Carotid endarterectomy	Accreditation status*	Overall evaluation score (higher is better)	Number of beds	Major medical school affiliation?	Number of residents	Computerized drug order system (1 to 5 scale, higher is preferred; see page 23 for details)
2.3	3.8	6.5	7.7	10.3	11.9	7.5	6.7	6.4	5.4	8.2	–	91	161	–	–	–
–	–	–	–	–	–	–	–	–	–	–	–[2]	–[2]	44	No	0	–
–	–	–		–	–	–	–	–	–	–	4	98	61	No	0	–
–	–	–	–	–	–	–	–	–	–	–	–[2]	–[2]	23	No	0	–
			★				★	★			4	86	215	No	5	–
									×		3	87	257	No	0	–
	–			–	×		–		–	–	4	89	200	No	4	–
–	–	–	–	–	–	–	–	–	–	–	–[2]	–[2]	22	No	0	–
–	–	–	–	–	–	–	–	–	–	–	–[2]	–[2]	72	No	0	–
–	–	–	–	–	–	–	–	–	–	–	–[2]	–[2]	34	No	0	–
–	–	–	–	–	–	–	–	–	–	–	–[2]	–[2]	30	No	0	–
–	–	–		–	–	–	–	–	–	–	4	95	50	No	0	–
	–	–	★	–	–	–	★	★	–	–	4	94	169	No	0	–
	–			–			–	–	–	–	4	96	150	No	1	–
	–			–			–	★	–	–	4	94	151	No	0	–
–	–	–	–	–	–	–	–	–	–	–	–[2]	–[2]	33	No	–	–
×	×		×		×	×	×			★	4	93	702	No	0	–
–	–	–	–	–	–	–	–	–	–	–	–[2]	–[2]	32	No	0	–
×	–					×	★				4	94	280	No	0	–
–	–	–		–	–	–	–	–	–	–	4	90	92	No	0	–
–	–	–	–	–	–	–	–	–	–	–	–[2]	–[2]	21	No	0	–
–	–	–		–	–	–	–	–	–	–	4	88	56	No	0	–
–	–	–	–	–	–	–	–	–	–	–	4	94	67	No	0	–
–	–	–	–	–	–	–	–	–	–	–	–[2]	–[2]	28	No	0	–
–	–	–		–	–	–	–	–	–	–	4	90	74	No	0	–
–	–	–	–	–	–	–	–	–	–	–	4	87	30	No	0	–
–	–	–	–	–	–	–	–	–	–	–	4	90	43	No	0	–
–	–	–		–	–		–	–	–	–	4	96	90	No	0	–
	–	–		–			–	–	–	–	5	97	102	No	0	–
–	–	–	★	–	–	–	–	–	–	–	–[2]	–[2]	117	No	0	–
–	–	–		–	–	–	–	–	–	–	–[2]	–[2]	40	No	0	–
											4	93	257	No	15	–
–	–	–	★	–	–	–	–	–	–	–	–[2]	–[2]	57	No	0	–
	×										4	94	502	No	0	–
–	–	–	–	–	–	–	–	–	–	–	4	98	59	No	0	–
–	–	–	–	–	–	–	–	–	–	–	4	93	43	No	0	–

***Accreditation Status:** 5=Accredited with commendation or with full standards compliance; 4=Accredited with requirements for improvement; 3=Conditional accreditation.

Detailed Ratings for All Areas

See more information on "Key Ratings for Metro Areas" table beginning on page 32

Blue is most favorable
Bold Italic is least favorable
Blank means neither better nor worse than average
"–" means insufficient data

	Death rates for all selected case types			Hospital outcomes: better (★) or worse (×) than average — Adjusted Death rates	Medical Cases										
	Number of cases	Actual death rate (%)	Adjusted death rate (%) (lower is better)	All selected cases	All selected medical cases	Heart attack	Congestive heart failure	Obstructive pulmonary disease	Pneumonia	Respiratory failure and arrest	Septicemia	Stroke	Gastrointestinal hemorrhage	Fluid, electrolyte, & acid-base disorders	Kidney failure
National Average	–	–	12.1	12.1	14.8	21.2	10.6	6.5	16.9	34.4	25.1	18.4	6.7	11.0	20.9
Alabama *(continued)*															
North Jackson, Bridgeport	636	9.6	11.1			–				–	–		–		–
Northeast Alabama Regional, Anniston	5,607	12.3	10.9	★	★							★	★		
Northport Medical Center, Northport	2,067	9.9	10.7	★	★						**✖**	★			
Parkway, Decatur	1,321	15.6	***14.2***	**✖**	**✖**				×						
Phenix Regional, Phenix City	2,064	16.5	***15.0***	**✖**	**✖**					×	**✖**	**✖**		**✖**	
Pickens County, Carrollton	1,230	13.2	12.7						**✖**	–				★	
Prattville Baptist, Prattville	1,036	12.8	11.0											★	–
Providence, Mobile	7,450	11.0	12.7	×	×			×		×					
Randolph, Roanoke	771	11.7	10.4										–		
Red Bay Hospital, Red Bay	537	11.4	14.4			–	**✖**			–	–		–		–
Riverview Regional, Gadsden	5,440	11.0	10.6	★	★									★	★
Russell, Alexander City	1,939	14.6	11.1										★	★	
Russellville Hospital, Russellville	516	12.4	***17.2***	**✖**	**✖**	–		–	**✖**	–	**✖**		–	–	–
St Clair Regional, Pell City	785	15.4	***14.8***	**✖**	**✖**	×	**✖**		**✖**	–	–		–		–
St Vincent's, Birmingham	6,035	9.4	11.6				**✖**		★						
Shelby Baptist, Alabaster	2,953	12.4	12.8												
Shoals, Muscle Shoals	696	9.2	10.9			–				–	–		–		
South Baldwin Regional, Foley	2,335	10.3	11.7					★							–
Southeast Alabama, Dothan	7,770	10.0	12.0					★							
Springhill, Mobile	3,557	11.7	12.0			×									
Stringfellow, Anniston	1,472	10.7	9.9	★	★				★					★	
Thomas, Fairhope	2,789	11.9	12.3								×				
Thomasville Infirmary, Thomasville	546	10.4	9.8			–		–		–	–				–
University of Alabama, Birmingham	6,256	10.8	***12.9***	**✖**	×		**✖**		**✖**		×	★			
University of South Alabama, Mobile	899	18.2	***14.7***	**✖**	**✖**			–			×			×	
USA Knollwood Park, Mobile	629	16.2	***16.1***	**✖**	**✖**	**✖**	×				×		–	–	–
Vaughan Regional, Selma	1,687	13.0	12.0				★					**✖**			
Vaughan Regional Parkway Campus, Selma	2,376	12.3	11.3				★			★		**✖**			
Walker Baptist, Jasper	3,382	14.9	12.8												
Washington County Infirmary, Chatom[1]	239	13.8	***18.9***	**✖**	**✖**	–	**✖**	–		–	–	–	–	–	–
Wedowee Hospital, Wedowee	378	11.4	14.0			–		×		–	–	–	–	–	–
Wiregrass, Geneva	1,521	8.8	8.0	★	★		★	★	★	–	★	★	★		
Woodland, Cullman	1,282	16.2	***15.6***	**✖**	**✖**						**✖**			**✖**	–

Footnotes are on page 350.

Hospital outcomes: better (★) or worse (×) than average											Results of accreditation review on full survey		Other facts			
Adjusted Death rates			Adjusted Adverse outcome rates													
Surgical cases			Surgical cases													
All selected surgical cases	Coronary artery bypass surgery	Large bowel surgery	All selected surgical cases	Coronary artery bypass surgery	Large bowel surgery	Gall bladder removal	Total knee replacement	Total hip replacement	Simple prostatectomy	Carotid endarterectomy	Accreditation status*	Overall evaluation score (higher is better)	Number of beds	Major medical school affiliation?	Number of residents	Computerized drug order system (1 to 5 scale, higher is preferred; see page 23 for details)
2.3	3.8	6.5	7.7	10.3	11.9	7.5	6.7	6.4	5.4	8.2	–	91	161	–	–	–
–	–	–	–	–	–	–	–	–	–	–	3	93	39	No	1	–
	–		✖	–		✖		–		✖	4	92	255	No	0	–
	–	–	★	–	–	–		–	–	–	5	96	196	No	0	–
–	–	–		–	–	–	–	–	–	–	4	96	94	No	0	–
	–		★	–			–	–	–	–	4	88	114	No	0	–
–	–	–	–	–	–	–	–	–	–	–	4	85	30	No	1	–
✖	–	–		–		–	–	–	–	–	4	93	54	No	0	–
						✖					4	88	349	No	0	–
–	–	–	–	–	–	–	–	–	–	–	–[2]	–[2]	66	No	0	–
–	–	–	–	–	–	–	–	–	–	–	–[2]	–[2]	25	No	0	–
					×	★					4	89	281	No	0	–
	–	–	★	–		–	–	–	–	–	4	87	81	No	0	–
–	–	–	–	–	–	–	–	–	–	–	4	98	100	No	0	–
–	–	–	–	–	–	–	–	–	–	–	–[2]	–[2]	51	No	0	–
				★		✖					4	92	255	No	0	–
×	–	×		–				–			4	83	228	No	10	–
–	–	–		–	–	–	–	–	–	–	5	94	128	No	5	–
	–	–		–			–	–	–	–	4	95	82	No	0	–
			★				★				4	87	353	No	0	–
							–	–	–	–	4	92	228	No	6	–
–	–	–	✖	–	–	✖	–	–	–	–	4	96	125	No	0	–
	–			–			★		–	–	4	92	150	No	4	–
–	–	–	–	–	–	–	–	–	–	–	–[2]	–[2]	27	No	0	–
						★		★	–		4	90	831	Yes	585	–
✖	–	–			–	–	–	–	–	–	4	93	187	Yes	13	–
–	–	–		–	–	–	–	–	–	–	4	91	150	Yes	4	–
–	–	–		–		–	–	–	✖	–	4	90	112	No	0	–
	–	–		–		★	–	–	★	–	4	96	130	No	0	–
	–	–		–		★		–	–	–	4	91	157	No	0	–
–	–	–	–	–	–	–	–	–	–	–	–[2]	–[2]	21	No	0	–
–	–	–	–	–	–	–	–	–	–	–	–[2]	–[2]	34	No	0	–
–	–	–		–	–	–	–	–	–	–	4	93	65	No	0	–
–	–	–		–	–	–	–	–	–	–	4	96	100	No	0	–

***Accreditation Status:** 5=Accredited with commendation or with full standards compliance; 4=Accredited with requirements for improvement; 3=Conditional accreditation.

Detailed Ratings for All Areas

See more information on "Key Ratings for Metro Areas" table beginning on page 32

Blue is most favorable
Bold Italic is least favorable
Blank means neither better nor worse than average
"–" means insufficient data

	Death rates for all selected case types			Hospital outcomes: better (★) or worse (✕) than average — Adjusted Death rates — Medical Cases											
	Number of cases	Actual death rate (%)	Adjusted death rate (%) (lower is better)	All selected cases	All selected medical cases	Heart attack	Congestive heart failure	Obstructive pulmonary disease	Pneumonia	Respiratory failure and arrest	Septicemia	Stroke	Gastrointestinal hemorrhage	Fluid, electrolyte, & acid-base disorders	Kidney failure
National Average	–	–	12.1	12.1	14.8	21.2	10.6	6.5	16.9	34.4	25.1	18.4	6.7	11.0	20.9
Alaska															
Alaska Native, Anchorage	793	8.8	11.8				✕						–	–	–
Alaska Regional, Anchorage	962	10.0	11.8					–					–	–	
Bartlett Regional, Juneau	714	7.8	9.2	★	★							★	–	–	–
Central Peninsula General, Soldotna	589	8.8	10.1			–		–			–			–	–
Fairbanks - Denali, Fairbanks	1,166	9.2	11.7						★				–		✖
Ketchikan General, Ketchikan	474	11.2	12.4			–				–	–		–	–	–
Norton Sound Regional, Nome	107	6.5	12.7			–	–	–	–	–	–	–	–	–	–
Providence Alaska, Anchorage	3,278	10.1	11.2				✖	★				★			
Providence Kodiak Island, Kodiak	121	4.1	6.2			–	–	–	–	–	–	–	–	–	–
SEARHC Mt Edgecumbe, Sitka	111	3.6	4.8	★	★	–	–	–	–	–	–	–	–	–	–
Sitka Community, Sitka	150	9.3	8.8			–	–	–	★	–	–		–	–	–
South Peninsula, Homer	234	6.4	6.7	★	★	–	–	–		–	–	★	–	–	–
Valley, Palmer	762	10.2	10.5										–	–	–
Wrangell Medical Center, Wrangell	70	14.3	12.5			–	–	–	–	–	–	–	–	–	–
Yukon Kuskokwim Delta Regional, Bethel	270	3.3	5.1	★	★	–	–	–	★	–	–	–	–	–	–
American Samoa															
LBJ Tropical, Pago Pago	218	17.0	***22.9***	✖	✖	–	–	–	✖	–	–	–	–	–	–
Arizona															
Phoenix Area															
Arizona Heart, Phoenix	645	6.2	11.9					–	–	–	–	–	–	–	–
Arizona Surgical, Phoenix	230	15.2	14.5			–		–		–	–	–	–	–	–
Arrowhead, Glendale	810	12.1	12.5					–						–	
Chandler Regional, Chandler	2,042	12.4	12.4										✕		
Del E Webb, Sun City West	3,563	10.1	12.1				✕							★	
Desert Samaritan, Mesa	6,261	10.2	11.6			★		✖	★		★			★	
Good Samaritan Regional, Phoenix	4,775	8.8	11.7								✕			★	
John C Lincoln - Deer Valley, Phoenix	925	10.9	11.3				★	–		✕			–	–	
John C Lincoln - North Mountain, Phoenix	5,178	11.7	***13.6***	✖	✖		✖								✕
Maricopa, Phoenix	2,038	22.3	***14.2***	✖	✖	✖		✕		✖		✖		✖	
Maryvale, Phoenix	2,692	12.3	12.1									✕	✕		
Mayo Clinic, Phoenix	1,775	3.8	8.7	★	★					–	–				★
Mesa General, Mesa	1,289	12.2	11.7												
Mesa Lutheran, Mesa	3,065	12.1	***13.8***	✖	✖	✖					✖				
Paradise Valley, Phoenix	2,155	15.5	***13.7***	✖	✖	✖								✖	

Footnotes are on page 350.

Hospital outcomes: better (★) or worse (×) than average											Results of accreditation review on full survey		Other facts			
Adjusted Death rates			Adjusted Adverse outcome rates													
Surgical cases			Surgical cases													
All selected surgical cases	Coronary artery bypass surgery	Large bowel surgery	All selected surgical cases	Coronary artery bypass surgery	Large bowel surgery	Gall bladder removal	Total knee replacement	Total hip replacement	Simple prostatectomy	Carotid endarterectomy	Accreditation status*	Overall evaluation score (higher is better)	Number of beds	Major medical school affiliation?	Number of residents	Computerized drug order system (1 to 5 scale, higher is preferred; see page 23 for details)
2.3	3.8	6.5	7.7	10.3	11.9	7.5	6.7	6.4	5.4	8.2	–	91	161	–	–	–
–	–	–		–	×	–		–	–	–	4	95	140	No	48	–
–	–	–	★	–	–	–		–	–	–	5	95	178	No	0	–
–	–	–	★	–	–	–	–	–	–	–	4	86	64	No	0	–
–	–	–	–	–	–	–	–	–	–	–	4	91	46	No	0	–
	–	–	★	–	★	–	–	–	–	–	4	86	119	No	0	–
–	–	–	–	–	–	–	–	–	–	–	4	93	36	No	0	–
–	–	–	–	–	–	–	–	–	–	–	–[2]	–[2]	34	No	0	–
									–		4	89	341	No	14	–
–	–	–	–	–	–	–	–	–	–	–	4	92	25	No	0	–
–	–	–	–	–	–	–	–	–	–	–	4	95	60	No	0	–
–	–	–	–	–	–	–	–	–	–	–	–[2]	–[2]	24	No	0	–
–	–	–	–	–	–	–	–	–	–	–	–[2]	–[2]	20	No	0	–
–	–	–	–	–	–	–	–	–	–	–	4	82	36	No	0	–
–	–	–	–	–	–	–	–	–	–	–	–[2]	–[2]	8	No	0	–
–	–	–	–	–	–	–	–	–	–	–	4	84	50	No	12	–
–	–	–	–	–	–	–	–	–	–	–	–[2]	–[2]	125	No	5	–
		–			–	–	–	–	–	★	–[2]	–[2]	59	No	–	–
–	–	–	–	–	–	–	–	–	–	–	4	92	20	No	1	–
–	–	–		–	–	–	–	–	–	–	4	92	115	No	0	–
	–	–		–			★	–	–	–	–[2]	–[2]	120	No	5	–
	–			–			✖			–	4	94	161	No	0	–
✖	×										4	95	385	No	1	–
						✖			★		4	93	537	Yes	221	–
	–	–			–	–	–	–	–	–	–[2]	–[2]	74	No	0	–
											–[2]	–[2]	239	No	8	–
✖	–	–	×	–	✖	–	–	–	–	–	4	88	491	Yes	103	–
	–	–		–		–	–	–	–	–	4	88	171	No	0	–
★		–								–	5	98	154	Yes	69	–
	–	–	★		★	–	–	–	–	–	4	93	130	No	0	–
✖					✖				–		4	97	189	No	0	–
	–	×		–		–	–	–	–	–	4	95	140	No	1	–

***Accreditation Status:** 5=Accredited with commendation or with full standards compliance; 4=Accredited with requirements for improvement; 3=Conditional accreditation.

Detailed Ratings for All Areas

See more information on "Key Ratings for Metro Areas" table beginning on page 32

Blue is most favorable
Bold Italic is least favorable
Blank means neither better nor worse than average
"–" means insufficient data

	Death rates for all selected case types				Hospital outcomes: better (★) or worse (×) than average — Adjusted Death rates — Medical Cases										
	Number of cases	Actual death rate (%)	Adjusted death rate (%) (lower is better)	All selected cases	All selected medical cases	Heart attack	Congestive heart failure	Obstructive pulmonary disease	Pneumonia	Respiratory failure and arrest	Septicemia	Stroke	Gastrointestinal hemorrhage	Fluid, electrolyte, & acid-base disorders	Kidney failure
National Average	–	–	12.1	12.1	14.8	21.2	10.6	6.5	16.9	34.4	25.1	18.4	6.7	11.0	20.9
Arizona *(continued)*															
Phoenix Area *(continued)*															
Phoenix Baptist, Phoenix	2,445	12.9	12.0												
Phoenix Children's, Phoenix	–	–	–	–	–	–	–	–	–	–	–	–	–	–	–
Phoenix Indian, Phoenix	225	8.0	9.6			–	–	–		–	–	–	–	–	–
Phoenix Memorial, Phoenix[1]	1,160	10.7	10.4	★		★							–		
St Joseph's, Phoenix	3,910	11.0	11.9							✖		★ (blue)			
St Luke's, Phoenix	1,310	7.1	***14.6***	✖				–			–		–	–	–
Scottsdale Healthcare - Osborn, Scottsdale	5,816	11.8	11.2	★	★ (blue)								✖		★ (blue)
Scottsdale Healthcare - Shea, Scottsdale	6,786	7.6	**10.6** (blue)	★ (blue)	★ (blue)					×	★	★	★ (blue)		
Tempe St Luke's, Tempe	776	14.2	13.3			✖		–					–	×	
Thunderbird Samaritan, Glendale[1]	4,233	13.5	***13.2***	✖	✖			✖				×			
Valley Lutheran, Mesa	8,804	11.7	12.3			×		✖							
Walter O Boswell, Sun City	10,507	11.5	***12.7***	✖	✖		✖	✖	×		★				
Wickenburg Regional, Wickenburg	366	8.2	**8.6** (blue)	★ (blue)	★	–	–	–			–		–	–	–
Other Areas															
Benson Hospital, Benson	198	10.1	13.8			–		–		–	–	–	–	–	–
Carondelet Holy Cross, Nogales	248	11.7	12.1			–		–		–	–	–	–	–	–
Carondelet St Joseph's, Tucson	2,745	14.0	***17.0***	✖	✖		✖	✖	✖			✖	✖		
Carondelet St Mary's, Tucson	6,158	11.2	***13.8***	✖	✖			✖	✖	✖		✖			
Casa Grande Regional, Casa Grande	1,568	10.7	11.7												
Chinle Comprehensive Care, Chinle	455	12.1	13.7			–		–		–	–	–	–		–
Cobre Valley, Globe	679	11.3	***15.9***	✖	✖	–				–	–		–		–
Copper Queen, Bisbee	272	9.2	12.5			–	–	–		–	–	–	–	–	–
El Dorado, Tucson	2,369	11.5	***14.1***	✖	✖		×		×			×			✖
Flagstaff Medical Center, Flagstaff	2,114	8.9	12.1			✖							–		
Fort Defiance Indian, Fort Defiance	233	6.4	7.8	★	★	–	–	–		–	–	–	–	–	–
Havasu Regional, Lake Havasu City	2,711	10.3	***13.5***	✖	✖				✖		×				
Hu Hu Kam, Sacaton	66	–	–	–	–	–	–	–	–	–	–	–	–	–	–
Indian Health Service Hopi, Polacca	70	7.1	7.9			–	–	–	★ (blue)	–	–	–	–	–	–
Kingman Regional, Kingman	3,433	11.6	***13.2***	✖	×					✖		×			
Kino, Tucson	1,203	26.6	***17.7***	✖	✖				✖	×	×	✖	✖		
La Paz Regional, Parker	962	7.7	**8.4** (blue)	★ (blue)	★ (blue)	–			★ (blue)	★			★		–
Mt Graham, Safford	886	12.2	***15.1***	✖	✖	–		✖				✖		×	–
Navapache Regional, Show Low	1,422	8.6	11.7					★				✖	–		

Footnotes are on page 350.

Hospital outcomes: better (★) or worse (×) than average											Results of accreditation review on full survey		Other facts			
Adjusted Death rates			Adjusted Adverse outcome rates													
Surgical cases			Surgical cases													
All selected surgical cases	Coronary artery bypass surgery	Large bowel surgery	All selected surgical cases	Coronary artery bypass surgery	Large bowel surgery	Gall bladder removal	Total knee replacement	Total hip replacement	Simple prostatectomy	Carotid endarterectomy	Accreditation status*	Overall evaluation score (higher is better)	Number of beds	Major medical school affiliation?	Number of residents	Computerized drug order system (1 to 5 scale, higher is preferred; see page 23 for details)
2.3	3.8	6.5	7.7	10.3	11.9	7.5	6.7	6.4	5.4	8.2	–	91	161	–	–	–
						★	✖		–	★	4	91	201	No	24	–
–	–	–	–	–	–	–	–	–	–	–	4	94	219	–	14	–
–	–	–	–	–	–	–	–	–	–	–	4	90	127	No	0	–
		–			–	–	–	–	–		4	93	167	No	0	–
							★	–		✖	–[2]	–[2]	570	Yes	150	–
✖	✖	–	✖	✖	–	–	✖	✖	–	–	4	91	243	No	0	–
				★		✖	×			✖	4	93	258	No	18	–
★	✖	★			★				★	×	4	93	251	No	0	–
–	–	–		–	–	–	–	–	–	–	4	94	110	No	1	–
		✖	×		×				✖		5	89	288	No	0	–
	–			–						–	4	96	232	No	0	–
★		★	×		★		✖	✖		★	4	93	273	No	0	–
–	–	–	–	–	–	–	–	–	–	–	4	91	20	No	0	–
–	–	–	–	–	–	–	–	–	–	–	4	85	22	No	0	–
–	–	–	–	–	–	–	–	–	–	–	4	95	80	No	0	–
	–	×				×		–			4	95	292	No	15	–
			★				★				4	91	385	No	46	–
	–	–	★	–	–		–	–	–	–	4	95	116	No	0	–
–	–	–	–	–	–	–	–	–	–	–	4	89	46	No	4	–
–	–	–		–	–	–	–	–	–	–	4	86	49	No	0	–
–	–	–	–	–	–	–	–	–	–	–	4	95	49	No	0	–
	–	–		–				–	–		4	94	166	No	0	–
★	–	–	★	–				–	–		4	90	146	No	0	–
–	–	–	–	–	–	–	–	–	–	–	4	99	52	No	0	–
	–		★	–				★		★	4	89	118	No	4	–
–	–	–	–	–	–	–	–	–	–	–	4	84	10	No	0	–
–	–	–	–	–	–	–	–	–	–	–	4	91	17	No	0	–
	–	✖	×	–				–	×	–	4	86	110	No	0	–
–	–	–	–	–	–	–	–	–	–	–	4	79	135	Yes	8	–
–	–	–	–	–	–	–	–	–	–	–	–[2]	–[2]	39	No	1	–
–	–	–		–		–	–	–	–	–	4	89	44	No	0	–
	–	–	★	–				–	★	–	4	94	54	No	0	–

***Accreditation Status:** 5=Accredited with commendation or with full standards compliance; 4=Accredited with requirements for improvement; 3=Conditional accreditation.

Detailed Ratings for All Areas

See more information on "Key Ratings for Metro Areas" table beginning on page 32

Blue is most favorable
Bold Italic is least favorable
Blank means neither better nor worse than average
"–" means insufficient data

	Death rates for all selected case types			Hospital outcomes: better (★) or worse (×) than average — Adjusted Death rates — Medical Cases											
	Number of cases	Actual death rate (%)	Adjusted death rate (%) (lower is better)	All selected cases	All selected medical cases	Heart attack	Congestive heart failure	Obstructive pulmonary disease	Pneumonia	Respiratory failure and arrest	Septicemia	Stroke	Gastrointestinal hemorrhage	Fluid, electrolyte, & acid-base disorders	Kidney failure
National Average	–	–	12.1	12.1	14.8	21.2	10.6	6.5	16.9	34.4	25.1	18.4	6.7	11.0	20.9
Arizona *(continued)*															
Other Areas *(continued)*															
Northern Cochise, Willcox	237	10.1	14.4			–	–	–		–	–	–	–	–	–
Northwest, Tucson	4,079	11.9	12.3					✖							
Page Hospital, Page	147	9.5	13.1			–	–	–	–	–	–	–	–	–	–
Payson Regional, Payson	860	11.4	12.2										–		–
Sierra Vista Regional, Sierra Vista	1,288	13.0	***16.4***	✖	✖			✖					✖		✖
Southeast Arizona, Douglas	328	14.6	***19.0***	✖	✖	–	–	–	✖	–	–	–	–	–	–
Tuba City Indian, Tuba City	453	7.9	9.1	★	★	–		–		–	–	–	–	–	–
Tucson General, Tucson	850	11.1	14.3	×	×					✖	–		–	–	–
Tucson Heart, Tucson	1,022	6.8	9.4	★	★			–		–	–		–	–	–
Tucson Medical Center, Tucson	6,269	10.8	***14.5***	✖	✖		✖	✖	✖	✖		×		✖	
University, Tucson	2,639	10.3	10.2	★	★				★			★			
Verde Valley, Cottonwood	2,609	12.8	***15.9***	✖	✖	✖		✖	✖			✖			✖
Western Arizona Regional, Bullhead City	843	8.8	12.3			–				★			–	–	–
White Mountain Regional, Springerville	355	5.1	5.1	★	★	–	★		★	–	–	–	–	–	–
Winslow Memorial, Winslow	384	7.6	9.2			–		–		–	–	–	–	–	–
Yavapai Regional, Prescott	3,519	10.4	12.7			✖					✖				
Yuma Regional, Yuma	5,951	10.3	11.0	★	★										★
Arkansas															
Arkansas Heart, Little Rock	1,491	6.3	10.7			★	✖	–	–	–	–	–	–	–	–
Arkansas Methodist, Paragould	2,691	14.7	***15.8***	✖	✖	✖	✖				✖		✖		×
Ashley County, Crossett	708	19.5	***18.9***	✖	✖	✖		–	✖		✖	✖	–		–
Baptist, Blytheville	1,458	16.9	***15.9***	✖	✖		×				✖			✖	–
Baptist, Forrest City	933	13.6	13.5										–		–
Baptist, Osceola	1,269	10.1	12.9						✖	–			–		–
Baptist Health, Arkadelphia	887	15.6	***16.4***	✖	✖	✖					✖		–	✖	–
Baptist Health, Heber Springs	394	16.2	12.8			–		–		–			–		–
Baptist Health, Little Rock	9,877	9.3	12.0				✖		★						
Baptist Health, North Little Rock[1]	4,835	11.7	12.7						✖	×				★	
Bates, Bentonville	397	11.3	15.5	×	×	–		–		–	–	–	–	–	–
Baxter Regional, Mountain Home	5,541	11.4	***14.4***	✖	✖	✖	✖	✖	✖					✖	
Booneville Community, Booneville	541	14.4	14.0					–		–	–	★	–	–	–
Bradley County, Warren	908	14.8	13.9	×	×		✖	–		–			–		–
Carroll Regional, Berryville	1,045	12.1	11.2			×	✖	–	★				★		–

Footnotes are on page 350.

Hospital outcomes: better (★) or worse (×) than average											Results of accreditation review on full survey		Other facts			
Adjusted Death rates			Adjusted Adverse outcome rates													
Surgical cases			Surgical cases													
All selected surgical cases	Coronary artery bypass surgery	Large bowel surgery	All selected surgical cases	Coronary artery bypass surgery	Large bowel surgery	Gall bladder removal	Total knee replacement	Total hip replacement	Simple prostatectomy	Carotid endarterectomy	Accreditation status*	Overall evaluation score (higher is better)	Number of beds	Major medical school affiliation?	Number of residents	Computerized drug order system (1 to 5 scale, higher is preferred; see page 23 for details)
2.3	3.8	6.5	7.7	10.3	11.9	7.5	6.7	6.4	5.4	8.2	–	91	161	–	–	–
–	–	–	–	–	–	–	–	–	–	–	4	94	24	No	0	–
			★					★			5	97	134	No	0	–
–	–	–	–	–	–	–	–	–	–	–	4	93	25	No	0	–
–	–	–		–	–	–	–	–	–	–	4	94	66	No	0	–
✖	–	–		–		–		–	–	–	4	92	65	No	0	–
–	–	–	–	–	–	–	–	–	–	–	4	91	75	No	0	–
–	–	–	–	–	–	–	–	–	–	–	4	90	69	No	17	–
–	–	–		–	–	–	–	–	★	–	–[2]	–[2]	80	No	0	–
		–			–	–	–	–	–		4	93	60	No	–	–
			✖				✖	✖	★		4	90	427	Yes	31	3
★			★			–	★		–		4	92	319	Yes	0	–
✖	–	✖		–	✖						4	88	99	No	0	–
	–	–		–		–	–	–	–		4	88	90	No	0	–
–	–	–	–	–	–	–	–	–	–	–	–[2]	–[2]	89	No	0	–
–	–	–	–	–	–	–	–	–	–	–	–[2]	–[2]	10	No	0	–
	–	✖		–	×		★		–	–	4	93	127	No	0	–
	–		★	–	★					★	4	90	237	No	0	–
		–	★	★	–	–	–	–	–		4	94	84	Yes	0	–
	–	–	✖	–		✖	–	–	–	–	4	83	129	No	0	–
–	–	–	–	–	–	–	–	–	–	–	–[2]	–[2]	40	No	0	–
–	–	–	–	–	–	–	–	–	–	–	4	94	96	No	0	–
–	–	–	–	–	–	–	–	–	–	–	4	93	86	No	0	–
–	–	–	–	–	–	–	–	–	–	–	4	95	59	No	0	–
–	–	–	–	–	–	–	–	–	–	–	4	94	57	No	0	–
–	–	–	–	–	–	–	–	–	–	–	4	92	24	No	0	–
							✖			★	5	98	620	No	0	–
	–		×	×							5	97	200	No	0	–
–	–	–		–	–	–	–	–	–	–	–[2]	–[2]	63	No	–	–
	–						×			★	–[2]	–[2]	163	No	0	–
–	–	–	–	–	–	–	–	–	–	–	–[2]	–[2]	26	No	0	–
–	–	–	–	–	–	–	–	–	–	–	–[2]	–[2]	56	No	0	–
–	–	–		–	–	–	–	–	–	–	4	87	31	No	0	–

***Accreditation Status:** 5=Accredited with commendation or with full standards compliance; 4=Accredited with requirements for improvement; 3=Conditional accreditation.

Detailed Ratings for All Areas

See more information on "Key Ratings for Metro Areas" table beginning on page 32

Blue is most favorable
Bold Italic is least favorable
Blank means neither better nor worse than average
"–" means insufficient data

	Death rates for all selected case types			Hospital outcomes: better (★) or worse (×) than average — Adjusted Death rates — Medical Cases											
	Number of cases	Actual death rate (%)	Adjusted death rate (%) (lower is better)	All selected cases	All selected medical cases	Heart attack	Congestive heart failure	Obstructive pulmonary disease	Pneumonia	Respiratory failure and arrest	Septicemia	Stroke	Gastrointestinal hemorrhage	Fluid, electrolyte, & acid-base disorders	Kidney failure
National Average	–	–	12.1	12.1	14.8	21.2	10.6	6.5	16.9	34.4	25.1	18.4	6.7	11.0	20.9
Arkansas *(continued)*															
Central Arkansas, Searcy	3,262	13.9	12.9								✖				
Chicot, Lake Village	1,222	11.0	12.0			–							–		–
Conway Regional, Conway	2,946	13.1	***13.3***	✖	✖	×		×			✖				
Crawford, Van Buren	1,954	13.2	12.1												
Crittenden, West Memphis	2,134	13.4	***14.5***	✖	✖	✖					✖			✖	✖
Dardanelle Hospital, Dardanelle	329	14.0	***18.3***	✖	✖	–	–	–		–	–	–	–	–	–
De Queen Regional, De Queen	1,099	17.0	***15.2***	✖	✖		×		×		✖				–
Delta, Dumas	535	13.8	12.2			–		–		–	–		–		–
DeWitt City, DeWitt	642	15.4	13.3			–	✖	–		★			–		–
Drew, Monticello	881	16.7	13.2				×								✖
Eastern Ozarks Regional, Cherokee Village	717	11.9	13.5			–				–	–		–		✖
Fulton County, Salem	721	17.1	***16.8***	✖	✖			×	✖	–	–	✖	–		✖
Gravette Medical Center, Gravette	1,101	11.4	12.5				×		★	–	–		–	✖	–
Harris, Newport	1,473	10.4	**9.3**	★	★	–			★						
Helena Regional, Helena	1,740	13.8	11.1			✖			★		✖			★	
Hot Spring County, Malvern	1,470	14.4	13.5	×	×	✖					✖	✖			–
Jefferson Regional, Pine Bluff	5,637	13.4	***14.7***	✖	✖			✖	✖				✖	✖	
John Ed Chambers, Danville	565	13.1	***15.6***	✖	✖				✖	–	–		–	–	–
Johnson Regional, Clarksville	1,340	13.9	13.5	×	×	✖			×	–					–
Little River, Ashdown	486	15.8	12.9					–		–			–	–	–
Magnolia Hospital, Magnolia	1,366	20.0	***17.0***	✖	✖	✖	✖				✖	✖			✖
Medical Center, Calico Rock	436	18.3	***18.8***	✖	✖	–	✖	–	✖	–	✖	–	–	–	–
Medical Center of South Arkansas, El Dorado	2,745	15.0	***14.9***	✖	✖	✖				★	✖	✖	✖		
Medical Park, Hope	1,736	16.7	11.6			✖	★	×							★
Mena Medical Center, Mena	1,175	15.1	***15.7***	✖	✖	✖	✖			–				–	–
National Park, Hot Springs	2,976	12.6	12.3								✖				
Newport Hospital, Newport	1,470	9.7	11.1					★					–		–
North Arkansas Regional, Harrison	3,126	11.5	**10.8**	★	★		★								
Northwest, Springdale[1]	5,157	12.3	***15.5***	✖	✖		✖					✖		✖	
Ouachita County, Camden	1,872	17.4	***16.4***	✖	✖		×		✖		✖	✖	✖		–
Ozark Health, Clinton	563	14.6	***17.7***	✖	✖	–		–	✖	–	–	✖	–	–	–
Piggott Community, Piggott	872	18.9	***16.5***	✖	✖	×	✖		✖		✖		–		–
Pike County, Murfreesboro	338	16.6	***17.2***	✖	✖	–		–		–	–	✖	–	–	–
Randolph County, Pocahontas	873	18.8	***17.5***	✖	✖	✖	✖		✖		×	×	–		–
Rebsamen, Jacksonville	1,383	14.5	***14.9***	✖	✖	×		✖	✖		✖				

Footnotes are on page 350.

Hospital outcomes: better (★) or worse (×) than average											Results of accreditation review on full survey		Other facts			
Adjusted Death rates			Adjusted Adverse outcome rates													
Surgical cases			Surgical cases													
All selected surgical cases	Coronary artery bypass surgery	Large bowel surgery	All selected surgical cases	Coronary artery bypass surgery	Large bowel surgery	Gall bladder removal	Total knee replacement	Total hip replacement	Simple prostatectomy	Carotid endarterectomy	Accreditation status*	Overall evaluation score (higher is better)	Number of beds	Major medical school affiliation?	Number of residents	Computerized drug order system (1 to 5 scale, higher is preferred; see page 23 for details)
2.3	3.8	6.5	7.7	10.3	11.9	7.5	6.7	6.4	5.4	8.2	–	91	161	–	–	–
	–	–	★				–	–	–		4	92	148	No	0	–
–	–	–		–	–	–	–	–	–	–	–[2]	–[2]	52	No	0	–
	–			–			✖	–		–	4	91	116	No	0	–
	–	–		–	–	–	–	–		–	4	87	103	No	0	–
	–	–		–		–	–	–	–	–	4	95	95	No	0	–
–	–	–	–	–	–	–	–	–	–	–	–[2]	–[2]	44	No	0	–
–	–	–	–	–	–	–	–	–	–	–	–[2]	–[2]	75	No	0	–
–	–	–	–	–	–	–	–	–	–	–	–[2]	–[2]	20	No	0	–
–	–	–	–	–	–	–	–	–	–	–	–[2]	–[2]	88	No	0	–
–	–	–	–	–	–	–	–	–	–	–	–[2]	–[2]	50	No	0	–
–	–	–	–	–	–	–	–	–	–	–	–[2]	–[2]	40	No	0	–
–	–	–	–	–	–	–	–	–	–	–	–[2]	–[2]	30	No	0	–
–	–	–	–	–	–	–	–	–	–	–	–[2]	–[2]	58	No	0	–
–	–	–	–	–	–	–	–	–	–	–	4	90	88	No	0	–
–	–	–	–	–	–	–	–	–	–	–	4	89	145	No	0	–
–	–	–	–	–	–	–	–	–	–	–	–[2]	–[2]	92	No	0	–
✖			✖			✖			×		4	88	356	No	0	–
–	–	–	–	–	–	–	–	–	–	–	–[2]	–[2]	41	No	0	–
–	–	–		–	–	–	–	–	–	–	–[2]	–[2]	90	No	0	–
–	–	–	–	–	–	–	–	–	–	–	–[2]	–[2]	42	No	0	–
–	–	–	–	–	–	–	–	–	–	–	4	97	62	No	0	–
–	–	–	–	–	–	–	–	–	–	–	–[2]	–[2]	26	No	0	–
	–			–		✖		–		–	4	95	162	No	0	–
–	–	–	–	–	–	–	–	–	–	–	4	83	71	No	0	–
–	–	–		–	–	–	–	–	–	–	–[2]	–[2]	42	No	0	–
★	★	★	★					–	–		–[2]	–[2]	166	No	0	–
–	–	–	–	–	–	–	–	–	–	–	–[2]	–[2]	86	No	0	–
★	–	★		–				–	–	–	4	91	111	No	0	–
											4	95	222	No	14	–
	–	–	✖	–			–	–	✖	–	4	93	118	No	4	–
–	–	–	–	–	–	–	–	–	–	–	–[2]	–[2]	32	No	2	–
–	–	–	–	–	–	–	–	–	–	–	–[2]	–[2]	35	No	2	–
–	–	–	–	–	–	–	–	–	–	–	–[2]	–[2]	32	No	0	–
–	–	–	–	–	–	–	–	–	–	–	4	95	50	No	0	–
–	–	–	–	–	–	–	–	–	–	–	4	90	113	No	0	–

***Accreditation Status:** 5=Accredited with commendation or with full standards compliance; 4=Accredited with requirements for improvement; 3=Conditional accreditation.

Detailed Ratings for All Areas

See more information on "Key Ratings for Metro Areas" table beginning on page 32

Blue is most favorable
Bold Italic is least favorable
Blank means neither better nor worse than average
"–" means insufficient data

	Death rates for all selected case types				Hospital outcomes: better (★) or worse (×) than average — Adjusted Death rates — Medical Cases										
	Number of cases	Actual death rate (%)	Adjusted death rate (%) (lower is better)	All selected cases	All selected medical cases	Heart attack	Congestive heart failure	Obstructive pulmonary disease	Pneumonia	Respiratory failure and arrest	Septicemia	Stroke	Gastrointestinal hemorrhage	Fluid, electrolyte, & acid-base disorders	Kidney failure
National Average	–	–	12.1	12.1	14.8	21.2	10.6	6.5	16.9	34.4	25.1	18.4	6.7	11.0	20.9
Arkansas *(continued)*															
Regional Med Ctr of NE Arkansas, Jonesboro	2,270	11.5	12.9												✖
St Anthony's, Morrilton	995	22.4	***19.7***	✖	✖		✖	–	✖		✖	✖	–		✖
St Bernards Regional, Jonesboro	8,542	12.9	***14.8***	✖	✖		✖	✖	✖		✖		✖		✖
St Edward Mercy, Fort Smith	6,157	11.2	11.8			★									
St Joseph's Regional, Hot Springs	6,566	12.6	12.4				✖		×	★	×				
St Mary Rogers, Rogers	2,795	11.3	12.2			×				★		✖			×
St Marys Regional, Russellville	2,875	14.0	12.1										★		×
St Vincent Infirmary, Little Rock	7,945	11.0	11.9												
St Vincent North, Sherwood	283	11.7	15.9	×		–	–	–		–	–	–	–	–	–
Saline, Benton	1,960	15.4	***15.7***	✖	✖					–	✖	✖	✖		
Siloam Springs Memorial, Siloam Springs	1,459	13.8	13.3				★	×							–
Southwest Regional, Little Rock	877	12.8	11.9										–		
Sparks Regional, Fort Smith	7,555	12.0	12.6	×		✖							×		✖
Stuttgart Regional, Stuttgart	1,630	14.5	***13.8***	✖	✖		✖	★				✖			
University Hospital of Arkansas, Little Rock	1,886	12.2	12.4							★					
Washington Regional, Fayetteville	4,574	12.4	***13.7***	✖	✖		✖	✖			✖	✖		★	
White County, Searcy	3,946	12.8	***14.1***	✖	✖	✖				✖	×				×
White River, Batesville[1]	3,678	12.9	***15.0***	✖	✖		✖	✖	✖					×	
California															
Los Angeles and Orange Counties															
Alhambra Hospital, Alhambra	1,581	11.8	8.4	★	★			★	★			★			★
Anaheim General, Anaheim	1,479	13.9	11.2			✖									
Anaheim Memorial, Anaheim	2,523	11.8	11.7												
Antelope Valley, Lancaster	3,063	13.9	12.2			★							✖		
Bellflower Medical Center, Bellflower	1,424	9.7	9.3	★	★			★		–					
Bellwood General, Bellflower	–	–	–	–	–	–	–	–	–	–	–	–	–	–	–
Beverly, Montebello	3,458	13.4	12.7						×				×	✖	
Brea Community, Brea	800	15.9	14.0	×		✖		✖					–	–	
Brotman, Culver City	3,062	12.3	9.0	★	★		★		★	★	★	★			★
California, Los Angeles	1,916	15.4	9.2	★	★		★		★			★			★
Cedars - Sinai, Los Angeles	12,665	10.2	9.4	★	★	★	★		★	★		★	★	★	★
Centinela, Inglewood	3,243	10.0	10.0	★	★		★		★			★			
Century City, Los Angeles	1,809	14.0	9.5	★	★				★			★	★		
Chapman, Orange	626	17.1	***14.9***	✖	✖	–					–		–	–	✖

Footnotes are on page 350.

Hospital outcomes: better (★) or worse (×) than average											Results of accreditation review on full survey		Other facts			
Adjusted Death rates			Adjusted Adverse outcome rates													
Surgical cases			Surgical cases													
All selected surgical cases	Coronary artery bypass surgery	Large bowel surgery	All selected surgical cases	Coronary artery bypass surgery	Large bowel surgery	Gall bladder removal	Total knee replacement	Total hip replacement	Simple prostatectomy	Carotid endarterectomy	Accreditation status*	Overall evaluation score (higher is better)	Number of beds	Major medical school affiliation?	Number of residents	Computerized drug order system (1 to 5 scale, higher is preferred; see page 23 for details)
2.3	3.8	6.5	7.7	10.3	11.9	7.5	6.7	6.4	5.4	8.2	–	91	161	–	–	–
	–	–	★	★		–	–	–	–	–	4	91	104	No	0	–
–	–	–	–	–	–	–	–	–	–	–	–[2]	–[2]	54	No	0	–
✖	×						★	★		✖	4	91	279	**Yes**	0	–
				★		★					4	93	343	No	0	–
★		★			★						4	92	218	No	0	–
	–		★	–	★			–	–	–	4	**87**	92	No	0	–
	–			–		×		–	–	–	4	92	135	No	0	–
		★	✖			×	✖		–		4	92	605	**Yes**	0	–
–	–	–	–	–	–	–	–	–	–	–	–[2]	–[2]	69	No	–	–
×	–	–		–		×	–	–	–	–	4	**86**	83	No	0	–
✖	–	–		–		–	–	–	–	–	4	**87**	52	No	0	–
–	–	–		–	–	–	–	–	–	–	4	**88**	76	No	0	–
			×			✖		✖			4	93	370	**Yes**	0	–
–	–	–	–	–	–	–	–	–	–	–	–[2]	–[2]	49	No	0	–
✖	–	–		–	×	–		×	–	–	5	93	285	**Yes**	0	–
								✖	–		4	**84**	201	No	0	–
	–	✖		–			★	–		✖	4	90	154	No	0	–
✖	–		×	–	✖	×	×				4	91	175	No	0	–
–	–	–		–	–	–	–	–	–	–	4	**86**	144	No	1	1
–	–	–		–	–	–	–	–	–	–	4	89	101	No	2	1
	–	–			★			–	–	–	4	93	375	No	34	2
×	–			–				–		–	4	93	336	No	0	1
–	–	–		–	–	–	–	–	–	–	4	**84**	145	No	1	1
–	–	–	–	–	–	–	–	–	–	–	4	90	110	–	1	–
	–						★	–	–	–	4	92	166	No	0	1
–	–	–		–	–	–	–	–	–	–	5	**98**	60	No	0	1
	–					–	–	–	–		4	**95**	244	No	0	1
–	–	–		–	–	–	–	–	–	–	4	93	230	No	24	2
★		★						★	✖	✖	4	**97**	849	**Yes**	285	4
	–	–				–				–	4	**96**	377	No	0	1
	–	–		–	★	–	–	–	–	–	4	**87**	156	No	1	1
–	–	–	–	–	–	–	–	–	–	–	4	92	40	No	0	1

***Accreditation Status:** 5=Accredited with commendation or with full standards compliance; 4=Accredited with requirements for improvement; 3=Conditional accreditation.

Detailed Ratings for All Areas

See more information on "Key Ratings for Metro Areas" table beginning on page 32

Blue is most favorable
Bold Italic is least favorable
Blank means neither better nor worse than average
"–" means insufficient data

	Death rates for all selected case types: Number of cases	Actual death rate (%)	Adjusted death rate (%) (lower is better)	All selected cases	Hospital outcomes: better (★) or worse (×) than average — Adjusted Death rates — Medical Cases: All selected medical cases	Heart attack	Congestive heart failure	Obstructive pulmonary disease	Pneumonia	Respiratory failure and arrest	Septicemia	Stroke	Gastrointestinal hemorrhage	Fluid, electrolyte, & acid-base disorders	Kidney failure
National Average	–	–	12.1	12.1	14.8	21.2	10.6	6.5	16.9	34.4	25.1	18.4	6.7	11.0	20.9
California *(continued)*															
Los Angeles and Orange Counties *(continued)*															
Children's, Orange	–	–	–	–	–	–	–	–	–	–	–	–	–	–	–
Childrens, Los Angeles	–	–	–	–	–	–	–	–	–	–	–	–	–	–	–
Citrus Valley, West Covina	2,698	11.7	10.9	★	★		**★**								
Citrus Valley Intercommunity, Covina	2,792	12.1	12.5						×					★	
City of Angels, Los Angeles	61	–	–	–	–	–	–	–	–	–	–	–	–	–	–
City of Hope National, Duarte	292	14.4	13.3			–	–	–		–		–	–		–
Coast Plaza Doctors, Norwalk	797	14.9	13.8	×						✖	✖		–		
Coastal Communities, Santa Ana	704	18.6	13.1			–		–					–		
Community, Gardena	472	13.1	9.8		★	–	–	–		–	–		–		–
Community, Huntington Park[1]	905	5.4	**6.6**	**★**	**★**	–	**★**	**★**	★			★	–	–	★
Daniel Freeman Marina, Marina Del Rey	1,458	13.6	**10.2**	**★**	**★**			★		**★**					
Daniel Freeman Memorial, Inglewood	4,520	11.7	**8.6**	**★**	**★**		**★**		**★**	**★**	**★**	★			**★**
Doctors, West Covina	230	3.0	**2.9**	**★**	**★**	–	–	–	–	**★**	–	–	–	–	–
Downey Regional, Downey	4,952	13.8	12.7	×	×			✖							
East Los Angeles Doctors, Los Angeles	612	8.7	**5.5**	**★**	**★**	–	**★**		**★**		★	**★**	–	–	
Encino - Tarzana Regional, Encino	1,844	15.9	12.4				×		**★**	×		✖			
Encino - Tarzana Regional, Tarzana	4,181	10.1	**9.8**	**★**	**★**	**★**			**★**		**★**	**★**			**★**
Foothill Presbyterian, Glendora	1,299	14.3	***14.9***	✖	✖				✖					✖	✖
Fountain Valley Regional, Fountain Valley	3,549	11.9	**9.7**	**★**	**★**	**★**			**★**			**★**			
Garden Grove Hospital, Garden Grove	1,940	17.4	12.0												
Garfield, Monterey Park	3,326	10.4	**6.7**	**★**	**★**		**★**		**★**		**★**	**★**	**★**	**★**	**★**
Glendale Adventist, Glendale	3,822	12.6	12.1				**★**				✖		✖		
Glendale Memorial, Glendale	4,778	10.9	**8.8**	**★**	**★**	**★**	**★**		**★**		**★**	**★**		**★**	★
Good Samaritan, Los Angeles	5,251	10.8	**9.5**	**★**	**★**	**★**	**★**	★	**★**		**★**			**★**	★
Granada Hills Community, Granada Hills	1,732	13.2	**8.1**	**★**	**★**		**★**	**★**	**★**			★	★	–	
Greater El Monte, South El Monte	865	14.0	**7.8**	**★**	**★**				**★**		**★**		–	–	
Henry Mayo Newhall, Valencia	2,589	11.4	**9.1**	**★**	**★**		**★**	**★**	**★**			✖		★	
Hoag Presbyterian, Newport Beach	7,246	11.6	**10.6**	**★**	**★**				**★**	**★**	**★**				
Hollywood Community, Hollywood	950	10.6	**6.9**	**★**	**★**	–	**★**		**★**		**★**		–	★	**★**
Huntington, Pasadena	5,391	12.4	**10.6**	**★**	**★**				**★**	×					
Huntington Beach Hospital, Huntington Beach	1,691	14.4	11.8											★	
Huntington East Valley, Glendora	671	13.9	**9.0**	**★**	**★**	✖		**★**	**★**	**★**			–		–
Irvine Regional, Irvine	1,325	14.3	11.5												
Kaiser Permanente, Anaheim	1,573	13.1	12.6						×					–	

Footnotes are on page 350.

Hospital outcomes: better (★) or worse (×) than average											Results of accreditation review on full survey		Other facts			
Adjusted Death rates			Adjusted Adverse outcome rates													
Surgical cases			Surgical cases													
All selected surgical cases	Coronary artery bypass surgery	Large bowel surgery	All selected surgical cases	Coronary artery bypass surgery	Large bowel surgery	Gall bladder removal	Total knee replacement	Total hip replacement	Simple prostatectomy	Carotid endarterectomy	Accreditation status*	Overall evaluation score (higher is better)	Number of beds	Major medical school affiliation?	Number of residents	Computerized drug order system (1 to 5 scale, higher is preferred; see page 23 for details)
2.3	3.8	6.5	7.7	10.3	11.9	7.5	6.7	6.4	5.4	8.2	–	91	161	–	–	–
–	–	–	–	–	–	–	–	–	–	–	–[2]	–[2]	192	–	42	–
–	–	–	–	–	–	–	–	–	–	–	4	89	286	–	85	–
	–	–		–			–	–	–	–	4	90	508	No	64	2
		–				–		–	–		–[2]	–[2]	252	No	7	1
–	–	–	–	–	–	–	–	–	–	–	4	91	292	No	–	1
–	–	–	–	–	–	–	–	–	–	–	4	93	137	No	0	2
–	–	–	–	–	–	–	–	–	–	–	3	80	101	Yes	1	1
–	–	–		–	–	–	–	–	–	–	4	96	132	No	0	1
–	–	–	–	–	–	–	–	–	–	–	4	81	22	No	0	1
–	–	–		–	–	–	–	–	–	–	4	91	226	No	5	1
–	–	–		–	–	–	–	–	–	–	4	87	118	No	0	1
						–	–	–	–	–	4	87	331	No	0	1
–	–	–	–	–	–	–	–	–	–	–	4	95	27	No	0	1
				★	★			–			4	91	222	No	8	1
–	–	–	–	–	–	–	–	–	–	–	4	92	127	No	1	1
	–	–		–		–			–	–	–[2]	–[2]	151	No	0	1
★		★	★		★		–	–		★	4	92	232	No	0	–
–	–	–		–	–	–	–	–	–	–	4	94	106	No	0	2
			★				★	–	–	–	4	100	396	No	0	1
	–	–		–		–	–	–	–	–	5	93	155	No	1	1
	–	–					–	–		–	4	90	211	No	0	1
		–					★		–		4	96	457	Yes	39	1
							×	–			4	90	290	No	0	4
✖	✖		✖	✖					✖		4	90	357	Yes	8	1
	–	–			–	–	–	–	–	–	–[2]	–[2]	139	No	3	1
–	–	–	–	–	–	–	–	–	–	–	4	83	102	No	0	1
	–	–	★	–		–	–	–	–	–	4	79	217	No	5	–
★	★			✖					★		4	95	350	No	0	4
–	–	–	–	–	–	–	–	–	–	–	5	86	160	No	1	1
										★	4	92	450	No	18	4
–	–	–		–	–	–	–	–	–	–	4	92	102	No	0	1
–	–	–	–	–	–	–	–	–	–	–	4	83	92	No	0	1
–	–	–		–		–	–	–	–	–	4	92	141	No	0	–
★	–		★	–		★	–	–	–	–	4	87	150	No	18	2

***Accreditation Status:** 5=Accredited with commendation or with full standards compliance; 4=Accredited with requirements for improvement; 3=Conditional accreditation.

Detailed Ratings for All Areas

See more information on "Key Ratings for Metro Areas" table beginning on page 32

Blue is most favorable
Bold Italic is least favorable
Blank means neither better nor worse than average
"–" means insufficient data

	Death rates for all selected case types				Hospital outcomes: better (★) or worse (×) than average — Adjusted Death rates — Medical Cases										
	Number of cases	Actual death rate (%)	Adjusted death rate (%) (lower is better)	All selected cases	All selected medical cases	Heart attack	Congestive heart failure	Obstructive pulmonary disease	Pneumonia	Respiratory failure and arrest	Septicemia	Stroke	Gastrointestinal hemorrhage	Fluid, electrolyte, & acid-base disorders	Kidney failure
National Average	–	–	12.1	12.1	14.8	21.2	10.6	6.5	16.9	34.4	25.1	18.4	6.7	11.0	20.9
California *(continued)*															
Los Angeles and Orange Counties *(continued)*															
Kaiser Permanente, Baldwin Park	15	60.0	***40.0***	✖	✖	–	–	–	–	–	–	–	–	–	–
Kaiser Permanente, Bellflower	3,792	11.8	***14.2***	✖	✖		×	✖	✖	✖	✖	★		✖	×
Kaiser Permanente, Harbor City	2,366	12.6	13.1		✖									×	×
Kaiser Permanente, Panorama City	3,059	12.4	12.3												
Kaiser Permanente, Woodland Hills	3,120	12.3	***13.5***	✖	✖			✖							
Kaiser Permanente Los Angeles, Los Angeles	3,344	10.3	***13.4***	✖	✖				×	✖	×				✖
Kaiser Permanente West Los Angeles, Los Angeles	3,479	13.9	13.0	×	✖				✖		✖				
La Palma Intercommunity, La Palma	789	9.3	**8.7**	**★**	**★**		**★**	–					–	–	–
LAC + USC, Los Angeles	765	12.4	10.1	★	★		**★**				✖		–	–	
LAC - Harbor - UCLA, Torrance	716	16.8	11.1				★	–	★		✖		–	–	
LAC - High Desert, Lancaster	33	–	–	–	–	–	–	–	–	–	–	–	–	–	–
Lakewood Regional, Lakewood	2,954	11.4	12.0			★									
Lancaster Community, Lancaster	2,138	11.3	**10.3**	**★**	**★**		★	★						★	
Lincoln, Los Angeles	160	0.6	2.7	★	–	–	–	–	–	–	–	–	–	–	–
Little Company of Mary, Torrance[1]	4,474	12.1	**10.9**	**★**	**★**							**★**		★	
Long Beach Memorial, Long Beach	3,332	14.3	12.9	×					✖						
Long Beach Memorial, Long Beach	5,549	11.0	11.7									**★**			
Los Alamitos Medical Center, Los Alamitos	3,319	15.2	11.8				★		×	×		**★**	×		
Los Angeles Community, Los Angeles[1]	855	5.1	**5.9**	**★**	**★**	–	**★**	**★**	**★**		**★**	–	–		
Los Angeles Metropolitan, Los Angeles	559	10.9	**8.5**	**★**	**★**	–	**★**					–	–		
Los Angeles Metropolitan - Hawthorne, Hawthorne[1]	–	–	–	–	–	–	–	–	–	–	–	–	–	–	–
Martin Luther King - Drew, Los Angeles	898	12.1	**8.9**	**★**	**★**				★	**★**			–		
Memorial, Gardena	1,208	17.7	12.6				**★**						–	×	✖
Methodist Hospital of Southern California, Arcadia	4,464	11.7	**9.8**	**★**	**★**		**★**		**★**			**★**	×		
Midway, Los Angeles	3,615	18.0	**9.8**	**★**	**★**				**★**		**★**	**★**			
Mission - Panorama, Panorama City	968	13.1	**7.6**	**★**	**★**			**★**	**★**						
Mission Regional, Mission Viejo	2,574	11.8	11.8												
Monrovia Community, Monrovia	1,115	12.6	11.6			–				–		✖	–	**★**	
Monterey Park Hospital, Monterey Park	1,470	7.6	**6.4**	**★**	**★**		**★**	★	**★**		**★**	★	–		**★**
Motion Picture and Television Fund, Woodland Hills	467	13.1	11.4					–		–	–		–		–
Northridge - Roscoe Blvd Campus, Northridge	3,688	11.7	**9.1**	**★**	**★**		**★**		**★**					**★**	
Northridge - Sherman Way Campus, Van Nuys	1,364	14.6	**8.9**	**★**	**★**		**★**		**★**	–		★	–		**★**
Orange Coast, Fountain Valley	2,399	14.2	12.1				✖								
Orthopaedic, Los Angeles	137	–	–	–	–	–	–	–	–	–	–	–	–	–	–

Footnotes are on page 350.

Hospital outcomes: better (★) or worse (×) than average											Results of accreditation review on full survey		Other facts			
Adjusted Death rates			Adjusted Adverse outcome rates													
Surgical cases			Surgical cases													
All selected surgical cases	Coronary artery bypass surgery	Large bowel surgery	All selected surgical cases	Coronary artery bypass surgery	Large bowel surgery	Gall bladder removal	Total knee replacement	Total hip replacement	Simple prostatectomy	Carotid endarterectomy	Accreditation status*	Overall evaluation score (higher is better)	Number of beds	Major medical school affiliation?	Number of residents	Computerized drug order system (1 to 5 scale, higher is preferred; see page 23 for details)
2.3	3.8	6.5	7.7	10.3	11.9	7.5	6.7	6.4	5.4	8.2	–	91	161	–	–	–
–	–	–	–	–	–	–	–	–	–	–	–[2]	–[2]	158	No	0	2
	–			–						–	4	93	282	No	10	2
★	–	★		–		★		–	–		4	87	189	No	0	2
	–			–		–			–		4	85	211	No	0	2
	–			–					–		4	87	140	No	18	2
		–				–			–	✖	4	89	384	Yes	0	2
	–			–				✖		–	4	90	180	No	0	2
–	–	–	–	–	–	–	–	–	–	–	4	88	139	No	3	1
–	–	–	–	–	–	–	–	–	–	–	4	85	756	No	804	1
–	–	–	–	–	–	–	–	–	–	–	5	91	336	Yes	361	1
–	–	–	–	–	–	–	–	–	–	–	5	98	25	No	0	1
								–	–	–	4	90	148	No	1	1
	–			–			–	–	–		4	87	117	No	0	1
–	–	–	–	–	–	–	–	–	–	–	4	83	61	No	0	1
			×		×					✖	4	93	227	No	28	1
✖	–					–					–[2]	–[2]	278	No	0	–
				★	✖				★		5	96	691	Yes	8	2
	–			–				–			4	91	173	No	1	1
–	–	–		–	–	–	–	–	–	–	4	86	186	No	1	1
–	–	–	–	–	–	–	–	–	–	–	4	83	173	No	1	–
–	–	–	–	–	–	–	–	–	–	–	–[2]	–[2]	–	–	–	–
–	–	–	–	–	–	–	–	–	–	–	4	82	257	No	321	–
✖	–	–	✖	–	–	–	–	–	–	–	4	90	107	No	1	1
★	★		★	★					–		4	92	409	No	34	4
	–			–			–	–	–	–	4	86	150	No	1	1
–	–	–	–	–	–	–	–	–	–	–	5	96	96	No	–	1
✖	✖					–	–	–	–		4	90	254	No	0	3
–	–	–	–	–	–	–	–	–	–	–	4	92	49	No	2	1
–	–	–		–	–	–		–		–	4	88	95	No	0	1
–	–	–	–	–	–	–	–	–	–	–	4	91	218	No	6	1
											4	93	382	No	20	2
–	–	–		–	–	–	–	–	–	–	4	93	171	No	2	2
✖	–	×		–			–	–	–	–	4	94	230	No	0	2
–	–	–		–	–	–		✖	–	–	4	87	73	No	3	1

***Accreditation Status:** 5=Accredited with commendation or with full standards compliance; 4=Accredited with requirements for improvement; 3=Conditional accreditation.

Detailed Ratings for All Areas

See more information on "Key Ratings for Metro Areas" table beginning on page 32

Blue is most favorable
Bold Italic is least favorable
Blank means neither better nor worse than average
"–" means insufficient data

	Death rates for all selected case types				Hospital outcomes: better (★) or worse (×) than average — Adjusted Death rates — Medical Cases											
	Number of cases	Actual death rate (%)	Adjusted death rate (%) (lower is better)	All selected cases	All selected medical cases	Heart attack	Congestive heart failure	Obstructive pulmonary disease	Pneumonia	Respiratory failure and arrest	Septicemia	Stroke	Gastrointestinal hemorrhage	Fluid, electrolyte, & acid-base disorders	Kidney failure
National Average	–	–	12.1	12.1	14.8	21.2	10.6	6.5	16.9	34.4	25.1	18.4	6.7	11.0	20.9
California *(continued)*															
Los Angeles and Orange Counties *(continued)*															
Pacific, Long Beach	1,245	20.1	**10.1**	**★**	**★**		**★**		**★**				–		
Pacific Alliance, Los Angeles	1,976	8.8	**6.9**	**★**	**★**			**★**	**★**			**★**	**★**		**★**
Pacifica, Sun Valley	736	17.5	12.5										–	×	–
Placentia Linda, Placentia	970	12.8	***15.1***	✖	✖				✖					×	–
Pomona Valley, Pomona	4,546	13.1	**9.6**	**★**	**★**	**★**		★	**★**	★	**★**			**★**	
Presbyterian Intercommunity, Whittier	4,720	11.7	12.1					✖		✖					★
Providence Holy Cross, Mission Hills	2,317	12.3	**9.0**	**★**	**★**	**★**	**★**		**★**						
Providence St Joseph, Burbank	8,314	11.6	**9.3**	**★**	**★**	**★**	**★**	★	**★**		**★**	**★**		**★**	**★**
Queen of Angels - Hollywood Presbyterian, LA	4,069	13.0	**7.5**	**★**	**★**		**★**	**★**	**★**	**★**	**★**	**★**		**★**	**★**
Robert F Kennedy, Hawthorne	1,494	14.2	**9.3**	**★**	**★**		**★**			✖	**★**				
Saddleback, Laguna Hills	4,402	14.7	***13.3***	✖	✖				✖	×			✖	×	✖
St Francis, Lynwood	2,893	14.1	**10.5**	**★**	**★**		**★**				★				
St Johns, Santa Monica	5,759	8.6	**8.0**	**★**	**★**	**★**	**★**		**★**	**★**	★	**★**		**★**	
St Joseph, Orange	4,737	10.9	12.5			**★**		✖	✖	✖					
St Jude, Fullerton	5,289	12.6	***13.5***	✖	✖		✖	✖	✖					✖	✖
St Luke, Pasadena	1,596	13.0	**7.7**	**★**	**★**		**★**		**★**	**★**	**★**			★	**★**
St Mary, Long Beach	2,698	11.3	**9.5**	**★**	**★**	**★**			★	★		**★**		**★**	**★**
St Vincent, Los Angeles	3,700	9.5	**8.3**	**★**	**★**		**★**		**★**	**★**	**★**	**★**			**★**
San Clemente Hospital, San Clemente	1,102	14.2	11.8						★				–		
San Dimas Community, San Dimas	997	17.0	12.9					✖		–			×		–
San Gabriel Valley, San Gabriel	3,294	14.7	**9.3**	**★**	**★**		**★**		**★**		**★**	**★**			**★**
San Pedro Peninsula, San Pedro	1,877	16.2	12.1												
Santa Ana Hospital, Santa Ana	388	8.2	11.5			–		–		–	–	–	–	–	–
Santa Marta, Los Angeles	1,378	8.2	**6.0**	**★**	**★**		**★**	**★**	**★**	**★**	**★**	**★**			**★**
Santa Monica UCLA, Santa Monica	2,973	12.3	**10.1**	**★**	**★**		**★**								
Santa Teresita, Duarte	637	14.0	11.3					✖			–	★	–	–	
Sherman Oaks Hospital, Sherman Oaks	1,704	17.0	***15.2***	✖	✖	✖			✖				✖		×
South Coast, Laguna Beach	1,128	12.4	12.1								★				×
Suburban, Paramount	897	13.5	11.9			–							–	–	
Temple, Los Angeles	2,209	5.3	**5.0**	**★**	**★**	**★**	**★**	**★**	**★**	**★**	**★**	**★**		**★**	**★**
Torrance Memorial, Torrance	5,627	12.1	11.6			★									
Tri-City Regional, Hawaiian Gardens	940	13.6	13.4			–				×			–		
Tustin Hospital, Tustin	82	1.2	2.5	★	★	–	–	–	–	–	–	–	–	–	–
UCLA, Los Angeles[1]	4,868	10.1	**9.9**	**★**	**★**		**★**		★		✖	**★**		**★**	

Footnotes are on page 350.

Hospital outcomes: better (★) or worse (✕) than average											Results of accreditation review on full survey		Other facts			
Adjusted Death rates			Adjusted Adverse outcome rates													
Surgical cases			Surgical cases													
All selected surgical cases	Coronary artery bypass surgery	Large bowel surgery	All selected surgical cases	Coronary artery bypass surgery	Large bowel surgery	Gall bladder removal	Total knee replacement	Total hip replacement	Simple prostatectomy	Carotid endarterectomy	Accreditation status*	Overall evaluation score (higher is better)	Number of beds	Major medical school affiliation?	Number of residents	Computerized drug order system (1 to 5 scale, higher is preferred; see page 23 for details)
2.3	3.8	6.5	7.7	10.3	11.9	7.5	6.7	6.4	5.4	8.2	–	91	161	–	–	–
–	–	–	–	–	–	–	–	–	–	–	4	**83**	92	No	29	1
	–	–	★	–	–	–	–	–	–	–	4	91	109	No	0	1
–	–	–	–	–	–	–	–	–	–	–	4	**82**	204	No	0	1
–	–	–	★	–	–	–	–	–	–	–	5	**96**	114	No	0	1
						✕		–	–		4	**94**	398	No	18	3
			★		★	★	✕		★		4	91	312	No	20	2
	–	–					–	–	–	–	4	90	207	No	0	1
			★	★			★		★		4	90	328	No	0	1
	–			–			–			–	4	**87**	398	No	0	1
–	–	–	–	–	–	–	–	–	–	–	4	91	195	No	4	2
		★	★					★	–		4	**94**	148	No	9	4
	–					–	–	–		–	4	93	414	No	42	2
★	★		★	★		★					4	92	271	No	11	1
		★	★								4	93	290	No	0	4
							✕		★		5	**97**	347	No	27	4
	–	–		–		–	–	–	–	–	–[2]	–[2]	102	No	0	1
	–					–	–	–		–	4	92	202	No	8	2
								–		–	4	**86**	290	No	20	2
–	–	–		–	–	–	–	–	–	–	4	**98**	71	No	0	1
–	–	–		–	–	–	–	–	–	–	4	**88**	93	No	0	2
	–	–	★	–					–	–	4	90	274	No	0	4
	–			–		–		–	–	–	4	92	309	No	12	1
–	–	–	★	–	–	–	–	–	★	–	4	91	90	No	0	1
–	–	–		–	–	–	–	–	–	–	4	**95**	83	No	0	1
	–	★	★		★	–	–	–			4	**84**	221	No	13	1
–	–	–	–	–	–	–	–	–	–	–	4	91	283	No	3	1
–	–	–		–	–	–		–	–	–	4	93	153	No	0	1
★	–	–	★	–	★	–	–	–	–	–	4	**98**	126	No	0	1
–	–	–	–	–	–	–	–	–	–	–	4	**94**	132	No	1	1
★	–	–		–	–	–	–	–	–	–	4	93	130	No	1	1
					✕						4	**87**	360	No	0	2
–	–	–		–	–	–	–	–	–	–	4	89	150	No	–	4
–	–	–	–	–	–	–	–	–	–	–	3	**80**	117	No	1	1
★	★					–		★			–[2]	–[2]	650	**Yes**	554	4

***Accreditation Status:** 5=Accredited with commendation or with full standards compliance; 4=Accredited with requirements for improvement; 3=Conditional accreditation.

Detailed Ratings for All Areas

See more information on "Key Ratings for Metro Areas" table beginning on page 32

Blue is most favorable
Bold Italic is least favorable
Blank means neither better nor worse than average
"–" means insufficient data

	Death rates for all selected case types			Hospital outcomes: better (★) or worse (×) than average — Adjusted Death rates — Medical Cases											
	Number of cases	Actual death rate (%)	Adjusted death rate (%) (lower is better)	All selected cases	All selected medical cases	Heart attack	Congestive heart failure	Obstructive pulmonary disease	Pneumonia	Respiratory failure and arrest	Septicemia	Stroke	Gastrointestinal hemorrhage	Fluid, electrolyte, & acid-base disorders	Kidney failure
National Average	–	–	12.1	12.1	14.8	21.2	10.6	6.5	16.9	34.4	25.1	18.4	6.7	11.0	20.9
California *(continued)*															
Los Angeles and Orange Counties *(continued)*															
University of California - Irvine, Orange	916	11.0	10.5					–		★			–		
USC - Kenneth Norris Cancer, Los Angeles	374	12.6	12.8			–	–	–		–	–	–	–		–
USC University, Los Angeles	1,177	3.7	7.4	★	★	–	★	–	★	–		★	–	–	★
Valley Care - Los Angeles County UCLA, Sylmar	238	21.0	14.6			–	–	–		–	–	–	–	–	–
Valley Presbyterian, Van Nuys	3,334	11.5	10.7	★	★		★								★
Verdugo Hills, Glendale	2,096	14.5	***13.8***	✖	✖	✖		×		×					
West Anaheim Medical Center, Anaheim	2,097	17.5	13.0												
West Hills, Canoga Park	3,033	13.6	11.6												
Western, Anaheim	779	14.5	12.8										–		
Western, Santa Ana	1,857	16.9	13.1	×					×				★		
White, Los Angeles	2,697	11.3	7.9	★	★		★		★		★	★			★
Whittier Hospital, Whittier	1,311	17.9	***14.0***	✖	✖			✖					×		✖
Riverside and San Bernardino Counties															
Arrowhead Regional, Colton	416	17.1	11.3			–		–		–			–	–	–
Barstow Community, Barstow	1,284	14.2	12.2												
Bear Valley, Big Bear Lake	140	13.6	16.0			–	–	–	–	–	–	–	–	–	–
Chino Valley, Chino	1,362	11.8	8.9	★	★		★		★				★		
Colorado River, Needles	726	9.9	12.6			–					–		–	–	–
Community, San Bernardino	1,412	17.4	12.0												
Corona Regional, Corona	1,773	15.3	12.1												
Desert Regional, Palm Springs	4,579	13.2	***13.1***	✖	×			✖	×	×			★		
Desert Valley, Victorville	748	15.9	***15.2***	✖	✖	✖					×	✖	–	–	
Doctors', Montclair	791	19.5	***16.2***	✖	✖	✖			✖						
Eisenhower, Rancho Mirage	8,869	9.3	11.6			★							✖		
Hemet Valley, Hemet	3,203	14.5	***14.9***	✖	✖			✖	✖		✖				
Hi-Desert, Joshua Tree	1,634	18.9	***14.8***	✖	✖		×		✖	✖					×
Inland Valley Regional, Wildomar	1,262	9.1	9.4	★	★				★				✖		
John F Kennedy, Indio	2,033	11.6	10.8	★	★										★
Kaiser Permanente, Fontana	4,722	12.7	***15.3***	✖	✖		×	✖	✖	✖	✖			✖	
Kaiser Permanente, Riverside	2,734	11.6	***15.1***	✖	✖	×		×	✖	✖			✖		
Loma Linda University (Anderson St), Loma Linda[1]	4,541	12.8	12.6		×				✖						
Loma Linda University (Barton Rd), Loma Linda	–	–	–	–	–	–	–	–	–	–	–	–	–	–	–
Menifee Valley, Sun City	1,715	12.6	11.2		★		★	★							★

Footnotes are on page 350.

Hospital outcomes: better (★) or worse (×) than average											Results of accreditation review on full survey		Other facts			
Adjusted Death rates			Adjusted Adverse outcome rates													
Surgical cases			Surgical cases													
All selected surgical cases	Coronary artery bypass surgery	Large bowel surgery	All selected surgical cases	Coronary artery bypass surgery	Large bowel surgery	Gall bladder removal	Total knee replacement	Total hip replacement	Simple prostatectomy	Carotid endarterectomy	Accreditation status*	Overall evaluation score (higher is better)	Number of beds	Major medical school affiliation?	Number of residents	Computerized drug order system (1 to 5 scale, higher is preferred; see page 23 for details)
2.3	3.8	6.5	7.7	10.3	11.9	7.5	6.7	6.4	5.4	8.2	–	91	161	–	–	–
	–	–			–	–	–	–	–	–	4	**96**	383	**Yes**	0	**5**
–	–	–		–		–	–	–	–	–	–[2]	–[2]	60	No	0	1
	–	–	★			–			–	–	4	91	285	**Yes**	0	1
–	–	–	–	–	–	–	–	–	–	–	4	93	213	No	2	–
	–		★			–	★		–		4	89	209	No	8	1
	–	–		–		–	★	–	–	–	–[2]	–[2]	63	No	0	1
	–	–				–	–	–	–	–	4	92	219	No	0	1
	–							–			4	93	212	No	0	2
	✖	–	×	✖	–	–	–	–	–	–	4	92	183	No	0	1
✖	✖	–			–	–	–	–	–	–	4	91	282	No	0	1
	–	–					–	–	–	–	4	**97**	344	**Yes**	66	2
–	–	–	–	–	–	–	–	–	–	–	4	93	181	No	2	1
–	–	–	–	–	–	–	–	–	–	–	4	***86***	304	No	119	1
–	–	–	–	–	–	–	–	–	–	–	4	***83***	56	No	0	1
–	–	–	–	–	–	–	–	–	–	–	4	***84***	9	No	0	1
–	–	–	★	–	–	–	–	–	–	–	4	**95**	114	No	1	2
–	–	–	–	–	–	–	–	–	–	–	4	***84***	49	No	0	1
	–	–		–		–	–	–	–	–	4	93	274	No	0	2
	–	–		–		–	–	–	–	–	4	***84***	210	No	0	1
✖	✖						✖		★		4	90	348	No	10	1
–	–	–		–	–	–	–	–	–	–	4	**94**	83	No	0	2
–	–	–	–	–	–	–	–	–	–	–	4	89	102	No	1	–
							✖		★	★	4	**97**	261	No	0	1
✖	–	✖	×	–	✖		–	–	–		4	89	395	No	39	1
✖	–	✖		–		–	–	–	–	–	4	91	42	No	0	–
✖	–	–		–		–	–	–	–	–	4	**94**	80	No	0	1
	–	–		–				–	–	–	4	93	130	No	0	1
	–			–					–	★	4	92	299	No	30	2
✖	–	–		–		–			–		4	92	188	No	18	2
			✖			★	✖	✖	✖		–[2]	–[2]	653	**Yes**	196	4
–	–	–	–	–	–	–	–	–	–	–	–[2]	–[2]	–	–	–	–
✖	–	✖		–		–	–	–	–	–	4	91	84	No	0	1

***Accreditation Status:** 5=Accredited with commendation or with full standards compliance; 4=Accredited with requirements for improvement; 3=Conditional accreditation.

Detailed Ratings for All Areas

See more information on "Key Ratings for Metro Areas" table beginning on page 32

Blue is most favorable
Bold Italic is least favorable
Blank means neither better nor worse than average
"–" means insufficient data

	Death rates for all selected case types			Hospital outcomes: better (★) or worse (×) than average — Adjusted Death rates											
					Medical Cases										
	Number of cases	Actual death rate (%)	Adjusted death rate (%) (lower is better)	All selected cases	All selected medical cases	Heart attack	Congestive heart failure	Obstructive pulmonary disease	Pneumonia	Respiratory failure and arrest	Septicemia	Stroke	Gastrointestinal hemorrhage	Fluid, electrolyte, & acid-base disorders	Kidney failure
National Average	–	–	12.1	12.1	14.8	21.2	10.6	6.5	16.9	34.4	25.1	18.4	6.7	11.0	20.9
California *(continued)*															
Riverside and San Bernardino Counties *(continued)*															
Moreno Valley Community, Moreno Valley	853	10.6	10.1	★	★		★ (blue)			–			–	–	★ (blue)
Mountains, Lake Arrowhead	168	7.1	8.0			–	–	–	–	–	–	–	–	–	–
Palo Verde, Blythe	689	12.5	***15.6***	✖	✖	×			×	–	×	✖	–		–
Parkview, Riverside	2,224	19.1	***14.8***	✖	✖	×	×	✖	✖		×				
Rancho Springs, Murrieta	1,619	9.1	10.5	★	★			★ (blue)	★		★ (blue)				
Redlands Community, Redlands	2,776	13.8	***15.2***	✖	✖		✖	×	✖		×				
Riverside Community, Riverside	2,806	13.4	12.9					✖	×						
Riverside County Regional, Moreno Valley	256	19.1	***16.7***	✖	✖	–	–	–	×	–	–	✖	–	–	–
St Bernardine, San Bernardino	2,880	12.7	12.4			★				×					
St Mary Regional, Apple Valley	2,418	10.9	12.5												
San Antonio, Upland	4,069	12.3	12.5					✖						✖	
San Gorgonio, Banning	1,305	20.0	***18.3***	✖	✖	×			✖		✖	✖	✖		
Victor Valley, Victorville	1,412	12.4	***14.2***	✖	✖	★			✖				✖	✖	
Sacramento Area															
Kaiser Permanente Sacramento, Sacramento	6,747	11.4	***14.5***	✖	✖			✖	✖	✖	✖				✖
Kaiser Permanente South Sacramento, Sacramento	2,413	13.8	***15.3***	✖	✖		✖	✖	✖	×		✖		✖	✖
Mercy, Folsom	1,222	14.0	12.5											★	
Mercy General, Sacramento	5,035	10.6	10.7 (blue)	★ (blue)	★ (blue)						★				
Mercy San Juan, Carmichael	8,271	16.3	12.5				×						★ (blue)		
Methodist, Sacramento	2,621	18.0	13.0	×	×			✖							
Sutter General, Sacramento	7,843	11.1	***13.4***	✖	✖		✖		✖				✖		✖
Sutter Memorial, Sacramento	–	–	–	–	–	–	–	–	–	–	–	–	–	–	–
University of California - Davis, Sacramento	2,764	12.6	12.4							★					
San Diego Area															
Alvarado, San Diego	4,273	12.9	11.6				★ (blue)			✖					
Children's, San Diego	–	–	–	–	–	–	–	–	–	–	–	–	–	–	–
Fallbrook Hospital, Fallbrook[1]	1,004	13.3	12.2										–		–
Grossmont, La Mesa	5,397	14.0	12.6		✖					✖		✖			
Kaiser Permanente, San Diego[1]	5,822	11.8	***13.6***	✖	✖		✖	✖	✖	✖		★ (blue)			✖
Palomar, Escondido	5,324	13.9	***13.2***	✖	✖			✖	✖	✖					
Paradise Valley, National City	2,206	11.4	7.4 (blue)	★ (blue)	★ (blue)		★ (blue)	★ (blue)	★ (blue)	★ (blue)	★ (blue)	★ (blue)	★ (blue)	★	★ (blue)
Pomerado, Poway	2,388	17.2	***14.1***	✖	✖			✖	✖	✖					
Scripps, Chula Vista	2,148	11.8	11.5												

Footnotes are on page 350.

Hospital outcomes: better (★) or worse (×) than average											Results of accreditation review on full survey		Other facts			
Adjusted Death rates			Adjusted Adverse outcome rates													
Surgical cases			Surgical cases													
All selected surgical cases	Coronary artery bypass surgery	Large bowel surgery	All selected surgical cases	Coronary artery bypass surgery	Large bowel surgery	Gall bladder removal	Total knee replacement	Total hip replacement	Simple prostatectomy	Carotid endarterectomy	Accreditation status*	Overall evaluation score (higher is better)	Number of beds	Major medical school affiliation?	Number of residents	Computerized drug order system (1 to 5 scale, higher is preferred; see page 23 for details)
2.3	3.8	6.5	7.7	10.3	11.9	7.5	6.7	6.4	5.4	8.2	–	91	161	–	–	–
–	–	–		–	–	–	–	–	–	–	4	92	72	No	0	1
–	–	–	–	–	–	–	–	–	–	–	4	81	14	No	0	–
–	–	–	–	–	–	–	–	–	–	–	–[2]	–[2]	35	No	0	1
✖	–	–		–		–	–	–	–	–	4	89	193	No	5	4
	–	–	★	–		–		–	–	–	4	95	49	No	0	1
	–		★	–			★	★			4	92	194	No	6	1
✖	✖		×	✖		–		–	–		4	97	329	No	5	4
–	–	–	–	–	–	–	–	–	–	–	4	94	282	Yes	18	1
		–	✖	×		–		–	–	–	4	89	268	No	0	2
✖	✖	✖		✖				–	–	✖	4	88	195	No	4	3
		×		✖					–		–[2]	–[2]	298	No	0	1
–	–	–		–	–	–	–	–	–	–	4	93	52	No	0	1
–	–	–		–	–	–	–	–	–	–	–[2]	–[2]	121	No	4	1
	–			–				✖	★		4	88	304	No	25	2
	–	–		–		–		–		–	4	94	175	Yes	276	2
	–	–		–		–	–	–	–	–	4	95	95	No	0	2
★	★		★	★		×		★		★	4	94	307	Yes	0	2
											4	92	352	No	34	2
	–	–		–		–		–	–	–	4	97	154	No	19	2
	★		×	★			✖	✖	★		4	84	754	No	–	2
–	–	–	–	–	–	–	–	–	–	–	–[2]	–[2]	283	–	0	–
	–	–		✖		–		–	–	–	4	91	464	Yes	529	3
			★					–		★	4	87	199	No	2	1
–	–	–	–	–	–	–	–	–	–	–	4	91	271	–	15	–
–	–	–	★	–	–	–	–	–	–	–	4	87	142	No	4	1
★	★	★									4	92	384	No	25	4
	–		★	–					★	★	5	94	310	No	29	2
									★		4	87	214	Yes	60	1
–	–	–		–	–		–	–	–	–	4	92	237	No	7	1
	–	–	★	–				★	–	–	–[2]	–[2]	238	No	6	1
	–	–		–			–	–	–	–	–[2]	–[2]	183	No	6	3

***Accreditation Status:** 5=Accredited with commendation or with full standards compliance; 4=Accredited with requirements for improvement; 3=Conditional accreditation.

Detailed Ratings for All Areas

See more information on "Key Ratings for Metro Areas" table beginning on page 32

Blue is most favorable
Bold Italic is least favorable
Blank means neither better nor worse than average
"–" means insufficient data

	Death rates for all selected case types			Hospital outcomes: better (★) or worse (×) than average — Adjusted Death rates — Medical Cases											
	Number of cases	Actual death rate (%)	Adjusted death rate (%) (lower is better)	All selected cases	All selected medical cases	Heart attack	Congestive heart failure	Obstructive pulmonary disease	Pneumonia	Respiratory failure and arrest	Septicemia	Stroke	Gastrointestinal hemorrhage	Fluid, electrolyte, & acid-base disorders	Kidney failure
National Average	–	–	12.1	12.1	14.8	21.2	10.6	6.5	16.9	34.4	25.1	18.4	6.7	11.0	20.9
California *(continued)*															
San Diego Area *(continued)*															
Scripps, Encinitas	2,146	12.6	11.7					✖							
Scripps Green, La Jolla	2,167	6.1	11.0					×			–	★	×		
Scripps Memorial, La Jolla	3,181	10.1	**10.5**	**★**	**★**	★			**★**						
Scripps Mercy, San Diego	4,638	10.9	**9.9**	**★**	**★**	**★**	**★**	**★**	**★**	×					**★**
Sharp, Chula Vista	4,023	11.4	**10.7**	**★**	**★**				★		**★**				
Sharp, Coronado	902	15.9	***14.3***	✖	✖				×				–		
Sharp Mary Birch Hospital for Women, San Diego	11	–	–	–	–	–	–	–	–	–	–	–	–	–	–
Sharp Memorial, San Diego	6,149	11.5	12.2									✖			
Tri-City, Oceanside	7,226	13.2	12.4										★		
UCSD - La Jolla/Thornton, La Jolla	–	–	–	–	–	–	–	–	–	–	–	–	–	–	–
University of California - San Diego, San Diego	2,024	10.8	12.8					×							
Villaview, San Diego	303	17.5	12.5			–		–		–	–	–	–	–	–
San Francisco Bay Area															
Alameda County, Oakland	880	16.3	10.2	★	**★**		**★**		★	**★**		✖			
Alameda Hospital, Alameda	1,944	16.3	13.0							–					
Alta Bates, Berkeley	4,485	11.7	**11.0**	**★**	★	**★**							**★**		
California Pacific - California Campus, San Francisco[1]	5,799	9.1	**10.3**	**★**	**★**	**★**	**★**								★
California Pacific - Davies Campus, San Francisco[1]	786	12.7	**9.0**	**★**	**★**		**★**	–				**★**	–		–
California Pacific - East Campus, San Francisco[1]	–	–	–	–	–	–	–	–	–	–	–	–	–	–	–
California Pacific - Pacific Campus, San Francisco[1]	–	–	–	–	–	–	–	–	–	–	–	–	–	–	–
Children's, Oakland	–	–	–	–	–	–	–	–	–	–	–	–	–	–	–
Chinese, San Francisco[1]	2,012	8.4	**9.1**	**★**	**★**		**★**				★	**★**			
Community, Los Gatos	2,234	11.7	11.4											★	×
Contra Costa Regional, Martinez	589	11.4	11.2							–			–		–
Doctors, Pinole	1,357	13.0	13.5	×				✖							
Doctors, San Pablo	2,780	15.9	12.9	×					×		×				
Eden, Castro Valley	2,974	13.9	***13.3***	✖	✖		×		✖						
El Camino, Mountain View	5,171	12.0	11.6				✖				**★**			★	
Good Samaritan, San Jose	4,899	11.4	11.6									★			
Healdsburg General, Healdsburg	746	13.9	14.0	×	×	✖		–		×					–
John Muir, Walnut Creek[1]	5,577	11.9	11.8												
Kaiser Permanente, Hayward[1]	3,393	17.1	12.4										**★**	×	
Kaiser Permanente, Oakland	3,566	13.0	***13.1***	✖	✖				✖		✖				

Footnotes are on page 350.

Hospital outcomes: better (★) or worse (×) than average											Results of accreditation review on full survey		Other facts			
Adjusted Death rates			Adjusted Adverse outcome rates													
Surgical cases			Surgical cases													
All selected surgical cases	Coronary artery bypass surgery	Large bowel surgery	All selected surgical cases	Coronary artery bypass surgery	Large bowel surgery	Gall bladder removal	Total knee replacement	Total hip replacement	Simple prostatectomy	Carotid endarterectomy	Accreditation status*	Overall evaluation score (higher is better)	Number of beds	Major medical school affiliation?	Number of residents	Computerized drug order system (1 to 5 scale, higher is preferred; see page 23 for details)
2.3	3.8	6.5	7.7	10.3	11.9	7.5	6.7	6.4	5.4	8.2	–	91	161	–	–	–
★	–	★	★	–				–	★	★	4	93	145	No	3	3
★		–	★			–					4	90	165	No	5	2
								★		★	4	***82***	431	No	42	3
							★				4	***88***	447	No	52	3
								✖	–		4	93	206	No	0	4
–	–	–	–	–	–	–	–	–	–	–	4	93	195	No	3	4
–	–	–	–	–	–	–	–	–	–	–	4	**95**	166	No	–	4
							✖				4	91	488	No	54	4
						★	✖	✖	★	★	3	92	397	No	0	1
–	–	–	–	–	–	–	–	–	–	–	–[2]	–[2]	–	–	–	–
	×	–			★	–			–	–	4	93	468	**Yes**	431	4
–	–	–	–	–	–	–	–	–	–	–	4	92	100	No	2	1
–	–	–	–	–	–	–	–	–	–	–	–[2]	–[2]	269	No	48	1
	–			–		–	–	–	–	–	4	***87***	100	No	0	–
								✖			4	***83***	468	No	42	2
★		★	★					★	★	★	4	90	470	**Yes**	67	2
–	–	–	–	–	–	–	–	–	–	–	4	90	341	No	3	–
–	–	–	–	–	–	–	–	–	–	–	4	90	–	–	–	–
–	–	–	–	–	–	–	–	–	–	–	4	90	754	–	147	–
–	–	–	–	–	–	–	–	–	–	–	4	***88***	204	–	77	–
	–	–		–			–	–		–	5	**97**	54	No	0	2
	–	×		–		–		–		–	–[2]	–[2]	143	No	0	1
–	–	–	–	–	–	–	–	–	–	–	4	91	117	No	27	1
✖	–	✖	✖	–	✖	–	✖	–	–	–	4	91	137	No	1	1
	–					–	–	–	–	–	4	93	286	No	5	1
	–		★	–		★		–		–	4	93	191	No	0	2
			★	×		★	★	★	★		4	**94**	264	No	0	1
			★							★	4	***86***	332	No	0	3
	–	–		–		–	–	–	–	–	4	89	49	No	0	1
	✖	★					★		★		4	**96**	296	No	4	2
	–			–					–		5	***86***	204	No	11	2
	–			–		–			–	–	4	***86***	264	No	10	2

***Accreditation Status:** 5=Accredited with commendation or with full standards compliance; 4=Accredited with requirements for improvement; 3=Conditional accreditation.

Detailed Ratings for All Areas

See more information on "Key Ratings for Metro Areas" table beginning on page 32

Blue is most favorable
Bold Italic is least favorable
Blank means neither better nor worse than average
"–" means insufficient data

	Death rates for all selected case types				Hospital outcomes: better (★) or worse (×) than average — Adjusted Death rates — Medical Cases										
	Number of cases	Actual death rate (%)	Adjusted death rate (%) (lower is better)	All selected cases	All selected medical cases	Heart attack	Congestive heart failure	Obstructive pulmonary disease	Pneumonia	Respiratory failure and arrest	Septicemia	Stroke	Gastrointestinal hemorrhage	Fluid, electrolyte, & acid-base disorders	Kidney failure
National Average	–	–	12.1	12.1	14.8	21.2	10.6	6.5	16.9	34.4	25.1	18.4	6.7	11.0	20.9
California *(continued)*															
San Francisco Bay Area *(continued)*															
Kaiser Permanente, Redwood City	2,039	12.0	12.6				×			✖		**★**			×
Kaiser Permanente, Richmond	–	–	–	–	–	–	–	–	–	–	–	–	–	–	–
Kaiser Permanente, San Francisco	3,788	10.7	12.3			**★**	★		✖		✖			✖	
Kaiser Permanente, San Rafael	1,826	14.1	***13.8***	✖	✖		✖		×			**★**			✖
Kaiser Permanente, Santa Clara	2,955	13.8	***13.5***	✖	✖						✖				
Kaiser Permanente, Santa Rosa	1,845	11.4	13.3				✖				**★**				
Kaiser Permanente, South San Francisco	2,052	14.3	***13.4***	✖	✖		✖	✖						✖	
Kaiser Permanente, Vallejo[1]	4,332	13.8	***13.1***	✖	✖				✖		×				
Kaiser Permanente, Walnut Creek	4,027	12.6	***13.7***	✖	✖				✖			×	✖		
Kaiser Permanente Santa Teresa, San Jose	1,969	13.0	12.7						✖						**★**
Lucile Packard Children's, Palo Alto	–	–	–	–	–	–	–	–	–	–	–	–	–	–	–
Marin General, Greenbrae	4,000	13.0	***14.1***	✖	✖		✖			✖		✖			
Menlo Park Surgical, Menlo Park	21	–	–	–	–	–	–	–	–	–	–	–	–	–	–
Mills - Peninsula, Burlingame[1]	5,697	12.9	12.8	×	✖	**★**			✖					★	✖
Mt Diablo, Concord	4,066	13.6	***14.2***	✖	✖		✖		✖	×			×	✖	
Nelson Holderman, Yountville[1]	520	15.4	***15.0***	✖	✖	–	✖				✖	–	–	–	–
Northbay, Fairfield[1]	1,161	18.1	***18.9***	✖	✖	×		✖	✖		✖	✖	×	✖	
Novato Community, Novato	1,116	16.7	***14.0***	✖	✖			–	✖	×	×				
O'Connor, San Jose	4,298	11.2	**10.6**	**★**	**★**	**★**	**★**					×		★	
Palm Drive, Sebastopol	946	11.6	10.7					–			**★**		**★**		
Petaluma Valley, Petaluma	1,720	15.3	11.9												×
Queen of the Valley, Napa	3,293	11.9	11.7												
Regional, San Jose	3,285	11.6	**9.8**	**★**	**★**		**★**		**★**	★		**★**			
St Francis, San Francisco	2,495	12.2	11.0												
St Helena, Deer Park	1,647	8.6	**9.9**	**★**	**★**			–	★	**★**				✖	–
St Louise Regional, Gilroy	793	15.8	13.5			–		–					–		–
St Luke's, San Francisco	1,582	11.9	**10.2**	**★**	**★**										
St Mary's, San Francisco	3,742	10.7	**10.2**	**★**	**★**										
St Rose, Hayward	2,701	13.4	**9.7**	**★**	**★**				**★**		**★**				
San Francisco General, San Francisco	1,350	12.7	11.4			✖	**★**				✖	✖			
San Jose Medical Center, San Jose	2,413	14.8	11.4											★	★
San Leandro Hospital, San Leandro	3,939	13.8	**10.7**	**★**	**★**		★		**★**			**★**	×		
San Mateo County General, San Mateo	399	15.3	11.8					–					–	–	–
San Ramon Regional, San Ramon	1,342	11.3	**9.5**	**★**	**★**						★		★		

Footnotes are on page 350.

Hospital outcomes: better (★) or worse (×) than average											Results of accreditation review on full survey		Other facts			
Adjusted Death rates			Adjusted Adverse outcome rates													
Surgical cases			Surgical cases													
All selected surgical cases	Coronary artery bypass surgery	Large bowel surgery	All selected surgical cases	Coronary artery bypass surgery	Large bowel surgery	Gall bladder removal	Total knee replacement	Total hip replacement	Simple prostatectomy	Carotid endarterectomy	Accreditation status*	Overall evaluation score (higher is better)	Number of beds	Major medical school affiliation?	Number of residents	Computerized drug order system (1 to 5 scale, higher is preferred; see page 23 for details)
2.3	3.8	6.5	7.7	10.3	11.9	7.5	6.7	6.4	5.4	8.2	–	91	161	–	–	–
	–		★	–		–		★	–	★	4	85	171	No	0	2
–	–	–	–	–	–	–	–	–	–	–	–[2]	–[2]	–	–	–	–
		–	★		★	–			–	★	–[2]	–[2]	236	No	10	2
	–			–		–			–	–	–[2]	–[2]	119	No	0	2
	–			–		–	★		★	–	4	89	249	Yes	5	2
	–	–	★	–		–	★		–	★	4	90	103	No	0	2
	–			–		–			–	–	–[2]	–[2]	79	No	0	2
★	–			–							4	88	224	No	0	2
	–			–		×					4	85	229	No	0	2
	–	–		–		–		–	–		4	93	218	No	2	2
–	–	–	–	–	–	–	–	–	–	–	4	90	214	–	0	–
			★				★	×			4	96	165	No	0	2
–	–	–	–	–	–	–	–	–	–	–	4	99	16	No	0	1
★		★	★	★					★	★	4	92	283	No	0	4
			★					–	–		4	97	303	No	–	2
–	–	–	–	–	–	–	–	–	–	–	–[2]	–[2]	540	No	33	–
–	–	–		–	–	–	–	–	–	–	4	96	110	No	0	1
–	–	–		–	–	–	–	–	–	–	4	95	22	No	0	2
		★									4	88	283	No	0	2
–	–	–		–	–	–	–	–	–	–	4	91	48	No	0	1
	–	–		–		–	–	–	–	–	4	83	82	No	0	4
										★	4	89	142	No	0	4
	–	–	★	–			–	–	–	–	4	93	192	No	2	3
	–	–	★	–	★	–			–	–	4	87	187	No	0	2
		–				–	–	×			–[2]	–[2]	168	No	4	–
–	–	–		–	–	–	–	–	–	–	4	88	93	No	0	2
	–	–		–		–	–	–	–	–	3	78	225	No	7	2
			×		★		×	×	–		4	88	232	No	68	2
	–	–		–		–	–	–	–	–	4	93	175	No	2	1
–	–	–		–	–	–	–	–	–	–	4	88	537	Yes	229	1
	–					–	–	–	–	–	5	97	327	No	6	2
	–		★	–				–	★		4	98	122	No	1	1
–	–	–	–	–	–	–	–	–	–	–	4	96	85	No	0	1
	–	–	★	–		–	–	–	–	–	4	92	95	No	0	1

***Accreditation Status:** 5=Accredited with commendation or with full standards compliance; 4=Accredited with requirements for improvement; 3=Conditional accreditation.

Detailed Ratings for All Areas

See more information on "Key Ratings for Metro Areas" table beginning on page 32

Blue is most favorable
Bold Italic is least favorable
Blank means neither better nor worse than average
"–" means insufficient data

	Death rates for all selected case types			Hospital outcomes: better (★) or worse (×) than average — Adjusted Death rates — Medical Cases											
	Number of cases	Actual death rate (%)	Adjusted death rate (%) (lower is better)	All selected cases	All selected medical cases	Heart attack	Congestive heart failure	Obstructive pulmonary disease	Pneumonia	Respiratory failure and arrest	Septicemia	Stroke	Gastrointestinal hemorrhage	Fluid, electrolyte, & acid-base disorders	Kidney failure
National Average	–	–	12.1	12.1	14.8	21.2	10.6	6.5	16.9	34.4	25.1	18.4	6.7	11.0	20.9
California *(continued)*															
San Francisco Bay Area *(continued)*															
Santa Clara Valley, San Jose	1,717	18.0	***13.4***	✖	✖		**★**		✖						
Santa Rosa Memorial, Santa Rosa	5,152	12.1	12.8	×	×	**★**	✖					✖			
Sequoia, Redwood City	4,178	10.0	**10.6**	**★**	★	**★**								**★**	
Seton, Daly City	4,560	10.6	**9.8**	**★**	**★**	**★**	★		**★**			**★**			
Sonoma Developmental Center, Eldridge	63	7.9	8.3			–	–	–	–	–	–	–	–	–	–
Sonoma Valley, Sonoma[1]	1,096	12.9	10.8											★	
Stanford Hospital, Stanford[1]	5,422	10.5	11.9							✖					
Summit, Oakland	8,583	11.6	**8.8**	**★**	**★**		**★**	★	**★**	★	**★**	**★**	**★**	**★**	★
Sutter, Santa Rosa	730	15.8	***15.2***	✖	✖	×		–				✖	–	–	
Sutter Delta, Antioch	1,910	14.5	11.8				★	**★**	✖						
Sutter Solano, Vallejo	1,658	16.9	***16.3***	✖	✖		✖		✖		✖	×	✖		
UCSF, San Francisco	2,864	12.9	12.2												
VacaValley, Vacaville[1]	909	20.2	***20.1***	✖	✖	✖		✖	✖	–				✖	–
Valley Care, Pleasanton	–	–	–	–	–	–	–	–	–	–	–	–	–	–	–
Valley Care - Valley Memorial, Livermore[1]	1,772	13.9	11.1		★				★						
Washington, Fremont[1]	4,629	11.0	**10.1**	**★**	**★**	★	**★**								**★**
Other Areas															
Adventist Health Redbud, Clearlake	969	15.2	13.9	×	×	–	✖								–
Arroyo Grande Community, Arroyo Grande	1,379	13.6	***14.3***	✖	✖		✖	✖		×				✖	
Bakersfield Heart, Bakersfield	506	8.1	9.1	★	★			–	★	–	–		–	–	–
Bakersfield Memorial, Bakersfield	4,563	13.1	12.3			**★**		×							
Barton, South Lake Tahoe	1,166	8.7	11.6								–		–		–
Biggs - Gridley, Gridley	587	9.5	10.6					★			–		–	–	–
Central Valley General, Hanford	842	16.2	***16.3***	✖	✖		×	✖	✖	–		✖	–		
Chowchilla District, Chowchilla	115	13.0	14.1			–	–	–		–	–	–	–	–	–
Coalinga Regional, Coalinga	231	12.6	13.0			–		–		–	–	–	–	–	–
Colusa Community, Colusa	450	11.3	12.8			–				–			–	–	–
Community, Clovis	1,279	17.8	***16.0***	✖	✖		✖		✖			✖			–
Community, Fresno	6,856	15.7	12.6							✖					
Community, Monterey	4,731	10.7	***13.5***	✖	✖	×		✖		×		✖			
Community of San Buenaventura, Ventura	4,268	10.8	***13.3***	✖	✖			×	✖						
Corcoran District, Corcoran	237	5.9	8.1			–	–	–		–	–	–	–	–	–
Dameron, Stockton[1]	3,570	14.6	***14.6***	✖	✖		✖		✖		✖	✖		×	

Footnotes are on page 350.

Hospital outcomes: better (★) or worse (✕) than average											Results of accreditation review on full survey		Other facts			
Adjusted Death rates			Adjusted Adverse outcome rates													
Surgical cases			Surgical cases													
All selected surgical cases	Coronary artery bypass surgery	Large bowel surgery	All selected surgical cases	Coronary artery bypass surgery	Large bowel surgery	Gall bladder removal	Total knee replacement	Total hip replacement	Simple prostatectomy	Carotid endarterectomy	Accreditation status*	Overall evaluation score (higher is better)	Number of beds	Major medical school affiliation?	Number of residents	Computerized drug order system (1 to 5 scale, higher is preferred; see page 23 for details)
2.3	3.8	6.5	7.7	10.3	11.9	7.5	6.7	6.4	5.4	8.2	–	91	161	–	–	–
–	–	–	★	–	–	–	–	–	–	–	4	**84**	377	**Yes**	128	2
	✖			✖					–	★	4	**86**	225	No	8	4
★		★	★	★				★		★	4	**88**	201	No	0	2
								–	✖		4	90	164	No	13	1
–	–	–	–	–	–	–	–	–	–	–	–[2]	–[2]	917	No	28	–
–	–	–		–		–	–	–	–	–	–[2]	–[2]	34	No	0	2
	✖		✖	✖	✖		✖				4	92	417	**Yes**	566	**5**
★		★	★		★						3	**77**	420	No	39	2
–	–	–	–	–	–	–	–	–	–	–	4	**94**	114	No	2	2
	–	–		–		–	–	–	–	–	4	93	111	No	4	2
–	–	–		–	–	–	–	–	–	–	4	**94**	102	No	0	2
						–		–	–		4	89	661	**Yes**	0	3
–	–	–	–	–	–	–	–	–	–	–	4	**96**	43	No	0	1
–	–	–	–	–	–	–	–	–	–	–	–[2]	–[2]	68	–	0	–
✖	–	–		–		–	–	–	–	–	4	**86**	110	No	3	4
								✖			4	**83**	279	**Yes**	0	1
–	–	–		–		–	–	–	–	–	4	**94**	40	No	0	–
	–	–		–		–	–	–	–	–	3	**83**	30	No	1	1
		–	★	★	–	–	–	–	–	–	4	**86**	47	No	–	1
							✕	–	✕		4	**87**	275	No	0	2
	–	–		–		–		–	–	–	5	93	81	No	0	1
–	–	–	–	–	–	–	–	–	–	–	–[2]	–[2]	55	No	0	–
–	–	–	–	–	–	–	–	–	–	–	4	**87**	40	No	0	–
–	–	–	–	–	–	–	–	–	–	–	–[2]	–[2]	23	No	0	–
–	–	–	–	–	–	–	–	–	–	–	–[2]	–[2]	24	No	0	1
–	–	–	–	–	–	–	–	–	–	–	3	**81**	38	No	0	–
✖	–	✖		–	✕	–	–	–	–	–	5	**99**	143	No	2	4
			★				★				4	**96**	375	No	37	4
	–			–		✖			–		5	93	197	No	0	1
						✕	✕		★		4	91	179	No	0	1
–	–	–	–	–	–	–	–	–	–	–	–[2]	–[2]	32	**Yes**	0	–
								–	–		4	**83**	188	No	5	1

***Accreditation Status:** 5=Accredited with commendation or with full standards compliance; 4=Accredited with requirements for improvement; 3=Conditional accreditation.

Detailed Ratings for All Areas

See more information on "Key Ratings for Metro Areas" table beginning on page 32

Blue is most favorable
Bold Italic is least favorable
Blank means neither better nor worse than average
"–" means insufficient data

	Death rates for all selected case types			Hospital outcomes: better (★) or worse (×) than average — Adjusted Death rates — Medical Cases											
	Number of cases	Actual death rate (%)	Adjusted death rate (%) (lower is better)	All selected cases	All selected medical cases	Heart attack	Congestive heart failure	Obstructive pulmonary disease	Pneumonia	Respiratory failure and arrest	Septicemia	Stroke	Gastrointestinal hemorrhage	Fluid, electrolyte, & acid-base disorders	Kidney failure
National Average	–	–	12.1	12.1	14.8	21.2	10.6	6.5	16.9	34.4	25.1	18.4	6.7	11.0	20.9
California *(continued)*															
Other Areas *(continued)*															
Delano Regional, Delano	1,278	13.7	12.8										–	✖	–
Doctors, Manteca	1,227	13.2	11.6							–			–		
Doctors, Modesto	5,719	13.4	12.6										×		✖
Dominican, Santa Cruz	4,389	13.9	12.8	×	×	★		✖	✖					×	
El Centro Regional, El Centro	2,302	11.3	11.4												
Emanuel, Turlock	2,666	15.1	***15.7***	✖	✖	×			✖	×					
Enloe, Chico	5,678	11.3	***12.9***	✖	✖			✖	✖						
Fairchild, Yreka	871	11.4	***15.1***	✖	✖	–	✖	–			–		–	–	
Feather River, Paradise	2,417	13.0	12.4												✖
Frank R Howard, Willits	649	10.6	11.4					–		–				–	–
Fremont, Yuba City[1]	2,941	8.9	11.3										★	★	
French, San Luis Obispo	1,595	9.5	13.4		×			–					✖		–
General, Eureka	844	14.1	12.8					–					–	–	
George L Mee, King City	390	7.7	9.1			–		–		–	–	–	–	–	–
Glenn, Willows	182	17.6	***19.0***	✖	✖	–	–	–	✖	–	–	–	–	–	–
Goleta Valley Cottage, Santa Barbara	543	14.4	***15.0***	✖	✖		×	–		–			–	–	–
Good Samaritan, Bakersfield	277	6.5	9.0			–	–	–		–	–	–	–	–	–
Hanford Community, Hanford	1,904	14.3	***13.9***	✖	✖						✖	×	✖		
Hazel Hawkins, Hollister	851	12.0	12.8					✖		–			–		–
Indian Valley, Greenville[1]	166	12.0	14.3			–	–	–	–	–	–	–	–	–	–
Jerold Phelps - Southern Humboldt, Garberville[1]	153	13.1	9.9			–	–	–			–	–	–	–	–
John C Fremont, Mariposa	255	11.4	13.9			–		–		–	–	–	–	–	–
Kaiser Permanente, Fresno	1,904	11.3	12.4			★			×						
Kaweah Delta, Visalia[1]	6,608	13.7	***13.4***	✖	✖	★	✖	✖	✖					✖	
Kern, Bakersfield	524	17.4	13.9					–		✖			–		
Kern Valley, Lake Isabella	596	13.9	13.4			–		✖			–		–		–
Kingsburg Medical Center, Kingsburg	102	4.9	5.3	★	★	–	–	–	–	–	–	–	–	–	–
Lassen, Susanville	381	12.3	14.0			–		–		✖	–	–	–	–	–
Lodi Memorial, Lodi[1]	3,094	13.8	***13.8***	✖	✖				✖			×	×		×
Lompoc Healthcare, Lompoc	683	13.3	***16.1***	✖	✖		×	–	✖		–		–		–
Los Robles Regional, Thousand Oaks	4,399	10.1	9.9	★	★	★			★		★	★			
Mad River, Arcata	1,190	11.8	13.0										–	★	–
Madera Community, Madera	1,820	15.2	***14.1***	✖	✖						✖			✖	
Marian, Santa Maria	3,706	13.2	***13.8***	✖	✖		×	✖	✖						

Footnotes are on page 350.

Hospital outcomes: better (★) or worse (×) than average											Results of accreditation review on full survey		Other facts			
Adjusted Death rates			Adjusted Adverse outcome rates													
Surgical cases			Surgical cases													
All selected surgical cases	Coronary artery bypass surgery	Large bowel surgery	All selected surgical cases	Coronary artery bypass surgery	Large bowel surgery	Gall bladder removal	Total knee replacement	Total hip replacement	Simple prostatectomy	Carotid endarterectomy	Accreditation status*	Overall evaluation score (higher is better)	Number of beds	Major medical school affiliation?	Number of residents	Computerized drug order system (1 to 5 scale, higher is preferred; see page 23 for details)
2.3	3.8	6.5	7.7	10.3	11.9	7.5	6.7	6.4	5.4	8.2	–	91	161	–	–	–
–	–	–		–	–	–	–	–	–	–	4	91	156	No	3	1
–	–	–		–	–	–	–	–	–	–	4	89	73	No	0	1
✖											4	**85**	392	No	0	1
						✖			–		4	89	234	No	0	2
	–	–		–				–		–	4	**84**	107	No	0	–
	–	–		–		✖	–	–	–		–[2]	–[2]	125	No	0	1
			★			×	★			★	4	**86**	291	No	0	3
–	–	–	★	–	–	–	–	–	–	–	4	**96**	20	No	0	–
	–	–	★	–		–		–	–		4	**96**	43	No	0	1
–	–	–		–	–	–	–	–	–	–	4	91	28	No	0	–
	–			–		×					4	91	90	No	0	1
		–	★		★	–	×	★	–		4	**87**	124	No	1	1
–	–	–		–	–	–	–	–	–		–[2]	–[2]	66	No	0	–
–	–	–	–	–	–	–	–	–	–	–	5	**97**	42	No	0	–
–	–	–	–	–	–	–	–	–	–	–	–[2]	–[2]	27	No	0	–
–	–	–		–	–	–	–	–	–	–	4	93	79	No	0	1
–	–	–	–	–	–	–	–	–	–	–	–[2]	–[2]	64	No	0	1
	–	–		–			–	–	–	–	4	**87**	40	No	2	–
	–	–	★	–		–	–	–	–	–	4	**98**	20	No	0	–
–	–	–	–	–	–	–	–	–	–	–	–[2]	–[2]	7	No	0	–
–	–	–	–	–	–	–	–	–	–	–	–[2]	–[2]	18	No	0	–
–	–	–	–	–	–	–	–	–	–	–	–[2]	–[2]	18	No	0	–
	–	–	★	–	★			–	–	–	4	91	121	No	0	2
					✖	✖		✖		★	4	89	206	No	0	1
–	–	–	–	–	–	–	–	–	–	–	4	**95**	171	No	90	1
–	–	–	–	–	–	–	–	–	–	–	–[2]	–[2]	27	No	0	–
–	–	–	–	–	–	–	–	–	–	–	–[2]	–[2]	35	No	0	1
–	–	–	–	–	–	–	–	–	–	–	–[2]	–[2]	28	No	0	–
	–		★	–	★		★				4	89	139	No	0	2
–	–	–	★	–	–	–	–	–	–	–	4	**87**	60	No	2	1
	✖			✖					★		4	93	213	No	0	3
✖	–	–		–		–	–	–	–	–	4	**84**	78	No	0	–
×	–	–		–			–	–	–	–	4	**96**	100	No	0	1
				★	✖				–		4	**95**	132	No	0	2

***Accreditation Status:** 5=Accredited with commendation or with full standards compliance; 4=Accredited with requirements for improvement; 3=Conditional accreditation.

Detailed Ratings for All Areas

See more information on "Key Ratings for Metro Areas" table beginning on page 32

Blue is most favorable
Bold Italic is least favorable
Blank means neither better nor worse than average
"–" means insufficient data

	Death rates for all selected case types			Hospital outcomes: better (★) or worse (×) than average											
				Adjusted Death rates											
				Medical Cases											
	Number of cases	Actual death rate (%)	Adjusted death rate (%) (lower is better)	All selected cases	All selected medical cases	Heart attack	Congestive heart failure	Obstructive pulmonary disease	Pneumonia	Respiratory failure and arrest	Septicemia	Stroke	Gastrointestinal hemorrhage	Fluid, electrolyte, & acid-base disorders	Kidney failure
National Average	–	–	12.1	12.1	14.8	21.2	10.6	6.5	16.9	34.4	25.1	18.4	6.7	11.0	20.9
California *(continued)*															
Other Areas *(continued)*															
Mark Twain St Joseph's, San Andreas	1,076	13.8	***14.1***	✖	✖									★	–
Marshall, Placerville	2,213	11.5	12.6							✖			★		
Mayers, Fall River Mills[1]	296	14.2	***17.7***	✖	✖	–		–	✖	–	–	–	–	✖	–
Memorial, Los Banos[1]	823	16.8	13.8	×	×				×	✖				–	
Memorial, Modesto[1]	3,933	13.2	11.8												
Mendocino Coast, Fort Bragg	885	16.2	***16.3***	✖	✖	×	✖	–	×	×				✖	–
Mercy, Bakersfield[1]	4,230	14.7	12.2												
Mercy, Mt Shasta	931	10.6	11.6					–					–	–	
Mercy, Redding	4,442	13.6	***14.8***	✖	✖		✖	✖	✖	✖					
Mercy Hospital and Health Services, Merced[1]	2,609	12.6	10.0	★	★				★			★		★	★
Mercy Medical Center, Merced	1,551	14.1	12.9				✖								
Mercy Westside, Taft	192	14.6	***17.8***	✖	✖	–	–	–	×	–	–	–	–	✖	–
Modoc, Alturas	146	13.7	11.9			–	–	–		–	–	–	–	–	–
Natividad, Salinas	594	10.8	11.3			–		–					–	–	–
Northern Inyo, Bishop	566	12.0	12.2					–		–			–		–
Oak Valley, Oakdale	905	13.8	12.4					–							
Ojai Valley, Ojai	530	18.3	***15.4***	✖	✖			–				✖	–	✖	–
Oroville Hospital, Oroville	2,791	12.5	12.5			✖	✖							★	
Pioneers, Brawley	1,291	10.9	10.3	★	★							★		★	
Plumas, Quincy	335	10.4	10.5			–		–		–	–	–	–	–	–
Redding Medical Center, Redding	5,719	9.0	11.3			★	✖	×				★			
Redwood, Fortuna	1,033	14.0	***14.8***	✖	✖	×		✖		–		✖		–	–
Rideout, Marysville	3,203	15.0	13.0	×	✖			×				✖	★		
Ridgecrest Regional, Ridgecrest	878	13.3	***16.2***	✖	✖	✖					–	×	×		–
St Agnes, Fresno	11,244	12.2	***12.9***	✖	✖		✖	✖	✖						
St Dominic's, Manteca	429	17.9	***17.2***	✖	✖	✖		–				–	–	✖	–
St Elizabeth, Red Bluff	2,072	11.9	11.4							×					
St Francis, Santa Barbara	1,056	11.0	12.5										–		–
St John's Pleasant Valley, Camarillo	1,378	15.2	12.2							×				★	
St John's Regional, Oxnard	3,324	12.1	10.6	★	★	★	★				★				
St Joseph, Eureka	2,220	11.2	12.7					✖		✖					
St Joseph's, Stockton	7,036	12.5	11.8			★									
Salinas Valley, Salinas[1]	5,393	8.9	10.2	★	★	★	★				★				
San Joaquin, Bakersfield	4,599	12.7	***13.0***	✖	✖				✖				✖		

Footnotes are on page 350.

Hospital outcomes: better (★) or worse (×) than average											Results of accreditation review on full survey		Other facts			
Adjusted Death rates			Adjusted Adverse outcome rates													
Surgical cases			Surgical cases													
All selected surgical cases	Coronary artery bypass surgery	Large bowel surgery	All selected surgical cases	Coronary artery bypass surgery	Large bowel surgery	Gall bladder removal	Total knee replacement	Total hip replacement	Simple prostatectomy	Carotid endarterectomy	Accreditation status*	Overall evaluation score (higher is better)	Number of beds	Major medical school affiliation?	Number of residents	Computerized drug order system (1 to 5 scale, higher is preferred; see page 23 for details)
2.3	3.8	6.5	7.7	10.3	11.9	7.5	6.7	6.4	5.4	8.2	–	91	161	–	–	–
–	–	–	★	–	–	–	–	–	–	–	4	97	30	No	0	–
	–			–				–			4	82	100	No	0	–
–	–	–	–	–	–	–	–	–	–	–	–[2]	–[2]	22	No	0	1
–	–	–	–	–	–	–	–	–	–	–	4	85	48	No	2	2
				★					–		4	91	296	No	15	2
–	–	–		–	–	–	–	–	–	–	4	84	54	No	0	–
✖	–	×		–	✖	✖	★		–	–	4	87	372	No	0	2
★	–	–	★	–	★	–	–	–	–	–	4	93	33	No	0	–
	★								★		4	92	202	No	25	2
	–			–				★		–	4	92	101	No	3	2
	–	–		–		–	–	–	–	–	4	79	158	No	4	2
–	–	–	–	–	–	–	–	–	–	–	4	89	21	No	0	2
–	–	–	–	–	–	–	–	–	–	–	–[2]	–[2]	87	No	0	–
–	–	–	–	–	–	–	–	–	–	–	4	96	129	Yes	6	1
–	–	–	★	–	–	–	–	–	–	–	4	90	30	No	0	–
–	–	–		–	–	–	–	–	–	–	4	87	33	No	0	–
–	–	–	–	–	–	–	–	–	–	–	4	88	38	No	0	1
	–		★	–			–	–	–	–	–[2]	–[2]	100	No	0	1
	–	–		–			–	–	–	–	4	87	99	No	0	–
–	–	–	–	–	–	–	–	–	–	–	4	92	18	No	0	–
★	★		★	★			★	★	–		4	86	188	No	0	1
–	–	–		–		–	–	–	–	–	4	93	35	No	0	–
★	–			–			–	–		–	–[2]	–[2]	78	No	0	1
–	–	–		–	–	–	–	–	–	–	4	93	80	No	0	2
			★			★			★	★	4	96	326	No	0	2
–	–	–	–	–	–	–	–	–	–	–	4	95	77	No	0	2
	–	–		–				–		–	4	92	61	No	0	–
	–	–	★	–	–	–	★		–	–	4	87	70	No	0	1
	–		★	–		–	–	–	–	–	4	82	180	No	0	5
								✖	–		–[2]	–[2]	230	No	0	5
	–	–	★		★	–	★		–		4	87	96	No	0	–
				★		×	✖		★		4	90	248	No	0	2
★			★	★						★	5	97	172	No	11	1
			★	★				–		★	4	91	178	No	6	1

***Accreditation Status:** 5=Accredited with commendation or with full standards compliance; 4=Accredited with requirements for improvement; 3=Conditional accreditation.

Detailed Ratings for All Areas

See more information on "Key Ratings for Metro Areas" table beginning on page 32

Blue is most favorable
Bold Italic is least favorable
Blank means neither better nor worse than average
"–" means insufficient data

	Death rates for all selected case types			Hospital outcomes: better (★) or worse (×) than average — Adjusted Death rates — Medical Cases											
	Number of cases	Actual death rate (%)	Adjusted death rate (%) (lower is better)	All selected cases	All selected medical cases	Heart attack	Congestive heart failure	Obstructive pulmonary disease	Pneumonia	Respiratory failure and arrest	Septicemia	Stroke	Gastrointestinal hemorrhage	Fluid, electrolyte, & acid-base disorders	Kidney failure
National Average	–	–	12.1	12.1	14.8	21.2	10.6	6.5	16.9	34.4	25.1	18.4	6.7	11.0	20.9
California *(continued)*															
Other Areas *(continued)*															
San Joaquin General, French Camp	747	14.3	***15.2***	✖	✖	✖		–	✖	–	✖		–		–
San Luis Obispo General, San Luis Obispo	88	17.0	15.9			–	–	–	–	–	–	–	–	–	–
Sanger General, Sanger	230	13.5	14.6			–		–	×	–	–	–	–	–	–
Santa Barbara Cottage, Santa Barbara	4,120	8.8	11.3												
Santa Paula Memorial, Santa Paula	546	16.5	***15.9***	✖	✖			–	✖	–		✖		★	–
Santa Ynez Valley Cottage, Solvang	209	9.6	8.6			–	–	–			–		–	–	–
Selma Community, Selma	785	18.6	***15.1***	✖	✖			–		–		✖	–		
Seneca, Chester	222	11.3	14.2			–	–	–		–	–	–	–	–	–
Sierra - Kings, Reedley	444	12.8	12.7			–		–		–	–		–		–
Sierra Nevada, Grass Valley	4,031	10.2	9.6	★	★				★			★	★	★	
Sierra View, Porterville	2,870	15.1	***14.5***	✖	✖			×	✖	✖					
Sierra Vista Regional, San Luis Obispo	1,673	11.2	***13.8***	✖	✖	✖		✖		✖					
Simi Valley Hospital, Simi Valley[1]	1,670	14.3	7.6	★	★		★		★	★	★	★		★	
Sonora Community, Sonora	1,791	10.2	9.4	★	★		★		★	★	★			★	
Southern Inyo, Lone Pine[1]	51	9.8	11.0			–	–	–	–	–	–	–	–	–	–
Surprise Valley, Cedarville	63	11.1	9.6			–	–	–	–	–	–	–	–	–	–
Sutter, Davis	968	15.3	***14.0***	✖	✖	✖		–			×	✖		–	–
Sutter, Roseville	4,219	14.2	12.5						×		✖				
Sutter, Tracy	1,074	11.7	12.0					✖					–		
Sutter Amador, Jackson	1,490	10.6	11.9			✖			★				★		–
Sutter Auburn Faith, Auburn	2,646	11.8	***13.9***	✖	✖	✖	×								
Sutter Coast, Crescent City	1,776	13.7	***14.0***	✖	✖				✖	✖					
Sutter Lakeside, Lakeport	1,495	12.4	13.4												
Sutter Maternity and Surgery Center, Santa Cruz	289	2.4	10.3			–	–	–	–	–	–	–	–	–	–
Tahoe Forest, Truckee	542	5.7	7.8	★	★	–		–		–			–	–	–
Trinity, Weaverville	360	12.2	15.6	×	×	–	–	✖		–	–	–	–	–	–
Tulare District, Tulare[1]	2,107	13.5	13.3	×	×	✖									
Tuolumne General, Sonora	676	13.5	14.0		×			–			★		–		–
Twin Cities, Templeton	2,112	12.4	12.9					✖							
Ukiah Valley, Ukiah[1]	1,829	12.8	13.1					★							
Ventura County, Ventura	430	14.2	***16.6***	✖	✖	–		✖		–	–	✖	–	–	
Watsonville Community, Watsonville	1,691	12.9	11.8										✖		
Woodland Memorial, Woodland[1]	1,566	13.5	12.7					★				×			

Footnotes are on page 350.

Hospital outcomes: better (★) or worse (×) than average											Results of accreditation review on full survey		Other facts			
Adjusted Death rates			Adjusted Adverse outcome rates													
Surgical cases			Surgical cases													
All selected surgical cases	Coronary artery bypass surgery	Large bowel surgery	All selected surgical cases	Coronary artery bypass surgery	Large bowel surgery	Gall bladder removal	Total knee replacement	Total hip replacement	Simple prostatectomy	Carotid endarterectomy	Accreditation status*	Overall evaluation score (higher is better)	Number of beds	Major medical school affiliation?	Number of residents	Computerized drug order system (1 to 5 scale, higher is preferred; see page 23 for details)
2.3	3.8	6.5	7.7	10.3	11.9	7.5	6.7	6.4	5.4	8.2	–	91	161	–	–	–
–	–	–	–	–	–	–	–	–	–	–	4	93	181	No	11	1
–	–	–	–	–	–	–	–	–	–	–	4	**84**	46	No	0	1
–	–	–	–	–	–	–	–	–	–	–	–[2]	–[2]	39	No	0	1
				×						★	4	**95**	295	**Yes**	43	4
–	–	–	–	–	–	–	–	–	–	–	4	**81**	34	No	0	1
–	–	–	–	–	–	–	–	–	–	–	4	**94**	20	No	0	1
–	–	–	–	–	–	–	–	–	–	–	4	92	47	No	0	1
–	–	–	–	–	–	–	–	–	–	–	–[2]	–[2]	10	No	0	–
–	–	–	–	–	–	–	–	–	–	–	4	**82**	39	No	0	–
	–			–			×			–	4	**94**	48	No	0	–
×	–	–	★	–		–		–	★	–	–[2]	–[2]	120	No	0	1
	–			–			–	–	–	–	4	91	160	No	1	1
–	–	–	★	–	–	–	–	–	–	–	4	91	225	No	10	1
	–	–		–				–	–	–	4	**98**	50	No	0	–
–	–	–	–	–	–	–	–	–	–	–	–[2]	–[2]	4	No	0	–
–	–	–	–	–	–	–	–	–	–	–	–[2]	–[2]	4	No	0	–
	–	–		–	★	–		–	–	–	4	91	48	No	1	2
	–			–			★				4	90	183	No	8	2
–	–	–		–	–	–	–	–	–	–	4	91	59	No	0	4
	–	–	★	–		–	★	–		–	4	**95**	85	No	0	2
	–			–		–			★	–	4	90	105	No	2	2
	–	–	★	–			★	–	–	–	4	93	59	No	0	2
	–	–		–		–		×	–	–	–[2]	–[2]	54	No	0	2
–	–	–		–	–	–	–	–	–	–	4	**94**	30	No	0	2
–	–	–	★	–	–	–	–	–	–	–	4	**84**	35	No	0	–
–	–	–	–	–	–	–	–	–	–	–	–[2]	–[2]	39	No	0	–
–	–	–		–		–	–	–	–	–	3	**87**	100	No	0	1
–	–	–	–	–	–	–	–	–	–	–	4	**83**	44	No	0	–
	–	–		–				–	–	–	4	**81**	72	No	0	–
	–	–	★	–		–	–	–	★	–	4	93	85	No	0	–
–	–	–	–	–	–	–	–	–	–	–	4	**83**	162	**Yes**	3	1
	–			–		–		–	–	–	4	**88**	117	No	1	1
	–	–		–		–	–	–	–	–	4	93	103	No	3	2

***Accreditation Status:** 5=Accredited with commendation or with full standards compliance; 4=Accredited with requirements for improvement; 3=Conditional accreditation.

Detailed Ratings for All Areas

See more information on "Key Ratings for Metro Areas" table beginning on page 32

Blue is most favorable
Bold Italic is least favorable
Blank means neither better nor worse than average
"–" means insufficient data

	Death rates for all selected case types				Hospital outcomes: better (★) or worse (×) than average — Adjusted Death rates — Medical Cases										
	Number of cases	Actual death rate (%)	Adjusted death rate (%) (lower is better)	All selected cases	All selected medical cases	Heart attack	Congestive heart failure	Obstructive pulmonary disease	Pneumonia	Respiratory failure and arrest	Septicemia	Stroke	Gastrointestinal hemorrhage	Fluid, electrolyte, & acid-base disorders	Kidney failure
National Average	–	–	12.1	12.1	14.8	21.2	10.6	6.5	16.9	34.4	25.1	18.4	6.7	11.0	20.9
Colorado															
Denver Area															
Centura St Anthony Central, Denver	4,161	16.6	***13.6***	✖	✖				✖	✖			✖		
Centura St Anthony North, Westminster	1,520	14.1	13.4	×						✖			✖		
Children's, Denver	–	–	–	–	–	–	–	–	–	–	–	–	–	–	–
Denver Health, Denver[1]	983	10.5	10.6				★								**★**
Exempla Lutheran, Wheat Ridge	4,621	12.1	***13.2***	✖	✖	★	✖	✖		✖					
Exempla St Joseph, Denver	6,346	9.6	***13.5***	✖	✖		✖	✖	✖				✖	×	
Littleton Adventist, Littleton[1]	–	–	–	–	–	–	–	–	–	–	–	–	–	–	–
Medical Center of Aurora, Aurora	3,303	14.1	11.8			**★**									
National Jewish, Denver	73	4.1	7.9			–	–	–	–	–	–	–	–	–	–
North Suburban, Thornton	1,588	16.6	***14.7***	✖	✖	×									
Platte Valley, Brighton	624	15.9	11.2												–
Porter Adventist, Denver[1]	5,171	11.8	12.1			★						✖			
Presbyterian - St Luke's, Denver	3,700	10.7	11.7						★	★			×		
Rose, Denver	3,076	10.9	11.8							**★**					
Swedish, Englewood	3,964	12.1	11.7								**★**				
University of Colorado, Denver	1,534	9.9	10.8			**★**				✖					
Other Areas															
Arkansas Valley Regional, La Junta	1,573	11.4	11.0								**★**				
Aspen Valley, Aspen[1]	121	2.5	**3.5**	**★**	**★**	–	–	–	–	–	–	–	–	–	–
Avista Adventist, Louisville	579	9.8	10.0			–		–		–	–		–	–	–
Boulder Community, Boulder	2,660	9.8	11.3			★							✖		
Clagett, Rifle[1]	184	12.0	11.6			–	–	–		–	–	–	–	–	–
Colorado Plains, Fort Morgan	896	11.6	10.9							–					–
Community, Grand Junction	992	9.2	11.6				★				–		–		–
Delta County, Delta	1,465	10.4	11.3						**★**		★				–
Estes Park Medical Center, Estes Park	220	10.5	13.1			–	–	–		–	–	–	–	–	–
Gunnison Valley, Gunnison	169	5.3	**6.6**	**★**	**★**	–	–	–	–	–	–	–	–	–	–
Heart of the Rockies Regional, Salida	761	11.0	12.5										–	–	–
Keefe, Cheyenne Wells	93	15.1	18.5	×	×	–	–	–	×	–	–	–	–	–	–
Kit Carson County, Burlington	260	12.7	11.3			–		–		–	–		–	–	–
Kremmling Memorial, Kremmling[1]	69	20.3	***23.9***	✖	✖	–	–	–	✖	–	–	–	–	–	–
Longmont United, Longmont	2,096	11.7	13.4	×	✖			×							
McKee, Loveland	2,218	10.1	12.1					✖						**★**	

Footnotes are on page 350.

Hospital outcomes: better (★) or worse (✕) than average											Results of accreditation review on full survey		Other facts			
Adjusted Death rates			Adjusted Adverse outcome rates													
Surgical cases			Surgical cases													
All selected surgical cases	Coronary artery bypass surgery	Large bowel surgery	All selected surgical cases	Coronary artery bypass surgery	Large bowel surgery	Gall bladder removal	Total knee replacement	Total hip replacement	Simple prostatectomy	Carotid endarterectomy	Accreditation status*	Overall evaluation score (higher is better)	Number of beds	Major medical school affiliation?	Number of residents	Computerized drug order system (1 to 5 scale, higher is preferred; see page 23 for details)
2.3	3.8	6.5	7.7	10.3	11.9	7.5	6.7	6.4	5.4	8.2	–	91	161	–	–	–
								★	✕	–	4	***82***	417	No	41	–
	–	–		–		–	–	–	–	–	–[2]	–[2]	106	No	0	–
–	–	–	–	–	–	–	–	–	–	–	4	**94**	198	–	7	–
–	–	–	–	–	–	–	–	–	–	–	4	90	303	**Yes**	157	–
			★			★		★	–	★	4	91	359	No	0	–
★			★	★					–		4	92	480	No	105	–
–	–	–	–	–	–	–	–	–	–	–	4	***86***	129	–	0	–
	–					★		–	–	–	4	93	334	No	6	3
–	–	–	–	–	–	–	–	–	–	–	5	**98**	24	No	0	–
✖	–	–		–		–	–	–	–	–	4	**94**	125	No	1	–
–	–	–	–	–	–	–	–	–	–	–	4	92	49	No	0	–
									–	✖	4	***86***	292	No	4	–
							★	✖	–		4	***88***	442	No	7	–
	✖							★	–	–	4	92	250	No	7	2
★	–	★	★	★	★	★		★	★	–	5	**94**	349	No	8	3
	–	–		✕	–	–		–	–	–	–[2]	–[2]	332	**Yes**	0	–
	–	–		–	–	–	–	–	★	–	–[2]	–[2]	67	No	0	–
–	–	–	–	–	–	–	–	–	–	–	–[2]	–[2]	41	No	0	–
–	–	–		–	–	–	–	–	–	–	4	***88***	58	No	0	–
★		★					★		–	–	4	89	197	No	0	–
–	–	–	–	–	–	–	–	–	–	–	–[2]	–[2]	75	No	0	–
–	–	–		–	–	–	–	–	–	–	4	***85***	50	No	0	–
	–	–	★	–		–	★	–	–	–	4	91	58	No	0	–
	–	✖		–				–	–	–	4	***87***	44	No	0	–
–	–	–	–	–	–	–	–	–	–	–	–[2]	–[2]	16	No	0	–
–	–	–	–	–	–	–	–	–	–	–	–[2]	–[2]	22	No	0	–
–	–	–		–	–	–	–	–	–	–	–[2]	–[2]	33	No	0	–
–	–	–	–	–	–	–	–	–	–	–	–[2]	–[2]	12	No	0	–
–	–	–	–	–	–	–	–	–	–	–	–[2]	–[2]	24	No	0	–
–	–	–	–	–	–	–	–	–	–	–	–[2]	–[2]	19	No	0	–
	–	–	★	–		–		–	–	–	4	***87***	107	No	0	–
	–			–			✕	★	–	–	4	**95**	92	No	0	–

***Accreditation Status:** 5=Accredited with commendation or with full standards compliance; 4=Accredited with requirements for improvement; 3=Conditional accreditation.

Detailed Ratings for All Areas

See more information on "Key Ratings for Metro Areas" table beginning on page 32

Blue is most favorable
Bold Italic is least favorable
Blank means neither better nor worse than average
"–" means insufficient data

	Death rates for all selected case types			Hospital outcomes: better (★) or worse (×) than average — Adjusted Death rates — Medical Cases											
	Number of cases	Actual death rate (%)	Adjusted death rate (%) (lower is better)	All selected cases	All selected medical cases	Heart attack	Congestive heart failure	Obstructive pulmonary disease	Pneumonia	Respiratory failure and arrest	Septicemia	Stroke	Gastrointestinal hemorrhage	Fluid, electrolyte, & acid-base disorders	Kidney failure
National Average	–	–	12.1	12.1	14.8	21.2	10.6	6.5	16.9	34.4	25.1	18.4	6.7	11.0	20.9
Colorado *(continued)*															
Other Areas *(continued)*															
Memorial, Colorado Springs	5,381	10.9	11.5				★				★	×	✖		
Memorial, Craig	423	11.8	13.7					–		–	–	–	–	–	–
Mercy, Durango	1,270	9.8	10.6			★					★				–
Montrose Memorial, Montrose	1,130	9.3	12.2							–	–	✖	–	–	–
Mt San Rafael, Trinidad	585	11.8	10.4					–	★					–	–
North Colorado, Greeley	4,843	10.2	11.8												
Parkview, Pueblo	3,121	10.1	9.2	★	★	★		★	★		★				★
Penrose - St Francis, Colorado Springs[1]	5,362	9.9	10.6	★	★	★			★		★				
Pioneers Hospital of Rio Blanco, Meeker	162	14.8	***17.9***	✖	✖	–	–	–		–	–	–	–	–	–
Poudre Valley, Fort Collins	4,425	9.9	***13.1***	✖		★		×				×			
Prowers, Lamar	720	12.2	10.0	★	★	–		–	★	–					–
St Mary - Corwin, Pueblo	2,599	13.1	***13.8***	✖	✖										
St Marys, Grand Junction	4,675	8.4	10.8	★	★	★								★	
St Thomas More Centura, Canon City	1,267	12.1	13.5		×	✖								×	–
St Vincent General, Leadville[1]	217	5.5	6.5	★	★	–		–		–	–	–	–	–	–
San Luis Valley Regional, Alamosa	1,033	10.4	13.7					×		–				★	–
Southeast Colorado, Springfield	335	14.0	***15.9***	✖	✖	–		–		–	–	–	–	–	–
Southwest, Cortez[1]	1,073	9.3	10.2	★	★			–						★	
Spanish Peaks Regional, Walsenburg	436	15.4	13.2			–		–		–	✖	–	–	–	–
Sterling Regional, Sterling	976	11.3	***15.5***	✖	✖	✖	✖			–				–	–
Vail Valley, Vail	138	7.2	13.9			–	–	–	–	–	–	–	–	–	–
Valley View, Glenwood Springs[1]	751	13.3	14.0	×				–		✖	–	✖			–
Weisbrod Memorial County, Eads	57	12.3	13.4			–	–	–	–	–	–	–	–	–	–
Yampa Valley, Steamboat Springs	258	5.0	7.6	★	★	–	–	–		–	–	–	–	–	–
Yuma District, Yuma	140	9.3	10.3			–	–	–	–	–	–	–	–	–	–
Connecticut															
Fairfield and New Haven Counties															
Bridgeport Hospital, Bridgeport	5,782	13.6	***13.1***	✖	✖		✖						✖	×	
Danbury Hospital, Danbury	5,833	13.1	10.0	★	★		★		★		★				★
Greenwich Hospital, Greenwich[1]	3,488	11.8	10.6	★	★				★		★				
Griffin, Derby	2,769	15.1	***13.8***	✖	✖							✖	✖	✖	
Hospital of St Raphael, New Haven	11,521	11.1	9.8	★	★	★	★		★	★	★		★		★
Masonic Geriatric, Wallingford	402	18.7	14.7	×	×	–		–	✖	–	–		–		–

Footnotes are on page 350.

Hospital outcomes: better (★) or worse (×) than average											Results of accreditation review on full survey		Other facts			
Adjusted Death rates			Adjusted Adverse outcome rates													
Surgical cases			Surgical cases													
All selected surgical cases	Coronary artery bypass surgery	Large bowel surgery	All selected surgical cases	Coronary artery bypass surgery	Large bowel surgery	Gall bladder removal	Total knee replacement	Total hip replacement	Simple prostatectomy	Carotid endarterectomy	Accreditation status*	Overall evaluation score (higher is better)	Number of beds	Major medical school affiliation?	Number of residents	Computerized drug order system (1 to 5 scale, higher is preferred; see page 23 for details)
2.3	3.8	6.5	7.7	10.3	11.9	7.5	6.7	6.4	5.4	8.2	–	91	161	–	–	–
			★						–		4	93	386	No	0	–
–	–	–	–	–	–	–	–	–	–	–	3	**86**	29	No	0	–
–	–	–	✖	–	–	–	✖	–	–	–	4	**85**	71	No	0	–
	–	–	★	–		–	–	–	–	–	4	**84**	62	No	0	–
–	–	–	–	–	–	–	–	–	–	–	4	93	31	No	0	–
	★								–		4	92	276	No	24	–
		–						★			5	**95**	260	No	0	–
			★					★			4	**85**	384	No	0	–
–	–	–	–	–	–	–	–	–	–	–	–[2]	–[2]	17	No	0	–
×					✖	✖	★			★	–[2]	–[2]	254	No	18	–
–	–	–	–	–	–	–	–	–	–	–	4	**87**	40	No	0	–
✖	–			–			★	×		–	4	91	261	No	10	–
			★				★	★	★		–[2]	–[2]	251	No	21	–
	–	–		–		–		–	–	–	4	**83**	40	No	0	–
–	–	–	–	–	–	–	–	–	–	–	–[2]	–[2]	38	No	0	–
–	–	–		–	–	–	–	–	–	–	4	**85**	85	No	0	–
–	–	–	–	–	–	–	–	–	–	–	–[2]	–[2]	25	No	0	–
✖	–	–		–	–	–	–	–	–	–	4	**97**	42	No	0	–
–	–	–	–	–	–	–	–	–	–	–	–[2]	–[2]	24	No	0	–
✖	–	–		–				–	–	–	4	**86**	36	No	0	–
–	–	–	–	–	–	–	–	–	–	–	4	**97**	49	No	0	–
–	–	–		–	–	–	–	–	–	–	4	93	63	No	0	–
–	–	–	–	–	–	–	–	–	–	–	–[2]	–[2]	8	No	0	–
–	–	–	–	–	–	–	–	–	–	–	4	**96**	74	No	0	–
–	–	–	–	–	–	–	–	–	–	–	–[2]	–[2]	11	No	0	–
			✖	✖			✖				5	**96**	345	**Yes**	–	–
★	–			–					–		5	93	271	**Yes**	57	–
	–			–					–		5	**96**	160	No	22	–
	–		✖	–			✖	–		–	4	92	160	**Yes**	25	–
★			✖	✖	✖		✖	✖			4	92	464	**Yes**	118	–
–	–	–	–	–	–	–	–	–	–	–	4	**97**	35	No	0	–

***Accreditation Status:** 5=Accredited with commendation or with full standards compliance; 4=Accredited with requirements for improvement; 3=Conditional accreditation.

Detailed Ratings for All Areas

See more information on "Key Ratings for Metro Areas" table beginning on page 32

Blue is most favorable
Bold Italic is least favorable
Blank means neither better nor worse than average
"–" means insufficient data

	Death rates for all selected case types				Hospital outcomes: better (★) or worse (×) than average — Adjusted Death rates — Medical Cases											
	Number of cases	Actual death rate (%)	Adjusted death rate (%) (lower is better)	All selected cases	All selected medical cases	Heart attack	Congestive heart failure	Obstructive pulmonary disease	Pneumonia	Respiratory failure and arrest	Septicemia	Stroke	Gastrointestinal hemorrhage	Fluid, electrolyte, & acid-base disorders	Kidney failure
National Average	–	–	12.1	12.1	14.8	21.2	10.6	6.5	16.9	34.4	25.1	18.4	6.7	11.0	20.9
Connecticut *(continued)*															
Fairfield and New Haven Counties *(continued)*															
Midstate, Meriden	3,977	13.9	***15.3***	✖	✖			✖	✖			✖	✖		
Milford Hospital, Milford	2,409	13.2	12.1									✖			
Norwalk Hospital, Norwalk[1]	5,132	11.8	12.3				✖	×				★		★	
St Mary's, Waterbury[1]	4,574	14.9	12.0												
St Vincent's, Bridgeport	7,003	12.2	11.5			★								✖	
Stamford Hospital, Stamford[1]	4,138	12.4	12.9	×				✖						✖	
Waterbury Hospital, Waterbury	5,358	13.8	***13.0***	✖	✖					✖			✖		
Yale - New Haven, New Haven	7,128	10.4	11.6			★						×			
Hartford Area															
Bradley, Southington	1,847	14.3	***13.7***	✖	✖			✖					✖		
Bristol Hospital, Bristol	3,514	13.5	11.6											★	
Connecticut Children's, Hartford	–	–	–	–	–	–	–	–	–	–	–	–	–	–	–
Hartford Hospital, Hartford	11,549	12.7	**11.0**	★	★	★		×	★	✖	★	✖			
Manchester Memorial, Manchester	3,538	13.6	***13.9***	✖	✖				✖				✖		
New Britain General, New Britain	5,980	13.4	**11.1**	★	★								★		
Rockville General, Rockville	1,798	12.5	***13.8***	✖	✖			×							
St Francis, Hartford	9,868	12.0	**11.3**	★		★								✖	★
University of Connecticut - John Dempsey, Farmington	2,131	12.0	10.7	★	★										★
Other Areas															
Charlotte Hungerford, Torrington	3,363	14.7	***13.6***	✖	✖	✖	×		✖						
Day Kimball, Putnam	2,249	10.2	11.0												
Johnson, Stafford Springs	1,948	14.6	***14.4***	✖	✖			✖	✖			×			
Lawrence and Memorial, New London	5,858	12.5	12.5		×		✖			✖	★				
Middlesex, Middletown	4,958	16.0	***16.1***	✖	✖		✖	✖	✖	✖	×	✖	✖	✖	
New Milford Hospital, New Milford	1,546	13.2	10.8						★						
Sharon Hospital, Sharon	1,375	10.9	11.5					✖			★				✖
William W Backus, Norwich	4,358	12.3	12.2										✖		
Windham, Willimantic[1]	2,505	11.8	11.4					×		★		★			
Delaware															
Delaware Valley Area															
Alfred I Dupont Hospital for Children, Wilmington	–	–	–	–	–	–	–	–	–	–	–	–	–	–	–
Christiana, Wilmington	–	–	–	–	–	–	–	–	–	–	–	–	–	–	–
Christiana Care, Newark[1]	14,443	10.8	**10.8**	★	★		★	★	★		★	★			

Footnotes are on page 350.

Hospital outcomes: better (★) or worse (×) than average											Results of accreditation review on full survey		Other facts			
Adjusted Death rates			Adjusted Adverse outcome rates													
Surgical cases			Surgical cases													
All selected surgical cases	Coronary artery bypass surgery	Large bowel surgery	All selected surgical cases	Coronary artery bypass surgery	Large bowel surgery	Gall bladder removal	Total knee replacement	Total hip replacement	Simple prostatectomy	Carotid endarterectomy	Accreditation status*	Overall evaluation score (higher is better)	Number of beds	Major medical school affiliation?	Number of residents	Computerized drug order system (1 to 5 scale, higher is preferred; see page 23 for details)
2.3	3.8	6.5	7.7	10.3	11.9	7.5	6.7	6.4	5.4	8.2	–	91	161	–	–	–
	–			–					–		4	**87**	94	No	0	–
	–			–			–	–	–	–	4	89	51	No	0	–
	–		×	–		✖		★		✖	4	**83**	286	**Yes**	60	–
	–			–	★		★	–	–		4	93	170	**Yes**	58	–
			✖								4	92	291	**Yes**	45	2
	–		✖	–			✖	–		✖	4	**94**	296	**Yes**	60	–
	–		✖	–				✖			4	**86**	247	**Yes**	53	–
★	★				✖			✖			4	**94**	722	**Yes**	478	–
	–	–		–	★	–	–	–	–	–	4	91	74	No	0	–
	–			–			✖	–	–	–	–[2]	–[2]	128	**Yes**	0	–
–	–	–	–	–	–	–	–	–	–	–	–[2]	–[2]	104	–	0	–
★	★								★	★	4	93	770	**Yes**	64	–
	–			–	★			–	–	✖	5	**94**	161	No	0	–
	–			–			✖				4	90	262	No	0	–
	–	–		–		–	–	–	–	✖	4	**94**	50	No	0	–
★	★			★				✖			4	92	545	No	31	–
		–	×		–	–	×		–	–	4	92	128	**Yes**	0	–
	–			–		✖			★		4	**85**	102	No	0	–
★	–	–	★	–		–	–	–	–	–	4	**95**	101	**Yes**	0	–
	–			–			–	–	–	–	4	90	89	No	0	–
★	–			–	★		✖				4	90	228	No	0	–
	–		★	–		★			★		4	89	124	No	24	–
	–	–	★	–		–	–	–	–	–	4	**94**	62	No	0	–
	–	–	★	–		–	★	–	–	–	4	89	85	No	0	–
	–			–			×				4	**95**	164	No	5	–
	–		★	–				–	–	–	4	90	78	No	0	–
–	–	–	–	–	–	–	–	–	–	–	4	**88**	152	–	2	–
–	–	–	–	–	–	–	–	–	–	–	–[2]	–[2]	–	–	–	–
		★	×				✖	×			5	**95**	767	**Yes**	199	–

***Accreditation Status:** 5=Accredited with commendation or with full standards compliance; 4=Accredited with requirements for improvement; 3=Conditional accreditation.

Detailed Ratings for All Areas

See more information on "Key Ratings for Metro Areas" table beginning on page 32

Blue is most favorable
Bold Italic is least favorable
Blank means neither better nor worse than average
"–" means insufficient data

	Death rates for all selected case types				Hospital outcomes: better (★) or worse (×) than average											
					Adjusted Death rates											
					Medical Cases											
	Number of cases	Actual death rate (%)	Adjusted death rate (%) (lower is better)	All selected cases	All selected medical cases	Heart attack	Congestive heart failure	Obstructive pulmonary disease	Pneumonia	Respiratory failure and arrest	Septicemia	Stroke	Gastrointestinal hemorrhage	Fluid, electrolyte, & acid-base disorders	Kidney failure
National Average	–	–	12.1	12.1	14.8	21.2	10.6	6.5	16.9	34.4	25.1	18.4	6.7	11.0	20.9
Delaware *(continued)*															
Delaware Valley Area *(continued)*															
St Francis, Wilmington[1]	4,536	12.8	12.0								✖				
Other Areas															
Bayhealth, Dover	6,031	13.4	***15.2***	✖	✖	×		✖	✖			×	✖	✖	
Beebe, Lewes	4,579	10.5	**10.9**	★	★					★				★	
Nanticoke, Seaford	2,457	11.6	12.1			✖	★					✖	×		
District of Columbia															
Children's National, Washington	–	–	–	–	–	–	–	–	–	–	–	–	–	–	–
Columbia Hospital for Women, Washington	104	–	–	–	–	–	–	–	–	–	–	–	–	–	–
District of Columbia General, Washington	1,152	16.0	12.2									✖			
George Washington University, Washington	2,371	10.4	**10.2**	★	★		★		★	×					
Georgetown University, Washington	2,879	11.3	**9.5**	★	★			★	★			★			
Greater Southeast, Washington	3,317	12.4	**8.6**	★	★		★		★		★	★			
Hadley, Washington	980	9.9	**9.2**	★	★	–	★		★						
Howard University, Washington	3,037	11.5	**7.6**	★	★	★	★	★	★	★	★	★		★	
Providence, Washington	5,677	9.4	**9.2**	★	★	★	★	★	★			★		★	
Sibley, Washington	5,358	8.9	**9.8**	★	★			★	★		★				
Washington Hospital Center, Washington	9,010	8.5	**9.0**	★	★	★	★	★	★		★	★		★	★
Florida															
Brevard, Orange, Seminole, and Volusia Counties															
Atlantic, Daytona Beach	792	15.5	11.5			×						★	✖	–	–
Bert Fish, New Smyrna Beach	2,743	12.3	**10.7**	★	★						★				★
Cape Canaveral, Cocoa Beach	3,655	10.8	**10.5**	★	★			★							
Central Florida Regional, Sanford	3,365	10.2	**8.8**	★	★	★	★		★	★	★				
Florida, Altamonte Springs	–	–	–	–	–	–	–	–	–	–	–	–	–	–	–
Florida, Apopka	–	–	–	–	–	–	–	–	–	–	–	–	–	–	–
Florida, Deland	3,247	14.1	**10.6**	★	★		★					★			
Florida, Orlando	22,027	10.7	**10.6**	★	★	★	★		★			★	★	★	
Florida - East Orlando, Orlando	–	–	–	–	–	–	–	–	–	–	–	–	–	–	–
Florida - Fish Memorial, Orange City	2,872	13.7	10.9	★	★		★								
Halifax, Daytona Beach	7,304	13.0	12.3									✖			
Health Central, Ocoee	2,123	14.6	12.1			✖				✖				★	
Holmes Regional, Melbourne	15,215	11.0	**11.0**	★	★	★									★
Memorial - Ormond Beach, Ormond Beach	5,122	11.9	**10.4**	★	★	★		★			★	★	★		

Footnotes are on page 350.

Hospital outcomes: better (★) or worse (×) than average											Results of accreditation review on full survey		Other facts			
Adjusted Death rates			Adjusted Adverse outcome rates													
Surgical cases			Surgical cases													
All selected surgical cases	Coronary artery bypass surgery	Large bowel surgery	All selected surgical cases	Coronary artery bypass surgery	Large bowel surgery	Gall bladder removal	Total knee replacement	Total hip replacement	Simple prostatectomy	Carotid endarterectomy	Accreditation status*	Overall evaluation score (higher is better)	Number of beds	Major medical school affiliation?	Number of residents	Computerized drug order system (1 to 5 scale, higher is preferred; see page 23 for details)
2.3	3.8	6.5	7.7	10.3	11.9	7.5	6.7	6.4	5.4	8.2	–	91	161	–	–	–
	–		★	–	★	★			✖	★	4	**87**	197	**Yes**	18	–
✖	–	✖	×	–					✖		4	**84**	348	No	0	–
	–		★	–							4	**86**	212	No	8	–
	–	✖	✖	–	✖		–	–	–		4	90	110	No	0	–
–	–	–	–	–	–	–	–	–	–	–	4	92	188	–	111	–
–	–	–		–	–	–	–	–	–	–	3	91	76	No	0	–
–	–	–	–	–	–	–	–	–	–	–	–[2]	–[2]	250	**Yes**	10	–
	–					–		–	–	–	4	91	277	**Yes**	0	–
★						–			–		4	**86**	345	**Yes**	190	–
	–			–		–	–	–	–	–	4	**84**	262	No	7	–
–	–	–	–	–	–	–	–	–	–	–	4	**96**	148	No	1	–
✖	✖	–	✖	✖		–	–	–		–	4	93	285	**Yes**	234	–
	–		✖	–	✖			–	✖	–	4	**94**	304	**Yes**	56	–
★	–	★	✖	–	★		✖	✖		★	4	92	202	**Yes**	0	–
		×	✖	✖	✖				×		4	**95**	791	No	209	–
–	–	–	–	–	–	–	–	–	–	–	4	89	214	No	0	–
	–			–		×	★	★	–	–	4	92	116	No	0	–
	–			–							4	90	125	No	4	–
											–[2]	–[2]	226	No	4	2
–	–	–	–	–	–	–	–	–	–	–	–[2]	–[2]	–	–	–	–
–	–	–	–	–	–	–	–	–	–	–	–[2]	–[2]	–	–	–	–
	–			–				–	–	–	4	91	156	No	0	–
★			★	★							4	**88**	1,352	No	89	–
–	–	–	–	–	–	–	–	–	–	–	–[2]	–[2]	–	–	–	–
	–			–			✖	–	–	–	4	**95**	97	No	0	–
					✖		★		–		4	**94**	475	**Yes**	25	–
–	–	–		–	✖	–	–	–	–	–	4	**95**	132	No	0	–
★										★	4	93	528	No	0	–
			★	★				★	–	★	–[2]	–[2]	188	No	9	–

***Accreditation Status:** 5=Accredited with commendation or with full standards compliance; 4=Accredited with requirements for improvement; 3=Conditional accreditation.

Detailed Ratings for All Areas

See more information on "Key Ratings for Metro Areas" table beginning on page 32

Blue is most favorable
Bold Italic is least favorable
Blank means neither better nor worse than average
"–" means insufficient data

	Death rates for all selected case types			Hospital outcomes: better (★) or worse (×) than average — Adjusted Death rates — Medical Cases											
	Number of cases	Actual death rate (%)	Adjusted death rate (%) (lower is better)	All selected cases	All selected medical cases	Heart attack	Congestive heart failure	Obstructive pulmonary disease	Pneumonia	Respiratory failure and arrest	Septicemia	Stroke	Gastrointestinal hemorrhage	Fluid, electrolyte, & acid-base disorders	Kidney failure
National Average	–	–	12.1	12.1	14.8	21.2	10.6	6.5	16.9	34.4	25.1	18.4	6.7	11.0	20.9
Florida *(continued)*															
Brevard, Orange, Seminole, and Volusia Counties *(continued)*															
Memorial - Peninsula, Ormond Beach	1,502	20.0	***13.5***	✖	✖			✖				✖	×		
Orlando Regional, Orlando[1]	11,376	11.7	**10.8**	**★**	**★**		**★**		**★**			**★**			
Orlando Regional Lucerne, Orlando	–	–	–	–	–	–	–	–	–	–	–	–	–	–	–
Parrish, Titusville	4,779	10.7	**10.8**	**★**	**★**		★		**★**	✖			**★**		
Sand Lake (Orlando Regional), Orlando	–	–	–	–	–	–	–	–	–	–	–	–	–	–	–
Wuesthoff, Rockledge[1]	5,921	10.7	11.2	★	**★**		★					★			**★**
Charlotte, Collier, and Lee Counties															
Bon Secours St Joseph, Port Charlotte	5,293	10.4	**9.9**	**★**	**★**			**★**	★		**★**	**★**	**★**		
Cape Coral Hospital, Cape Coral	6,939	12.5	***12.8***	✖	✖	✖			✖						✖
Charlotte Regional, Punta Gorda	5,312	8.8	**10.3**	**★**	**★**	**★**						**★**			
East Pointe, Lehigh Acres	1,348	14.3	11.9							×					
Fawcett, Port Charlotte	5,916	11.7	12.1												
Gulf Coast, Fort Myers	1,092	11.6	13.1					×				×	–	✖	–
Healthpark, Fort Myers	–	–	–	–	–	–	–	–	–	–	–	–	–	–	–
Lee, Fort Myers[1]	13,185	9.6	11.4	★		**★**				×					✖
Naples Community, Naples	15,344	9.4	**10.9**	**★**	**★**	**★**	**★**				**★**				
Southwest Florida Regional, Fort Myers	7,217	9.6	***13.4***	✖	✖		✖	×							
Hillsborough, Manatee, Pinellas, Polk, and Sarasota Counties															
All Children's, St Petersburg	–	–	–	–	–	–	–	–	–	–	–	–	–	–	–
Bartow Memorial, Bartow	1,185	15.4	***14.6***	✖	✖								✖	–	✖
Bayfront, St Petersburg	3,797	14.0	11.7			✖	★		**★**					✖	
Blake, Bradenton	9,326	12.1	***12.7***	✖	×					✖	**★**			✖	
Bon Secours - Venice, Venice[1]	8,084	11.8	12.5		×		✖	×		✖				×	
Brandon Regional, Brandon	4,338	11.9	**10.0**	**★**	**★**	×	**★**		**★**	**★**	**★**	**★**			
Doctors, Sarasota	4,953	12.9	**10.9**	**★**	**★**		**★**				**★**				**★**
Edward White, St Petersburg	2,369	14.7	**10.7**	**★**	**★**										
Englewood Community, Englewood	3,895	11.3	**10.3**	**★**	**★**					**★**	**★**			★	
H Lee Moffitt Cancer Center, Tampa[1]	551	14.7	14.3	×	✖	–	–	–		–		–			–
Heart of Florida Regional, Davenport	2,314	11.4	12.2				★					✖			
Helen Ellis, Tarpon Springs	4,471	11.8	**10.2**	**★**	**★**			★	**★**		★				★
Lake Wales Medical Center, Lake Wales[1]	1,722	15.0	***13.9***	✖	✖						×			×	×
Lakeland Regional, Lakeland	16,149	10.7	12.0			**★**			✖						×
Largo Medical Center, Largo	6,970	12.3	**10.7**	**★**	**★**	**★**					**★**				

Footnotes are on page 350.

Hospital outcomes: better (★) or worse (×) than average											Results of accreditation review on full survey		Other facts			
Adjusted Death rates			Adjusted Adverse outcome rates													
Surgical cases			Surgical cases													
All selected surgical cases	Coronary artery bypass surgery	Large bowel surgery	All selected surgical cases	Coronary artery bypass surgery	Large bowel surgery	Gall bladder removal	Total knee replacement	Total hip replacement	Simple prostatectomy	Carotid endarterectomy	Accreditation status*	Overall evaluation score (higher is better)	Number of beds	Major medical school affiliation?	Number of residents	Computerized drug order system (1 to 5 scale, higher is preferred; see page 23 for details)
2.3	3.8	6.5	7.7	10.3	11.9	7.5	6.7	6.4	5.4	8.2	–	91	161	–	–	–
–	–	–		–	–	–	–	–	–	–	–[2]	–[2]	119	No	8	–
											4	91	1,183	Yes	146	–
–	–	–	–	–	–	–	–	–	–	–	–[2]	–[2]	267	–	6	–
	–		★	–				★			5	96	210	No	0	–
–	–	–	–	–	–	–	–	–	–	–	–[2]	–[2]	–	–	–	–
							×				4	93	215	No	13	–
	–		★	–						★	4	89	313	No	19	–
	–		★	–						★	–[2]	–[2]	212	No	7	–
	×			×				★		★	4	86	148	No	1	–
	–	–	×	–		×	–	–	–	–	4	92	75	No	0	–
	–		★	–			★			★	4	97	216	No	0	2
	–	–		–		–	–		–	–	4	96	120	No	0	–
–	–	–	–	–	–	–	–	–	–	–	–[2]	–[2]	–	–	–	–
★	★		★	★			★	★			4	88	647	No	82	–
				★			★				4	94	434	No	0	–
×				★							4	92	400	No	9	–
–	–	–	–	–	–	–	–	–	–	–	4	97	216	–	12	–
–	–	–		–	–	–	–	–	–	–	4	82	56	No	0	–
									–		5	96	287	Yes	34	–
	×			×		×	★				4	97	256	No	0	–
★	–	★		–	★	★	×	×			4	86	161	No	0	–
	–			–				–			4	87	255	No	0	–
	–			–					–	★	4	88	147	No	0	–
	–		★	–		–	★	–	–		4	92	124	No	0	2
	–			–							4	93	100	No	1	–
	–	★	★	–		–	–	–	–	–	4	94	117	No	0	–
	–	×		–		–	–	–	–	–	5	98	51	No	0	–
	–			–	★				–		4	96	109	No	0	–
	–	–	★	–			–	–	–	–	–[2]	–[2]	154	No	–	–
★		★			★	×	×				4	95	615	No	0	–
★		★	★	★	★	★				★	5	96	230	No	4	2

***Accreditation Status:** 5=Accredited with commendation or with full standards compliance; 4=Accredited with requirements for improvement; 3=Conditional accreditation.

Detailed Ratings for All Areas

See more information on "Key Ratings for Metro Areas" table beginning on page 32

Blue is most favorable
Bold Italic is least favorable
Blank means neither better nor worse than average
"–" means insufficient data

	Death rates for all selected case types			Hospital outcomes: better (★) or worse (×) than average											
				Adjusted Death rates											
					Medical Cases										
	Number of cases	Actual death rate (%)	Adjusted death rate (%) (lower is better)	All selected cases	All selected medical cases	Heart attack	Congestive heart failure	Obstructive pulmonary disease	Pneumonia	Respiratory failure and arrest	Septicemia	Stroke	Gastrointestinal hemorrhage	Fluid, electrolyte, & acid-base disorders	Kidney failure
National Average	–	–	12.1	12.1	14.8	21.2	10.6	6.5	16.9	34.4	25.1	18.4	6.7	11.0	20.9
Florida *(continued)*															
Hillsborough, Manatee, Pinellas, Polk, and Sarasota Counties *(continued)*															
Manatee, Bradenton	8,503	13.4	***12.7***	✖							✖				
Mease, Dunedin	3,979	14.6	11.9												
Mease Countryside, Safety Harbor	5,086	13.0	12.0						★						
Memorial, Tampa	2,942	13.8	11.6					×	★		★				
Morton Plant Mease, Clearwater	10,946	9.7	10.2	★	★	★			★		★	★			
Northside, St Petersburg[1]	4,520	15.7	11.3	★	★			★	★		★				
Palms of Pasadena, St Petersburg	5,926	9.5	10.0	★	★		★	★		★	★	★	★		
Regency, Winter Haven	–	–	–	–	–	–	–	–	–	–	–	–	–	–	–
St Anthony's, St Petersburg	5,409	13.2	10.1	★	★				★			★		★	
St Joseph's, Tampa	9,735	12.5	10.0	★	★		★		★	★	★	★			★
St Joseph's Women's, Tampa	–	–	–	–	–	–	–	–	–	–	–	–	–	–	–
St Petersburg Medical Center, St Petersburg	2,492	16.2	11.3		★			★	★						★
Sarasota Memorial, Sarasota	15,481	10.6	11.7			★		✖					×	×	
South Bay, Sun City Center	3,639	13.1	11.4						★						
South Florida Baptist, Plant City	1,699	11.7	10.8		★		★				★				
Sun Coast, Largo	–	–	–	–	–	–	–	–	–	–	–	–	–	–	–
Tampa General, Tampa	3,069	10.2	11.9												
Town and Country, Tampa	1,476	12.9	12.3			✖									–
University, Tampa	5,085	14.2	11.4		★						★				
University - Carrollwood, Tampa	1,251	14.5	11.0			✖			★						–
Winter Haven Hospital, Winter Haven	9,307	11.2	12.1				★					★			✖
South Florida															
Aventura Hospital, Aventura	5,632	18.4	12.0						★			✖			
Baptist, Miami	6,362	11.8	9.4	★	★		★		★	★		★		★	
Bethesda, Boynton Beach	6,091	14.7	11.4				★							✖	
Boca Raton Community, Boca Raton	12,211	12.0	10.4	★	★		★		★	★	★	★	★		
Broward General, Fort Lauderdale	2,175	13.8	10.8	★	★										
Cedars, Miami	7,277	11.2	9.9	★	★	★	★		★	★		★			★
Cleveland Clinic, Fort Lauderdale	2,098	11.4	11.0					★							
Columbia, West Palm Beach	1,599	20.5	12.3								★				
Coral Gables Hospital, Coral Gables	4,229	10.9	10.0	★	★			★	★	★	★	★			
Coral Springs Medical Center, Coral Springs	1,448	12.8	10.9		★								–		
Delray Medical Center, Delray Beach	8,450	10.7	10.0	★	★	★	★		★		★				

Footnotes are on page 350.

Hospital outcomes: better (★) or worse (×) than average											Results of accreditation review on full survey		Other facts			
Adjusted Death rates			Adjusted Adverse outcome rates													
Surgical cases			Surgical cases													
All selected surgical cases	Coronary artery bypass surgery	Large bowel surgery	All selected surgical cases	Coronary artery bypass surgery	Large bowel surgery	Gall bladder removal	Total knee replacement	Total hip replacement	Simple prostatectomy	Carotid endarterectomy	Accreditation status*	Overall evaluation score (higher is better)	Number of beds	Major medical school affiliation?	Number of residents	Computerized drug order system (1 to 5 scale, higher is preferred; see page 23 for details)
2.3	3.8	6.5	7.7	10.3	11.9	7.5	6.7	6.4	5.4	8.2	–	91	161	–	–	–
✖	✖										5	**95**	502	No	0	–
	–			–		✖		–	–		4	91	258	No	7	–
	–			–					–		–[2]	–[2]	100	No	3	–
	–		★	–			–	–	–		4	90	140	No	0	–
							✖			★	4	93	742	No	116	–
✖		✖					–	–	–		5	**97**	288	No	9	–
★	–	★	★	–	★		★				4	**94**	307	No	4	–
–	–	–	–	–	–	–	–	–	–	–	–[2]	–[2]	–	–	–	–
	–			–				★			5	**96**	340	No	21	–
✖	✖		×					✖			4	**95**	883	No	0	–
–	–	–	–	–	–	–	–	–	–	–	–[2]	–[2]	–	–	–	–
✖	–	✖		–			–	–			4	**94**	140	No	0	2
★		★	★						★	★	4	**97**	568	No	0	–
	–			–	★	★	×	–	–	★	4	**86**	112	No	1	–
✖	–			–		–	–		–		5	93	96	No	0	–
–	–	–	–	–	–	–	–	–	–	–	–[2]	–[2]	241	–	8	–
	×			✖		–			–		4	**88**	691	**Yes**	197	–
	–	–	★	–			–	–	–	–	4	92	185	No	3	–
								★	–		5	**98**	357	No	0	–
–	–	–		–	–	–	–	–	–	–	–[2]	–[2]	112	No	4	–
×	–		×	–	✖				✖	★	4	89	506	No	0	–
	–	×		–	✖		–	–	✖	–	4	**94**	407	No	31	2
			×			✖	★	★	–		5	**98**	457	No	0	–
	–			–							4	**97**	362	No	0	–
	–		×	–	×	★	✖				4	92	355	No	33	–
		–		✖		–	–	–	–	–	4	**94**	525	No	19	–
×		✖	✖	×	✖			✖	✖		4	**94**	493	No	9	–
★	–	★	★	–	★	–	–	–	–		4	**97**	120	No	4	–
	–	–		–		–	–	–	–	–	4	**96**	250	No	4	–
	–			–		★	–			–	4	90	150	No	1	–
✖	–	✖		–	×	–	–	–	–	–	4	**95**	182	No	0	–
			★	★							5	**98**	313	No	6	–

***Accreditation Status:** 5=Accredited with commendation or with full standards compliance; 4=Accredited with requirements for improvement; 3=Conditional accreditation.

Detailed Ratings for All Areas

See more information on "Key Ratings for Metro Areas" table beginning on page 32

Blue is most favorable
Bold Italic is least favorable
Blank means neither better nor worse than average
"–" means insufficient data

	Death rates for all selected case types			Hospital outcomes: better (★) or worse (×) than average — Adjusted Death rates — Medical Cases											
	Number of cases	Actual death rate (%)	Adjusted death rate (%) (lower is better)	All selected cases	All selected medical cases	Heart attack	Congestive heart failure	Obstructive pulmonary disease	Pneumonia	Respiratory failure and arrest	Septicemia	Stroke	Gastrointestinal hemorrhage	Fluid, electrolyte, & acid-base disorders	Kidney failure
National Average	–	–	12.1	12.1	14.8	21.2	10.6	6.5	16.9	34.4	25.1	18.4	6.7	11.0	20.9
Florida *(continued)*															
South Florida *(continued)*															
Fishermen's, Marathon	847	11.0	***14.5***	✖	✖					–		×	–		–
Florida, Fort Lauderdale	6,071	16.2	**11.1**	★	★	★			★		★			✖	
Glades General, Belle Glade	308	16.2	14.7			–		–		–	–	–	–	–	–
Good Samaritan, West Palm Beach	4,763	11.2	**10.8**	★	★				★				★		
Healthsouth Doctors', Coral Gables	2,127	10.3	**9.8**	★	★			★	★						
Hialeah Hospital, Hialeah	3,521	16.3	**9.6**	★	★		★		★	★	★				
Hollywood Medical Center, Hollywood	1,829	15.2	12.8											✖	
Holy Cross, Fort Lauderdale	6,664	10.2	**10.7**	★	★										★
Homestead Hospital, Homestead	1,065	16.5	12.5										✖	×	
Imperial Point, Fort Lauderdale	1,291	15.6	11.6												
Jackson Memorial, Miami	2,123	11.0	**10.4**	★	★		★					★			★
Jackson South, Miami	1,698	23.5	***16.0***	✖	✖	×		×	✖		✖			✖	
JFK, Atlantis	8,653	14.7	11.9			★			★						
Jupiter Medical Center, Jupiter	4,033	10.2	**9.0**	★	★		★		★		★	★		★	★
Kendall, Miami	5,451	15.0	**9.5**	★	★		★		★	★	★	★			★
Larkin, South Miami	1,684	13.2	**8.8**	★	★				★		★				
Lower Keys, Key West	1,115	13.2	13.6	×					×						–
Mariners, Tavernier	607	10.9	11.8			–		–			–		–	–	–
Memorial - Pembroke, Pembroke Pines	1,264	15.7	13.0			✖		×							
Memorial Regional, Hollywood	5,599	14.8	12.5			★	×						×	✖	
Memorial West, Pembroke Pines	2,354	10.6	**9.5**	★	★		★		★						
Mercy, Miami	6,863	10.1	**8.5**	★	★	★	★		★	★	★	★	★		
Miami Children's, Miami	–	–	–	–	–	–	–	–	–	–	–	–	–	–	–
Miami Jewish Home for the Aged, Miami	359	22.0	***16.0***	✖	✖	–	–	–	✖	–	–	–	–	–	–
Mt Sinai, Miami Beach	7,033	10.7	**10.1**	★	★	★	★		★			★	★		
Mt Sinai & Miami Heart Institute, Miami Beach	4,181	10.6	**8.5**	★	★	★	★		★	★	★	★	★	★	
North Broward, Pompano Beach	3,799	18.4	***14.9***	✖	✖		✖	✖	✖		✖		✖	✖	✖
North Ridge, Fort Lauderdale	5,852	8.9	**9.3**	★	★	★	★	★	★	★	★				
North Shore, Miami	1,918	16.2	12.0												
Northwest, Margate	3,141	16.4	**10.7**	★	★			✖	★	★	★				
Palm Beach Gardens Med Ctr, Palm Beach Gardens	5,222	9.4	**10.7**	★	★							★	★		
Palm Springs General, Hialeah	5,399	11.9	**9.9**	★	★			★	★		★	★	★	★	
Palmetto General, Hialeah	4,041	14.1	**9.2**	★	★	★	★		★			★		★	★
Palms West, Loxahatchee	1,315	11.7	**9.9**	★	★				★	★					

Footnotes are on page 350.

Hospital outcomes: better (★) or worse (×) than average											Results of accreditation review on full survey		Other facts			
Adjusted Death rates			Adjusted Adverse outcome rates													
Surgical cases			Surgical cases													
All selected surgical cases	Coronary artery bypass surgery	Large bowel surgery	All selected surgical cases	Coronary artery bypass surgery	Large bowel surgery	Gall bladder removal	Total knee replacement	Total hip replacement	Simple prostatectomy	Carotid endarterectomy	Accreditation status*	Overall evaluation score (higher is better)	Number of beds	Major medical school affiliation?	Number of residents	Computerized drug order system (1 to 5 scale, higher is preferred; see page 23 for details)
2.3	3.8	6.5	7.7	10.3	11.9	7.5	6.7	6.4	5.4	8.2	–	91	161	–	–	–
–	–	–		–	–	–	–	–	–	–	4	***81***	58	No	0	–
						★	–	–			4	**97**	459	No	7	–
–	–	–	–	–	–	–	–	–	–	–	4	***86***	73	No	0	–
	–			–			✖				–[2]	–[2]	341	No	0	–
★	–	–		–		–			–	–	4	**95**	157	No	1	–
	–	–		–	–	★	–	–	–	–	5	93	411	No	7	–
✖	–	✖		–		–	–	–	–	–	4	**97**	238	No	3	–
★		★			★		★				4	90	437	No	45	–
–	–	–	★	–	–	–	–	–	–	–	4	93	100	No	3	–
–	–	–		–	–	–	–	–	–	–	4	**96**	160	No	0	–
✖	–	✖				–	–	–	–	–	4	90	1,329	**Yes**	919	–
–	–	–	–	–	–	–	–	–	–	–	5	**96**	233	No	4	–
										★	4	**96**	364	No	0	2
	–			–		✖					4	***88***	156	No	0	–
	–						–	–	–	–	4	**97**	316	No	15	–
–	–	–	–	–	–	–	–	–	–	–	4	**98**	112	No	1	–
	–	–		–		–	–	–	–	–	4	93	169	No	1	–
–	–	–	–	–	–	–	–	–	–	–	4	91	42	No	0	–
–	–	–		–	–	–	–	–	–	–	4	**99**	190	No	0	–
								–	✖		4	**94**	672	No	0	–
	–			–	★		–	–	–	–	5	**97**	174	No	0	–
								★		–	4	90	339	No	0	–
–	–	–	–	–	–	–	–	–	–	–	4	93	238	–	89	–
–	–	–	–	–	–	–	–	–	–	–	4	**96**	32	No	1	–
											4	***82***	544	**Yes**	129	–
		★			★				–		–[2]	–[2]	278	No	7	–
×	–	–		–		–	–	–		–	4	**94**	316	No	0	–
★	★										4	92	391	No	5	–
–	–	–		–	–	–	–	–	–	–	4	**94**	197	No	2	–
	–			–		★	–	–	–	–	4	92	150	No	2	–
			✖			✖	✖		–		4	91	204	No	4	–
	–	×	★	–		★		–		–	4	89	190	No	0	–
	–			–	★				–	–	3	93	360	No	8	–
	–	–		–		–	–	–	–	–	4	93	117	No	1	2

***Accreditation Status:** 5=Accredited with commendation or with full standards compliance; 4=Accredited with requirements for improvement; 3=Conditional accreditation.

Detailed Ratings for All Areas

See more information on "Key Ratings for Metro Areas" table beginning on page 32

Blue is most favorable
Bold Italic is least favorable
Blank means neither better nor worse than average
"–" means insufficient data

	Death rates for all selected case types				Hospital outcomes: better (★) or worse (×) than average — Adjusted Death rates — Medical Cases										
	Number of cases	Actual death rate (%)	Adjusted death rate (%) (lower is better)	All selected cases	All selected medical cases	Heart attack	Congestive heart failure	Obstructive pulmonary disease	Pneumonia	Respiratory failure and arrest	Septicemia	Stroke	Gastrointestinal hemorrhage	Fluid, electrolyte, & acid-base disorders	Kidney failure
National Average	–	–	12.1	12.1	14.8	21.2	10.6	6.5	16.9	34.4	25.1	18.4	6.7	11.0	20.9
Florida *(continued)*															
South Florida *(continued)*															
Pan American, Miami	3,736	15.1	7.9	★	★		★	★	★		★	★	★		
Parkway Regional, North Miami Beach	3,922	22.6	***15.0***	✖	✖	✖	✖	✖	✖		✖	✖		✖	×
Plantation General, Plantation	929	17.3	10.9				★		★						
St Mary's, West Palm Beach	2,217	15.3	12.8										✖		
South Miami, Miami	3,023	10.2	8.5	★	★	★	★		★			★		★	
South Shore, Miami Beach	2,059	22.2	11.7				★								
University, Tamarac	4,512	17.2	12.4				★	✖						✖	
University of Miami - Sylvester Cancer Center, Miami[1]	154	16.9	10.9			–	–	–		–		–	–		–
Wellington Regional, West Palm Beach	1,088	18.5	11.9										–	✖	
West Boca, Boca Raton	2,737	15.5	11.1	★	★		★								
Westchester General, Miami	420	10.0	9.9		★	–				–	–	–	–		
Westside Regional, Plantation	3,753	15.2	11.1	★	★		★								
Other Areas															
Baptist, Jacksonville[1]	3,601	12.2	11.9												
Baptist, Pensacola	5,346	12.8	11.7				★								
Baptist - Beaches, Jacksonville Beach	1,636	13.3	11.7												–
Baptist - Nassau, Fernandina Beach	752	15.6	***16.3***	✖	✖	–			✖	–	✖	×	✖		–
Bay, Panama City	6,157	11.7	11.5		★	★		✖				★			
Brooksville Regional, Brooksville	3,073	13.5	11.7				★								
Calhoun - Liberty, Blountstown	369	13.0	12.9			–		–		–	–	–	–	–	–
Citrus, Inverness	7,147	12.6	12.7	×	✖				✖				✖		✖
Community Hospital, New Port Richey	8,270	13.1	10.8	★	★	✖	★		★	★	★				★
Desoto, Arcadia	1,128	11.0	10.5										–		–
Doctor's, Perry	1,310	10.5	10.8										–		
Doctors, Bonifay	715	19.0	***14.8***	✖	✖		✖			×		×	–	–	
East Pasco, Zephyrhills	3,972	12.4	12.0			×				★		✖			
Ed Fraser & Baker, MacClenny	66	7.6	6.9			–	–	–	–	–	–	–	–	–	–
Flagler, Saint Augustine	4,269	10.9	9.9	★	★				★		★				★
Florida - Heartland, Sebring	5,465	12.3	11.3	★	★		★				★		★	★	★
Florida - Waterman, Eustis	5,996	12.8	10.2	★	★				★	★	★				★
Fort Walton Beach Medical Center, Fort Walton Beach	4,556	12.0	12.0												
Gadsden, Quincy	221	16.7	***17.3***	✖	✖	–		–	×	–	–	–	–		–
George E Weems, Apalachicola	272	11.4	11.7			–		–			–	–	–	–	–

Footnotes are on page 350.

Hospital outcomes: better (★) or worse (×) than average											Results of accreditation review on full survey		Other facts			
Adjusted Death rates			Adjusted Adverse outcome rates													
Surgical cases			Surgical cases													
All selected surgical cases	Coronary artery bypass surgery	Large bowel surgery	All selected surgical cases	Coronary artery bypass surgery	Large bowel surgery	Gall bladder removal	Total knee replacement	Total hip replacement	Simple prostatectomy	Carotid endarterectomy	Accreditation status*	Overall evaluation score (higher is better)	Number of beds	Major medical school affiliation?	Number of residents	Computerized drug order system (1 to 5 scale, higher is preferred; see page 23 for details)
2.3	3.8	6.5	7.7	10.3	11.9	7.5	6.7	6.4	5.4	8.2	–	91	161	–	–	–
	–			–			–	–	–	–	4	90	146	No	0	–
✖	–	✖	✖	–	✖	✖	–	–	–	–	4	92	392	No	9	–
–	–	–	✖	–	–	–	–	–	–	–	4	96	264	No	4	–
	–			–		–			–	–	–[2]	–[2]	460	No	0	–
	–								–		4	94	318	No	37	–
–	–	–		–	–	–	–	–	–	–	4	87	155	Yes	4	–
	–			–			–	–			5	96	271	No	0	–
–	–	–	–	–	–	–	–	–	–	–	4	96	40	Yes	0	–
–	–	–		–		–	–	–	–	–	4	92	93	Yes	0	–
	–			–		×	–	–	–	–	5	97	150	No	1	–
–	–	–	–	–	–	–	–	–	–	–	–[2]	–[2]	160	No	9	–
	–			–			–	–			5	97	204	No	0	–
×		✖						✖	–		5	97	519	No	0	–
	–		★					–			4	94	435	No	0	–
	–	–	★	–		–	–	–	–	–	4	95	82	No	0	–
–	–	–		–	–	–	–	–	–	–	3	92	32	No	0	–
✖	✖							–			4	92	315	No	0	–
	–			–				–	–	–	4	83	91	No	0	–
–	–	–	–	–	–	–	–	–	–	–	–[2]	–[2]	30	No	1	–
★	–			–		★	✖	★			4	86	171	No	0	–
	–			–		★	✖	✖			4	93	414	No	7	–
–	–	–		–	–	–	–	–	–	–	–[2]	–[2]	49	No	0	–
–	–	–	–	–	–	–	–	–	–	–	–[2]	–[2]	46	No	1	–
–	–	–	–	–	–	–	–	–	–	–	4	93	28	No	0	–
	–		★	–	★	✖	★				4	91	127	No	0	–
–	–	–	–	–	–	–	–	–		–	–[2]	–[2]	25	No	–	–
	–			–					–		4	86	246	No	0	–
	–		✖	–	×	✖			–		4	92	175	Yes	0	–
	–			–					–		4	87	133	No	0	–
	–			–							4	94	247	No	0	–
–	–	–	–	–	–	–	–	–	–	–	–[2]	–[2]	51	No	0	–
–	–	–	–	–	–	–	–	–	–	–	–[2]	–[2]	29	No	0	–

***Accreditation Status:** 5=Accredited with commendation or with full standards compliance; 4=Accredited with requirements for improvement; 3=Conditional accreditation.

Detailed Ratings for All Areas

See more information on "Key Ratings for Metro Areas" table beginning on page 32

Blue is most favorable
Bold Italic is least favorable
Blank means neither better nor worse than average
"–" means insufficient data

	Death rates for all selected case types			Hospital outcomes: better (★) or worse (×) than average — Adjusted Death rates — Medical Cases												
	Number of cases	Actual death rate (%)	Adjusted death rate (%) (lower is better)	All selected cases	All selected medical cases	Heart attack	Congestive heart failure	Obstructive pulmonary disease	Pneumonia	Respiratory failure and arrest	Septicemia	Stroke	Gastrointestinal hemorrhage	Fluid, electrolyte, & acid-base disorders	Kidney failure
National Average	–	–	12.1	12.1	14.8	21.2	10.6	6.5	16.9	34.4	25.1	18.4	6.7	11.0	20.9
Florida *(continued)*															
Other Areas *(continued)*															
Gulf Breeze Hospital, Gulf Breeze	1,594	8.0	7.7	★	★		★	★	★		★		★		★
Gulf Coast, Panama City	4,037	11.6	12.9	×			✖								
Gulf Pines, Port St Joe	479	15.9	***15.4***	✖	✖	–		–		–	–	✖	–	–	–
Healthmark Regional, Defuniak Springs	859	17.8	***14.6***	✖	✖					✖			–		
Hendry Regional, Clewiston	573	16.8	***15.7***	✖	✖			×				✖	–	✖	–
Highlands Regional, Sebring	4,075	12.0	***13.2***	✖	✖	✖			×	×					
Indian River, Vero Beach	7,829	10.0	12.4			✖									×
Jackson County, Marianna	1,856	13.3	10.8	★	★	✖									
Jay Hospital, Jay	774	8.9	10.7			–				–	–		–	★	–
Lake City Medical Center, Lake City	2,236	11.9	10.3	★	★	×				★					
Lawnwood Regional, Fort Pierce	5,486	12.7	10.3	★	★				★	★	★	★	×		
Leesburg Regional, Leesburg	10,428	10.9	11.9					✖				★	×		
Madison County, Madison	462	13.2	11.5			–		–		–	–	–	–		
Martin, Stuart[1]	8,058	10.2	10.3	★	★				★				★		
Memorial, Jacksonville	6,502	13.1	12.1			★		★							
Memorial - Flagler, Bunnell[1]	1,040	15.9	12.3					★							
Munroe Regional, Ocala	12,678	10.0	11.0	★	★	★			★						
Nature Coast Regional, Williston[1]	635	20.0	***14.9***	✖	✖	✖				–		✖	–		–
North Bay, New Port Richey	1,830	16.5	12.2								★			✖	
North Florida Regional, Gainesville	8,088	10.1	11.2	★	★		×			★	★	★			
North Okaloosa, Crestview	2,235	10.5	10.5	★	★			★				★			
Northwest Florida, Chipley	950	13.7	12.0			×	★						–	–	
Oak Hill, Spring Hill	7,068	10.3	10.1	★	★		★	★			★	★			
Ocala Regional, Ocala	7,940	10.2	11.4											✖	
Orange Park Medical Center, Orange Park	3,700	16.4	12.3							×					★
Osceola Regional, Kissimmee	2,214	13.3	12.1												
Pasco Regional, Dade City	1,417	13.3	***13.7***	✖		✖		✖					–		
Putnam, Palatka	4,507	11.1	11.5												
Raulerson, Okeechobee	3,249	11.4	10.6	★	★			★			★				–
Regional, Hudson/Bayonet Point	7,317	12.5	11.1	★	★	★					★				
Sacred Heart, Pensacola[1]	6,229	10.6	12.6												
St Lucie, Port St Lucie	5,402	11.8	10.8	★	★			★	★	★	★				
St Luke's, Jacksonville[1]	5,842	7.8	10.7	★	★										
St Vincent's, Jacksonville	8,919	10.9	10.9	★	★	★	★		★						★

Footnotes are on page 350.

Hospital outcomes: better (★) or worse (×) than average											Results of accreditation review on full survey		Other facts			
Adjusted Death rates			Adjusted Adverse outcome rates													
Surgical cases			Surgical cases													
All selected surgical cases	Coronary artery bypass surgery	Large bowel surgery	All selected surgical cases	Coronary artery bypass surgery	Large bowel surgery	Gall bladder removal	Total knee replacement	Total hip replacement	Simple prostatectomy	Carotid endarterectomy	Accreditation status*	Overall evaluation score (higher is better)	Number of beds	Major medical school affiliation?	Number of residents	Computerized drug order system (1 to 5 scale, higher is preferred; see page 23 for details)
2.3	3.8	6.5	7.7	10.3	11.9	7.5	6.7	6.4	5.4	8.2	–	91	161	–	–	–
★	–	–	★	–		–		–	–	–	–[2]	–[2]	48	No	0	–
×	–			–			★		★	–	4	93	165	No	0	–
–	–	–	–	–	–	–	–	–	–	–	–[2]	–[2]	45	No	0	–
–	–	–	–	–	–	–	–	–	–	–	–[2]	–[2]	34	No	0	–
–	–	–	–	–	–	–	–	–	–	–	4	**96**	32	No	0	–
✖	–	✖		–					–		4	**96**	126	No	1	–
★	–		✖	–			✖	✖	–	★	4	93	280	No	10	–
–	–	–	✖	–	–	–	✖	–	–	–	4	***82***	85	No	0	–
–	–	–	–	–	–	–	–	–	–	–	–[2]	–[2]	31	No	0	–
–	–	–		–	–		–	–	–	–	4	91	70	No	0	–
			✖	×			✖	–			4	90	342	No	7	–
			★	★				✖	–	★	4	89	294	No	0	–
–	–	–	–	–	–	–	–	–	–	–	–[2]	–[2]	30	No	0	–
	–			–			✖		★		–[2]	–[2]	324	No	0	–
	✖		✖	✖	×		✖		–		4	91	333	No	8	4
–	–	–	✖	–	–	–	✖	–	–	–	–[2]	–[2]	73	No	0	–
★	★		★	★						★	4	**96**	323	No	0	–
–	–	–	–	–	–	–	–	–	–	–	–[2]	–[2]	40	No	0	–
	–	×		–		–	–	–	–	–	4	91	122	No	0	–
	✖										4	**94**	266	No	6	–
	–	–		–		–		–	–	–	4	91	95	No	0	–
–	–	–	–	–	–	–	–	–	–	–	4	90	76	No	0	–
	–			–		×					–[2]	–[2]	204	No	0	–
★	★		★	★			★	★			4	93	210	No	0	3
	–			–				–	–		4	91	196	No	2	–
	–	–		–				–	–	–	4	91	156	No	1	–
✖	–	–		–			–	–	–	–	4	***81***	120	No	0	–
	–			–				–		×	4	***85***	141	No	0	–
	–	–	×	–		×	✖	–	–	–	4	***88***	101	No	0	–
★	★		★	★						★	4	**95**	256	No	0	–
	✖			✖	×			★			4	90	431	**Yes**	0	–
	–			–				×			4	**94**	150	No	1	–
★	★			★			×				4	93	223	**Yes**	0	–
	✖					★			–		5	**94**	344	No	36	–

***Accreditation Status:** 5=Accredited with commendation or with full standards compliance; 4=Accredited with requirements for improvement; 3=Conditional accreditation.

Detailed Ratings for All Areas

See more information on "Key Ratings for Metro Areas" table beginning on page 32

Blue is most favorable
Bold Italic is least favorable
Blank means neither better nor worse than average
"–" means insufficient data

	Death rates for all selected case types			Hospital outcomes: better (★) or worse (×) than average — Adjusted Death rates — Medical Cases											
	Number of cases	Actual death rate (%)	Adjusted death rate (%) (lower is better)	All selected cases	All selected medical cases	Heart attack	Congestive heart failure	Obstructive pulmonary disease	Pneumonia	Respiratory failure and arrest	Septicemia	Stroke	Gastrointestinal hemorrhage	Fluid, electrolyte, & acid-base disorders	Kidney failure
National Average	–	–	12.1	12.1	14.8	21.2	10.6	6.5	16.9	34.4	25.1	18.4	6.7	11.0	20.9
Florida *(continued)*															
Other Areas *(continued)*															
Santa Rosa, Milton[1]	1,404	12.7	***14.3***	**✖**	**✖**				×	**✖**					–
Sebastian River, Sebastian	3,178	8.2	8.0	★	★		★		★	★	★	★		★	
Seven Rivers, Crystal River	4,771	12.4	10.7	★	★		★	★							
Shands, Jacksonville	3,083	13.3	12.4				★								
Shands, Starke	591	21.5	***18.2***	**✖**	**✖**	**✖**		**✖**	**✖**	–	–	**✖**	–	**✖**	–
Shands at AGH, Gainesville	2,276	12.5	11.3												
Shands at Lake Shore, Lake City	1,486	10.7	10.6	★	★		★							**✖**	
Shands at the University of Florida, Gainesville	4,053	10.4	12.4												
South Lake, Clermont	1,509	12.7	11.4						★						
Spring Hill Regional, Spring Hill	1,168	9.8	9.9	★	★				★		★			**✖**	–
Sun Coast, Clermont	3,224	13.3	8.6	★	★		★	★	★	★	★				
Tallahassee Community, Tallahassee	3,545	15.0	11.4		★			★	★			★			×
Tallahassee Memorial, Tallahassee	7,520	10.4	12.3									★		**✖**	
Trinity, Jasper	458	10.0	11.1			–		–		–		–	–	–	–
Twin Cities, Niceville	1,582	13.3	11.9							×					
West Florida, Pensacola	6,143	11.4	11.7							**✖**	★	★			
Georgia															
Atlanta Area															
Atlanta Medical Center, Atlanta	3,327	14.8	12.5					★						**✖**	
Children's Healthcare at Egleston, Atlanta	–	–	–	–	–	–	–	–	–	–	–	–	–	–	–
Children's Healthcare at Scottish Rite, Atlanta	–	–	–	–	–	–	–	–	–	–	–	–	–	–	–
Crawford Long - Emory University, Atlanta	5,723	9.1	10.2	★	★		★					★			★
Decatur Hospital, Decatur	–	–	–	–	–	–	–	–	–	–	–	–	–	–	–
Dekalb, Decatur	6,425	14.9	***14.0***	**✖**	**✖**		**✖**		**✖**		**✖**		**✖**		
Emory - Adventist, Smyrna	835	15.2	12.1										–	–	
Emory Dunwoody, Atlanta	898	12.7	10.2	★	★								–	–	**✖**
Emory Eastside, Snellville	2,596	14.3	12.5										×	×	
Emory Northlake Regional, Tucker	1,147	16.9	10.9												×
Emory Parkway, Lithia Springs	857	15.9	12.9							**✖**	★	×	–		
Emory University, Atlanta	5,168	9.1	11.0	★	★	★	★		★	**✖**					
Fayette Community, Fayetteville	1,087	16.2	***14.9***	**✖**	**✖**		×				×	**✖**			**✖**
Grady, Atlanta[1]	5,216	13.8	12.8	×			★		×	×	**✖**				★
Gwinnett, Lawrenceville	5,556	12.1	11.5					★							

Footnotes are on page 350.

Hospital outcomes: better (★) or worse (×) than average											Results of accreditation review on full survey		Other facts			
Adjusted Death rates			Adjusted Adverse outcome rates													
Surgical cases			Surgical cases													
All selected surgical cases	Coronary artery bypass surgery	Large bowel surgery	All selected surgical cases	Coronary artery bypass surgery	Large bowel surgery	Gall bladder removal	Total knee replacement	Total hip replacement	Simple prostatectomy	Carotid endarterectomy	Accreditation status*	Overall evaluation score (higher is better)	Number of beds	Major medical school affiliation?	Number of residents	Computerized drug order system (1 to 5 scale, higher is preferred; see page 23 for details)
2.3	3.8	6.5	7.7	10.3	11.9	7.5	6.7	6.4	5.4	8.2	–	91	161	–	–	–
	–	–	✖	–		–	✖	–	–	–	4	**98**	96	No	0	–
	–	★		–				–	–		4	**96**	133	No	1	–
	–			–							4	89	128	No	1	–
✖	×	–				–	–	–	–	–	4	91	678	**Yes**	162	–
–	–	–	–	–	–	–	–	–	–	–	4	**94**	30	No	0	–
	–		★			–		–	–	–	5	93	269	No	9	–
–	–	–		–	–	–	–	–	–	–	4	93	83	No	0	–
×	✖		✖	✖					–		4	**96**	558	**Yes**	0	–
–	–	–		–	–	–	–	–	–	–	4	**96**	68	No	0	–
	–	–	★	–	–	–			–	–	–[2]	–[2]	75	No	0	–
	–			–					–		–[2]	–[2]	300	**Yes**	21	–
✖	✖			✖			★		–		4	**94**	180	No	1	–
×	✖						★	✖			4	92	514	No	32	–
–	–	–	–	–	–	–	–	–	–	–	–[2]	–[2]	20	No	0	–
	–	–	★	–			★	–	–	–	4	**97**	65	No	0	–
✖	✖			×	×		★		–		4	**94**	491	No	0	4
✖	✖			✖				–	–		4	89	450	No	10	1
–	–	–	–	–	–	–	–	–	–	–	–[2]	–[2]	206	–	3	–
–	–	–	–	–	–	–	–	–	–	–	–[2]	–[2]	165	–	2	–
			×					–	×		5	**96**	397	**Yes**	0	4
–	–	–	–	–	–	–	–	–	–	–	4	93	84	–	4	–
×	–			–					–		4	90	394	No	5	3
–	–	–	–	–	–	–	–	–	–	–	4	**96**	30	No	0	–
–	–	–		–	–	–	–	–	–	–	4	93	140	No	0	2
	–			–				–	–	–	5	**87**	131	No	0	2
–	–	–		–	–	–	–	–	–	–	4	93	112	No	9	2
	–	–		–		–	–	–	–	–	4	**83**	182	No	0	4
	×		✖	✖		✖			–	✖	5	**96**	473	**Yes**	0	4
–	–	–		–	–	–	–	–	–	–	4	92	100	No	–	4
✖	–	✖	✖	–		–	–	–	–	–	4	**83**	762	**Yes**	0	1
✖	–	×		–					–		4	**97**	390	No	75	4

***Accreditation Status:** 5=Accredited with commendation or with full standards compliance; 4=Accredited with requirements for improvement; 3=Conditional accreditation.

Detailed Ratings for All Areas

See more information on "Key Ratings for Metro Areas" table beginning on page 32

Blue is most favorable
Bold Italic is least favorable
Blank means neither better nor worse than average
"–" means insufficient data

	Death rates for all selected case types			Hospital outcomes: better (★) or worse (×) than average — Adjusted Death rates											
					Medical Cases										
	Number of cases	Actual death rate (%)	Adjusted death rate (%) (lower is better)	All selected cases	All selected medical cases	Heart attack	Congestive heart failure	Obstructive pulmonary disease	Pneumonia	Respiratory failure and arrest	Septicemia	Stroke	Gastrointestinal hemorrhage	Fluid, electrolyte, & acid-base disorders	Kidney failure
National Average	–	–	12.1	12.1	14.8	21.2	10.6	6.5	16.9	34.4	25.1	18.4	6.7	11.0	20.9
Georgia *(continued)*															
Atlanta Area *(continued)*															
Henry, Stockbridge	2,726	13.7	***14.2***	✖	✖	✖	✖								
Hughes Spalding Children's, Atlanta	–	–	–	–	–	–	–	–	–	–	–	–	–	–	–
Joan Glancy, Duluth	–	–	–	–	–	–	–	–	–	–	–	–	–	–	–
North Fulton Regional, Roswell	2,858	13.7	***13.3***	✖	✖			×		✖				✖	
Northside, Atlanta	3,235	10.5	11.6												
Northside - Cherokee, Canton	1,541	18.3	***15.6***	✖	✖	✖			✖	✖	×	✖			
Piedmont, Atlanta	7,612	9.0	11.7			★									
Rockdale, Conyers[1]	2,477	14.7	***14.1***	✖	✖				✖	✖				×	
St Joseph's, Atlanta	10,462	8.6	11.3	★	★	★	✖							×	
Shepherd Center, Atlanta	–	–	–	–	–	–	–	–	–	–	–	–	–	–	–
South Fulton, East Point	4,665	15.1	10.3	★	★		★		★				★		
Southern Regional, Riverdale	5,251	14.2	***13.1***	✖	✖						✖			✖	
Southwest, Atlanta	703	15.1	11.0			★	★	–					–		
Wellstar Cobb, Austell	5,345	12.6	***12.9***	✖	×	×		✖		✖					
Wellstar Douglas, Douglasville	1,650	15.6	***14.2***	✖	✖		✖		✖	×					
Wellstar Kennestone, Marietta	7,925	12.6	11.7			✖				★					
Wesley Woods Center of Emory University, Atlanta	446	12.3	12.5			–		–		–	–	–	–		–
Other Areas															
Appling, Baxley[1]	471	14.2	14.9	×	✖	–	–	–		–		×	–	–	–
Athens Regional, Athens	6,701	10.0	11.7			★						★		×	
Bacon County, Alma[1]	665	11.0	12.2			–		–		–			–		–
Baptist, Cumming	1,339	16.1	***14.2***	✖	✖		✖					×			×
Baptist Worth County, Sylvester	541	15.0	***17.0***	✖	✖	–	✖	–		–	–	✖	–	×	–
Barrow, Winder	760	15.8	13.4			✖		–			✖		–		–
Berrien County, Nashville	802	11.7	10.8			–				–			–		–
BJC, Commerce	970	17.7	***16.2***	✖	✖	×	✖		✖				–		✖
Brooks County, Quitman	774	12.0	10.8					★	★	–			–		–
Burke, Waynesboro	831	14.1	***15.6***	✖	✖	✖		–	✖	–			–		–
Camden, St Marys	548	14.8	***15.3***	✖	✖		×	–		–			✖		–
Candler, Savannah	6,651	12.7	9.3	★	★		★	★	★	★		★	★		
Candler County, Metter	835	13.7	***14.5***	✖	✖	–		–		–	✖		–		
Central State, Milledgeville[1]	320	10.0	7.8	★	★	–	–	–	★	–	–	–	–		–
Charlton, Folkston	379	17.9	14.8	×	×			✖		–		–	–		–

Footnotes are on page 350.

Hospital outcomes: better (★) or worse (×) than average											Results of accreditation review on full survey		Other facts			
Adjusted Death rates			Adjusted Adverse outcome rates													
Surgical cases			Surgical cases													
All selected surgical cases	Coronary artery bypass surgery	Large bowel surgery	All selected surgical cases	Coronary artery bypass surgery	Large bowel surgery	Gall bladder removal	Total knee replacement	Total hip replacement	Simple prostatectomy	Carotid endarterectomy	Accreditation status*	Overall evaluation score (higher is better)	Number of beds	Major medical school affiliation?	Number of residents	Computerized drug order system (1 to 5 scale, higher is preferred; see page 23 for details)
2.3	3.8	6.5	7.7	10.3	11.9	7.5	6.7	6.4	5.4	8.2	–	91	161	–	–	–
×	–	×		–		×	–	–	–		4	92	118	No	0	–
–	–	–	–	–	–	–	–	–	–	–	–[2]	–[2]	–	–	–	–
–	–	–	–	–	–	–	–	–	–	–	–[2]	–[2]	–	–	–	–
	–	–	★	–				–	–	–	4	**98**	167	No	0	1
×	–	×		–	×		★			–	5	**97**	386	No	53	2
–	–	–		–	×	–	–	–	–	–	–[2]	–[2]	84	No	0	1
							★	★			4	91	415	No	0	4
	–		★	–			–	–	–		4	**95**	107	No	0	4
			×	×			×				5	**94**	346	No	0	2
–	–	–	–	–	–	–	–	–	–	–	4	93	–	–	–	–
	–			–	★			–	–		–[2]	–[2]	369	No	25	1
	–		★	–		★		–			4	92	319	No	0	2
–	–	–	–	–	–	–	–	–	–	–	3	89	100	No	2	1
	–	×		–	×				–		4	**94**	311	No	21	2
–	–	–		–	–	–	–	–	–	–	4	92	67	No	0	2
★	–			–					★		4	93	403	No	49	2
–	–	–	–	–	–	–	–	–	–	–	4	91	94	No	0	4
–	–	–	–	–	–	–	–	–	–	–	4	**97**	39	No	0	–
★	★										4	**96**	315	No	0	–
–	–	–	–	–	–	–	–	–	–	–	4	93	38	No	2	–
–	–	–		–	–	–	–	–	–	–	4	89	41	No	0	2
–	–	–	–	–	–	–	–	–	–	–	4	***88***	49	No	0	–
–	–	–	–	–	–	–	–	–	–	–	4	***86***	56	No	0	–
–	–	–	–	–	–	–	–	–	–	–	4	91	45	No	0	–
–	–	–	–	–	–	–	–	–	–	–	4	92	66	No	0	–
–	–	–	–	–	–	–	–	–	–	–	4	92	35	No	0	–
–	–	–	–	–	–	–	–	–	–	–	4	**94**	40	No	0	–
–	–	–	–	–	–	–	–	–	–	–	4	92	40	No	0	–
★	–			–			–	–	×		4	93	300	No	0	–
–	–	–		–	–	–	–	–	–	–	4	91	42	No	0	–
–	–	–	–	–	–	–	–	–	–	–	–[2]	–[2]	1,258	No	1	–
–	–	–	–	–	–	–	–	–	–	–	–[2]	–[2]	36	No	0	–

***Accreditation Status:** 5=Accredited with commendation or with full standards compliance; 4=Accredited with requirements for improvement; 3=Conditional accreditation.

Detailed Ratings for All Areas

See more information on "Key Ratings for Metro Areas" table beginning on page 32

Blue is most favorable
Bold Italic is least favorable
Blank means neither better nor worse than average
"–" means insufficient data

	Death rates for all selected case types			Hospital outcomes: better (★) or worse (×) than average — Adjusted Death rates	Medical Cases										
	Number of cases	Actual death rate (%)	Adjusted death rate (%) (lower is better)	All selected cases	All selected medical cases	Heart attack	Congestive heart failure	Obstructive pulmonary disease	Pneumonia	Respiratory failure and arrest	Septicemia	Stroke	Gastrointestinal hemorrhage	Fluid, electrolyte, & acid-base disorders	Kidney failure
National Average	–	–	12.1	12.1	14.8	21.2	10.6	6.5	16.9	34.4	25.1	18.4	6.7	11.0	20.9
Georgia *(continued)*															
Other Areas *(continued)*															
Chastatee Regional, Dahlonega	756	12.4	12.3			–		–					–	–	
Chatuge Regional, Hiawassee[1]	639	17.1	***15.0***	✖	✖	✖		–				✖	–	–	–
Cobb, Royston[1]	1,578	12.5	11.5											★	
Coffee Regional, Douglas	1,959	12.2	11.8												
Coliseum, Macon	3,112	11.4	12.2												
Colquitt Regional, Moultrie	1,880	13.7	***14.5***	✖	✖	✖	✖								
Crisp Regional, Cordele	1,394	13.4	***14.8***	✖	✖			×	✖	–	✖				✖
Doctors, Augusta	3,444	13.3	10.7	★	★						★		★		
Doctors, Columbus	2,501	15.4	***14.4***	✖	✖			✖	✖		✖		✖		
Dodge County, Eastman	1,586	17.0	***13.8***	✖	✖	✖	✖	–							
Donalsonville Hospital, Donalsonville	695	6.2	8.4	★	★	–	★		★	–	–		–		–
Dooly, Vienna	210	15.7	13.8			–		–		–	–	–	–	–	–
Dorminy, Fitzgerald	1,298	12.2	13.3				✖			–					×
Early, Blakely[1]	228	17.5	15.7	×	×	–	×	–		–		–	–	–	–
East Georgia Regional, Statesboro	2,868	12.2	9.0	★	★	×		★	★	★	★	★	★	★	
Elbert Memorial, Elberton	1,283	14.0	11.0			★									–
Emanuel County, Swainsboro	1,262	15.5	***14.3***	✖	✖		✖						–		
Emory, Cartersville	1,701	15.8	***15.2***	✖	✖				✖		✖	✖		✖	
Emory Peachtree Regional, Newnan	1,213	12.8	11.1									✖		★	
Evans, Claxton	976	12.1	***14.3***	✖	✖	–			✖	–	–		–		–
Fairview Park, Dublin	3,289	12.7	12.3										★		
Fannin Regional, Blue Ridge	1,161	13.9	12.2			✖									
Flint River, Montezuma	680	19.3	***16.7***	✖	✖		✖	–		–		×	–		–
Floyd, Rome	3,083	15.1	***16.1***	✖	✖	✖	✖		✖		×	✖		✖	✖
Georgia Baptist Meriwether, Warm Springs	506	16.6	***15.8***	✖	✖	–		–		–		✖	–	×	–
Gordon, Calhoun	1,417	14.5	12.4												✖
Grady General, Cairo	868	13.1	12.2					–						–	–
Habersham County, Demorest	1,333	14.3	***14.4***	✖	✖		×	×				×			–
Hamilton, Dalton	4,265	11.9	11.4										★		
Hancock, Sparta	382	13.6	13.4			–		–		–	✖	–	–		–
Hart County, Hartwell	1,102	15.9	13.3							–	✖				×
Higgins General, Bremen[1]	811	17.9	***15.6***	✖	✖	✖		–		–		✖	–	✖	
Houston, Warner Robins[1]	2,858	12.7	12.6					★			×				
Hughston Sports Medicine, Columbus	1,414	0.2	5.2		–	–	–	–	–	–	–	–	–	–	–

Footnotes are on page 350.

Hospital outcomes: better (★) or worse (✖) than average											Results of accreditation review on full survey		Other facts			
Adjusted Death rates			Adjusted Adverse outcome rates													
Surgical cases			Surgical cases													
All selected surgical cases	Coronary artery bypass surgery	Large bowel surgery	All selected surgical cases	Coronary artery bypass surgery	Large bowel surgery	Gall bladder removal	Total knee replacement	Total hip replacement	Simple prostatectomy	Carotid endarterectomy	Accreditation status*	Overall evaluation score (higher is better)	Number of beds	Major medical school affiliation?	Number of residents	Computerized drug order system (1 to 5 scale, higher is preferred; see page 23 for details)
2.3	3.8	6.5	7.7	10.3	11.9	7.5	6.7	6.4	5.4	8.2	–	91	161	–	–	–
–	–	–		–	–	–	–	–	–	–	4	86	49	No	0	–
–	–	–	–	–	–	–	–	–	–	–	4	84	142	No	0	–
–	–	–	–	–	–	–	–	–	–	–	4	85	71	No	0	–
✖	–	–		–	✖	–	–	–	–	–	4	97	88	No	0	–
	–			–				–	–		4	92	180	No	0	2
	–	–		–		–	–	–		–	4	93	84	No	0	–
–	–	–		–	–	–	–	–	–	–	4	91	65	No	7	–
	–			–				–	–		4	91	216	No	0	2
	–	–		–		✖	–	–		–	4	94	171	No	0	–
–	–	–	–	–	–	–	–	–	–	–	4	84	87	No	0	–
–	–	–	–	–	–	–	–	–	–	–	4	98	65	No	0	–
–	–	–	–	–	–	–	–	–	–	–	–[2]	–[2]	25	No	0	–
–	–	–	–	–	–	–	–	–	–	–	4	87	60	No	0	–
–	–	–	–	–	–	–	–	–	–	–	4	97	32	No	0	–
	–	–		–		–		–	–	–	–[2]	–[2]	158	No	0	–
–	–	–		–	–	–	–	–	–	–	4	95	42	No	0	–
–	–	–	–	–	–	–	–	–	–	–	4	96	42	No	0	–
	–	–		–			–	–	–	–	4	88	80	No	0	2
–	–	–		–	–	–	–	–	–	–	4	91	144	No	1	2
–	–	–	–	–	–	–	–	–	–	–	4	99	35	No	0	–
	–			–		★	–	–			3	82	190	No	0	2
–	–	–	–	–	–	–	–	–	–	–	–[2]	–[2]	32	No	0	–
–	–	–	–	–	–	–	–	–	–	–	4	88	49	No	0	–
	–	–		–		–	–	–			4	93	216	No	20	–
–	–	–	–	–	–	–	–	–	–	–	–[2]	–[2]	38	No	0	–
–	–	–		–	–	–	–	–	–	–	4	93	54	No	0	–
–	–	–	–	–	–	–	–	–	–	–	4	92	49	No	0	–
	–	–		–		–	–	–	–	–	4	88	53	No	0	–
	–			–	★			–		–	4	97	282	No	0	–
–	–	–	–	–	–	–	–	–	–	–	–[2]	–[2]	35	No	0	–
–	–	–		–	–	–	–	–	–	–	4	81	82	No	1	–
–	–	–	–	–	–	–	–	–	–	–	4	98	36	No	0	–
	–		✖	–		✖		–		–	4	91	186	Yes	0	–
	–	–	✖	–	–	–	✖	✖	–	–	4	91	100	No	0	–

***Accreditation Status:** 5=Accredited with commendation or with full standards compliance; 4=Accredited with requirements for improvement; 3=Conditional accreditation.

Detailed Ratings for All Areas

See more information on "Key Ratings for Metro Areas" table beginning on page 32

Blue is most favorable
Bold Italic is least favorable
Blank means neither better nor worse than average
"–" means insufficient data

	Death rates for all selected case types				Hospital outcomes: better (★) or worse (×) than average — Adjusted Death rates — Medical Cases										
	Number of cases	Actual death rate (%)	Adjusted death rate (%) (lower is better)	All selected cases	All selected medical cases	Heart attack	Congestive heart failure	Obstructive pulmonary disease	Pneumonia	Respiratory failure and arrest	Septicemia	Stroke	Gastrointestinal hemorrhage	Fluid, electrolyte, & acid-base disorders	Kidney failure
National Average	–	–	12.1	12.1	14.8	21.2	10.6	6.5	16.9	34.4	25.1	18.4	6.7	11.0	20.9
Georgia *(continued)*															
Other Areas *(continued)*															
Hutcheson, Fort Oglethorpe	3,789	15.9	11.7					**★**							
Irwin County, Ocilla	324	13.0	12.8			–		–		–	–	×	–	–	–
Jeff Davis, Hazlehurst	556	18.3	***16.9***	✖	✖	–		–	✖	–			–	✖	–
Jefferson, Louisville	640	18.4	***15.6***	✖	✖	–		–		–		×		×	–
John D Archbold, Thomasville	4,537	10.7	11.2			**★**						✖	★		**★**
Lanier Park, Gainesville	2,623	10.2	***14.7***	✖	✖	×	✖					✖			
Liberty Regional, Hinesville	541	15.5	14.5	×	×	–		–					–	×	–
Louis Smith, Lakeland	408	13.2	13.9			–		–		–	–	✖	–		–
Macon Northside, Macon	1,611	11.9	11.7												**★**
McDuffie Regional, Thomson	1,058	17.6	***15.3***	✖	✖	–		–	×	–	✖				–
Meadows Regional, Vidalia	1,715	14.8	11.6												
The Medical Center, Columbus	2,724	17.4	***13.3***	✖	×	×				×					
Medical Center of Central Georgia, Macon	8,660	10.7	12.6					✖		★	×				
Medical College of Georgia, Augusta[1]	1,779	11.0	12.3								✖	**★**			**★**
Memorial, Adel	1,059	10.0	10.3	★				★			★		–		–
Memorial, Bainbridge[1]	1,175	12.0	12.1										–		
Memorial Health, Savannah[1]	5,365	10.5	**10.2**	**★**	**★**	★	**★**	★	**★**						
Middle Georgia, Macon	2,046	12.6	12.3			×					✖				
Minnie G Boswell, Greensboro	412	19.9	***18.8***	✖	✖	–		–	✖	–		✖	–	✖	–
Mitchell County, Camilla	305	17.0	14.5			–	–	–	✖	–		–	–	–	–
Monroe County, Forsyth	695	23.7	***24.1***	✖	✖		✖	–	✖	–	✖	✖	✖	✖	–
Mountainside, Jasper	796	14.2	13.9	×		–							–	–	–
Murray, Chatsworth	694	13.7	11.1			–	✖		**★**				–		✖
Newnan Hospital, Newnan	2,400	12.3	12.6			✖									
Newton General, Covington	2,112	15.5	***15.6***	✖	✖		✖	✖	✖						
North Georgia, Ellijay	988	9.0	10.1	★	★	–		★		–	–		–		–
Northeast Georgia, Gainesville	5,284	13.2	***14.1***	✖	✖	✖		✖	✖	✖				✖	
Oconee Regional, Milledgeville	1,939	14.4	**10.6**	**★**	**★**			**★**		**★**					**★**
Palmyra, Albany[1]	2,249	11.5	11.5							✖					
Perry Hospital, Perry[1]	1,040	10.1	10.0	★	★			–	★	–			–		–
Phoebe Putney, Albany	6,403	11.2	**10.6**	**★**	**★**	★			**★**		★				
Polk, Cedartown	786	12.8	12.1			–				–			–		–
Rabun County, Clayton	691	12.9	**9.8**	**★**	**★**	–		–	★	**★**			–		
Redmond Regional, Rome	6,830	11.6	***12.8***	✖	✖	**★**	✖	✖	✖					×	

Footnotes are on page 350.

Hospital outcomes: better (★) or worse (×) than average											Results of accreditation review on full survey		Other facts			
Adjusted Death rates			Adjusted Adverse outcome rates													
Surgical cases			Surgical cases													
All selected surgical cases	Coronary artery bypass surgery	Large bowel surgery	All selected surgical cases	Coronary artery bypass surgery	Large bowel surgery	Gall bladder removal	Total knee replacement	Total hip replacement	Simple prostatectomy	Carotid endarterectomy	Accreditation status*	Overall evaluation score (higher is better)	Number of beds	Major medical school affiliation?	Number of residents	Computerized drug order system (1 to 5 scale, higher is preferred; see page 23 for details)
2.3	3.8	6.5	7.7	10.3	11.9	7.5	6.7	6.4	5.4	8.2	–	91	161	–	–	–
	–			–			–	–	–	×	4	89	179	No	0	2
–	–	–	–	–	–	–	–	–	–	–	4	**96**	64	No	0	–
–	–	–	–	–	–	–	–	–	–	–	4	**96**	50	No	0	–
–	–	–	–	–	–	–	–	–	–	–	4	**94**	37	No	0	–
	–		×	–			×	–			4	92	264	No	0	–
	–	–	★	–		–		★	–	★	4	91	109	No	0	–
–	–	–	–	–	–	–	–	–	–	–	4	89	28	No	0	–
–	–	–	–	–	–	–	–	–	–	–	4	***84***	40	No	0	–
	–			–		–		–	–	–	4	91	103	No	0	2
–	–	–		–	–	–	–	–	–	–	4	**94**	35	No	0	–
–	–	–		–	–	–	–	–	–	–	4	**97**	73	No	0	–
✖	–	✖		–		×	–	–	–	–	–[2]	–[2]	409	No	42	–
×			✖				✖		✖		4	***83***	495	**Yes**	90	–
	–	–	✖			–	✖	–	–	–	4	***88***	461	**Yes**	157	–
–	–	–	–	–	–	–	–	–	–	–	4	93	60	No	1	–
–	–	–		–	–	–	–	–	–	–	4	**97**	80	No	0	–
			★				★		–		4	**95**	378	**Yes**	47	–
	–	–		–			–	–	–		3	91	119	No	1	2
–	–	–	–	–	–	–	–	–	–	–	4	91	26	No	0	–
–	–	–	–	–	–	–	–	–	–	–	4	93	23	No	0	–
–	–	–	–	–	–	–	–	–	–	–	4	92	37	No	0	–
–	–	–	–	–	–	–	–	–	–	–	4	**95**	26	No	0	1
–	–	–	–	–	–	–	–	–	–	–	4	90	33	No	0	–
★	–			–		✖	★	–	–	–	4	91	100	No	0	–
–	–	–	★	–	★	–	–	–	–	–	5	**99**	90	No	0	–
–	–	–	–	–	–	–	–	–	–	–	4	**94**	50	No	0	–
	–	✖		–					–	★	4	91	288	No	14	–
	–	–		–		–	–	–	–	–	4	91	147	No	0	–
	–		★	–		★	★			–	4	***86***	163	No	0	–
–	–	–	–	–	–	–	–	–	–	–	4	89	45	No	0	–
					×						4	91	411	No	19	–
–	–	–	–	–	–	–	–	–	–	–	4	***88***	40	No	0	–
–	–	–	–	–	–	–	–	–	–	–	–[2]	–[2]	21	No	0	–
										★	4	***87***	199	No	0	–

***Accreditation Status:** 5=Accredited with commendation or with full standards compliance; 4=Accredited with requirements for improvement; 3=Conditional accreditation.

Detailed Ratings for All Areas

See more information on "Key Ratings for Metro Areas" table beginning on page 32

Blue is most favorable
Bold Italic is least favorable
Blank means neither better nor worse than average
"–" means insufficient data

	Death rates for all selected case types			Hospital outcomes: better (★) or worse (×) than average — Adjusted Death rates — Medical Cases											
	Number of cases	Actual death rate (%)	Adjusted death rate (%) (lower is better)	All selected cases	All selected medical cases	Heart attack	Congestive heart failure	Obstructive pulmonary disease	Pneumonia	Respiratory failure and arrest	Septicemia	Stroke	Gastrointestinal hemorrhage	Fluid, electrolyte, & acid-base disorders	Kidney failure
National Average	–	–	12.1	12.1	14.8	21.2	10.6	6.5	16.9	34.4	25.1	18.4	6.7	11.0	20.9
Georgia *(continued)*															
Other Areas *(continued)*															
St Francis, Columbus	5,631	12.5	***13.0***	**×**	**×**					**×**				**×**	
St Joseph, Augusta	2,503	10.6	13.2	×	**×**			×							
St Joseph's, Savannah[1]	5,420	8.9	11.3												
St Marys, Athens[1]	2,952	12.6	***14.0***	**×**	**×**	**×**					×			×	
Satilla Regional, Waycross	3,408	12.5	11.6												
Smith, Hahira	445	12.1	11.5			–		–		–			–	–	–
South Georgia, Valdosta	5,226	12.0	11.4							**×**			★		
Southeast Georgia Regional, Brunswick[1]	5,209	10.8	**10.2**	**★**	**★**		**★**					**×**		**★**	★
Spalding Regional, Griffin	4,029	13.5	***14.8***	**×**	**×**				**×**		**×**			**×**	**×**
Stephens County, Toccoa	2,223	12.2	12.1								×				★
Stewart - Webster, Richland	402	12.7	12.0			–		–		–	–		–	**★**	–
Sumter Regional, Americus	1,887	16.2	***14.7***	**×**	**×**	**×**	**×**		×					**×**	
Sylvan Grove, Jackson	265	18.5	***15.7***	**×**	**×**	–	×	–			–	–	–	–	–
Tanner, Carrollton	3,555	15.3	***13.2***	**×**	**×**	**×**					**×**				
Tanner, Villa Rica	679	8.2	**8.9**	**★**	**★**	–	–		★	–	**★**		–	–	–
Tattnall, Reidsville	243	10.7	10.9			–	–	–		–	–	–	–	–	–
Taylor Regional, Hawkinsville	1,055	13.5	13.3			×				–					–
Tift Regional, Tifton	3,561	12.2	11.5				**★**								
Union General, Blairsville	1,132	14.0	12.1									**×**			×
University, Augusta[1]	9,334	12.0	***12.9***	**×**	×	**★**		×	×		**×**	**×**			
Upson Regional, Thomaston	2,509	14.4	***16.1***	**×**	**×**	**×**	×		**×**		×	**×**	×	**×**	**×**
Walton, Monroe[1]	1,518	16.7	***16.1***	**×**	**×**	**×**				–		**×**		**×**	
Washington County Regional, Sandersville	1,214	15.0	***13.8***	**×**	**×**	×			**×**						–
Wayne, Jesup	1,410	15.3	12.4									**×**			
Wellstar Paulding, Dallas	636	14.2	13.8					–				×	–		–
West Georgia, La Grange[1]	4,011	15.0	***14.3***	**×**	**×**	**×**			**×**	**★**	**×**				
Wheeler County, Glenwood	449	10.7	9.6			–	★	–		–			–	–	–
Wills, Washington	853	14.4	13.2			**×**									–
Guam															
Guam Memorial Authority, Oka Tumuning[1]	1,133	16.9	***16.5***	**×**	**×**		**×**	**×**	**×**				×	–	
Hawaii															
Castle, Kailua	1,838	12.6	12.6					★		×					
Hilo Medical Center, Hilo	2,420	12.4	12.3					**×**							

Footnotes are on page 350.

Hospital outcomes: better (★) or worse (×) than average											Results of accreditation review on full survey		Other facts			
Adjusted Death rates			Adjusted Adverse outcome rates													
Surgical cases			Surgical cases													
All selected surgical cases	Coronary artery bypass surgery	Large bowel surgery	All selected surgical cases	Coronary artery bypass surgery	Large bowel surgery	Gall bladder removal	Total knee replacement	Total hip replacement	Simple prostatectomy	Carotid endarterectomy	Accreditation status*	Overall evaluation score (higher is better)	Number of beds	Major medical school affiliation?	Number of residents	Computerized drug order system (1 to 5 scale, higher is preferred; see page 23 for details)
2.3	3.8	6.5	7.7	10.3	11.9	7.5	6.7	6.4	5.4	8.2	–	91	161	–	–	–
							–	–			4	97	217	No	0	–
	–		✖	–			✖	✖	–		–[2]	–[2]	145	No	0	–
							★		–		4	94	216	No	0	–
	–			–	★		✖		–	–	4	87	172	No	0	–
	–			–			★	–	✖	–	4	99	116	No	4	–
–	–	–	–	–	–	–	–	–	–	–	–[2]	–[2]	71	No	0	–
	–			–						★	4	89	335	No	0	–
	–			–			★			✖	4	94	300	No	0	–
	–			–				–	–	–	4	92	158	No	1	–
	–			–			–	–	–	–	4	87	96	No	0	–
–	–	–	–	–	–	–	–	–	–	–	–[2]	–[2]	32	No	0	–
✖	–	–		–		✖	–	–	–	–	4	98	132	No	0	–
–	–	–	–	–	–	–	–	–	–	–	–[2]	–[2]	28	No	0	–
✖	–	✖		–	✖	–	★	–	–	–	4	87	156	No	0	–
–	–	–	–	–	–	–	–	–	–	–	4	94	36	No	0	–
–	–	–	–	–	–	–	–	–	–	–	–[2]	–[2]	25	No	0	–
–	–	–		–	–	–	–	–	–	–	4	91	55	No	0	–
	–		★	–			★			–	4	86	176	No	0	–
–	–	–		–	–	–	–	–	–	–	–[2]	–[2]	45	No	0	–
✖	✖	✖	✖	✖			✖				4	83	495	Yes	0	–
	–			–			–	–			4	90	115	No	0	–
–	–	–		–	–	–	–	–	–	–	4	91	57	No	0	1
–	–	–		–	–		–	–	–	–	4	84	56	No	0	–
–	–	–	–	–	–	–	–	–	–	–	4	86	110	No	0	–
–	–	–	–	–	–	–	–	–	–	–	4	96	34	No	1	2
×	–	✖	✖	–	✖		–	–	–		4	92	194	No	0	–
–	–	–	–	–	–	–	–	–	–	–	–[2]	–[2]	40	No	0	–
–	–	–	–	–	–	–	–	–	–	–	4	87	38	No	0	–
–	–	–	–	–	–	–	–	–	–	–	–[2]	–[2]	159	No	–	–
	–	–	×	–		–	✖	–	–	–	4	96	147	No	0	–
	–	–		–		×	–	–	–	–	4	84	56	No	0	–

***Accreditation Status:** 5=Accredited with commendation or with full standards compliance; 4=Accredited with requirements for improvement; 3=Conditional accreditation.

Detailed Ratings for All Areas

See more information on "Key Ratings for Metro Areas" table beginning on page 32

Blue is most favorable
Bold Italic is least favorable
Blank means neither better nor worse than average
"–" means insufficient data

	Death rates for all selected case types			Hospital outcomes: better (★) or worse (✕) than average — Adjusted Death rates — Medical Cases											
	Number of cases	Actual death rate (%)	Adjusted death rate (%) (lower is better)	All selected cases	All selected medical cases	Heart attack	Congestive heart failure	Obstructive pulmonary disease	Pneumonia	Respiratory failure and arrest	Septicemia	Stroke	Gastrointestinal hemorrhage	Fluid, electrolyte, & acid-base disorders	Kidney failure
National Average	–	–	12.1	12.1	14.8	21.2	10.6	6.5	16.9	34.4	25.1	18.4	6.7	11.0	20.9
Hawaii *(continued)*															
Kahuku Hospital, Kahuku	56	17.9	18.9			–	–	–	–	–	–	–	–	–	–
Kaiser Moanalua, Honolulu	2,657	10.9	11.9						✕			**★**			
Kapiolani Medical Center at Pali Momi, Aiea	2,031	11.0	11.0			✕	**★**					★			
Kauai Veterans, Waimea	394	8.4	**6.6**	**★**	**★**			–	★	–	**★**		–	–	–
Kona, Kealakekua	915	10.6	10.1	★	★		★	–	**★**					–	✕
Kuakini, Honolulu	4,241	10.8	**10.0**	**★**	**★**	★					**★**	**★**			**★**
Maui, Wailuku	2,202	10.9	**10.4**	**★**	**★**										
Molokai General, Kaunakakai	67	11.9	11.5			–	–	–	–	–	–	–	–	–	–
North Hawaii, Kamuela	493	8.1	**8.8**	**★**	★	–		–		–	–		–	–	–
Queen's, Honolulu	5,841	9.8	**9.9**	**★**	**★**		**★**		**★**	★	**★**	**★**			
St Francis, Honolulu	2,791	10.4	**9.1**	**★**	**★**		**★**		**★**			**★**			
St Francis - West, Ewa Beach	1,930	12.1	**9.0**	**★**	**★**		**★**		**★**		★				
Straub, Honolulu[1]	3,248	10.1	**8.8**	**★**	**★**	**★**			**★**		**★**	**★**	**★**	★	
Wahiawa General, Wahiawa	1,025	14.3	13.1			✕									–
Wilcox, Lihue	1,543	9.5	**8.6**	**★**	**★**				**★**		**★**	**★**		**★**	
Idaho															
Bannock Regional, Pocatello	1,539	12.0	***15.1***	**✖**	**✖**		**✖**	**✖**		**✖**				**★**	–
Benewah, St Maries	284	16.9	14.9		**✖**	–	–	–	**✖**	–	–		–	–	–
Bingham, Blackfoot[1]	525	11.4	14.8	✕	✕		**✖**	–		–	–		–	–	–
Bonner General, Sandpoint	726	8.7	12.1							–	–		–	–	–
Cassia Regional, Burley	1,076	10.3	12.3			–				–	–				–
Clearwater Valley, Orofino	448	11.2	13.8			–		**✖**	**★**	–	–	–	–	–	–
Eastern Idaho Regional, Idaho Falls	4,124	10.3	12.5				**✖**								
Franklin County, Preston	184	14.7	14.1			–	–	–		–	–	–	–	–	–
Gritman, Moscow	823	9.8	11.2								–				–
Kootenai, Coeur d'Alene	4,089	10.0	12.0												
Lost Rivers, Arco	150	12.7	13.3			–	–	–		–	–	–	–	–	–
Madison, Rexburg	792	9.7	12.9					–		–	–		–	–	–
Magic Valley Regional, Twin Falls	2,214	11.0	***14.9***	**✖**	**✖**		**✖**					**✖**	**✖**		
Mercy, Nampa	2,354	11.0	12.3												
Minidoka, Rupert	427	8.7	11.0			–				–	–		–	–	–
Pocatello Regional, Pocatello	1,148	10.5	13.9	✕	✕			–		**✖**		✕	✕		
St Alphonsus Regional, Boise	5,577	9.3	12.9	✕	**✖**					**✖**					
St Joseph Regional, Lewiston	2,720	10.2	12.7				✕		✕						
St Luke's Regional, Boise	5,343	8.3	11.9												

Footnotes are on page 350.

Hospital outcomes: better (★) or worse (×) than average											Results of accreditation review on full survey		Other facts			
Adjusted Death rates			Adjusted Adverse outcome rates													
Surgical cases			Surgical cases													
All selected surgical cases	Coronary artery bypass surgery	Large bowel surgery	All selected surgical cases	Coronary artery bypass surgery	Large bowel surgery	Gall bladder removal	Total knee replacement	Total hip replacement	Simple prostatectomy	Carotid endarterectomy	Accreditation status*	Overall evaluation score (higher is better)	Number of beds	Major medical school affiliation?	Number of residents	Computerized drug order system (1 to 5 scale, higher is preferred; see page 23 for details)
2.3	3.8	6.5	7.7	10.3	11.9	7.5	6.7	6.4	5.4	8.2	–	91	161	–	–	–
–	–	–	–	–	–	–	–	–	–	–	4	**88**	24	No	0	–
	–	–			×	–	–	–	–	–	4	92	162	**Yes**	9	–
	–	–		–			✖	–	–	–	4	**97**	75	No	0	–
–	–	–	–	–	–	–	–	–	–	–	4	**87**	49	No	0	–
–	–	–	★	–	–	–	–	–	–	–	4	**95**	53	No	0	–
			✖	✖		×	✖	–	–	–	5	**96**	150	**Yes**	0	–
	–	–		–			–	–	–	–	4	91	194	No	0	–
–	–	–	–	–	–	–	–	–	–	–	4	92	15	No	0	–
–	–	–	–	–	–	–	–	–	–	–	4	90	35	No	–	–
		★		✖							4	**96**	423	**Yes**	2	–
	✖	★	✖	✖	✖		–	–	×	–	4	93	203	**Yes**	0	–
	–	–		–	–		–	–	–	–	4	**96**	102	No	0	–
★	★	–		★	✖		✖	–			4	89	139	No	2	–
–	–	–	★	–	–	–	–	–	–	–	4	93	69	No	0	–
–	–	–	★	–	–		–	–	–	–	4	**87**	71	No	0	–
	–	–		–				–	–	–	4	**94**	120	No	0	–
–	–	–	–	–	–	–	–	–	–	–	–[2]	–[2]	25	No	0	–
–	–	–		–	–	–	–	–	–	–	4	**85**	37	No	0	–
	–	–	★	–		–	–	–	–	–	4	**94**	48	No	0	–
–	–	–		–	–	–	×	–	–	–	4	91	87	No	0	–
–	–	–	–	–	–	–	–	–	–	–	–[2]	–[2]	18	No	0	–
	×		★		★		★			★	4	**96**	273	No	0	2
–	–	–	–	–	–	–	–	–	–	–	–[2]	–[2]	20	No	0	–
	–	–	★	–		–	–	–	–	–	4	**86**	53	No	0	–
★	–		★	–			★	★			4	91	225	No	0	–
–	–	–	–	–	–	–	–	–	–	–	–[2]	–[2]	10	No	0	–
–	–	–		–	–	–		–	–	–	–[2]	–[2]	52	No	0	–
	–			–					–	–	4	89	160	No	0	–
	–		×	–			✖		–	–	–[2]	–[2]	132	No	0	–
–	–	–	–	–	–	–	–	–	–	–	–[2]	–[2]	29	No	0	–
–	–	–		–	–	–		–	–	–	5	**98**	87	No	0	–
			★				★				4	91	281	No	0	–
	–			–					–		4	93	140	No	0	–
										★	4	**96**	326	No	37	–

***Accreditation Status:** 5=Accredited with commendation or with full standards compliance; 4=Accredited with requirements for improvement; 3=Conditional accreditation.

Detailed Ratings for All Areas

See more information on "Key Ratings for Metro Areas" table beginning on page 32

Blue is most favorable
Bold Italic is least favorable
Blank means neither better nor worse than average
"–" means insufficient data

	Death rates for all selected case types				Hospital outcomes: better (★) or worse (×) than average — Adjusted Death rates — Medical Cases											
	Number of cases	Actual death rate (%)	Adjusted death rate (%) (lower is better)	All selected cases	All selected medical cases	Heart attack	Congestive heart failure	Obstructive pulmonary disease	Pneumonia	Respiratory failure and arrest	Septicemia	Stroke	Gastrointestinal hemorrhage	Fluid, electrolyte, & acid-base disorders	Kidney failure
National Average	–	–	12.1	12.1	14.8	21.2	10.6	6.5	16.9	34.4	25.1	18.4	6.7	11.0	20.9
Idaho *(continued)*															
St Mary's, Cottonwood	443	9.3	10.8			–		–		–	–		–	–	–
Syringa General, Grangeville	255	7.5	8.8			–	–	–		–	–	–	–	–	–
Twin Falls Clinic and Hospital, Twin Falls	1,603	11.8	13.2				✖				★				
Walter Knox, Emmett	312	14.4	10.9			–		–		–	–		–	–	–
West Valley, Caldwell	1,647	10.9	***13.9***	✖	✖			–				×			✖
Wood River, Sun Valley	369	8.4	11.5			–		–	★	–	–	–	–	–	–
Illinois															
Chicago Area															
Advocate Bethany, Chicago	899	8.7	**7.5**	**★**	**★**	★	**★**			**★**	**★**		–		–
Advocate Christ and Hope Children's, Oak Lawn	11,735	13.8	12.1									✖	★	★	
Advocate Good Samaritan, Downers Grove	5,764	11.6	**10.6**	**★**	**★**				**★**		★	**★**			
Advocate Good Shepherd, Barrington	3,030	12.9	12.1							★					
Advocate Illinois Masonic, Chicago[1]	2,652	11.8	**10.2**	**★**	**★**		★		**★**						**★**
Advocate Lutheran/Lutheran Children's, Park Ridge[1]	9,846	10.4	**9.6**	**★**	**★**	**★**	**★**		**★**	**★**		**★**	**★**		
Advocate Ravenswood, Chicago	2,430	12.9	10.9	★	**★**		**★**		★						
Advocate South Suburban, Hazel Crest	5,303	12.7	**9.7**	**★**	**★**		**★**		**★**			**★**	★		**★**
Advocate Trinity, Chicago	2,824	9.4	**7.7**	**★**	**★**		**★**	**★**	**★**			**★**	★		
Alexian Brothers, Elk Grove Village	4,858	11.4	11.5							**★**					
Catholic Health Partners Columbus, Chicago	1,270	9.6	**8.1**	**★**	**★**			–	**★**	–		**★**	–		
Central DuPage, Winfield	5,511	10.9	***13.4***	✖	✖		✖	✖		✖	✖	★			
Children's, Chicago	–	–	–	–	–	–	–	–	–	–	–	–	–	–	–
Condell, Libertyville	3,425	13.9	***13.5***	✖	✖					✖					
Cook County, Chicago	1,857	5.1	**7.5**	**★**	**★**		**★**	**★**	**★**		–	★		★	**★**
Delnor, Geneva	2,866	10.7	13.2	×	✖	✖			✖						★
Edgewater, Chicago	2,479	10.6	**5.8**	**★**	**★**		**★**	**★**	**★**	**★**	**★**	★	**★**	**★**	**★**
Edward, Naperville[1]	4,305	13.7	12.5												
Elmhurst Memorial, Elmhurst	6,833	11.2	**10.6**	**★**	**★**						★	★			
Evanston Northwestern, Evanston	10,392	10.5	11.9			**★**	✖	★				★	×		
Glenbrook, Glenview	–	–	–	–	–	–	–	–	–	–	–	–	–	–	–
Glenoaks, Glendale Heights	720	23.1	***16.7***	✖	✖	×	✖		×			✖	×	–	–
Gottlieb, Melrose Park	3,236	10.4	**9.2**	**★**	**★**	**★**			**★**			**★**			
Grant, Chicago	1,386	10.0	**9.7**	**★**	**★**		**★**		**★**						
Harvard Memorial, Harvard	388	12.4	13.3					–		–	–		–	–	–
Highland Park Hospital, Highland Park	2,344	11.9	12.4				✖		×			**★**			

Footnotes are on page 350.

Hospital outcomes: better (★) or worse (×) than average											Results of accreditation review on full survey		Other facts			
Adjusted Death rates			Adjusted Adverse outcome rates													
Surgical cases			Surgical cases													
All selected surgical cases	Coronary artery bypass surgery	Large bowel surgery	All selected surgical cases	Coronary artery bypass surgery	Large bowel surgery	Gall bladder removal	Total knee replacement	Total hip replacement	Simple prostatectomy	Carotid endarterectomy	Accreditation status*	Overall evaluation score (higher is better)	Number of beds	Major medical school affiliation?	Number of residents	Computerized drug order system (1 to 5 scale, higher is preferred; see page 23 for details)
2.3	3.8	6.5	7.7	10.3	11.9	7.5	6.7	6.4	5.4	8.2	–	91	161	–	–	–
–	–	–	–	–	–	–	–	–	–	–	–[2]	–[2]	28	No	0	–
–	–	–	–	–	–	–	–	–	–	–	–[2]	–[2]	16	No	0	–
	–			–		–		–	–	–	–[2]	–[2]	38	No	0	–
–	–	–	–	–	–	–	–	–	–	–	–[2]	–[2]	17	No	0	–
	–		★	–				–	★	–	–[2]	–[2]	106	No	0	–
–	–	–		–	–	–	–	–	–	–	–[2]	–[2]	64	No	0	–
–	–	–	–	–	–	–	–	–	–	–	4	90	102	No	0	–
		✖			✖						4	93	620	**Yes**	200	–
							✖				–[2]	–[2]	238	No	0	–
	–	★		–	★			–		–	4	93	154	No	0	–
	–	–				–	–	–	–	–	5	90	326	**Yes**	200	–
★		★			★		✖	✖	★		4	92	573	**Yes**	165	–
×	–					–	–	–	–	–	–[2]	–[2]	324	No	57	–
	–			–				★			–[2]	–[2]	194	No	0	–
	–		★	–	★		–	–	–	–	4	92	217	No	0	–
	★			★				✖			4	**95**	346	No	16	–
–	–	–		–	–	–	–	–	–	–	4	89	128	**Yes**	24	–
	✖			✖							4	91	321	No	0	–
–	–	–	–	–	–	–	–	–	–	–	4	91	218	–	14	–
	–			–		✖	★	–	–	–	5	**98**	183	No	0	–
–	–	–		–	–	–	–	–	–	–	4	***86***	593	**Yes**	454	–
	–			–					✖	–	4	**95**	118	No	0	–
	–			–		–	–	–	–	–	4	92	213	No	6	–
						×			–		4	91	151	No	0	–
★											4	***88***	305	No	0	–
			✖				✖	✖			4	**95**	562	**Yes**	0	–
–	–	–	–	–	–	–	–	–	–	–	–[2]	–[2]	–	–	–	–
–	–	–	–	–	–	–	–	–	–	–	4	89	116	No	9	–
	★		★				–	–	–		4	**98**	176	No	0	–
	–	–			–	–	–	–		–	4	***84***	116	No	3	–
–	–	–	–	–	–	–	–	–	–	–	4	89	81	No	0	–
	–		★	–		–		★			–[2]	–[2]	234	No	–	–

***Accreditation Status:** 5=Accredited with commendation or with full standards compliance; 4=Accredited with requirements for improvement; 3=Conditional accreditation.

Detailed Ratings for All Areas

See more information on "Key Ratings for Metro Areas" table beginning on page 32

Blue is most favorable
Bold Italic is least favorable
Blank means neither better nor worse than average
"–" means insufficient data

	Death rates for all selected case types			Hospital outcomes: better (★) or worse (×) than average — Adjusted Death rates											
					Medical Cases										
	Number of cases	Actual death rate (%)	Adjusted death rate (%) (lower is better)	All selected cases	All selected medical cases	Heart attack	Congestive heart failure	Obstructive pulmonary disease	Pneumonia	Respiratory failure and arrest	Septicemia	Stroke	Gastrointestinal hemorrhage	Fluid, electrolyte, & acid-base disorders	Kidney failure
National Average	–	–	12.1	12.1	14.8	21.2	10.6	6.5	16.9	34.4	25.1	18.4	6.7	11.0	20.9
Illinois *(continued)*															
Chicago Area *(continued)*															
Hinsdale Hospital, Hinsdale	5,369	11.8	11.5												
Holy Cross, Chicago	5,415	13.1	11.5												**★**
Holy Family, Des Plaines	4,212	12.8	12.4												✖
Ingalls, Harvey	5,736	11.4	**10.6**	**★**	**★**	**★**		★		★		**★**	✖		
Jackson Park, Chicago[1]	997	11.7	**9.2**	**★**	**★**	–	**★**	**★**					✖		★
La Grange Memorial, La Grange	5,573	12.1	**10.0**	**★**	**★**	**★**	**★**	**★**			**★**	★		**★**	
La Rabida Children's, Chicago	–	–	–	–	–	–	–	–	–	–	–	–	–	–	–
Lake Forest Hospital, Lake Forest	1,926	9.6	11.6												
Little Company of Mary, Evergreen Park[1]	5,509	12.8	12.0					★							**★**
Loretto, Chicago	734	12.0	**7.9**	**★**	**★**		**★**		**★**		**★**		–	–	
Louis A Weiss, Chicago	3,131	13.6	**10.2**	**★**	**★**				★		**★**			★	★
Loyola University, Maywood	5,280	9.8	11.3		★							★	★	×	
MacNeal, Berwyn	5,719	15.0	12.1				✖	**★**		✖					
Memorial, Woodstock	2,099	13.4	***13.6***	✖	✖			✖							
Mercy, Chicago	4,109	12.6	11.9				**★**				×			✖	
Methodist, Chicago	1,633	12.1	**8.7**	**★**	**★**		**★**		**★**		**★**			**★**	**★**
Michael Reese, Chicago	3,026	12.7	**10.4**	**★**	**★**	**★**	★		**★**		✖	**★**			★
Midwestern Regional, Zion	315	15.6	***16.2***	✖	✖	–		–		–		–	–	–	–
Mt Sinai, Chicago	1,545	11.6	**8.6**	**★**	**★**		**★**	**★**	**★**			**★**			★
Northern Illinois, McHenry	3,317	13.4	***13.9***	✖	✖		✖		×						★
Northwest, Arlington Heights	9,073	12.5	12.5		×		×		✖						
Northwestern, Chicago	7,007	8.9	**9.7**	**★**	**★**	**★**					★	**★**		**★**	
Norwegian - American, Chicago	932	9.4	11.3			–		**★**		–			–		
Oak Park Hospital, Oak Park	2,168	12.2	**9.9**	**★**	**★**		**★**	**★**				★			
Our Lady of the Resurrection, Chicago	5,700	14.4	***12.9***	✖	✖	✖		✖							
Palos Community, Palos Heights	9,075	11.5	11.9						★						
Provena Mercy, Aurora	2,781	13.3	***13.9***	✖	✖			✖	×		✖	×	★	✖	
Provena St Joseph, Elgin	2,211	13.7	12.8											✖	
Provena St Joseph, Joliet	8,164	11.0	11.8									★			
Provident of Cook County, Chicago	719	12.8	10.0	★	★		★	**★**							**★**
Resurrection, Chicago	10,319	12.8	***13.4***	✖	✖	✖		★	✖				✖		
Roseland, Chicago	980	17.0	12.8			✖	**★**				✖		–		×
Rush - Copley, Aurora[1]	2,206	12.1	12.6						×						
Rush - Presbyterian - St Lukes, Chicago	5,485	7.2	**8.3**	**★**	**★**		**★**		**★**		**★**	**★**	★	★	**★**

Footnotes are on page 350.

Hospital outcomes: better (★) or worse (×) than average											Results of accreditation review on full survey		Other facts			
Adjusted Death rates			Adjusted Adverse outcome rates													
Surgical cases			Surgical cases													
All selected surgical cases	Coronary artery bypass surgery	Large bowel surgery	All selected surgical cases	Coronary artery bypass surgery	Large bowel surgery	Gall bladder removal	Total knee replacement	Total hip replacement	Simple prostatectomy	Carotid endarterectomy	Accreditation status*	Overall evaluation score (higher is better)	Number of beds	Major medical school affiliation?	Number of residents	Computerized drug order system (1 to 5 scale, higher is preferred; see page 23 for details)
2.3	3.8	6.5	7.7	10.3	11.9	7.5	6.7	6.4	5.4	8.2	–	91	161	–	–	–
	×		✖	✖							4	**88**	331	No	10	–
	–			–				–			4	**86**	245	**Yes**	0	–
✖	–	✖	✖	–			✖	✖	–		4	92	183	No	7	–
	★						✖				4	90	409	No	0	–
–	–	–	–	–	–	–	–	–	–	–	4	92	236	No	5	–
				★			✖	✖			4	**87**	158	No	20	–
–	–	–	–	–	–	–	–	–	–	–	5	**96**	–	–	–	–
	–	–		–		–	✖	✖	–	–	4	91	126	No	0	–
	–			–				✖			4	90	494	No	–	–
–	–	–	–	–	–	–	–	–	–	–	4	**86**	223	No	1	–
	–		✖	×		–	✖	✖	–	–	4	**88**	205	**Yes**	8	–
							×	✖			4	**95**	523	**Yes**	525	–
	–			–	★						4	**86**	275	**Yes**	59	–
	–		★	–			★	–	–	–	4	**87**	98	No	0	–
	–					–		–	✖	–	4	91	311	No	89	–
	–			–		–	–	–	–	–	4	92	189	No	4	–
	–	–		–		–		–	–	–	4	**79**	523	No	15	–
–	–	–	–	–	–	–	–	–	–	–	5	**97**	70	No	2	–
–	–	–		–	–	–	–	–	–	–	4	93	296	**Yes**	14	–
	–			–					–		4	**88**	133	No	0	–
				★			✖				4	91	395	No	0	–
★	★							★	✖	✖	4	**97**	642	**Yes**	363	–
–	–	–		–	–	–	–	–	–	–	4	**97**	230	No	8	–
	–			–		–	★		–	–	4	92	129	No	0	–
	–		★	–		★	–	–			4	**98**	216	No	0	–
	–			–			★	★	✖		4	93	340	No	0	–
								–	–		4	90	180	No	5	–
	–			–		–	×	✖	–		4	**88**	183	No	0	–
						★					–[2]	–[2]	369	No	0	–
–	–	–	–	–	–	–	–	–	–	–	4	89	113	No	0	–
✖								★	✖		5	**96**	369	**Yes**	110	–
–	–	–	–	–	–	–	–	–	–	–	4	93	128	No	0	–
	–			–				–	–		4	93	132	**Yes**	0	–
★											4	**87**	669	**Yes**	625	–

***Accreditation Status:** 5=Accredited with commendation or with full standards compliance; 4=Accredited with requirements for improvement; 3=Conditional accreditation.

Detailed Ratings for All Areas

See more information on "Key Ratings for Metro Areas" table beginning on page 32

Blue is most favorable
Bold Italic is least favorable
Blank means neither better nor worse than average
"–" means insufficient data

	Death rates for all selected case types				Hospital outcomes: better (★) or worse (×) than average — Adjusted Death rates — Medical Cases										
	Number of cases	Actual death rate (%)	Adjusted death rate (%) (lower is better)	All selected cases	All selected medical cases	Heart attack	Congestive heart failure	Obstructive pulmonary disease	Pneumonia	Respiratory failure and arrest	Septicemia	Stroke	Gastrointestinal hemorrhage	Fluid, electrolyte, & acid-base disorders	Kidney failure
National Average	–	–	12.1	12.1	14.8	21.2	10.6	6.5	16.9	34.4	25.1	18.4	6.7	11.0	20.9
Illinois *(continued)*															
Chicago Area *(continued)*															
Rush North Shore, Skokie	5,072	11.7	**9.6**	**★**	**★**		**★**	**★**	**★**			★	★	★	
Sacred Heart, Chicago	1,077	3.2	**5.7**	**★**	**★**	–	**★**	★	–	–		–	–	–	
St Alexius, Hoffman Estates	3,270	16.9	11.6					×							
St Anthony, Chicago	1,618	11.9	**8.9**	**★**	**★**		**★**	**★**			**★**				
St Bernard, Chicago	1,310	15.5	11.3			✖	**★**		**★**						
St Elizabeth, Chicago	1,980	10.4	**8.6**	**★**	**★**		**★**		**★**		**★**				**★**
St Francis, Blue Island	5,564	10.5	**9.7**	**★**	**★**	**★**	**★**	★		**★**		**★**	★		
St Francis, Evanston	5,669	13.3	**11.0**	**★**	**★**										**★**
St James, Chicago Heights	4,986	12.6	**11.0**	**★**	**★**							**★**		×	★
St James, Olympia Fields[1]	1,764	16.0	11.8												
St Joseph, Chicago	4,342	11.6	**10.2**	**★**	**★**	**★**	**★**	**★**	**★**						
St Mary of Nazareth, Chicago	2,195	7.5	**7.3**	**★**	**★**		**★**	**★**	**★**					**★**	
Sherman, Elgin	4,685	10.6	11.8												
Silver Cross, Joliet	4,274	12.4	11.3											**★**	
South Shore, Chicago	1,448	10.4	**8.4**	**★**	**★**		**★**	★				**★**	–		
Swedish Covenant, Chicago	4,504	15.0	11.6			✖	**★**			✖				**★**	★
Thorek, Chicago	1,352	8.8	**8.8**	**★**	**★**		**★**	★				★	–		
University of Chicago, Chicago	3,944	10.4	12.0						★			★		✖	
University of Illinois, Chicago	1,442	7.4	**7.8**	**★**	**★**		**★**		**★**			**★**		**★**	★
Victory, Waukegan[1]	3,343	10.2	**10.6**	**★**	**★**						**★**	★			**★**
Vista Health Provena St Therese, Waukegan	2,063	15.4	***13.7***	✖	✖	✖									
West Suburban, Oak Park	3,273	10.2	**9.9**	**★**	**★**		**★**		★			**★**			
Westlake, Melrose Park	3,098	9.1	**7.6**	**★**	**★**	★	**★**	**★**	**★**		**★**	**★**	**★**	**★**	
Other Areas															
Abraham Lincoln Memorial, Lincoln	1,233	13.3	12.8				★			–					
Alton Memorial, Alton	2,716	12.7	***14.2***	✖	✖			✖	✖				×		
Anderson, Maryville	2,747	15.2	***16.0***	✖	✖	✖	✖		✖		✖	✖			
Blessing, Quincy	6,281	11.5	11.9												
Bromenn, Normal	3,188	11.3	12.7				✖								
Carle Foundation, Urbana	4,541	9.7	12.4				×	✖							
Carlinville Area, Carlinville	1,271	11.0	**10.0**	**★**	**★**			★			★	**★**		**★**	
CGH, Sterling	3,411	11.7	***13.1***	✖	×	×	×								
Clay County, Flora	912	12.6	***14.8***	✖	✖				✖	–	–				–

Footnotes are on page 350.

Hospital outcomes: better (★) or worse (×) than average											Results of accreditation review on full survey		Other facts			
Adjusted Death rates			Adjusted Adverse outcome rates													
Surgical cases			Surgical cases													
All selected surgical cases	Coronary artery bypass surgery	Large bowel surgery	All selected surgical cases	Coronary artery bypass surgery	Large bowel surgery	Gall bladder removal	Total knee replacement	Total hip replacement	Simple prostatectomy	Carotid endarterectomy	Accreditation status*	Overall evaluation score (higher is better)	Number of beds	Major medical school affiliation?	Number of residents	Computerized drug order system (1 to 5 scale, higher is preferred; see page 23 for details)
2.3	3.8	6.5	7.7	10.3	11.9	7.5	6.7	6.4	5.4	8.2	–	91	161	–	–	–
★	★			★			✖			–	4	91	213	Yes	102	–
–	–	–		–	–	–	–	–		–	4	**88**	96	No	0	–
	–	–		–				–	–	–	4	90	171	No	0	–
–	–	–		–	–	–	–	–	–	–	4	**87**	163	No	0	–
–	–	–	–	–	–	–	–	–	–	–	4	89	194	No	5	–
	–	–	✖	–	–	–	–	–		–	4	**98**	224	No	18	–
				★						✖	4	91	256	No	0	–
							✖				4	**82**	283	No	94	–
	–			–						✖	4	93	332	No	18	–
✖	–					–	–	–	–	–	–[2]	–[2]	164	No	4	–
	✖			✖			×	–			4	**84**	408	Yes	74	–
			★			★	–	–	–	–	4	90	305	No	26	–
											4	92	238	No	0	–
	–			–				–	–	✖	4	89	227	No	0	–
–	–	–	★	–	–	–	–	–	–	–	4	**86**	125	No	3	–
	–			–				✖		–	3	90	265	No	12	–
–	–	–		–	–	–	–	–	–	–	4	89	137	No	3	–
✖	✖		✖	✖		–	✖	✖	–	✖	4	**95**	533	Yes	549	–
	–	–				–	–	–	–	–	4	90	432	Yes	29	–
✖	–			–				–	✖	–	4	91	102	No	0	–
×	–	–		–		–		–	–	–	5	**95**	229	No	0	–
		–	★				★		★	–	4	**80**	134	No	56	–
			★				–	–		★	4	**88**	230	Yes	39	–
–	–	–		–	–	–	–	–	–	–	4	**96**	60	No	0	–
	–			–		–	✖	–	–	–	4	**94**	138	No	0	1
	–			–				–	–		4	**82**	115	No	0	1
	–			–			★	★		✖	–[2]	–[2]	179	No	16	–
	–			–	★					–	–[2]	–[2]	242	No	0	–
			✖		×					✖	4	**99**	211	Yes	17	–
–	–	–	–	–	–	–	–	–	–	–	4	91	33	No	0	–
	–		★	–			★	–	–	–	4	89	143	No	0	–
–	–	–		–	–	–	–	–	–	–	4	**87**	31	No	0	–

***Accreditation Status:** 5=Accredited with commendation or with full standards compliance; 4=Accredited with requirements for improvement; 3=Conditional accreditation.

Detailed Ratings for All Areas

See more information on "Key Ratings for Metro Areas" table beginning on page 32

Blue is most favorable
Bold Italic is least favorable
Blank means neither better nor worse than average
"–" means insufficient data

	Death rates for all selected case types				Hospital outcomes: better (★) or worse (×) than average — Adjusted Death rates — Medical Cases										
	Number of cases	Actual death rate (%)	Adjusted death rate (%) (lower is better)	All selected cases	All selected medical cases	Heart attack	Congestive heart failure	Obstructive pulmonary disease	Pneumonia	Respiratory failure and arrest	Septicemia	Stroke	Gastrointestinal hemorrhage	Fluid, electrolyte, & acid-base disorders	Kidney failure
National Average	–	–	12.1	12.1	14.8	21.2	10.6	6.5	16.9	34.4	25.1	18.4	6.7	11.0	20.9
Illinois *(continued)*															
Other Areas *(continued)*															
Community Hospital, Ottawa	2,055	11.4	11.6								★			**★**	
Community Med Ctr Western Illinois, Monmouth	971	10.4	9.4	**★**	**★**			–			**★**	**★**			
Crawford, Robinson	800	18.6	***19.9***	✖	✖	×	✖		✖	✖	✖	✖	–		–
Crossroads, Mt Vernon	1,180	8.6	8.8	**★**	**★**		**★**	**★**	**★**						–
Decatur Memorial, Decatur	5,077	10.6	***14.5***	✖	✖		✖	✖	✖			✖			✖
Doctors, Springfield	1,481	10.6	11.9					×		✖					–
Edward A Utlaut, Greenville[1]	819	14.3	12.1					–		–		✖			
Fayette County, Vandalia[1]	1,059	13.0	12.5								–		✖		
Ferrell, Eldorado	885	16.5	***14.8***	✖	✖				✖	–			–		
Franklin, Benton	737	17.2	***18.8***	✖	✖	✖	✖	–			✖	✖	–	–	–
Freeport Memorial, Freeport	3,105	12.0	***14.9***	✖	✖	✖	✖		✖			✖			✖
Galena - Stauss, Galena	250	18.0	***18.0***	✖	✖	–	–	–		–	×	–	–	–	–
Galesburg Cottage, Galesburg	3,259	10.6	11.6											**★**	**★**
Gibson Area, Gibson City	865	10.9	11.8			**★**				–					–
Good Samaritan Regional, Mt Vernon	3,048	10.2	9.4	**★**	**★**				**★**		**★**				**★**
Graham, Canton[1]	1,700	15.2	***14.8***	✖	✖		✖				×	✖	✖		–
Hamilton, McLeansboro[1]	795	11.3	***14.8***	✖	✖			**★**		–	–	✖	–		–
Hammond - Henry, Geneseo	662	15.0	***17.2***	✖	✖	✖	×	–	✖	–	★	✖	✖	–	–
Hardin County General, Rosiclare	613	9.8	9.0	**★**	**★**	–				–	–		–		–
Harrisburg Medical Center, Harrisburg	1,769	14.7	***15.8***	✖	✖				✖				✖		✖
Herrin Hospital, Herrin	2,240	11.9	12.4					×				★			
Hillsboro Area, Hillsboro	997	14.0	***14.1***	✖	✖	–				–	✖		✖		–
Hoopeston Community, Hoopeston	382	16.2	***20.5***	✖	✖	–		–	✖	–	–	–	–		–
Hopedale Hospital, Hopedale[1]	510	9.2	12.7			–		–		–	–		–	–	
Illini, Pittsfield	1,021	13.0	11.2										★		
Illini, Silvis	3,363	12.1	12.2			×		**★**							
Illinois Valley, Peru	1,790	10.9	***14.4***	✖	✖	✖		✖		–				✖	✖
Iroquois, Watseka[1]	1,997	11.8	10.6	**★**	★				**★**						✖
Jersey, Jerseyville[1]	1,288	14.5	***14.3***	✖	✖	✖	✖	–					–		–
John and Mary Kirby, Monticello	252	13.5	14.6			–	–	–	✖	–	–	–	–	–	–
Katherine Shaw Bethea, Dixon	1,943	13.3	***16.4***	✖	✖		✖		✖			✖		✖	–
Kewanee Hospital, Kewanee	1,424	15.4	***15.0***	✖	✖	✖		✖		✖		✖			–
Kishwaukee, Dekalb	1,809	10.9	13.2		×					✖					
Lawrence County, Lawrenceville	897	15.2	***15.6***	✖	✖	✖		–		–	–	✖	–		✖

Footnotes are on page 350.

Hospital outcomes: better (★) or worse (×) than average											Results of accreditation review on full survey		Other facts			
Adjusted Death rates			Adjusted Adverse outcome rates													
Surgical cases			Surgical cases													
All selected surgical cases	Coronary artery bypass surgery	Large bowel surgery	All selected surgical cases	Coronary artery bypass surgery	Large bowel surgery	Gall bladder removal	Total knee replacement	Total hip replacement	Simple prostatectomy	Carotid endarterectomy	Accreditation status*	Overall evaluation score (higher is better)	Number of beds	Major medical school affiliation?	Number of residents	Computerized drug order system (1 to 5 scale, higher is preferred; see page 23 for details)
2.3	3.8	6.5	7.7	10.3	11.9	7.5	6.7	6.4	5.4	8.2	–	91	161	–	–	–
★	–	–		–		–	–	–	–	–	4	89	113	No	0	–
–	–	–	–	–	–	–	–	–	–	–	–[2]	–[2]	109	No	–	–
–	–	–	–	–	–	–	–	–	–	–	4	88	45	Yes	0	–
–	–	–		–	–	–	–	–	–	–	4	92	37	No	0	–
	–		✖	–		✖	✖		×		4	93	174	No	13	–
	–	–		–		–	–	–	–	–	–[2]	–[2]	68	No	0	–
–	–	–	–	–	–	–	–	–	–	–	4	96	192	No	1	–
–	–	–	–	–	–	–	–	–	–	–	4	96	41	No	0	–
–	–	–	–	–	–	–	–	–	–	–	–[2]	–[2]	36	No	0	–
–	–	–	–	–	–	–	–	–	–	–	4	92	34	No	0	–
	–			–					★	–	4	89	148	No	0	–
–	–	–	–	–	–	–	–	–	–	–	–[2]	–[2]	25	No	0	–
✖	–		✖	–		✖	✖		–	–	5	87	154	No	0	–
×	–	–		–		–	–	–	–	–	3	91	40	No	0	–
	–	★	★	–	★			–			–[2]	–[2]	127	No	0	–
	–			–		–	–	–	–	–	4	92	70	No	3	–
–	–	–	–	–	–	–	–	–	–	–	4	94	31	No	0	–
–	–	–		–	–	–	–	–	–	–	4	91	38	No	0	–
–	–	–	–	–	–	–	–	–	–	–	4	82	48	No	0	–
✖	–	–		–		–	–	–	–	–	4	94	80	No	0	–
	–	–		–		–		–	–	–	4	95	79	No	0	–
–	–	–	–	–	–	–	–	–	–	–	4	97	60	No	0	–
–	–	–	–	–	–	–	–	–	–	–	–[2]	–[2]	25	No	0	–
	–	–		–	–	–	–	–	–	–	–[2]	–[2]	119	No	2	–
–	–	–	–	–	–	–	–	–	–	–	4	86	45	No	0	–
	–		★	–		✖	★	★	–		4	88	105	No	0	–
	–	–	✖	–		–	✖	✖	–	–	4	91	88	No	0	–
–	–	–		–	–	–	–	–	–	–	4	85	112	No	2	–
	–	–	★	–		–	–	–	–	–	4	94	67	No	0	–
–	–	–	–	–	–	–	–	–	–	–	4	88	16	No	0	–
	–		★	–		–		–	–		–[2]	–[2]	85	No	0	–
★	–	–	★	–		–	–	–	–	–	4	87	49	No	0	–
	–	–	★	–	★	–				–	4	91	114	No	0	–
–	–	–	–	–	–	–	–	–	–	–	–[2]	–[2]	58	No	0	–

***Accreditation Status:** 5=Accredited with commendation or with full standards compliance; 4=Accredited with requirements for improvement; 3=Conditional accreditation.

Detailed Ratings for All Areas

See more information on "Key Ratings for Metro Areas" table beginning on page 32

Blue is most favorable
Bold Italic is least favorable
Blank means neither better nor worse than average
"–" means insufficient data

	Death rates for all selected case types				Hospital outcomes: better (★) or worse (×) than average — Adjusted Death rates — Medical Cases											
	Number of cases	Actual death rate (%)	Adjusted death rate (%) (lower is better)	All selected cases	All selected medical cases	Heart attack	Congestive heart failure	Obstructive pulmonary disease	Pneumonia	Respiratory failure and arrest	Septicemia	Stroke	Gastrointestinal hemorrhage	Fluid, electrolyte, & acid-base disorders	Kidney failure
National Average	–	–	12.1	12.1	14.8	21.2	10.6	6.5	16.9	34.4	25.1	18.4	6.7	11.0	20.9
Illinois *(continued)*															
Other Areas *(continued)*															
Marion Memorial, Marion	2,599	10.9	11.3						★						
Marshall Browning, Du Quoin	682	14.7	***16.1***	✖	✖	–			✖	–			–		–
Mason, Havana	589	16.1	13.3			–		–		–			×	–	–
Massac Memorial, Metropolis	1,080	14.4	13.1			✖		★				✖	–		✖
McDonough, Macomb	2,220	11.2	***14.8***	✖	✖	✖	✖			–		✖			
Memorial, Belleville[1]	6,939	9.9	10.8	★	★	★	★								
Memorial, Carbondale	2,625	12.8	***13.2***	✖	×			✖	×		×				
Memorial, Chester	667	12.9	12.5			–				–	–			×	–
Memorial, Springfield[1]	8,396	10.1	11.6		★	★	×			★		★		✖	
Methodist Medical Center of Illinois, Peoria	6,474	11.4	12.6				×		✖						
Morris Hospital, Morris	2,238	9.6	9.9	★	★						★	★			
Morrison Community, Morrison	125	18.4	***20.5***	✖	✖	–	–	–		–	–	–	–	–	–
Northwest Suburban, Belvidere	109	18.3	16.7			–	–	–		–	–	–	–	–	–
OSF St Anthony, Rockford	5,207	9.8	10.4	★	★	★	✖	★	★	★	★	★			
OSF St Francis, Peoria	7,040	10.6	12.0			★	✖	★							
OSF St James, Pontiac	1,317	13.4	12.4			✖									
OSF St Joseph, Bloomington	2,659	10.6	12.5			★	✖			✖		★			
OSF St Mary, Galesburg	2,721	11.0	12.9			✖									
Pana Community, Pana	644	10.6	12.3			–				–	–		–		–
Paris Community, Paris	731	14.2	13.6				✖	–					–	–	–
Passavant Area, Jacksonville	3,103	13.9	***13.8***	✖	✖	✖			✖					×	
Pekin Memorial, Pekin	2,485	14.8	***13.9***	✖	✖				×			×		✖	✖
Perry, Princeton	1,622	11.0	12.2			✖		✖		–					–
Proctor, Peoria	4,298	11.1	12.9	×			✖						✖		
Provena Covenant, Urbana	4,715	11.8	***13.2***	✖	✖		✖			✖					
Provena St Mary's, Kankakee	3,126	12.8	12.2												
Provena United Samaritans, Danville	4,984	12.6	***14.8***	✖	✖	✖	✖		×			×	✖	✖	✖
Red Bud Regional, Red Bud	799	15.0	***16.5***	✖	✖	–		✖		–	–			–	–
Richland, Olney	1,671	12.1	9.6	★	★			★	★	★					
Riverside, Kankakee	3,761	10.8	11.4			✖									
Rochelle Community, Rochelle	660	15.5	***14.6***	✖	×	–		–		–				×	–
Rockford Memorial, Rockford	6,088	11.2	12.2				✖								
St Anthony's, Alton	2,722	13.5	***13.6***	✖	✖			✖	✖						
St Anthony's, Effingham	3,548	11.2	***14.1***	✖	✖	✖	✖						×	×	

Footnotes are on page 350.

Hospital outcomes: better (★) or worse (×) than average											Results of accreditation review on full survey		Other facts			
Adjusted Death rates			Adjusted Adverse outcome rates													
Surgical cases			Surgical cases													
All selected surgical cases	Coronary artery bypass surgery	Large bowel surgery	All selected surgical cases	Coronary artery bypass surgery	Large bowel surgery	Gall bladder removal	Total knee replacement	Total hip replacement	Simple prostatectomy	Carotid endarterectomy	Accreditation status*	Overall evaluation score (higher is better)	Number of beds	Major medical school affiliation?	Number of residents	Computerized drug order system (1 to 5 scale, higher is preferred; see page 23 for details)
2.3	3.8	6.5	7.7	10.3	11.9	7.5	6.7	6.4	5.4	8.2	–	91	161	–	–	–
	–	–	★	–		★			–	–	4	91	84	No	0	–
–	–	–	–	–	–	–	–	–	–	–	4	92	33	No	0	–
–	–	–	–	–	–	–	–	–	–	–	5	**98**	36	No	0	–
–	–	–		–	–	–	–	–	–	–	4	***83***	38	No	0	–
×	–	×		–			–	★	–	✖	4	93	104	No	0	–
			★				★		–		4	**99**	341	No	0	1
	–			–			★	–	–		4	**96**	132	No	18	–
–	–	–	–	–	–	–	–	–	–	–	4	92	43	No	0	–
✖	×		✖	✖							4	***82***	453	**Yes**	107	–
											5	93	300	**Yes**	31	–
	–	–	★	–				–	–	–	4	93	82	No	0	–
–	–	–	–	–	–	–	–	–	–	–	–[2]	–[2]	21	No	0	–
–	–	–	–	–	–	–	–	–	–	–	4	**95**	69	No	0	–
										★	4	93	221	**Yes**	0	–
			✖	✖	✖		✖		✖	✖	4	***84***	532	**Yes**	136	–
	–	–		–		–	–	–	–	–	4	93	65	No	0	–
							–	–	–		4	91	141	No	0	–
	–		★	–						–	4	91	127	No	0	–
–	–	–	–	–	–	–	–	–	–	–	4	**96**	30	No	0	–
–	–	–	–	–	–	–	–	–	–	–	4	91	49	No	0	–
	–			–		–		–		–	4	93	105	No	0	–
	–	–		–		–	✖	–	–		4	92	97	No	0	–
	–	–	★	–			–	–	–	–	–[2]	–[2]	72	No	0	–
		×	✖				✖				4	90	129	No	0	–
✖	✖										4	93	246	**Yes**	0	–
	–			–	✖	–			–	–	4	93	150	No	0	–
✖	–	✖		–						–	–[2]	–[2]	259	No	25	–
✖	–	–		–	–	–	–	–	–	–	4	**94**	35	No	0	–
–	–	–		–	–	–	–	–	–	–	4	***86***	62	No	0	–
	–		★			★	★		–	–	4	**94**	278	No	0	–
–	–	–	✖	–	✖	–	–	–	–	–	4	***86***	30	No	0	–
								✖	–	★	4	89	344	No	3	–
	–	✖		–		–		–	–	–	4	**96**	254	No	0	1
×	–	✖		–			★		–	–	5	**96**	133	No	0	–

***Accreditation Status:** 5=Accredited with commendation or with full standards compliance; 4=Accredited with requirements for improvement; 3=Conditional accreditation.

Detailed Ratings for All Areas

See more information on "Key Ratings for Metro Areas" table beginning on page 32

Blue is most favorable
Bold Italic is least favorable
Blank means neither better nor worse than average
"–" means insufficient data

	Death rates for all selected case types			Hospital outcomes: better (★) or worse (×) than average — Adjusted Death rates	Medical Cases										
	Number of cases	Actual death rate (%)	Adjusted death rate (%) (lower is better)	All selected cases	All selected medical cases	Heart attack	Congestive heart failure	Obstructive pulmonary disease	Pneumonia	Respiratory failure and arrest	Septicemia	Stroke	Gastrointestinal hemorrhage	Fluid, electrolyte, & acid-base disorders	Kidney failure
National Average	–	–	12.1	12.1	14.8	21.2	10.6	6.5	16.9	34.4	25.1	18.4	6.7	11.0	20.9
Illinois *(continued)*															
Other Areas *(continued)*															
St Elizabeth, Granite City	2,149	13.7	11.6							★ (blue)					
St Elizabeth's, Belleville	6,493	11.8	11.5								✖				
St Francis, Litchfield	1,601	12.7	***13.6***	✖	×	×				–					
St John's, Springfield	9,378	8.9	11.6			★ (blue)		✖			★				
St Joseph, Murphysboro	1,108	10.8	10.7							–			★		
St Joseph's, Breese	1,251	11.0	11.8			–				✖			–		
St Joseph's, Highland	898	14.1	***16.2***	✖	✖	✖	✖	–	✖	–	–		–		–
St Margaret's, Spring Valley	1,587	10.1	13.7	×	✖	✖				–	✖				
St Mary's, Centralia	3,833	11.7	**9.8**	★ (blue)	★ (blue)		★ (blue)	★	★ (blue)	★ (blue)				★ (blue)	
St Mary's, Decatur	3,221	11.8	11.9			✖					★ (blue)				
St Mary's, East St Louis	896	11.3	**9.4**	★ (blue)	★ (blue)	–	★			★					
St Mary's, Streator	2,879	9.2	**8.7**	★ (blue)	★ (blue)				★ (blue)		★ (blue)			★ (blue)	
St Vincent, Taylorville	1,559	10.5	**10.2**	★ (blue)	★ (blue)										
Salem Township, Salem	1,059	9.8	10.5				★			–					–
Sarah Bush Lincoln, Mattoon	3,736	12.4	12.3							×					
Sarah D Culbertson, Rushville	596	18.1	***15.4***	✖	✖		✖	–		✖	✖		–	–	
Shelby, Shelbyville	1,628	7.7	**7.7**	★ (blue)	★ (blue)	×	★ (blue)	★ (blue)	★ (blue)	★	★ (blue)	★			★ (blue)
Sparta Community, Sparta[1]	758	14.1	***14.3***	✖	×			–		–					
Swedish American, Rockford[1]	5,609	10.3	11.4			★									
Touchette Regional, Centreville	390	12.3	13.1			–		–	✖	–	–		–	–	–
Trinity West, Rock Island	6,949	11.3	***12.9***	✖	✖		✖		✖						
Union County, Anna	903	14.2	***14.8***	✖	✖	–		–		–			–		–
Valley West, Sandwich	826	15.1	***17.2***	✖	✖		✖	×		✖	✖				–
Wabash General, Mt Carmel[1]	1,154	10.1	**9.8**	★ (blue)	★ (blue)				★				–		–
Washington County, Nashville	377	14.6	13.1					–		–	–		–		–
White County, Carmi	277	19.9	***18.0***	✖	✖	✖		–	✖	–	–	×	–	–	–
Wood River Township, Wood River	162	15.4	16.1		×	–	–	–	–	–	–	✖	–	–	–
Indiana															
Indianapolis Area															
Clarian Health Partners, Indianapolis	13,654	10.2	**10.2**	★ (blue)	★ (blue)	★ (blue)		★ (blue)	★ (blue)		★ (blue)	★ (blue)		★	
Community East, Indianapolis[1]	10,256	11.2	**9.8**	★ (blue)	★ (blue)	★ (blue)			★ (blue)	★ (blue)	★ (blue)	★ (blue)		★ (blue)	★ (blue)
Community North, Indianapolis	–	–	–	–	–	–	–	–	–	–	–	–	–	–	–
Community South, Indianapolis	2,692	13.5	13.0			✖			×				✖		★

Footnotes are on page 350.

Hospital outcomes: better (★) or worse (×) than average											Results of accreditation review on full survey		Other facts			
Adjusted Death rates			Adjusted Adverse outcome rates													
Surgical cases			Surgical cases													
All selected surgical cases	Coronary artery bypass surgery	Large bowel surgery	All selected surgical cases	Coronary artery bypass surgery	Large bowel surgery	Gall bladder removal	Total knee replacement	Total hip replacement	Simple prostatectomy	Carotid endarterectomy	Accreditation status*	Overall evaluation score (higher is better)	Number of beds	Major medical school affiliation?	Number of residents	Computerized drug order system (1 to 5 scale, higher is preferred; see page 23 for details)
2.3	3.8	6.5	7.7	10.3	11.9	7.5	6.7	6.4	5.4	8.2	–	91	161	–	–	–
	–	–	✖	–	★	–	✖	–	–	–	4	90	196	No	0	1
★	★			★		×		★			4	**96**	289	No	0	1
	–	–		–		–	–	–	–	–	4	90	62	No	0	–
		✖	✖		✖		✖	✖	✖		4	91	525	**Yes**	110	–
–	–	–		–	–	–	–	–	–	–	4	***88***	40	No	0	–
★	–	–	★	–		–	–	–	–	–	4	93	57	No	0	–
–	–	–		–	–	–	✖	–	–	–	4	***87***	76	No	0	–
	–	–		–		–		–	✖	–	4	***85***	90	No	0	–
	–			–		★	–	–	–	–	4	92	276	No	0	–
	–			–					–	–	4	**95**	131	No	1	–
–	–	–	–	–	–	–	–	–	–	–	4	**97**	119	No	0	1
	–	–		–			–	–	–	–	5	93	140	No	0	–
–	–	–		–	–	–	–	–	–	–	4	**96**	101	No	0	–
–	–	–		–	–	–	–	–	–	–	5	**99**	31	No	0	–
	–			–		×				–	4	89	133	No	0	–
–	–	–	–	–	–	–	–	–	–	–	–[2]	–[2]	28	No	0	–
–	–	–	–	–	–	–	–	–	–	–	4	89	37	No	0	–
–	–	–		–	–	–	–	–	–	–	4	**94**	35	No	0	–
★											4	89	291	No	0	–
–	–	–	–	–	–	–	–	–	–	–	4	93	189	No	–	1
	–			★						★	4	***84***	309	No	0	–
–	–	–		–	–	–	–	–	–	–	4	89	36	No	0	–
–	–	–		–	–	–	–	–	–	–	–[2]	–[2]	35	No	0	–
–	–	–	–	–	–	–	–	–	–	–	4	89	56	No	0	–
–	–	–	–	–	–	–	–	–	–	–	4	**96**	21	No	0	–
–	–	–	–	–	–	–	–	–	–	–	–[2]	–[2]	112	No	2	–
–	–	–	–	–	–	–	–	–	–	–	–[2]	–[2]	60	No	0	–
✖					✖						4	91	1,385	**Yes**	–	–
	×	★	✖	✖					–	✖	4	***87***	999	No	181	4
–	–	–	–	–	–	–	–	–	–	–	4	***87***	–	–	–	–
×	–			–			–	–	–	–	4	***88***	117	No	2	4

***Accreditation Status:** 5=Accredited with commendation or with full standards compliance; 4=Accredited with requirements for improvement; 3=Conditional accreditation.

Detailed Ratings for All Areas

See more information on "Key Ratings for Metro Areas" table beginning on page 32

Blue is most favorable
Bold Italic is least favorable
Blank means neither better nor worse than average
"–" means insufficient data

	Death rates for all selected case types				Hospital outcomes: better (★) or worse (×) than average — Adjusted Death rates — Medical Cases										
	Number of cases	Actual death rate (%)	Adjusted death rate (%) (lower is better)	All selected cases	All selected medical cases	Heart attack	Congestive heart failure	Obstructive pulmonary disease	Pneumonia	Respiratory failure and arrest	Septicemia	Stroke	Gastrointestinal hemorrhage	Fluid, electrolyte, & acid-base disorders	Kidney failure
National Average	–	–	12.1	12.1	14.8	21.2	10.6	6.5	16.9	34.4	25.1	18.4	6.7	11.0	20.9
Indiana *(continued)*															
Indianapolis Area *(continued)*															
Indiana University, Indianapolis	–	–	–	–	–	–	–	–	–	–	–	–	–	–	–
St Francis, Beech Grove[1]	9,988	11.1	12.1			★									
St Vincent, Indianapolis[1]	14,260	10.9	11.3	★	★	★			★						
Westview, Indianapolis	1,148	10.4	10.5												–
Winona, Indianapolis	1,173	14.5	11.4								✖	★			
Wishard, Indianapolis	2,623	12.7	10.7	★	★				★		×				★
Women's, Indianapolis	44	–	–	–	–	–	–	–	–	–	–	–	–	–	–
Other Areas															
Adams County, Decatur	1,294	11.5	12.8				×			–					×
Ball, Muncie	7,863	11.8	***12.7***	✖	×		×					×			
Bedford Regional, Bedford	1,537	13.6	13.3			×			✖						
Bloomington Hospital, Bloomington[1]	5,921	11.1	12.5			★	✖			✖					
Bloomington of Orange County, Paoli	772	14.4	13.5					–		–	–		–	–	–
Bluffton Regional, Bluffton	1,576	7.9	10.6							★			–	✖	
Cameron, Angola	456	11.6	***16.0***	✖	✖	–	✖	–		–	–		–	–	–
Clark, Jeffersonville	4,168	13.9	***13.3***	✖	✖		✖								
Columbus Regional, Columbus	4,129	10.9	12.9	×				×						✖	✖
Community, Munster[1]	7,933	9.5	11.9			★									★
Community of Anderson & Madison County, Anderson	3,084	10.2	10.8	★	★		★								
Community of Noble County, Kendallville	73	4.1	6.3			–	–	–	–	–	–	–	–	–	–
Daviess, Washington	1,233	10.9	11.1												
Deaconess, Evansville	8,942	10.6	11.7				×				★			★	
Deaconess St Joseph's, Huntingburg	916	13.0	13.6					–		–		✖	–		
Dearborn County, Lawrenceburg	1,859	11.6	12.0							–					✖
Decatur County, Greensburg	1,020	11.0	13.4							–					–
DeKalb, Auburn	1,135	15.1	***17.2***	✖	✖	✖	✖			–	–	✖	✖		
Dukes, Peru	918	11.3	13.2									✖	–	–	–
Dunn, Bedford	1,701	13.9	12.8							×					
Elkhart General, Elkhart	5,366	9.7	11.7								★				
Fayette, Connersville[1]	2,033	11.8	9.0	★	★		★		★	★			★	★	×
Floyd, New Albany[1]	4,306	12.0	12.5			✖						×			
Gibson General, Princeton	930	11.8	11.4			×									
Good Samaritan, Vincennes	5,613	10.1	12.7		×			✖				★			

Footnotes are on page 350.

Hospital outcomes: better (★) or worse (×) than average											Results of accreditation review on full survey		Other facts			
Adjusted Death rates			Adjusted Adverse outcome rates													
Surgical cases			Surgical cases													
All selected surgical cases	Coronary artery bypass surgery	Large bowel surgery	All selected surgical cases	Coronary artery bypass surgery	Large bowel surgery	Gall bladder removal	Total knee replacement	Total hip replacement	Simple prostatectomy	Carotid endarterectomy	Accreditation status*	Overall evaluation score (higher is better)	Number of beds	Major medical school affiliation?	Number of residents	Computerized drug order system (1 to 5 scale, higher is preferred; see page 23 for details)
2.3	3.8	6.5	7.7	10.3	11.9	7.5	6.7	6.4	5.4	8.2	–	91	161	–	–	–
–	–	–	–	–	–	–	–	–	–	–	–[2]	–[2]	–	–	–	–
				★		✖			✖	★	4	89	361	No	36	–
✖	✖			✖				✖			4	**88**	752	**Yes**	155	–
–	–	–		–		–	–	–	–	–	–[2]	–[2]	67	No	0	–
–	–	–		–	–	–	–	–	–	–	–[2]	–[2]	169	No	4	–
×	–	–		–		–	–	–	–	–	4	**86**	253	**Yes**	0	–
–	–	–	–	–	–	–	–	–	–	–	4	**87**	102	No	0	4
–	–	–		–		–	–	–	–	–	4	89	65	No	0	–
							✖	★			4	**88**	311	No	98	–
–	–	–		–	–	–	–	–	–	–	4	93	60	No	0	–
								–		✖	5	**86**	284	No	0	–
–	–	–	–	–	–	–	–	–	–	–	3	**87**	48	No	0	–
★	–	–		–		–		–	–	–	4	**94**	76	No	0	–
–	–	–	–	–	–	–	–	–	–	–	–[2]	–[2]	30	No	0	–
×	–	×		–			★	–	–		4	**86**	177	No	0	–
	–			–					–	–	4	**99**	197	No	0	–
						★				✖	4	**96**	292	No	14	–
	–	–		–				–	–	–	4	91	207	No	–	4
–	–	–	–	–	–	–	–	–	–	–	4	**96**	43	No	0	–
✖	–	–	×	–		–	–	–	–	–	4	**86**	56	No	0	–
			★			✖	★				4	**87**	287	No	18	2
–	–	–		–	–	–	–	–	–	–	4	**88**	60	No	0	–
	–	–	★	–	★		–	–	–	–	4	**83**	74	No	0	–
–	–	–	–	–	–	–	–	–	–	–	4	**97**	67	No	0	–
	–	–		–		–	–	–	–	–	4	**84**	45	No	0	–
–	–	–		–	–	–	–	–	–	–	4	**96**	40	No	0	–
	–	–		–		–	–	–	–	–	4	93	112	No	4	–
		★	★	★	★						4	**85**	269	No	0	–
	–	–	★	–		–		–	–	–	–[2]	–[2]	111	No	3	–
	–			–	★		✖			✖	4	90	154	No	0	–
–	–	–	–	–	–	–	–	–	–	–	4	93	64	No	0	–
			★	★	★						4	92	240	No	0	–

***Accreditation Status:** 5=Accredited with commendation or with full standards compliance; 4=Accredited with requirements for improvement; 3=Conditional accreditation.

Detailed Ratings for All Areas

See more information on "Key Ratings for Metro Areas" table beginning on page 32

Blue is most favorable
Bold Italic is least favorable
Blank means neither better nor worse than average
"–" means insufficient data

	Death rates for all selected case types			Hospital outcomes: better (★) or worse (×) than average — Adjusted Death rates											
					Medical Cases										
	Number of cases	Actual death rate (%)	Adjusted death rate (%) (lower is better)	All selected cases	All selected medical cases	Heart attack	Congestive heart failure	Obstructive pulmonary disease	Pneumonia	Respiratory failure and arrest	Septicemia	Stroke	Gastrointestinal hemorrhage	Fluid, electrolyte, & acid-base disorders	Kidney failure
National Average	–	–	12.1	12.1	14.8	21.2	10.6	6.5	16.9	34.4	25.1	18.4	6.7	11.0	20.9
Indiana *(continued)*															
Other Areas *(continued)*															
Goshen General, Goshen	2,514	11.8	13.1		×								✖		✖
Greene County General, Linton	1,195	12.4	***15.3***	✖	✖				✖	–			–		–
Hancock, Greenfield[1]	2,023	12.5	13.3	×	✖										
Harrison County, Corydon	1,026	12.2	11.3							–					–
Hendricks, Danville	2,967	12.6	12.9												
Henry County, New Castle	1,916	14.3	***16.9***	✖	✖	✖	✖	✖	✖			✖		✖	✖
Howard, Kokomo	2,183	12.0	12.0												
Huntington Memorial, Huntington	776	12.0	13.4							–			–		–
Jasper County, Rensselaer	709	14.5	13.8		×	✖			★	–	–	✖	✖		–
Jay County, Portland	806	12.2	13.5				✖			–			–		–
Johnson, Franklin	1,983	13.2	12.1										★		
King's Daughters', Madison[1]	2,989	12.5	***13.7***	✖	✖	✖	✖								
Kosciusko, Warsaw	1,643	14.0	***14.2***	✖	✖							✖		✖	–
La Porte Hospital, La Porte[1]	2,528	11.6	10.2	★	★			★	★						
Lafayette Home, Lafayette[1]	3,485	11.2	12.8		×	✖	×				★		✖	✖	
Lagrange Community, Lagrange	395	13.9	15.0	×		–		–	×		–		–	–	–
Lutheran of Indiana, Fort Wayne	7,555	10.4	12.1			★	✖					★			
Major, Shelbyville	1,659	12.3	***14.5***	✖	✖		✖		✖						
Margaret Mary, Batesville	1,105	12.1	13.9	×	✖		×			–				–	–
Marion General, Marion	4,047	13.0	***13.5***	✖	✖	✖	✖	★		✖					
Medical Center of Southern Indiana, Charlestown	1,013	13.4	***14.6***	✖	✖				×				–		
Memorial, Jasper	2,565	9.6	9.7	★	★			★	★						
Memorial, Logansport	1,637	11.1	***14.9***	✖	✖		✖			×	–		×		
Memorial, Seymour	2,211	14.1	***15.7***	✖	✖				✖			✖			✖
Memorial, South Bend	6,110	10.0	12.8	×	✖	★	✖			×		✖			
Methodist - Southlake Campus, Merrillville	5,440	11.5	11.9											✖	
Methodist Northlake, Gary[1]	3,388	13.9	10.4	★	★	★	★					★			★
Morgan, Martinsville	1,693	13.5	11.3								★			★	
Parkview, Fort Wayne	10,218	11.4	12.3				✖								×
Perry County, Tell City	742	13.1	***16.1***	✖	✖					–	–	✖	–		–
Porter, Valparaiso	6,126	10.5	11.7										★		
Putnam County, Greencastle	995	14.5	13.6							–	–		–		
Reid, Richmond[1]	7,032	10.4	10.3	★	★	✖		★	★					★	
Riverview, Noblesville	2,048	11.1	13.4	×			✖								×

Footnotes are on page 350.

Hospital outcomes: better (★) or worse (×) than average — Adjusted Death rates, Surgical cases: All selected surgical cases	Adjusted Death rates, Surgical cases: Coronary artery bypass surgery	Adjusted Death rates, Surgical cases: Large bowel surgery	Adjusted Adverse outcome rates, Surgical cases: All selected surgical cases	Adjusted Adverse outcome rates, Surgical cases: Coronary artery bypass surgery	Adjusted Adverse outcome rates, Surgical cases: Large bowel surgery	Adjusted Adverse outcome rates, Surgical cases: Gall bladder removal	Adjusted Adverse outcome rates, Surgical cases: Total knee replacement	Adjusted Adverse outcome rates, Surgical cases: Total hip replacement	Adjusted Adverse outcome rates, Surgical cases: Simple prostatectomy	Adjusted Adverse outcome rates, Surgical cases: Carotid endarterectomy	Results of accreditation review on full survey: Accreditation status*	Results of accreditation review on full survey: Overall evaluation score (higher is better)	Other facts: Number of beds	Other facts: Major medical school affiliation?	Other facts: Number of residents	Other facts: Computerized drug order system (1 to 5 scale, higher is preferred; see page 23 for details)
2.3	3.8	6.5	7.7	10.3	11.9	7.5	6.7	6.4	5.4	8.2	–	91	161	–	–	–
	–	–	★	–		–			★	–	4	91	113	No	0	–
–	–	–	–	–	–	–	–	–	–	–	4	92	40	No	0	–
	–		★	–	★	–		–	–	–	4	89	80	No	0	–
–	–	–		–		–	–	–	–	–	4	91	47	No	0	–
×	–	✖	✖	–	✖	✖	–	–	–	–	4	89	127	No	0	–
	–	–		–				–	–	–	4	92	107	No	0	4
	–	–		–			–	–	★	–	4	90	109	No	0	–
–	–	–	–	–	–	–	–	–	–	–	4	**85**	37	No	0	–
–	–	–	–	–	–	–	–	–	–	–	–[2]	–[2]	48	No	0	–
–	–	–		–	–	–	–	–	–	–	4	**95**	65	No	0	–
✖	–	✖		–	×		–	–	–	–	4	92	77	No	0	–
	–			–			–		–	–	3	92	86	No	0	–
	–	–	★	–		–		–	–	–	–[2]	–[2]	72	No	0	–
	–	–	★	–	★		–		★	–	4	**85**	172	No	0	–
★	–		★	–			★	★		–	4	**86**	394	No	0	–
–	–	–	–	–	–	–	–	–	–	–	4	**88**	53	No	0	–
✖	×										4	**88**	377	No	0	–
–	–	–	★	–	–	–	–	–	–	–	4	89	54	No	0	–
–	–	–		–	–	–	–	–	–	–	4	**94**	47	No	0	–
	–			–					–	–	4	93	191	No	0	–
–	–	–	–	–	–	–	–	–	–	–	4	**85**	80	No	0	–
	–		★	–					–	–	4	92	100	No	0	–
	–	–	★	–		–		–	–	–	–[2]	–[2]	83	No	0	–
	–	–		–				–	–	–	4	**94**	112	No	0	–
				★	✖						4	**84**	405	No	28	–
		✖		★	✖					✖	–[2]	–[2]	356	No	–	–
	–			–		–	–	–	–	–	4	91	563	No	12	–
–	–	–		–	–	–	–	–	–	–	4	92	86	No	0	–
							✖		★		4	**87**	477	No	1	4
–	–	–	–	–	–	–	–	–	–	–	4	91	38	No	0	–
										✖	4	**97**	260	No	0	–
–	–	–	–	–	–	–	–	–	–	–	4	**85**	85	No	0	–
	–			–			✖	★			4	**88**	211	No	0	–
✖	–	–		–		–		–	–	–	4	**94**	86	No	0	–

***Accreditation Status:** 5=Accredited with commendation or with full standards compliance; 4=Accredited with requirements for improvement; 3=Conditional accreditation.

Detailed Ratings for All Areas

See more information on "Key Ratings for Metro Areas" table beginning on page 32

Blue is most favorable
Bold Italic is least favorable
Blank means neither better nor worse than average
"–" means insufficient data

	Death rates for all selected case types			Hospital outcomes: better (★) or worse (×) than average — Adjusted Death rates — Medical Cases											
	Number of cases	Actual death rate (%)	Adjusted death rate (%) (lower is better)	All selected cases	All selected medical cases	Heart attack	Congestive heart failure	Obstructive pulmonary disease	Pneumonia	Respiratory failure and arrest	Septicemia	Stroke	Gastrointestinal hemorrhage	Fluid, electrolyte, & acid-base disorders	Kidney failure
National Average	–	–	12.1	12.1	14.8	21.2	10.6	6.5	16.9	34.4	25.1	18.4	6.7	11.0	20.9
Indiana *(continued)*															
Other Areas *(continued)*															
St Anthony, Crown Point	4,339	11.2	12.4			**★**					★		×	×	
St Anthony, Michigan City[1]	3,223	12.8	***13.5***	✖	✖				×	✖				×	
St Catherine, East Chicago	3,171	8.7	**8.2**	**★**	**★**		**★**	**★**	★			**★**		**★**	**★**
St Clare, Crawfordsville	1,653	14.4	***16.1***	✖	✖	✖		✖	✖		✖				
St Elizabeth, Lafayette[1]	4,229	13.5	***13.7***	✖	✖		×					✖			
St Francis, Mooresville[1]	1,603	0.4	**4.7**	**★**	**★**	–	–	–	–	–	–	–	–	–	–
St John's, Anderson[1]	4,149	11.5	**10.0**	**★**	**★**	**★**				★	**★**				★
St Joseph, Fort Wayne	3,472	12.4	11.4		★										**★**
St Joseph, Kokomo	2,917	14.4	**10.7**	**★**	**★**					★	★				**★**
St Joseph, Mishawaka	2,352	11.2	13.2	×	×	★									
St Joseph's Regional, Plymouth	1,293	12.2	***14.4***	✖	✖	✖				×		×			
St Joseph's Regional, South Bend	6,922	10.5	***13.2***	✖	✖		✖								
St Margaret Mercy, Dyer	1,767	13.9	11.7												
St Margaret Mercy, Hammond[1]	6,718	12.4	11.8			**★**									
St Mary, Hobart	4,365	11.2	11.7			★									
St Mary's, Evansville	6,751	10.1	12.3					✖					✖		
St Mary's Warrick, Boonville	914	12.8	10.4		★			–	★	–			–	–	
St Vincent, Frankfort	765	12.3	13.2							–			–		–
St Vincent, Williamsport	530	11.3	12.5					–		–	**★**	**★**	–	–	–
St Vincent Clay, Brazil	756	15.7	12.4												
St Vincent Mercy, Elwood	726	13.6	***14.8***	✖	✖				✖	–			–		–
Scott County, Scottsburg	743	16.6	***16.8***	✖	✖	✖			✖	–	×		–		
Starke, Knox	800	13.0	14.3	×	×			–				×	–		–
Sullivan County, Sullivan	1,171	15.5	***15.2***	✖	✖		✖			–	✖	✖			–
Terre Haute Regional, Terre Haute	3,263	11.9	10.9	★	★	★							★		
Tipton County, Tipton	966	12.3	***15.3***	✖	✖	–	✖			–	✖		–		–
Union, Terre Haute	7,190	13.6	12.2			**★**	×	✖			✖				
Wabash County, Wabash	939	14.2	***14.7***	✖	✖		✖			×				✖	–
Washington County, Salem	696	11.6	14.5	×	×			–		–	–		–	–	×
West Central, Clinton	1,132	14.5	12.7						✖						
White County, Monticello	853	11.4	***14.6***	✖	✖				✖	–	–	×	–	–	✖
Whitley, Columbia City	507	14.6	14.7	×	✖	✖		–	✖	✖			–		–
Wirth Regional, Oakland City	240	16.7	14.3			–		–		–		–	–	–	–
Witham, Lebanon	1,095	14.8	13.6	×	×										

Footnotes are on page 350.

Hospital outcomes: better (★) or worse (×) than average											Results of accreditation review on full survey		Other facts			
Adjusted Death rates			Adjusted Adverse outcome rates													
Surgical cases			Surgical cases													
All selected surgical cases	Coronary artery bypass surgery	Large bowel surgery	All selected surgical cases	Coronary artery bypass surgery	Large bowel surgery	Gall bladder removal	Total knee replacement	Total hip replacement	Simple prostatectomy	Carotid endarterectomy	Accreditation status*	Overall evaluation score (higher is better)	Number of beds	Major medical school affiliation?	Number of residents	Computerized drug order system (1 to 5 scale, higher is preferred; see page 23 for details)
2.3	3.8	6.5	7.7	10.3	11.9	7.5	6.7	6.4	5.4	8.2	–	91	161	–	–	–
							★				4	91	228	No	0	–
×	–			–				–		✖	4	91	207	No	0	–
★		★	★		★	–	✖	–	–		4	**95**	188	No	0	–
	–	–		–		–	–	–	–	–	4	91	72	No	0	–
✖	✖		×							×	4	**86**	159	No	–	–
	–	–	★	–		–	★	★	–	–	4	91	60	No	0	–
	–			–		–		–	–		4	**82**	176	No	0	–
✖						–			–		4	92	191	No	1	–
	–			–		–	–	–		–	4	92	154	No	0	–
	–			–		✖	✖	–	–		4	93	100	No	14	–
★	–	–	★	–			–	–	–	–	5	**98**	36	No	0	–
			★				★	★			4	91	310	No	27	–
	–	–		–		–	–	–	–	–	–[2]	–[2]	376	No	–	–
	★		★	★					–		4	93	643	No	73	–
						–	✖	–		×	4	**98**	146	No	0	–
			★	★		✖					4	**83**	650	**Yes**	23	–
–	–	–	–	–	–	–	–	–	–	–	4	**87**	28	No	0	–
–	–	–		–	–	–	–	–	–	–	4	92	53	No	0	–
–	–	–	–	–	–	–	–	–	–	–	4	**94**	16	No	0	–
–	–	–		–	–	–	–	–	–	–	4	**87**	36	No	0	–
–	–	–	–	–	–	–	–	–	–	–	4	**88**	40	No	0	–
–	–	–	–	–	–	–	–	–	–	–	4	89	45	No	0	–
–	–	–	–	–	–	–	–	–	–	–	4	**86**	35	No	0	–
–	–	–		–	–	–	–	–	–	–	4	**77**	37	No	0	–
							–	–	–	×	4	89	204	No	0	–
–	–	–	★	–	–	–	–	–	–	–	4	91	37	No	0	–
×						×		★			4	92	261	No	18	–
	–	–		–		–	–	–	–	–	4	**86**	50	No	0	–
–	–	–	–	–	–	–	–	–	–	–	4	89	58	No	0	–
–	–	–	–	–	–	–	–	–	–	–	4	92	27	No	0	–
–	–	–	–	–	–		–	–	–	–	4	**94**	59	No	0	–
–	–	–	–	–	–	–	–	–	–	–	4	**96**	41	No	0	–
–	–	–	–	–	–	–	–	–	–	–	–[2]	–[2]	20	No	0	–
–	–	–		–	–	–	–	–	–	–	4	93	49	No	0	–

***Accreditation Status:** 5=Accredited with commendation or with full standards compliance; 4=Accredited with requirements for improvement; 3=Conditional accreditation.

Detailed Ratings for All Areas

See more information on "Key Ratings for Metro Areas" table beginning on page 32

Blue is most favorable
Bold Italic is least favorable
Blank means neither better nor worse than average
"–" means insufficient data

	Death rates for all selected case types			Hospital outcomes: better (★) or worse (×) than average — Adjusted Death rates — Medical Cases											
	Number of cases	Actual death rate (%)	Adjusted death rate (%) (lower is better)	All selected cases	All selected medical cases	Heart attack	Congestive heart failure	Obstructive pulmonary disease	Pneumonia	Respiratory failure and arrest	Septicemia	Stroke	Gastrointestinal hemorrhage	Fluid, electrolyte, & acid-base disorders	Kidney failure
National Average	–	–	12.1	12.1	14.8	21.2	10.6	6.5	16.9	34.4	25.1	18.4	6.7	11.0	20.9
Indiana *(continued)*															
Other Areas *(continued)*															
Woodlawn, Rochester	831	9.5	13.0					×		–			–		–
Iowa															
Allen, Waterloo	4,890	8.9	12.2												★
Audubon County, Audubon	294	11.2	12.6			–	–	–		–	–		–	–	–
Avera Holy Family, Estherville	719	10.4	9.2	★	★								–	–	
Boone County, Boone	1,014	16.8	***17.4***	✖	✖	×	✖	✖	×	–		✖		✖	–
Broadlawns, Des Moines	565	11.7	11.0			–					–	–	–	–	★
Buena Vista Regional, Storm Lake	895	14.6	12.9							–			★		
Burgess, Onawa	1,115	12.1	10.9				✖	★	★	–					
Cass County, Atlantic	909	12.3	***14.8***	✖	✖	✖		✖		–	–	✖		–	–
Central, Elkader	190	12.6	11.2			–	–	–		–	–	–	–	–	–
Clarinda Regional, Clarinda	430	16.3	***19.3***	✖	✖	–		–	✖	–	–	✖	–	–	–
Clarke County, Osceola	474	11.6	12.0			–		–		–			–	–	–
Community, Sumner	322	14.6	13.7			–	×	–		–	–	–	–	–	–
Covenant, Waterloo	4,296	11.2	12.3												★
Crawford County, Denison	567	15.5	***15.2***	✖	✖	×				–	–	✖	–	✖	–
Dallas County, Perry	526	10.5	9.2	★	★	–	★	–		–			–	–	–
Davis County, Bloomfield	497	8.2	10.6			–		–		–	–		–	–	–
Decatur County, Leon	394	21.3	***22.1***	✖	✖	–		–	✖	–	–	×	–	✖	–
DeWitt Community, DeWitt	249	10.4	10.7			–	–	–		–	–	–	–	–	–
Dickinson County, Spirit Lake	936	8.9	13.2							–	–				–
Ellsworth Municipal, Iowa Falls	614	13.7	14.5	×	×			–		–	–		–	–	–
Finley, Dubuque	2,987	9.8	10.8	★											
Floyd County, Charles City	780	12.8	13.6							–	–		–	–	–
Floyd Valley, Le Mars	775	12.4	12.3					–		–			–	–	–
Fort Madison Community, Fort Madison	1,311	11.9	***15.1***	✖	✖		✖	✖	×	–	–		×		–
Genesis, Davenport	8,610	9.5	11.9			★	✖								✖
Grape, Hamburg	397	14.4	***16.3***	✖	✖	–	×	–		–	–	✖	–	–	–
Great River, West Burlington	3,295	10.3	13.2	×	✖				×						–
Greater Community, Creston	844	12.3	13.1			×				✖			–	–	–
Greene County, Jefferson	489	15.5	***15.9***	✖	✖		✖	–		–			–	–	–
Grinnell Regional, Grinnell	1,580	10.8	11.7							–					–
Guthrie County, Guthrie Center	282	12.8	13.4					–		–	–	–	–	–	–

Footnotes are on page 350.

Hospital outcomes: better (★) or worse (✕) than average											Results of accreditation review on full survey		Other facts			
Adjusted Death rates			Adjusted Adverse outcome rates													
Surgical cases			Surgical cases													
All selected surgical cases	Coronary artery bypass surgery	Large bowel surgery	All selected surgical cases	Coronary artery bypass surgery	Large bowel surgery	Gall bladder removal	Total knee replacement	Total hip replacement	Simple prostatectomy	Carotid endarterectomy	Accreditation status*	Overall evaluation score (higher is better)	Number of beds	Major medical school affiliation?	Number of residents	Computerized drug order system (1 to 5 scale, higher is preferred; see page 23 for details)
2.3	3.8	6.5	7.7	10.3	11.9	7.5	6.7	6.4	5.4	8.2	–	91	161	–	–	–
–	–	–		–	–	–	–	–	–	–	4	***82***	35	No	0	–
			★			✖	★		★		4	**99**	172	No	0	–
–	–	–	–	–	–	–	–	–	–	–	–[2]	–[2]	29	No	0	–
–	–	–	–	–	–	–	–	–	–	–	–[2]	–[2]	35	No	0	–
–	–	–		–	–	–	–	–	–	–	4	***88***	57	No	0	–
–	–	–	–	–	–	–	–	–	–	–	4	***80***	107	No	31	–
–	–	–		–	–	–	–	–	–	–	4	***85***	30	No	0	–
–	–	–		–		–	–	–	–	–	–[2]	–[2]	48	No	0	–
–	–	–		–	–	–	–	–	–	–	–[2]	–[2]	72	No	0	–
–	–	–	–	–	–	–	–	–	–	–	–[2]	–[2]	16	No	0	–
–	–	–	–	–	–	–	–	–	–	–	–[2]	–[2]	27	No	0	–
–	–	–	–	–	–	–	–	–	–	–	–[2]	–[2]	48	No	0	–
–	–	–	–	–	–	–	–	–	–	–	–[2]	–[2]	13	No	0	–
✖	–			–							4	***86***	239	No	0	–
–	–	–	–	–	–	–	–	–	–	–	–[2]	–[2]	28	No	0	–
–	–	–	–	–	–	–	–	–	–	–	–[2]	–[2]	33	No	0	–
–	–	–	–	–	–	–	–	–	–	–	–[2]	–[2]	35	No	0	–
–	–	–	–	–	–	–	–	–	–	–	–[2]	–[2]	49	No	0	–
–	–	–	–	–	–	–	–	–	–	–	4	**97**	8	No	0	–
–	–	–		–	–	–			–	–	4	***84***	49	No	0	–
–	–	–		–	–	–	–	–	–	–	4	***88***	40	No	0	–
	–		✖	–		–	✖	✖			4	**94**	107	No	0	–
–	–	–	–	–	–	–	–	–	–	–	–[2]	–[2]	31	No	0	–
–	–	–		–		–	–	–	–	–	–[2]	–[2]	44	No	0	–
–	–	–		–	–	–	–	–	–	–	4	**94**	50	**Yes**	0	–
	✕			✖			★			★	4	90	402	No	0	–
–	–	–	–	–	–	–	–	–	–	–	–[2]	–[2]	28	No	0	–
	–		★	–							4	93	199	No	0	–
	–	–		–		–	–	–	–	–	–[2]	–[2]	49	No	0	–
–	–	–	–	–	–	–	–	–	–	–	–[2]	–[2]	53	No	0	–
✖	–	✖		–		–	★	–	–	–	–[2]	–[2]	46	No	0	–
–	–	–	–	–	–	–	–	–	–	–	–[2]	–[2]	26	No	0	–

***Accreditation Status:** 5=Accredited with commendation or with full standards compliance; 4=Accredited with requirements for improvement; 3=Conditional accreditation.

Detailed Ratings for All Areas

See more information on "Key Ratings for Metro Areas" table beginning on page 32

Blue is most favorable
Bold Italic is least favorable
Blank means neither better nor worse than average
"–" means insufficient data

	Death rates for all selected case types				Hospital outcomes: better (★) or worse (×) than average — Adjusted Death rates — Medical Cases											
	Number of cases	Actual death rate (%)	Adjusted death rate (%) (lower is better)	All selected cases	All selected medical cases	Heart attack	Congestive heart failure	Obstructive pulmonary disease	Pneumonia	Respiratory failure and arrest	Septicemia	Stroke	Gastrointestinal hemorrhage	Fluid, electrolyte, & acid-base disorders	Kidney failure
National Average	–	–	12.1	12.1	14.8	21.2	10.6	6.5	16.9	34.4	25.1	18.4	6.7	11.0	20.9
Iowa *(continued)*															
Hamilton County, Webster City	1,157	10.0	10.0	★	★				★	–					×
Hegg, Rock Valley	223	16.6	14.5			–	–	–		–		–	–	–	–
Henry County, Mt Pleasant	720	14.0	***14.8***	✖	×		✖	–		–				–	–
Horn, Ida Grove	480	14.6	***16.4***	✖	✖	✖		–		–	–		–	–	–
Humboldt County, Humboldt	321	8.4	11.5			–		–		–	–	–	–	–	–
Iowa Lutheran, Des Moines	3,935	11.5	11.7				×	★			★				
Iowa Methodist, Des Moines	8,812	9.2	11.4			★									
Jackson County, Maquoketa	623	15.2	14.2	×				–		–		✖	–	–	–
Jefferson County, Fairfield	769	13.3	13.3							–		✖		–	
Jennie Edmundson, Council Bluffs	2,597	11.1	***14.4***	✖	✖	✖	✖						✖		
Keokuk Area, Keokuk	1,806	11.7	11.2						★						✖
Keokuk County, Sigourney	81	11.1	10.1			–	–	–	–	–	–	–	–	–	–
Knoxville Area, Knoxville	674	13.1	13.9			×			×	–	–		–		–
Kossuth Regional, Algona	376	16.2	***16.4***	✖	✖	–		–		–	–	✖	–	–	–
Loring, Sac City	690	10.7	11.9					★		–					–
Lucas County, Chariton	449	13.6	11.2			–	✖	–			–		–	–	–
Madison County, Winterset	611	19.0	***16.2***	✖	✖	–	✖	–	✖	–					–
Mahaska, Oskaloosa	835	15.7	***17.4***	✖	✖		✖	✖	×	–	–	×		–	✖
Manning Regional, Manning[1]	249	16.1	***22.6***	✖	✖	–	✖	–		–	–	–	–	–	–
Marshalltown Medical and Surgical, Marshalltown	2,318	13.0	13.0		×							✖			
Mary Greeley, Ames	4,473	8.7	9.2	★	★		★		★		★		★		
Mercy, Cedar Rapids	5,285	9.2	11.3								★				
Mercy, Centerville	849	16.0	***14.8***	✖	✖			✖		–	–			×	–
Mercy, Clinton	3,634	12.0	12.0								★	✖			
Mercy, Des Moines	13,067	11.2	11.5	★	★	★									
Mercy, Dubuque	4,048	11.0	***14.5***	✖	✖		✖	×	✖	×			×		
Mercy, Iowa City	4,776	9.0	10.8	★	★	★	✖				★		★	★	×
Mercy, New Hampton	419	16.9	***16.7***	✖	✖			–		–	–	✖	–	–	–
Mercy, Sioux City	6,067	10.7	11.2	★							★				
Mercy - North Iowa, Mason City	6,562	9.4	***13.4***	✖	✖		✖	×	✖				✖		
Mercy Hospital of Franciscan Sisters, Oelwein	628	11.0	11.1			–			★	–		✖	–	★	–
Merrill Pioneer, Rock Rapids	283	12.7	***18.5***	✖	✖	–		–	✖	–	–	✖	–	–	–
Metropolitan, Des Moines	1,978	13.3	11.8				★								★
Monroe County, Albia	421	12.8	***16.4***	✖	✖	–	✖	–		–	–	–	–	–	–
Montgomery County, Red Oak	1,151	10.7	11.7					✖		–	★		–	–	–

Footnotes are on page 350.

Hospital outcomes: better (★) or worse (×) than average											Results of accreditation review on full survey		Other facts			
Adjusted Death rates			Adjusted Adverse outcome rates													
Surgical cases			Surgical cases													
All selected surgical cases	Coronary artery bypass surgery	Large bowel surgery	All selected surgical cases	Coronary artery bypass surgery	Large bowel surgery	Gall bladder removal	Total knee replacement	Total hip replacement	Simple prostatectomy	Carotid endarterectomy	Accreditation status*	Overall evaluation score (higher is better)	Number of beds	Major medical school affiliation?	Number of residents	Computerized drug order system (1 to 5 scale, higher is preferred; see page 23 for details)
2.3	3.8	6.5	7.7	10.3	11.9	7.5	6.7	6.4	5.4	8.2	–	91	161	–	–	–
–	–	–	–	–	–	–	–	–	–	–	4	89	40	No	0	–
–	–	–	–	–	–	–	–	–	–	–	–[2]	–[2]	28	No	0	–
–	–	–		–	–	–	–	–	–	–	–[2]	–[2]	50	No	0	–
–	–	–	–	–	–	–	–	–	–	–	–[2]	–[2]	36	No	0	–
–	–	–	–	–	–	–	–	–	–	–	–[2]	–[2]	49	No	0	–
	✖							–			–[2]	–[2]	216	No	23	–
★					✖		★	✖		★	4	92	464	Yes	63	–
–	–	–	–	–	–	–	–	–	–	–	4	96	43	No	0	–
–	–	–	–	–	–	–	–	–	–	–	–[2]	–[2]	31	No	0	–
✖	–	×		–			✖		–	–	3	91	95	No	0	–
	–	–		–		–	–	–	–	–	4	97	93	No	0	–
–	–	–	–	–	–	–	–	–	–	–	–[2]	–[2]	25	No	0	–
–	–	–	–	–	–	–	–	–	–	–	4	94	38	No	0	–
–	–	–	–	–	–	–	–	–	–	–	–[2]	–[2]	24	No	0	–
–	–	–	–	–	–	–	–	–	–	–	–[2]	–[2]	33	No	0	–
–	–	–	–	–	–	–	–	–	–	–	–[2]	–[2]	44	No	0	–
–	–	–	–	–	–	–	–	–	–	–	–[2]	–[2]	31	No	0	–
–	–	–		–	–	–	–	–	–	–	4	86	53	No	0	–
–	–	–	–	–	–	–	–	–	–	–	–[2]	–[2]	29	No	0	–
	–		×	–		–	✖	✖	–	–	4	92	85	No	0	–
	–		✖	–		★	✖	✖			4	88	177	No	0	–
	–	★	✖	–			✖	✖			4	87	280	No	0	–
–	–	–		–	–	–	–	–	–	–	4	84	37	No	0	–
	–			–			–	–	–	–	4	96	152	No	0	–
								✖			4	88	556	No	23	–
				★			✖			★	4	93	316	No	0	–
										✖	4	88	228	No	0	–
–	–	–	–	–	–	–	–	–	–	–	4	90	23	No	0	–
									★		–[2]	–[2]	264	No	0	–
★	★		★	★	★	×	✖				4	93	225	No	26	–
–	–	–	–	–	–	–	–	–	–	–	4	89	25	No	0	–
–	–	–	–	–	–	–	–	–	–	–	–[2]	–[2]	16	No	0	–
✖	–	✖		–	–	–	–	–	–	–	–[2]	–[2]	140	Yes	33	–
–	–	–	–	–	–	–	–	–	–	–	–[2]	–[2]	38	No	0	–
–	–	–		–	–	–	–	–	–	–	–[2]	–[2]	40	No	2	–

***Accreditation Status:** 5=Accredited with commendation or with full standards compliance; 4=Accredited with requirements for improvement; 3=Conditional accreditation.

Detailed Ratings for All Areas

See more information on "Key Ratings for Metro Areas" table beginning on page 32

Blue is most favorable
Bold Italic is least favorable
Blank means neither better nor worse than average
"–" means insufficient data

	Death rates for all selected case types				Hospital outcomes: better (★) or worse (×) than average — Adjusted Death rates — Medical Cases											
	Number of cases	Actual death rate (%)	Adjusted death rate (%) (lower is better)	All selected cases	All selected medical cases	Heart attack	Congestive heart failure	Obstructive pulmonary disease	Pneumonia	Respiratory failure and arrest	Septicemia	Stroke	Gastrointestinal hemorrhage	Fluid, electrolyte, & acid-base disorders	Kidney failure
National Average	–	–	12.1	12.1	14.8	21.2	10.6	6.5	16.9	34.4	25.1	18.4	6.7	11.0	20.9
Iowa *(continued)*															
Northwest Iowa, Sheldon	472	10.8	12.4					–		–	–		–	–	–
Orange City Health System, Orange City[1]	591	10.2	11.8			–		–		–	–		–		–
Osceola, Sibley	335	13.1	15.0		×	–		–	✖	–	–		–	–	–
Ottumwa Regional, Ottumwa	2,851	10.8	10.5	★	★		★			★					★
Palo Alto, Emmetsburg[1]	665	15.6	***15.9***	✖	✖			–	✖	–			–		–
Pella Regional, Pella	702	8.1	11.1					–		–			–	–	–
Peoples Memorial Buchanan County, Independence	264	11.7	14.9			–	–	–		–	–	–	–	–	–
Regional Health Services of Howard County, Cresco	309	15.9	14.4			–		–		–	–	✖	–	–	–
Regional Northeast Iowa/Delaware Co, Manchester	538	12.5	13.7				×	–		–			–	–	–
Ringgold County, Mount Ayr	386	10.4	11.2			–		–		–	–		–	–	–
St Anthony Regional, Carroll	1,077	12.3	13.9	×	×					–	–			–	✖
St Luke's Methodist, Cedar Rapids	6,057	9.6	10.7	★	★					★	★				
St Luke's Regional, Sioux City[1]	4,719	8.7	12.9		×		✖				★				
Sartori, Cedar Falls	949	14.1	13.4		×			–						✖	–
Shelby County Myrtue, Harlan	912	12.3	11.1					–		–					–
Shenandoah Medical Center, Shenandoah	582	13.9	***15.3***	✖	✖			–	✖	–	–		–	–	–
Sioux Center Community, Sioux Center[1]	216	12.5	16.0			–	–	–		–	–	–	–	–	–
Sioux Valley, Cherokee	628	11.0	13.0					–		–	–	✖	–	–	–
Skiff, Newton	1,299	10.4	12.3							–					–
Southwest Iowa, Council Bluffs	2,039	9.4	***14.0***	✖	✖				×	×					–
Spencer Municipal, Spencer	1,478	9.2	12.3							–	★			–	–
Stewart, Lake City	1,010	10.7	13.9	×	×	×				–	–		–	–	–
Story County, Nevada[1]	146	13.7	13.4			–	–	–		–	–	–	–	–	–
Trinity - North Campus, Davenport[1]	628	15.0	12.9					–		–			–		–
Trinity Regional, Fort Dodge	3,414	12.7	***14.8***	✖	✖	✖	✖				✖	✖			
Unity, Muscatine	1,270	12.4	***14.1***	✖	✖			✖				×	×		–
University of Iowa, Iowa City[1]	2,756	6.9	9.7	★	★	★						★			
Van Buren County, Keosauqua	419	13.6	8.9	★	★	–		–		★			–	–	–
Virginia Gay, Vinton	337	14.2	12.3			–	★	–	★	–	–		–	–	–
Washington County, Washington	964	11.8	11.7							–			★	–	–
Waverly Municipal, Waverly	522	14.8	***17.5***	✖	✖		×	–		–	–	✖	✖	–	–
Wayne County, Corydon	554	14.1	13.5					–			–		–	–	✖
Winneshiek County, Decorah	664	9.8	11.3					★		–	–		–	–	–

Footnotes are on page 350.

Hospital outcomes: better (★) or worse (×) than average											Results of accreditation review on full survey		Other facts			
Adjusted Death rates			Adjusted Adverse outcome rates													
Surgical cases			Surgical cases													
All selected surgical cases	Coronary artery bypass surgery	Large bowel surgery	All selected surgical cases	Coronary artery bypass surgery	Large bowel surgery	Gall bladder removal	Total knee replacement	Total hip replacement	Simple prostatectomy	Carotid endarterectomy	Accreditation status*	Overall evaluation score (higher is better)	Number of beds	Major medical school affiliation?	Number of residents	Computerized drug order system (1 to 5 scale, higher is preferred; see page 23 for details)
2.3	3.8	6.5	7.7	10.3	11.9	7.5	6.7	6.4	5.4	8.2	–	91	161	–	–	–
–	–	–	–	–	–	–	–	–	–	–	–[2]	–[2]	24	No	0	–
–	–	–	–	–	–	–	–	–	–	–	–[2]	–[2]	30	No	0	–
–	–	–	★	–	–	–	–	–	–	–	–[2]	–[2]	32	No	0	–
	–		★	–					–	–	4	***86***	75	No	0	–
–	–	–	★	–	–	–	–	–	–	–	–[2]	–[2]	32	No	0	–
–	–	–	★	–		–	–	–	–	–	4	89	47	No	0	–
–	–	–	–	–	–	–	–	–	–	–	–[2]	–[2]	50	No	0	–
–	–	–	–	–	–	–	–	–	–	–	–[2]	–[2]	32	No	0	–
–	–	–		–	–	–	–	–	–	–	–[2]	–[2]	35	No	0	–
–	–	–		–	–	–	–	–	–	–	–[2]	–[2]	36	No	0	–
–	–	–		–		–	–	–	–	–	–[2]	–[2]	63	No	0	–
			×		×		×	×		★	4	91	356	No	0	–
	–		×	–		★	×	×	★	★	4	***85***	193	No	0	–
	–	–		–		–		–	–	–	4	91	46	No	0	–
–	–	–	–	–	–	–	–	–	–	–	–[2]	–[2]	52	No	0	–
–	–	–	–	–	–	–	–	–	–	–	–[2]	–[2]	31	No	0	–
–	–	–	–	–	–	–	–	–	–	–	–[2]	–[2]	21	No	0	–
–	–	–		–	–	–	–	–	–	–	–[2]	–[2]	40	No	0	–
	–	–		–		–		–	–	–	4	90	52	No	0	–
	–	–		–		–		×	–	–	4	90	189	No	0	–
	–	–		–		–				–	–[2]	–[2]	71	No	0	–
–	–	–	★	–	–	–	–	–	–	–	–[2]	–[2]	53	No	0	–
–	–	–	–	–	–	–	–	–	–	–	–[2]	–[2]	18	No	0	–
–	–	–		–		–	–	–	–	–	4	***86***	105	No	6	–
	–			–		★	×			–	4	93	161	No	2	–
	–	–		–		–	–	–	–	–	4	**97**	58	No	0	–
	×		×	×		–	★		–		4	92	707	**Yes**	387	–
–	–	–	–	–	–	–	–	–	–	–	–[2]	–[2]	40	No	0	–
–	–	–	–	–	–	–	–	–	–	–	–[2]	–[2]	29	No	0	–
–	–	–	–	–	–	–	–	–	–	–	–[2]	–[2]	48	No	0	–
–	–	–		–	–	–	–	–	–	–	4	**96**	38	No	0	–
–	–	–	–	–	–	–	–	–	–	–	–[2]	–[2]	28	No	0	–
–	–	–		–	–	–	–	–	–	–	4	***88***	83	No	0	–

***Accreditation Status:** 5=Accredited with commendation or with full standards compliance; 4=Accredited with requirements for improvement; 3=Conditional accreditation.

Detailed Ratings for All Areas

See more information on "Key Ratings for Metro Areas" table beginning on page 32

Blue is most favorable
Bold Italic is least favorable
Blank means neither better nor worse than average
"–" means insufficient data

	Death rates for all selected case types				Hospital outcomes: better (★) or worse (×) than average — Adjusted Death rates — Medical Cases										
	Number of cases	Actual death rate (%)	Adjusted death rate (%) (lower is better)	All selected cases	All selected medical cases	Heart attack	Congestive heart failure	Obstructive pulmonary disease	Pneumonia	Respiratory failure and arrest	Septicemia	Stroke	Gastrointestinal hemorrhage	Fluid, electrolyte, & acid-base disorders	Kidney failure
National Average	–	–	12.1	12.1	14.8	21.2	10.6	6.5	16.9	34.4	25.1	18.4	6.7	11.0	20.9
Kansas															
Kansas City Area															
Bethany, Kansas City	2,167	14.4	11.3												
Children's Mercy South, Overland Park	–	–	–	–	–	–	–	–	–	–	–	–	–	–	–
Menorah, Overland Park	1,489	8.9	11.5												
Olathe Medical Center, Olathe	3,146	10.2	11.3							✖					
Overland Park Regional, Overland Park	2,427	10.4	9.9	★	★		★	★		★			★		
Providence, Kansas City	3,328	10.6	10.4	★	★	★		★			★				
St Luke's South, Overland Park	119	5.0	6.8		★	–	–	–	–	–	–	–	–	–	–
Shawnee Mission Medical Center, Shawnee Mission	5,718	10.4	10.9	★	★	★			★						
University of Kansas, Kansas City[1]	1,414	11.0	13.3											✖	
Other Areas															
Allen County, Iola	907	13.2	***15.5***	✖	✖		×		✖	–	–	✖	–	★	–
Atchison Hospital, Atchison[1]	1,053	8.0	9.3	★	★		★	–						★	
Augusta Medical Complex, Augusta	309	20.1	13.2			–		–		–	–		–	–	–
Bob Wilson - Grant County, Ulysses	347	15.0	13.9					–		–	–	–	–	–	–
Central Kansas, Great Bend	1,735	11.9	***15.8***	✖	✖	✖		–	✖						
Citizens, Colby	589	11.4	14.5	×		–		✖		–	–	–	–		–
Clara Barton, Hoisington	242	12.4	***18.0***	✖	✖	–	–	–		–	–	–	–	–	–
Clay County, Clay Center	641	14.0	***15.3***	✖	✖			–	✖	–	–		–		–
Cloud County, Concordia	875	12.9	13.7					–	✖	–	–		–	–	–
Coffey County, Burlington	554	8.7	7.9	★	★	–		★	★	–	–	–	–		–
Coffeyville Regional, Coffeyville	2,084	10.6	9.5	★	★		★		★						×
Community, Onaga	693	11.0	9.2	★	★			–	★		–		–		–
Community Memorial, Marysville	890	13.0	13.4					–		–	–	✖	–		
Cushing, Leavenworth	953	8.5	9.5	★	★					–					–
Decatur County, Oberlin[1]	433	11.1	12.4			–		–		–	–		–	–	–
Fredonia Regional, Fredonia	436	11.9	11.2			–	★	–			–		–		–
Geary, Junction City	878	14.2	***16.6***	✖	✖			✖	✖	–	✖	✖	–		–
Goodland Regional, Goodland	431	11.4	14.2			–				–	–	–	–	–	–
Gove County, Quinter	553	6.3	7.2	★	★			–	★	–	–	–	–	★	–
Greeley County, Tribune	264	12.5	14.4			–		–		–	–	–	–		–
Greenwood County, Eureka	684	11.1	9.9	★	★			★	★	–	–	×	–		–
Halstead Hospital, Halstead	1,363	7.0	10.3		★				★		★				–
Hanover Hospital, Hanover	242	12.4	9.5			★	–	–		–	–	–	–	–	–

Footnotes are on page 350.

Hospital outcomes: better (★) or worse (✖) than average											Results of accreditation review on full survey		Other facts			
Adjusted Death rates			Adjusted Adverse outcome rates													
Surgical cases			Surgical cases													
All selected surgical cases	Coronary artery bypass surgery	Large bowel surgery	All selected surgical cases	Coronary artery bypass surgery	Large bowel surgery	Gall bladder removal	Total knee replacement	Total hip replacement	Simple prostatectomy	Carotid endarterectomy	Accreditation status*	Overall evaluation score (higher is better)	Number of beds	Major medical school affiliation?	Number of residents	Computerized drug order system (1 to 5 scale, higher is preferred; see page 23 for details)
2.3	3.8	6.5	7.7	10.3	11.9	7.5	6.7	6.4	5.4	8.2	–	91	161	–	–	–
	–	–		–		–	–	–	–	–	4	93	226	Yes	5	–
–	–	–	–	–	–	–	–	–	–	–	–[2]	–[2]	–	–	–	–
★	–	–				–		–	–		4	99	158	No	0	–
★	–		★		★				–		4	91	182	Yes	0	–
★	–	★	★		★	–	✖		–		5	97	269	No	0	–
									–		4	94	179	No	0	–
–	–	–	–	–	–	–	–	–	–	–	4	95	342	No	0	–
					★		✖				4	91	341	No	30	–
	–	–				–	–	–	–		–[2]	–[2]	387	Yes	379	–
–	–	–		–	–	–	–	–	–	–	–[2]	–[2]	49	No	0	–
–	–	–		–	–	–	–	–	–	–	3	81	40	No	0	–
–	–	–	–	–	–	–	–	–	–	–	–[2]	–[2]	40	No	0	–
–	–	–	–	–	–	–	–	–	–	–	–[2]	–[2]	30	No	0	–
	–	✖	✖	–		–	✖		–	–	4	95	96	No	0	–
–	–	–	–	–	–	–	–	–	–	–	–[2]	–[2]	40	No	–	–
–	–	–	–	–	–	–	–	–	–	–	–[2]	–[2]	28	No	0	–
–	–	–	★	–		★	–	–	–	–	–[2]	–[2]	32	No	0	–
–	–	–	–	–	–	–	–	–	–	–	–[2]	–[2]	31	No	0	–
–	–	–	–	–	–	–	–	–	–	–	–[2]	–[2]	22	No	0	–
	–	–		–		–	–	–	–	–	4	88	87	No	0	–
–	–	–	–	–	–	–	–	–	–	–	–[2]	–[2]	98	No	0	–
–	–	–		–	–	–	–	–	–	–	–[2]	–[2]	49	No	0	–
–	–	–	–	–	–	–	–	–	–	–	4	91	58	No	0	–
–	–	–	–	–	–	–	–	–	–	–	–[2]	–[2]	24	No	0	–
–	–	–	–	–	–	–	–	–	–	–	–[2]	–[2]	42	No	0	–
–	–	–	★	–	★	–	–	–	–	–	4	80	69	No	0	–
–	–	–	–	–	–	–	–	–	–	–	–[2]	–[2]	49	No	0	–
–	–	–	–	–	–	–	–	–	–	–	–[2]	–[2]	21	No	0	–
–	–	–	–	–	–	–	–	–	–	–	–[2]	–[2]	16	No	0	–
–	–	–	–	–	–	–	–	–	–	–	–[2]	–[2]	46	No	0	–
	–	–				–					–[2]	–[2]	120	No	0	–
–	–	–	–	–	–	–	–	–	–	–	–[2]	–[2]	18	No	0	–

***Accreditation Status:** 5=Accredited with commendation or with full standards compliance; 4=Accredited with requirements for improvement; 3=Conditional accreditation.

Detailed Ratings for All Areas

See more information on "Key Ratings for Metro Areas" table beginning on page 32

Blue is most favorable
Bold Italic is least favorable
Blank means neither better nor worse than average
"–" means insufficient data

	Death rates for all selected case types			Hospital outcomes: better (★) or worse (×) than average											
				Adjusted Death rates											
				Medical Cases											
	Number of cases	Actual death rate (%)	Adjusted death rate (%) (lower is better)	All selected cases	All selected medical cases	Heart attack	Congestive heart failure	Obstructive pulmonary disease	Pneumonia	Respiratory failure and arrest	Septicemia	Stroke	Gastrointestinal hemorrhage	Fluid, electrolyte, & acid-base disorders	Kidney failure
National Average	–	–	12.1	12.1	14.8	21.2	10.6	6.5	16.9	34.4	25.1	18.4	6.7	11.0	20.9
Kansas *(continued)*															
Other Areas *(continued)*															
Harper District 5, Harper	316	13.9	13.2					–		–	–		–	–	–
Hays Medical Center, Hays	2,578	9.3	12.5							×					–
Herington Municipal, Herington	390	8.5	**8.7**	**★**	★	–		–	**★**	–	–	–	–	–	–
Hiawatha Community, Hiawatha	591	16.2	***15.2***	✖	✖	–	✖	–		–	–		–	✖	–
Hillsboro Community, Hillsboro	223	17.0	13.7			–		–		–	–		–	–	–
Hodgeman County, Jetmore	220	10.5	9.8			–		–		–	–	–	–	–	–
Hospital District 1 of Crawford County, Girard	724	13.4	***15.9***	✖	✖		✖	–		–	–		–		–
Hospital District 6 of Harper County, Anthony	166	10.8	9.4			–	–	–		–	–	–	–	–	–
Hutchinson Hospital, Hutchinson	4,201	11.7	12.4				✖	**★**							
Kansas Heart, Wichita	450	2.2	9.0		–	–	–	–	–	–	–	–	–	–	–
Kingman Community, Kingman[1]	394	13.2	10.3					–		–			–	–	–
Kiowa County, Greensburg	145	8.3	7.4	★	★	–	–	–		–	–	–	–	–	–
Labette County, Parsons	1,782	11.8	***15.6***	✖	✖	✖		–	✖			×	✖		
Lawrence Memorial, Lawrence	2,646	11.4	13.2	×	✖			×		✖					
Lincoln County, Lincoln	416	6.0	**6.9**	**★**	**★**	–		–	★	–	–	–	–	–	–
Lindsborg Community, Lindsborg	343	11.7	13.0			–		–		–	–	✖	–	–	–
Medicine Lodge Memorial, Medicine Lodge	495	7.9	9.4	★		–		–		–	–	–	–	–	–
Memorial, Abilene	540	14.3	13.1					–		–	–		–	–	–
Memorial, McPherson	833	12.8	12.9							–	–		★		–
Mercy, Fort Scott[1]	1,925	13.0	***15.2***	✖	✖				✖			✖	×		✖
Mercy, Independence[1]	1,124	15.1	***14.7***	✖	✖	×		–	✖	–					–
Mercy, Manhattan[1]	1,926	11.2	12.9							✖					
Mercy, Moundridge	224	12.5	12.3			–	–	–		–	–	–	–	–	–
Miami County, Paola	572	13.5	13.8			–				–	×		–		–
Minneola District, Minneola	287	12.2	9.6					–		–	–	–	–	–	–
Mitchell County, Beloit	940	12.4	***14.5***	✖	✖				✖				–	–	–
Morris County, Council Grove	559	11.8	12.5				✖			–	–		–		–
Morton County, Elkhart[1]	595	8.6	**9.3**	**★**	**★**	–		–	**★**	–	–		–		–
Mt Carmel Regional, Pittsburg	2,115	12.1	***14.2***	✖	✖	✖									–
Neosho Regional, Chanute	1,225	14.9	***15.7***	✖	✖		✖	✖	✖						
Ness County, Ness City[1]	216	8.8	**6.9**	**★**	**★**	–	–	–	**★**	–	–		–	–	–
Newman Regional, Emporia	2,193	10.4	12.6			✖								✖	–
Newton Medical Center, Newton	1,747	8.5	10.6					✖				**★**			–
Norton County, Norton	292	10.6	12.4			–	×	–	**★**	–	–		–	–	–

Footnotes are on page 350.

Hospital outcomes: better (★) or worse (×) than average											Results of accreditation review on full survey		Other facts			
Adjusted Death rates			Adjusted Adverse outcome rates													
Surgical cases			Surgical cases													
All selected surgical cases	Coronary artery bypass surgery	Large bowel surgery	All selected surgical cases	Coronary artery bypass surgery	Large bowel surgery	Gall bladder removal	Total knee replacement	Total hip replacement	Simple prostatectomy	Carotid endarterectomy	Accreditation status*	Overall evaluation score (higher is better)	Number of beds	Major medical school affiliation?	Number of residents	Computerized drug order system (1 to 5 scale, higher is preferred; see page 23 for details)
2.3	3.8	6.5	7.7	10.3	11.9	7.5	6.7	6.4	5.4	8.2	–	91	161	–	–	–
–	–	–	–	–	–	–	–	–	–	–	–[2]	–[2]	38	No	0	–
	–		×				×				4	**96**	171	No	0	–
–	–	–	–	–	–	–	–	–	–	–	–[2]	–[2]	20	No	0	–
–	–	–	–	–	–	–	–	–	–	–	–[2]	–[2]	43	No	0	–
–	–	–	–	–	–	–	–	–	–	–	–[2]	–[2]	26	No	0	–
–	–	–	–	–	–	–	–	–	–	–	–[2]	–[2]	16	No	0	–
–	–	–		–	–	–	–	–	–	–	–[2]	–[2]	38	No	0	–
–	–	–	–	–	–	–	–	–	–	–	–[2]	–[2]	30	No	0	–
							★	–			–[2]	–[2]	144	No	0	–
		–	★	★	–	–	–	–	–	★	–[2]	–[2]	32	No	0	4
–	–	–	–	–	–	–	–	–	–	–	–[2]	–[2]	45	No	0	–
–	–	–	–	–	–	–	–	–	–	–	–[2]	–[2]	38	No	0	–
	–	–	×	–		–	×	–	–		–[2]	–[2]	58	No	0	–
	–		★	–		–	★		–	–	4	89	133	No	0	–
–	–	–	–	–	–	–	–	–	–	–	–[2]	–[2]	14	No	0	–
–	–	–	–	–	–	–	–	–	–	–	–[2]	–[2]	12	No	0	–
–	–	–	–	–	–	–	–	–	–	–	–[2]	–[2]	42	No	0	–
–	–	–	–	–	–	–	–	–	–	–	–[2]	–[2]	57	No	0	–
–	–	–	★	–	–	–	–	–	–	–	–[2]	–[2]	41	No	0	–
	–	–		–		–	–	–		–	4	**88**	71	No	0	–
	–	–		–	–	–	×	–	–	–	4	93	40	No	0	–
	–	–		–		–				–	4	**87**	114	No	0	–
–	–	–	–	–	–	–	–	–	–	–	–[2]	–[2]	21	No	0	–
–	–	–	–	–	–	–	–	–	–	–	4	92	20	No	0	–
–	–	–	–	–	–	–	–	–	–	–	–[2]	–[2]	15	No	0	–
–	–	–		–	–	–	–	–	–	–	–[2]	–[2]	49	No	0	–
–	–	–	–	–	–	–	–	–	–	–	–[2]	–[2]	28	No	0	–
–	–	–	–	–	–	–	–	–	–	–	–[2]	–[2]	40	No	0	–
×	–	×		–			×	–	–	–	4	89	126	No	0	–
×	–	–		–		–	–	–	–	–	4	93	60	No	0	–
–	–	–	–	–	–	–	–	–	–	–	–[2]	–[2]	20	No	0	–
	–	–		–		–	★	★	–	×	4	**97**	92	No	0	–
★	–	–		–	★			×	–	–	–[2]	–[2]	55	No	0	–
–	–	–	–	–	–	–	–	–	–	–	–[2]	–[2]	24	No	0	–

***Accreditation Status:** 5=Accredited with commendation or with full standards compliance; 4=Accredited with requirements for improvement; 3=Conditional accreditation.

Detailed Ratings for All Areas

See more information on "Key Ratings for Metro Areas" table beginning on page 32

Blue is most favorable
Bold Italic is least favorable
Blank means neither better nor worse than average
"–" means insufficient data

	Death rates for all selected case types			Hospital outcomes: better (★) or worse (×) than average — Adjusted Death rates											
				Medical Cases											
	Number of cases	Actual death rate (%)	Adjusted death rate (%) (lower is better)	All selected cases	All selected medical cases	Heart attack	Congestive heart failure	Obstructive pulmonary disease	Pneumonia	Respiratory failure and arrest	Septicemia	Stroke	Gastrointestinal hemorrhage	Fluid, electrolyte, & acid-base disorders	Kidney failure
National Average	–	–	12.1	12.1	14.8	21.2	10.6	6.5	16.9	34.4	25.1	18.4	6.7	11.0	20.9
Kansas *(continued)*															
Other Areas *(continued)*															
Osborne County, Osborne	316	10.4	9.4			–	★	–		–	–	–	–	–	–
Phillips County, Phillipsburg	441	12.0	10.2			–		–		–	–	–	–	–	–
Pratt Regional, Pratt	1,203	9.3	12.5					–			×				–
Ransom, Ottawa	1,158	13.2	13.2			✖				✖					–
Republic County, Belleville	689	13.5	13.5					–		–	–		–	–	–
Rush County, La Crosse	277	14.8	14.1			–		–		–	–	–	–	–	–
Russell Regional, Russell	557	11.1	11.0			✖		✖		–	–		–	★	–
Sabetha Community, Sabetha	276	12.3	10.6			–		–		–	–		–	–	–
St Catherine, Garden City	1,368	9.0	12.2												
St Francis, Topeka	5,555	11.0	11.3	★	★	★					★				
St John, Leavenworth	712	11.5	11.7				★	–		–			–		–
St Luke, Marion[1]	384	12.0	14.1					–		–	–	–	–	–	–
Salina Regional, Salina	4,541	10.0	***13.6***	✖	✖			✖	✖						
Scott County, Scott City	407	11.3	11.4			–		–	★	–	–	–	–		–
Sheridan County, Hoxie	135	14.1	12.5			–	–	–		–	–	–	–	–	–
Smith County, Smith Center	245	12.2	***17.1***	✖	✖	–		–	✖	–	–	–	–	–	–
South Central Kansas Regional, Arkansas City	757	16.8	***17.5***	✖	✖	✖		–		×	×	×	–		–
Southwest, Liberal	1,228	10.3	11.5					★				×			–
Stanton County, Johnson	51	9.8	11.3			–	–	–	–	–	–	–	–	–	–
Stevens County, Hugoton	185	13.0	13.4			–	–	–	✖	–	–	–	–	–	–
Stormont - Vail, Topeka	5,022	10.8	***13.3***	✖	✖		✖		×						✖
Sumner Regional, Wellington	555	14.4	***15.2***	✖	✖	–	✖	–		–			–	–	–
Susan B Allen, El Dorado	1,169	11.5	12.1			×				–					–
Trego County - Lemke, Wakeeney	417	7.9	9.3			–		–		–	–		–	–	–
Via Christi Regional, Wichita	15,479	11.5	***14.0***	✖	✖		✖		✖	×	×		✖		×
Via Christi Riverside, Wichita	1,415	11.8	13.1							✖					
Wamego City, Wamego	342	13.2	13.6			–		–		–	–		–	–	–
Washington County, Washington	244	10.2	10.0			–	–	–		–	–	–	–	–	–
Wesley, Wichita	7,480	11.1	***13.5***	✖	✖		✖	✖					×		
Western Plains, Dodge City[1]	1,401	10.9	12.1			–		–							–
William Newton, Winfield	920	12.1	14.0	×	×			–		–			✖		✖
Wilson County, Neodesha	236	21.2	***22.7***	✖	✖	–	✖	–	✖	–	–	×	–	–	–

Footnotes are on page 350.

Hospital outcomes: better (★) or worse (×) than average											Results of accreditation review on full survey		Other facts			
Adjusted Death rates			Adjusted Adverse outcome rates													
Surgical cases			Surgical cases													
All selected surgical cases	Coronary artery bypass surgery	Large bowel surgery	All selected surgical cases	Coronary artery bypass surgery	Large bowel surgery	Gall bladder removal	Total knee replacement	Total hip replacement	Simple prostatectomy	Carotid endarterectomy	Accreditation status*	Overall evaluation score (higher is better)	Number of beds	Major medical school affiliation?	Number of residents	Computerized drug order system (1 to 5 scale, higher is preferred; see page 23 for details)
2.3	3.8	6.5	7.7	10.3	11.9	7.5	6.7	6.4	5.4	8.2	–	91	161	–	–	–
–	–	–	–	–	–	–	–	–	–	–	–[2]	–[2]	29	No	0	–
–	–	–		–	–	–	–	–	–	–	–[2]	–[2]	29	No	0	–
×	–			–					–	–	–[2]	–[2]	69	No	0	–
–	–	–	–	–	–	–	–	–	–	–	4	90	46	No	0	–
–	–	–	★	–	–	–	–	–	–	–	4	**94**	48	No	0	–
–	–	–	–	–	–	–	–	–	–	–	–[2]	–[2]	24	No	0	–
–	–	–	–	–	–	–	–	–	–	–	4	93	39	No	0	–
–	–	–	–	–	–	–	–	–	–	–	–[2]	–[2]	27	No	0	–
	–	–	★	–				★	–	–	4	90	93	No	0	–
	✖			✖			★	★			4	89	269	**Yes**	0	–
–	–	–		–	–	–	–	–	–	–	4	**94**	30	No	0	–
–	–	–	–	–	–	–	–	–	–	–	–[2]	–[2]	22	No	0	–
	–			–			★		★		4	90	215	**Yes**	0	–
–	–	–	–	–	–	–	–	–	–	–	–[2]	–[2]	27	No	0	–
–	–	–	–	–	–	–	–	–	–	–	–[2]	–[2]	18	No	0	–
–	–	–	–	–	–	–	–	–	–	–	–[2]	–[2]	26	No	0	–
–	–	–	★	–	–	–	–	–	–	–	–[2]	–[2]	45	No	0	–
★	–	★		–	★	–		–		–	3	***84***	87	No	0	–
–	–	–	–	–	–	–	–	–	–	–	–[2]	–[2]	17	No	0	–
–	–	–	–	–	–	–	–	–	–	–	–[2]	–[2]	17	No	0	–
							★	★			4	***84***	295	**Yes**	0	–
–	–	–	–	–	–	–	–	–	–	–	–[2]	–[2]	67	No	0	–
	–	–		–		–	–	–	–	–	4	89	61	No	0	–
–	–	–	–	–	–	–	–	–	–	–	–[2]	–[2]	28	No	0	–
											–[2]	–[2]	942	**Yes**	124	4
	–	–	★	–		–	–	–	–	–	–[2]	–[2]	103	No	18	2
–	–	–	–	–	–	–	–	–	–	–	–[2]	–[2]	24	No	0	–
–	–	–	–	–	–	–	–	–	–	–	–[2]	–[2]	27	No	0	–
	×										4	**94**	534	No	0	2
	–	–	★	–		–	★		–	–	4	93	90	No	0	–
	–	–		–		–	–	–	–	–	–[2]	–[2]	49	No	0	–
–	–	–	–	–	–	–	–	–	–	–	–[2]	–[2]	38	No	0	–

***Accreditation Status:** 5=Accredited with commendation or with full standards compliance; 4=Accredited with requirements for improvement; 3=Conditional accreditation.

Detailed Ratings for All Areas

See more information on "Key Ratings for Metro Areas" table beginning on page 32

Blue is most favorable
Bold Italic is least favorable
Blank means neither better nor worse than average
"–" means insufficient data

	Death rates for all selected case types			Hospital outcomes: better (★) or worse (×) than average — Adjusted Death rates	Medical Cases										
	Number of cases	Actual death rate (%)	Adjusted death rate (%) (lower is better)	All selected cases	All selected medical cases	Heart attack	Congestive heart failure	Obstructive pulmonary disease	Pneumonia	Respiratory failure and arrest	Septicemia	Stroke	Gastrointestinal hemorrhage	Fluid, electrolyte, & acid-base disorders	Kidney failure
National Average	–	–	12.1	12.1	14.8	21.2	10.6	6.5	16.9	34.4	25.1	18.4	6.7	11.0	20.9
Kentucky															
Baptist East, Louisville	11,170	11.0	12.4												
Baptist Regional, Corbin	4,082	12.4	11.7			✖				★					
Berea Hospital, Berea	1,256	12.1	12.2					★					–	★	
Bluegrass, Versailles	416	16.6	***17.9***	✖	✖	–	×	–		–	–	✖	–	–	–
Bourbon, Paris	932	8.5	8.3	★	★		★			★			–		–
Breckinridge, Hardinsburg	804	11.9	13.6			×				–	–		–		
Caldwell County, Princeton	768	17.8	***16.3***	✖	✖	–	✖	✖		–	–		–		
Caritas, Louisville	6,736	12.8	11.2	★	★	✖	★			★					
Carroll County, Carrollton	597	15.9	11.9			✖		–		–	–		–	–	
Casey County, Liberty	405	10.1	10.5			–		–		–		–	–	×	–
Caverna, Horse Cave	443	16.5	***18.2***	✖	✖	–	✖	–		–	–	–	–	✖	–
Central Baptist, Lexington	5,715	9.2	12.6			★									
Clark Regional, Winchester	1,210	17.0	12.8					–					×		
Clinton County, Albany	858	9.2	13.6			–		★		–	–		–		–
Crittenden County, Marion[1]	1,779	11.8	10.3	★	★	✖			★					★	★
Cumberland County, Burkesville	533	9.2	11.2			–		–		–	–	×	–		–
Ephraim McDowell Regional, Danville	3,054	11.7	***13.7***	✖	✖				✖	×	×				
Flaget, Bardstown	1,222	12.5	***15.1***	✖	✖	×					–	✖	–		–
Fleming County, Flemingsburg	1,157	10.0	10.3	★	★		★			–			–	★	✖
Fort Logan, Stanford	731	12.2	10.5					–		–			–	★	–
Frankfort Regional, Frankfort	2,452	13.5	12.4					★							
Georgetown Community, Georgetown	905	12.8	11.2										–		
Greenview Regional, Bowling Green	2,792	12.5	11.7			✖				★					
Hardin, Elizabethtown	6,746	10.1	10.5	★	★				★	★					★
Harlan ARH, Harlan	3,052	8.9	9.7	★	★		★		★						
Harrison, Cynthiana	1,326	12.0	12.7								–		✖		–
Hazard ARH Regional, Hazard	4,231	10.2	8.7	★	★	✖	★		★	★		★	★	★	★
Highlands Regional, Prestonsburg	3,204	11.4	11.8			✖		★						★	
Jackson Purchase, Mayfield	2,762	11.5	9.6	★	★		★	★	★	★					
Jane Todd Crawford, Greensburg	373	14.7	15.2	×	×	–		–		–	–	–	–		–
Jenkins Community, Jenkins	347	6.9	9.3			–	★			–	–	–	–	–	–
Jennie Stuart, Hopkinsville	3,089	13.1	***14.8***	✖	✖		✖		✖					×	✖
Jewish, Louisville[1]	9,598	10.3	11.1	★	★				★			★			
Jewish, Shelbyville	1,877	13.9	***14.7***	✖	✖				✖		×	✖	✖		
Kentucky River, Jackson	2,361	10.8	11.2				★	★			×				–

Footnotes are on page 350.

Hospital outcomes: better (★) or worse (✖) than average											Results of accreditation review on full survey		Other facts			
Adjusted Death rates			Adjusted Adverse outcome rates													
Surgical cases			Surgical cases													
All selected surgical cases	Coronary artery bypass surgery	Large bowel surgery	All selected surgical cases	Coronary artery bypass surgery	Large bowel surgery	Gall bladder removal	Total knee replacement	Total hip replacement	Simple prostatectomy	Carotid endarterectomy	Accreditation status*	Overall evaluation score (higher is better)	Number of beds	Major medical school affiliation?	Number of residents	Computerized drug order system (1 to 5 scale, higher is preferred; see page 23 for details)
2.3	3.8	6.5	7.7	10.3	11.9	7.5	6.7	6.4	5.4	8.2	–	91	161	–	–	–
							✖				4	95	384	No	0	–
	–	–	★	–		★	–	–	–	–	4	91	240	No	0	–
–	–	–	–	–	–	–	–	–	–	–	4	88	48	No	0	–
–	–	–	–	–	–	–	–	–	–	–	–[2]	–[2]	50	No	–	–
–	–	–	–	–	–	–	–	–	–	–	4	93	58	No	0	–
–	–	–	–	–	–	–	–	–	–	–	–[2]	–[2]	27	No	0	–
–	–	–	–	–	–	–	–	–	–	–	4	91	38	No	0	–
	–			–							4	92	180	No	0	–
–	–	–	–	–	–	–	–	–	–	–	–[2]	–[2]	37	No	0	–
–	–	–	–	–	–	–	–	–	–	–	–[2]	–[2]	24	No	–	–
–	–	–	–	–	–	–	–	–	–	–	–[2]	–[2]	28	No	0	–
✖	✖		✖	✖	×	★			–	×	4	96	343	No	0	–
–	–	–		–	–	–	–	–	–	–	4	96	75	No	0	–
–	–	–	–	–	–	–	–	–	–	–	–[2]	–[2]	42	No	0	–
–	–	–	–	–	–	–	–	–	–	–	4	95	50	No	0	–
–	–	–	–	–	–	–	–	–	–	–	–[2]	–[2]	31	No	0	–
★	–		★	–				–	–	–	4	94	152	No	0	–
–	–	–		–		–	–	–	–	–	4	84	52	No	0	–
–	–	–	–	–	–	–	–	–	–	–	4	76	43	No	0	–
–	–	–	–	–	–	–	–	–	–	–	–[2]	–[2]	43	No	0	–
	–			–	×			–	–	–	4	89	146	No	0	–
–	–	–	–	–	–	–	–	–	–	–	4	96	58	No	0	–
	–			–							4	91	211	No	0	3
	–	✖						–			4	94	247	No	0	–
–	–	–		–	–	–	–	–	–	–	4	83	105	No	0	–
–	–	–		–	–	–	–	–	–	–	4	94	61	No	0	–
	–	–		–	–		–	–		–	4	85	288	No	0	–
×	–	–		–		–	–	–		–	4	88	148	No	0	–
	–			–		–	–	–	–	–	4	87	92	No	0	–
–	–	–	–	–	–	–	–	–	–	–	–[2]	–[2]	44	No	0	–
–	–	–	–	–	–	–	–	–	–	–	4	88	60	No	0	–
✖	–	✖		–		✖	–	–			4	83	139	No	0	–
			✖		✖				✖		4	90	435	No	0	–
	–	–		–			–	–	–	–	4	92	50	No	0	–
–	–	–	–	–	–	–	–	–	–	–	4	93	49	No	0	–

***Accreditation Status:** 5=Accredited with commendation or with full standards compliance; 4=Accredited with requirements for improvement; 3=Conditional accreditation.

Detailed Ratings for All Areas

See more information on "Key Ratings for Metro Areas" table beginning on page 32

Blue is most favorable
Bold Italic is least favorable
Blank means neither better nor worse than average
"–" means insufficient data

	Death rates for all selected case types			Hospital outcomes: better (★) or worse (×) than average — Adjusted Death rates	Medical Cases										
	Number of cases	Actual death rate (%)	Adjusted death rate (%) (lower is better)	All selected cases	All selected medical cases	Heart attack	Congestive heart failure	Obstructive pulmonary disease	Pneumonia	Respiratory failure and arrest	Septicemia	Stroke	Gastrointestinal hemorrhage	Fluid, electrolyte, & acid-base disorders	Kidney failure
National Average	–	–	12.1	12.1	14.8	21.2	10.6	6.5	16.9	34.4	25.1	18.4	6.7	11.0	20.9
Kentucky *(continued)*															
King's Daughters', Ashland	7,783	9.8	**11.2**	**★**	**★**	**★**				**★**					**★**
Knox County, Barbourville	919	12.5	12.7					★	✖		×		–		
Lake Cumberland Regional, Somerset	4,224	12.4	12.9	×											
Livingston, Salem	728	7.6	9.4	★	**★**	–			★	–	–		–	★	–
Logan, Russellville	1,134	13.5	12.2							**★**					–
Lourdes, Paducah	5,424	11.1	***14.5***	✖	✖		✖	×	✖			✖		✖	
Marshall County, Benton	799	13.5	10.8					–		–					✖
Mary Breckinridge, Hyden	692	8.7	**7.3**	**★**	**★**	–	★	**★**	**★**	–	–		–	–	–
Mary Chiles, Mt Sterling[1]	1,051	14.4	12.8									✖		–	
Marymount, London	2,082	11.1	**10.4**	**★**	**★**			★	**★**						
McDowell ARH, McDowell[1]	774	7.8	10.1			–						–	–		–
Meadowview Regional, Maysville	2,247	13.6	***14.2***	✖	✖				✖			✖			
The Medical Center, Bowling Green	6,024	12.4	**11.1**	**★**	**★**				★	**★**					
Medical Center, Franklin	672	15.5	***15.8***	✖	✖			–		–		✖	–		✖
Memorial, Manchester	1,553	10.8	**10.2**	**★**	**★**					**★**					
Methodist, Henderson	3,045	12.2	12.7			✖		★						★	×
Middlesboro ARH, Middlesboro	1,759	11.9	12.3				×			✖	✖		★	**★**	×
Monroe County, Tompkinsville	1,235	9.6	11.2						★	–	×		–	**★**	×
Muhlenberg, Greenville	1,811	12.7	13.3	×			✖			–				×	–
Murray - Calloway County, Murray	2,905	9.8	***14.1***	✖	✖	✖			✖		✖		**★**		✖
Norton, Louisville[1]	5,147	10.0	12.9	×	×			✖					×		
Norton Audubon, Louisville	6,834	11.1	11.6						**★**	**★**		✖			
Norton Southwest, Louisville	2,179	11.5	**10.2**	**★**	**★**				**★**	**★**					
Norton Spring View, Lebanon	1,351	14.7	11.5										–		
Norton Suburban, Louisville	5,718	12.5	11.9			✖			★				×		
Ohio County, Hartford	918	20.2	***18.4***	✖	✖		✖	–	✖		✖	✖	–		–
Our Lady of Bellefonte, Ashland	4,189	10.6	**10.4**	**★**	**★**				★	**★**			✖		**★**
Owen County, Owenton[1]	658	10.3	**8.5**	**★**	**★**	–		–		–	★		–	★	★
Owensboro Mercy, Owensboro	8,337	11.3	***13.6***	✖	✖			✖	✖			✖			
Parkway Regional, Fulton	1,030	13.3	13.7	×	×					–	×		✖		–
Pattie A Clay, Richmond	2,415	12.3	**9.6**	**★**	**★**				**★**	**★**					
Paul B Hall Regional, Paintsville	1,665	12.7	11.4												
Pikeville Methodist, Pikeville	3,086	12.9	12.8					★		✖		✖			
Pineville Community, Pineville[1]	2,239	6.0	**7.7**	**★**	**★**		**★**	**★**	**★**						
Regional Med Ctr of Hopkins County, Madisonville	4,465	13.1	***14.4***	✖	✖		✖	✖	✖		✖	✖			✖

Footnotes are on page 350.

Hospital outcomes: better (★) or worse (×) than average											Results of accreditation review on full survey		Other facts			
Adjusted Death rates			Adjusted Adverse outcome rates													
Surgical cases			Surgical cases													
All selected surgical cases	Coronary artery bypass surgery	Large bowel surgery	All selected surgical cases	Coronary artery bypass surgery	Large bowel surgery	Gall bladder removal	Total knee replacement	Total hip replacement	Simple prostatectomy	Carotid endarterectomy	Accreditation status*	Overall evaluation score (higher is better)	Number of beds	Major medical school affiliation?	Number of residents	Computerized drug order system (1 to 5 scale, higher is preferred; see page 23 for details)
2.3	3.8	6.5	7.7	10.3	11.9	7.5	6.7	6.4	5.4	8.2	–	91	161	–	–	–
			✖				✖	✖	–		4	91	331	No	0	–
–	–	–	–	–	–	–	–	–	–	–	4	***81***	42	No	0	–
✖	–	✖		–	×		–	–			4	90	215	No	0	–
–	–	–	–	–	–	–	–	–	–	–	–[2]	–[2]	26	No	0	–
–	–	–	–	–	–	–	–	–	–	–	4	***85***	55	No	0	–
	★	×		★					✖	★	4	91	389	No	23	–
–	–	–		–		–	–	–	–	–	4	93	46	No	0	–
–	–	–	–	–	–	–	–	–	–	–	–[2]	–[2]	40	No	5	–
–	–	–	–	–	–	–	–	–	–	–	4	***87***	63	No	0	–
	–	–	★	–			–	–	–	–	4	91	71	No	0	–
–	–	–	–	–	–	–	–	–	–	–	4	**96**	40	No	0	–
	–	–		–		–	–	–	–	–	4	***88***	91	No	0	–
					×						4	**95**	401	No	0	–
–	–	–	–	–	–	–	–	–	–	–	–[2]	–[2]	13	No	0	–
–	–	–	–	–	–	–	–	–	–	–	4	***88***	47	No	0	–
	–		★	–		★	–	–		–	4	***83***	181	No	0	–
–	–	–		–	–	–	–	–	–	–	4	91	96	No	0	–
–	–	–	–	–	–	–	–	–	–	–	4	91	49	No	0	–
	–	–		–	×		–	–	–	–	4	***86***	135	No	3	–
	–	–	×	–	★	✖			–	✖	4	93	125	No	0	–
									–	×	4	91	670	**Yes**	0	–
×	✖									✖	4	92	203	No	0	–
–	–	–		–	–		–	–	–	–	4	93	85	No	0	–
	–	–		–		–	–	–	–	–	4	89	47	No	0	–
	–			–							4	**94**	230	No	0	–
–	–	–	–	–	–	–	–	–	–	–	4	91	49	No	0	–
	–			–			–	–	–	–	4	**96**	194	No	6	–
–	–	–	–	–	–	–	–	–	–	–	–[2]	–[2]	50	No	0	–
✖			✖						✖	✖	4	***84***	317	No	0	–
–	–	–	★	–	–	–	–	–	–	–	4	**99**	38	No	0	–
	–			–			–	–	–	–	4	92	105	No	0	–
–	–	–	–	–	–	–	–	–	–	–	5	**98**	72	No	0	–
	–			–			–	–	–	–	4	92	181	No	0	–
–	–	–		–	–	–	–	–	–	–	4	91	120	No	0	–
	–			★			×	–			4	**94**	301	No	15	–

***Accreditation Status:** 5=Accredited with commendation or with full standards compliance; 4=Accredited with requirements for improvement; 3=Conditional accreditation.

Detailed Ratings for All Areas

See more information on "Key Ratings for Metro Areas" table beginning on page 32

Blue is most favorable
Bold Italic is least favorable
Blank means neither better nor worse than average
"–" means insufficient data

	Death rates for all selected case types				Hospital outcomes: better (★) or worse (×) than average — Adjusted Death rates — Medical Cases										
	Number of cases	Actual death rate (%)	Adjusted death rate (%) (lower is better)	All selected cases	All selected medical cases	Heart attack	Congestive heart failure	Obstructive pulmonary disease	Pneumonia	Respiratory failure and arrest	Septicemia	Stroke	Gastrointestinal hemorrhage	Fluid, electrolyte, & acid-base disorders	Kidney failure
National Average	–	–	12.1	12.1	14.8	21.2	10.6	6.5	16.9	34.4	25.1	18.4	6.7	11.0	20.9
Kentucky *(continued)*															
Rockcastle, Mt Vernon[1]	737	11.7	13.4			–				–	–		–		–
Russell County, Russell Springs	791	13.0	12.0							–		×	–		
St Claire, Morehead	2,719	13.7	***13.8***	✖	✖	✖		×			✖				
St Elizabeth - Grant County, Williamstown	326	13.5	***18.8***	✖	✖	–	✖	–	✖	–	–	–	–	–	–
St Joseph, Lexington	7,809	10.1	11.9									★ (blue)			
St Joseph East, Lexington	618	11.3	***14.9***	✖	✖		✖	–		–	–		–	–	–
St Luke East, Fort Thomas	4,174	13.1	9.6	★ (blue)	★ (blue)	★ (blue)	★ (blue)		★ (blue)	★ (blue)			★	★ (blue)	
St Luke West, Florence	2,228	11.6	9.0	★ (blue)	★ (blue)		★ (blue)		★ (blue)	★ (blue)		★ (blue)			★ (blue)
Samaritan, Lexington	2,025	10.5	11.1					★					★		
T J Samson, Glasgow	3,716	11.8	***13.2***	✖	×		✖			×					
Taylor County, Campbellsville	1,623	14.0	13.4	×	×						×				
Three Rivers, Louisa	1,416	14.6	***17.1***	✖	✖	✖	✖	✖		✖		✖	–		✖
Tri-County Baptist, La Grange	1,329	12.2	12.2												
Twin Lakes Regional, Leitchfield	1,272	13.6	***16.3***	✖	✖		✖		✖	×	×		×		–
University of Kentucky, Lexington	2,635	13.8	12.1												
University of Louisville, Louisville	1,092	13.0	9.5	★ (blue)	★ (blue)	★	★ (blue)	★ (blue)				×	–		
Wayne County, Monticello	691	11.6	10.9					–					–		–
Western Baptist, Paducah	6,571	9.4	11.2	★		★									
Westlake Regional, Columbia	1,222	11.9	9.6	★ (blue)	★ (blue)		★ (blue)		★ (blue)			★ (blue)	–		
Whitesburg Appalachian Regional, Whitesburg	2,199	10.6	13.1				★		✖	✖	✖			★ (blue)	✖
Williamson ARH, South Williamson	2,375	7.2	8.7	★ (blue)	★ (blue)		★ (blue)	★ (blue)		★ (blue)				★ (blue)	
Louisiana															
New Orleans Area															
Lakeland, New Orleans	1,794	13.3	11.4						★ (blue)						
Med Ctr of LA - University Campus, New Orleans	–	–	–	–	–	–	–	–	–	–	–	–	–	–	–
Med Ctr of LA at New Orleans, New Orleans	1,465	13.1	12.5								✖				
Memorial - Baptist Campus, New Orleans	8,121	10.6	10.0	★ (blue)	★ (blue)		★ (blue)		★ (blue)		★				
Memorial - Mercy Campus, New Orleans[1]	–	–	–	–	–	–	–	–	–	–	–	–	–	–	–
Ochsner Foundation, New Orleans	5,533	11.0	12.6				✖							✖	★
Pendleton Methodist, New Orleans	2,663	12.0	11.1						★ (blue)						
St Charles General, New Orleans	1,307	7.0	6.4	★ (blue)	★ (blue)		★ (blue)	★ (blue)	★ (blue)		★	★	★ (blue)		
St Claude, New Orleans	292	12.0	10.3			–	★	–			–	–	–	–	
Touro Infirmary, New Orleans	3,756	12.4	11.9											✖	
Tulane University, New Orleans	1,438	9.4	10.7					★		✖					

Footnotes are on page 350.

Hospital outcomes: better (★) or worse (×) than average											Results of accreditation review on full survey		Other facts			
Adjusted Death rates			Adjusted Adverse outcome rates													
Surgical cases			Surgical cases													
All selected surgical cases	Coronary artery bypass surgery	Large bowel surgery	All selected surgical cases	Coronary artery bypass surgery	Large bowel surgery	Gall bladder removal	Total knee replacement	Total hip replacement	Simple prostatectomy	Carotid endarterectomy	Accreditation status*	Overall evaluation score (higher is better)	Number of beds	Major medical school affiliation?	Number of residents	Computerized drug order system (1 to 5 scale, higher is preferred; see page 23 for details)
2.3	3.8	6.5	7.7	10.3	11.9	7.5	6.7	6.4	5.4	8.2	–	91	161	–	–	–
–	–	–	–	–	–	–	–	–	–	–	4	95	26	No	0	–
–	–	–	–	–	–	–	–	–	–	–	–[2]	–[2]	45	No	0	–
	–	–	★	–			–	–		–	4	90	133	Yes	0	–
–	–	–	–	–	–	–	–	–	–	–	–[2]	–[2]	20	No	0	–
											4	92	339	No	0	–
–	–	–		–	–	–	–	–	–	–	4	***81***	166	No	–	–
	–			–		–	★	–	–	–	4	92	185	No	0	–
	–	–		–		–	–	–	–	–	–[2]	–[2]	144	No	0	–
	–			–		–	×		–		4	***87***	173	No	0	–
✖	–	×		–			★		–		4	***85***	170	No	0	–
	–	–		–			–	–	–	–	4	***84***	90	No	0	–
–	–	–		–	–	–	–	–	–	–	5	**99**	90	No	0	–
–	–	–		–	–	–	–	–	–	–	5	**94**	75	No	0	–
–	–	–		–	–	–	–	–	–	–	4	**98**	75	No	0	–
			✖	✖		–	–	–	–	–	4	**94**	396	Yes	0	–
–	–	–		–	–	–	–	–	–	–	4	93	271	Yes	0	–
–	–	–	–	–	–	–	–	–	–	–	4	90	30	No	0	–
	★			★							4	**94**	247	No	0	–
–	–	–	–	–	–	–	–	–	–	–	4	***87***	80	No	0	–
–	–	–		–	–	–	–	–	–	–	4	**97**	69	No	0	–
–	–	–		–	–	–	–	–	–	–	4	***86***	98	No	0	–
✖	–	–				–	–	–	–	–	4	**95**	140	No	0	–
–	–	–	–	–	–	–	–	–	–	–	–[2]	–[2]	643	–	0	–
×	–	–		–		–	–	–	–	–	–[2]	–[2]	694	Yes	350	–
		✖									4	90	389	No	0	–
–	–	–	–	–	–	–	–	–	–	–	–[2]	–[2]	–	–	–	–
			★	★		★		★		★	4	92	356	No	203	–
				×			–	–	–		4	**94**	251	No	8	–
–	–	–	–	–	–	–	–	–	–	–	4	**96**	163	No	1	–
–	–	–	–	–	–	–	–	–	–	–	4	***83***	136	No	1	–
	–					–	×	–			5	93	283	Yes	8	–
	–	–				–		–	–		4	92	336	Yes	0	–

***Accreditation Status:** 5=Accredited with commendation or with full standards compliance; 4=Accredited with requirements for improvement; 3=Conditional accreditation.

Detailed Ratings for All Areas

See more information on "Key Ratings for Metro Areas" table beginning on page 32

Blue is most favorable
Bold Italic is least favorable
Blank means neither better nor worse than average
"–" means insufficient data

	Death rates for all selected case types				Hospital outcomes: better (★) or worse (×) than average — Adjusted Death rates — Medical Cases										
	Number of cases	Actual death rate (%)	Adjusted death rate (%) (lower is better)	All selected cases	All selected medical cases	Heart attack	Congestive heart failure	Obstructive pulmonary disease	Pneumonia	Respiratory failure and arrest	Septicemia	Stroke	Gastrointestinal hemorrhage	Fluid, electrolyte, & acid-base disorders	Kidney failure
National Average	–	–	12.1	12.1	14.8	21.2	10.6	6.5	16.9	34.4	25.1	18.4	6.7	11.0	20.9
Louisiana *(continued)*															
Other Areas															
Abbeville General, Abbeville	1,534	14.7	***16.8***	***×***	***×***	***×***	***×***		***×***	–				***×***	
Abram Kaplan Memorial, Kaplan	446	13.5	13.7			–		–		–			–	–	–
Acadia - St Landry, Church Point	182	18.7	***20.0***	***×***	***×***	–	–	–	***×***	–	–	–	–	–	–
Allen Parish, Kinder	246	11.8	10.4			–		–		–	★	–	–	–	–
American Legion, Crowley	1,690	15.1	***16.1***	***×***	***×***	×			***×***	***×***	×				
Avoyelles, Marksville	1,166	14.9	11.1									×			
Baton Rouge General, Baton Rouge	5,456	13.5	**10.0**	**★**	**★**		**★**	**★**	**★**			**★**		★	
Beauregard, Deridder	1,628	10.6	12.1				***×***						★		–
Bogalusa Community, Bogalusa	2,206	11.0	11.5			***×***	**★**								
Bunkie General, Bunkie	396	9.6	11.1			–		–		–	–	–	–		–
Byrd Regional, Leesville	1,372	10.9	10.8				×		**★**						
Caldwell, Columbia	321	2.8	**3.6**	**★**	**★**	–	**★**	–	–	–	–	–	–	–	–
Chalmette Medical Center, Chalmette	3,360	12.9	12.2			***×***			**★**		***×***				
Christus, Coushatta[1]	561	9.4	11.4			–	***×***	–	**★**	–		–	–	**★**	–
Christus St Frances Cabrini, Alexandria	5,216	14.2	***13.9***	***×***	***×***		***×***	***×***	***×***	×					
Christus St Patrick, Lake Charles	5,455	11.8	12.2												
Christus Schumpert Highland, Shreveport	1,650	11.1	10.8		★										
Christus Schumpert St Mary Place, Shreveport[1]	7,570	11.0	11.4		**★**		**★**								
Citizens, Columbia	730	10.0	**8.6**	**★**	**★**	–		**★**			**★**	–	–		
Dauterive, New Iberia	1,654	12.3	12.1										**★**	***×***	
Dequincy Memorial, Dequincy	439	9.8	10.1			–				–		–	–	★	–
DeSoto Regional, Mansfield	799	11.6	11.1			–		–		–					–
Doctors of Jefferson, Metairie	1,577	10.3	10.5	★	**★**										
Doctors', Opelousas	1,413	12.7	***14.0***	***×***	***×***				×			***×***			–
Doctors', Shreveport	1,396	9.5	10.4	★	**★**		★						–		★
E A Conway, Monroe	502	10.4	14.5			–		–		–	–	–	–		–
Earl K Long, Baton Rouge	271	8.5	11.6			–		–	–	–	–	–	–	–	–
East Carroll Parish, Lake Providence	162	17.9	***19.2***	***×***	***×***	–	–	–		–	–	–	–	–	–
East Jefferson General, Metairie	8,444	10.9	11.3	★	★				**★**					×	
Eunice Community, Eunice	743	10.9	13.5			–		–		–	***×***		–		–
Franklin, Winnsboro	1,722	15.3	***17.4***	***×***	***×***			***×***	***×***	–				***×***	–
Franklin Foundation, Franklin	826	14.5	***15.1***	***×***	***×***		***×***	–					–		–
Glenwood Regional, West Monroe	3,190	11.0	12.5				***×***								
Hardtner, Olla	423	6.9	**7.1**	**★**	**★**	–		–	**★**	–	–		–	–	–

Footnotes are on page 350.

Hospital outcomes: better (★) or worse (×) than average											Results of accreditation review on full survey		Other facts			
Adjusted Death rates			Adjusted Adverse outcome rates													
Surgical cases			Surgical cases													
All selected surgical cases	Coronary artery bypass surgery	Large bowel surgery	All selected surgical cases	Coronary artery bypass surgery	Large bowel surgery	Gall bladder removal	Total knee replacement	Total hip replacement	Simple prostatectomy	Carotid endarterectomy	Accreditation status*	Overall evaluation score (higher is better)	Number of beds	Major medical school affiliation?	Number of residents	Computerized drug order system (1 to 5 scale, higher is preferred; see page 23 for details)
2.3	3.8	6.5	7.7	10.3	11.9	7.5	6.7	6.4	5.4	8.2	–	91	161	–	–	–
	–	–		–			–	–	–	–	5	99	85	No	0	–
–	–	–	–	–	–	–	–	–	–	–	–[2]	–[2]	40	No	0	–
–	–	–	–	–	–	–	–	–	–	–	–[2]	–[2]	39	No	0	–
–	–	–	–	–	–	–	–	–	–	–	–[2]	–[2]	24	No	0	–
	–	–		–			–	–		–	–[2]	–[2]	178	No	0	–
–	–	–		–		–	–	–	–	–	4	98	47	No	0	2
					★		★	–	–		–[2]	–[2]	423	No	19	–
–	–	–	–	–	–	–	–	–	–	–	4	95	93	No	0	–
–	–	–	–	–	–	–	–	–	–	–	4	97	70	No	0	–
–	–	–	–	–	–	–	–	–	–	–	–[2]	–[2]	41	No	0	–
–	–	–		–	–	–	–	–	–	–	4	96	59	No	0	–
–	–	–	–	–	–	–	–	–	–	–	–[2]	–[2]	31	No	0	–
	–	–		–			–	–	–	–	5	96	138	No	1	–
–	–	–	–	–	–	–	–	–	–	–	–[2]	–[2]	49	No	0	–
									–		4	96	227	No	10	–
×		×			×			–			4	92	336	No	0	–
	×	–			×	–	–	–	–	–	–[2]	–[2]	158	No	2	–
	×						×				4	93	36	Yes	0	–
–	–	–	–	–	–	–	–	–	–	–	–[2]	–[2]	40	No	0	–
×	–	–		–		–	×	–	–		4	90	86	No	0	3
–	–	–	–	–	–	–	–	–	–	–	–[2]	–[2]	41	No	0	–
–	–	–	–	–	–	–	–	–	–	–	–[2]	–[2]	49	No	0	–
	–	–	×	×		–	×	–	–	–	4	94	120	No	0	–
	–			–		–		–	–	–	4	92	105	No	1	–
×	–	×		–		–		–	–	–	4	90	99	No	0	–
–	–	–	–	–	–	–	–	–	–	–	4	96	174	Yes	30	–
–	–	–	–	–	–	–	–	–	–	–	4	92	204	Yes	103	–
–	–	–	–	–	–	–	–	–	–	–	–[2]	–[2]	29	No	0	–
		★									4	87	389	No	13	–
–	–	–		–	–	–	–	–	–	–	4	87	62	No	0	–
–	–	–		–	–	–	–	–	×	–	–[2]	–[2]	47	No	0	–
–	–	–	–	–	–	–	–	–	–	–	–[2]	–[2]	42	No	0	–
	–	★		–	★			–	–	–	4	94	262	No	–	–
–	–	–	–	–	–	–	–	–	–	–	–[2]	–[2]	41	No	0	–

***Accreditation Status:** 5=Accredited with commendation or with full standards compliance; 4=Accredited with requirements for improvement; 3=Conditional accreditation.

Detailed Ratings for All Areas

See more information on "Key Ratings for Metro Areas" table beginning on page 32

Blue is most favorable
Bold Italic is least favorable
Blank means neither better nor worse than average
"–" means insufficient data

	Death rates for all selected case types			Hospital outcomes: better (★) or worse (×) than average — Adjusted Death rates — Medical Cases											
	Number of cases	Actual death rate (%)	Adjusted death rate (%) (lower is better)	All selected cases	All selected medical cases	Heart attack	Congestive heart failure	Obstructive pulmonary disease	Pneumonia	Respiratory failure and arrest	Septicemia	Stroke	Gastrointestinal hemorrhage	Fluid, electrolyte, & acid-base disorders	Kidney failure
National Average	–	–	12.1	12.1	14.8	21.2	10.6	6.5	16.9	34.4	25.1	18.4	6.7	11.0	20.9
Louisiana *(continued)*															
Other Areas *(continued)*															
Homer Memorial, Homer	1,339	13.4	11.7			✖		★		–					
Hood, Amite	613	11.7	12.7			×		–		–	–	–	–		–
Huey P Long, Pineville	132	10.6	14.4			–	–	–	–	–	–	–	–	–	–
Iberia, New Iberia	1,816	12.8	***14.1***	✖	✖	✖								✖	
Jackson Parish, Jonesboro	654	15.7	13.2			–			✖	–	★		–		
Jennings American Legion, Jennings	1,638	15.1	***18.7***	✖	✖	✖	✖		✖		✖	✖	×		×
Kenner Regional, Kenner	1,133	15.9	12.4						×						
Lady of the Sea General, Cut Off	747	16.9	***14.5***	✖	✖	×		–		×					–
Lafayette General, Lafayette	4,156	12.1	12.5				✖								
Lake Charles Memorial, Lake Charles	4,102	12.5	12.0							✖			✖		
Lakeside, Metairie	66	–	–	–	–	–	–	–	–	–	–	–	–	–	–
Lakeview Regional, Covington	1,614	12.8	11.5												
Lakewood, Morgan City	1,334	14.5	***15.7***	✖	✖				✖		✖	×			–
Lane, Zachary	2,119	15.4	***16.3***	✖	✖	×		×	✖	–	✖	×	✖		
LaSalle General, Jena	1,655	6.9	6.9	★	★	–	★	★	★	–			–		–
Leonard J Chaubert, Houma	546	11.5	12.9			–					–	–	–		–
Lincoln General, Ruston	3,243	13.4	10.7	★	★		★								
LSU Health Sciences Center, Shreveport	1,847	12.7	12.9				★				×		✖		
LSUMC/HCSD - Lallie Kemp, Independence	452	10.4	13.3			–		–		–	–	–	–	–	–
Madison Parish, Tallulah	464	15.1	13.8			–		–		–	–	✖	–	–	
Meadowcrest, Gretna	2,706	15.5	13.1	×	×	×					✖			✖	★
Medical Center of Southwest Louisiana, Lafayette	2,238	8.5	11.0				✖		★						
Minden Medical Center, Minden	1,590	13.3	10.6	★	★										–
Morehouse General, Bastrop	1,802	12.1	***13.9***	✖	✖	×				×	×				
Natchitoches Parish, Natchitoches[1]	1,333	13.1	12.2					–					–		
North Caddo, Vivian	689	11.3	***14.8***	✖	×	–		–		–	–	–	–	✖	–
North Monroe Medical Center, Monroe	2,971	12.4	13.1	×		✖	✖								
North Oaks, Hammond	4,355	13.0	***13.5***	✖	✖					×	✖		×		
Northshore Regional, Slidell	2,326	11.3	11.8						★					✖	
Oakdale Community, Oakdale	1,621	10.6	8.6	★	★				★		★				
Opelousas General, Opelousas	2,600	13.6	12.0								✖				★
Our Lady of Lourdes Regional, Lafayette	5,704	10.4	11.1	★	★					★	★				
Our Lady of the Lake Regional, Baton Rouge	9,184	12.1	12.5				✖								
Pointe Coupee General, New Roads	677	15.7	***15.1***	✖	✖	–		–		–	–		–		–

Footnotes are on page 350.

Hospital outcomes: better (★) or worse (×) than average											Results of accreditation review on full survey		Other facts			
Adjusted Death rates			Adjusted Adverse outcome rates													
Surgical cases			Surgical cases													
All selected surgical cases	Coronary artery bypass surgery	Large bowel surgery	All selected surgical cases	Coronary artery bypass surgery	Large bowel surgery	Gall bladder removal	Total knee replacement	Total hip replacement	Simple prostatectomy	Carotid endarterectomy	Accreditation status*	Overall evaluation score (higher is better)	Number of beds	Major medical school affiliation?	Number of residents	Computerized drug order system (1 to 5 scale, higher is preferred; see page 23 for details)
2.3	3.8	6.5	7.7	10.3	11.9	7.5	6.7	6.4	5.4	8.2	–	91	161	–	–	–
–	–	–	–	–	–	–	–	–	–	–	–[2]	–[2]	60	No	0	–
–	–	–	–	–	–	–	–	–	–	–	–[2]	–[2]	40	No	0	–
–	–	–	–	–	–	–	–	–	–	–	4	90	123	No	6	–
	–	–		–	★	–	–	–	–	–	4	91	78	No	0	–
–	–	–	–	–	–	–	–	–	–	–	–[2]	–[2]	49	No	0	–
–	–	–		–	–	–	–	–	–	–	4	91	53	No	0	–
	–					–	–	–	–	–	4	90	213	No	3	–
–	–	–	–	–	–	–	–	–	–	–	4	93	55	No	0	–
										★	4	***88***	318	No	0	–
✖		✖			×				–		4	**97**	301	No	16	–
–	–	–	–	–	–	–	–	–	–	–	4	92	75	No	1	2
	–	–			–	–	–	–	–		5	**97**	126	No	3	–
–	–	–		–	–	–	–	–	–	–	4	89	111	No	0	–
–	–	–		–		–	–	–	–	–	4	**94**	87	No	0	–
–	–	–	–	–	–	–	–	–	–	–	–[2]	–[2]	60	No	0	–
–	–	–	–	–	–	–	–	–	–	–	4	**96**	123	No	27	–
	–			–				–		–	4	89	111	No	0	–
	–	–		✖	–	–	–	–	–	–	4	90	413	**Yes**	352	–
–	–	–	–	–	–	–	–	–	–	–	4	**95**	68	No	0	–
–	–	–	–	–	–	–	–	–	–	–	–[2]	–[2]	47	No	0	–
	–	–					–	–	–	–	4	**97**	157	No	0	–
		–				–		–	–		4	92	138	No	0	2
–	–	–	★	–	–	–	–	–	–	–	4	**97**	130	No	0	–
	–	–		–		–	–	–	–	–	–[2]	–[2]	95	No	0	–
–	–	–	–	–	–	–	–	–	–	–	4	**95**	54	No	0	–
–	–	–	–	–	–	–	–	–	–	–	–[2]	–[2]	35	**Yes**	0	–
✖	–			–			★	–	–	–	4	93	186	No	1	–
	–							–	–	–	4	93	215	No	0	–
	★	–		★		–		–	–		4	***84***	147	No	1	–
–	–	–	–	–	–	–	–	–	–	–	4	**94**	54	No	0	3
	–	–		–		–		–		–	4	91	134	No	0	–
											4	**96**	220	No	0	–
		✖					★	★			4	***88***	668	No	0	–
–	–	–	–	–	–	–	–	–	–	–	–[2]	–[2]	27	No	0	–

***Accreditation Status:** 5=Accredited with commendation or with full standards compliance; 4=Accredited with requirements for improvement; 3=Conditional accreditation.

Detailed Ratings for All Areas

See more information on "Key Ratings for Metro Areas" table beginning on page 32

Blue is most favorable
Bold Italic is least favorable
Blank means neither better nor worse than average
"–" means insufficient data

	Death rates for all selected case types				Hospital outcomes: better (★) or worse (×) than average — Adjusted Death rates — Medical Cases											
	Number of cases	Actual death rate (%)	Adjusted death rate (%) (lower is better)	All selected cases	All selected medical cases	Heart attack	Congestive heart failure	Obstructive pulmonary disease	Pneumonia	Respiratory failure and arrest	Septicemia	Stroke	Gastrointestinal hemorrhage	Fluid, electrolyte, & acid-base disorders	Kidney failure
National Average	–	–	12.1	12.1	14.8	21.2	10.6	6.5	16.9	34.4	25.1	18.4	6.7	11.0	20.9
Louisiana *(continued)*															
Other Areas *(continued)*															
Prevost, Donaldsonville	145	23.4	***19.6***	✖	✖	–	–	–		–	✖	–	–	–	–
Rapides Regional, Alexandria	6,054	12.0	11.2	★	**★**					**★**		**★**			
Richardson, Rayville	1,071	13.4	***14.6***	✖	✖	✖				–	✖		–		–
Richland Parish, Delhi	957	8.5	10.0	★	★	–	★			–			–	★	–
River Parishes, La Place	820	15.0	***15.6***	✖	✖			–	✖			×	–		–
River West, Plaquemine	809	17.7	***14.0***	✖	×			×					–	✖	–
Riverland, Ferriday	1,146	16.3	12.0					–					–	**★**	
Riverside, Franklinton	968	10.2	**9.8**	**★**	**★**	×				–			–		–
Sabine, Many	1,072	13.2	10.9							–			–	★	
St Anne General, Raceland	631	12.2	**9.1**	**★**	**★**	–		–	**★**			–			
St Charles Parish, Luling	593	13.3	12.2					–				–	–		–
St Elizabeth, Gonzales	989	17.1	13.5										–	★	–
St Francis, Monroe	5,891	8.7	**9.6**	**★**	**★**	**★**	★	**★**	★			**★**			**★**
St James Parish, Lutcher	195	19.5	***17.1***	✖	✖	–	–	–	✖	–	–	–	–	–	–
St Tammany Parish, Covington	2,598	10.2	12.4												
Savoy, Mamou	1,912	10.3	10.5	★	**★**				**★**						
Slidell Memorial, Slidell	2,741	8.8	**10.1**	**★**	**★**		**★**		**★**						
South Cameron Memorial, Cameron	128	7.8	7.8			–	–	–	★	–	–	–	–	–	–
Springhill Medical Center, Springhill	1,311	15.0	10.9			✖	★				★				
Summit, Baton Rouge	922	19.2	***16.3***	✖	✖		✖		✖				–		✖
Terrebonne General, Houma	4,409	9.9	12.1						×					✖	
Thibodaux Regional, Thibodaux	2,820	12.8	***13.6***	✖	✖				✖		✖				
Tri-Ward General, Bernice	284	16.2	***17.3***	✖	✖	–	–	–		–	✖	–	–	–	–
University, Lafayette	359	8.9	9.7			–	–	–		–		–	–	–	–
Ville Platte Medical Center, Ville Platte	1,361	12.9	13.0			–	×								
W O Moss Regional, Lake Charles	175	5.7	9.1			–	–	–	–	–	–	–	–	–	–
Washington St Tammany Regional, Bogalusa	278	10.4	14.8			–	×	–		–	–	–	–	–	–
West Calcasieu Cameron, Sulphur	2,003	12.2	11.6												
West Carroll, Oak Grove	1,111	9.8	12.4			–			**★**	✖			–	×	–
West Feliciana Parish, St Francisville	64	15.6	15.3			–	–	–	–	–	–	–	–	–	–
West Jefferson, Marrero	4,635	12.2	11.6			★								✖	
Willis Knighton, Shreveport	8,841	9.4	12.2								×		**★**	★	
Willis Knighton Bossier, Bossier City	1,772	7.9	**8.4**	**★**	**★**						**★**	**★**	–	**★**	★
Winn Parish, Winnfield	1,490	12.2	**10.3**	**★**	**★**				**★**	–					

Footnotes are on page 350.

Hospital outcomes: better (★) or worse (×) than average											Results of accreditation review on full survey		Other facts			
Adjusted Death rates			Adjusted Adverse outcome rates													
Surgical cases			Surgical cases													
All selected surgical cases	Coronary artery bypass surgery	Large bowel surgery	All selected surgical cases	Coronary artery bypass surgery	Large bowel surgery	Gall bladder removal	Total knee replacement	Total hip replacement	Simple prostatectomy	Carotid endarterectomy	Accreditation status*	Overall evaluation score (higher is better)	Number of beds	Major medical school affiliation?	Number of residents	Computerized drug order system (1 to 5 scale, higher is preferred; see page 23 for details)
2.3	3.8	6.5	7.7	10.3	11.9	7.5	6.7	6.4	5.4	8.2	–	91	161	–	–	–
–	–	–	–	–	–	–	–	–	–	–	4	88	35	No	0	–
✖	✖	×					★	–			4	96	320	No	0	2
–	–	–	–	–	–	–	–	–	–	–	–[2]	–[2]	49	No	0	–
–	–	–	–	–	–	–	–	–	–	–	–[2]	–[2]	42	No	0	–
–	–	–		–	–	–	–	–	–	–	4	93	106	No	0	–
–	–	–	–	–	–	–	–	–	–	–	4	94	72	No	0	–
–	–	–	–	–	–	–	–	–	–	–	–[2]	–[2]	49	No	0	–
–	–	–	–	–	–	–	–	–	–	–	4	88	48	No	0	–
–	–	–	–	–	–	–	–	–	–	–	5	99	48	No	0	–
–	–	–	–	–	–	–	–	–	–	–	–[2]	–[2]	58	No	0	–
–	–	–	–	–	–	–	–	–	–	–	4	92	56	No	0	–
–	–	–	–	–	–	–	–	–	–	–	4	96	75	No	0	–
			★							✖	4	90	341	No	0	–
–	–	–	–	–	–	–	–	–	–	–	4	99	26	No	0	–
✖	✖		✖	✖		–	✖	–	–		4	92	133	No	0	–
	–	–		–			–	–	–	–	4	95	205	No	0	–
	✖	–			✖	–	–	–	–		5	97	173	No	0	–
–	–	–	–	–	–	–	–	–	–	–	–[2]	–[2]	33	No	0	–
–	–	–	★	–	–	–	–	–	–	–	4	97	63	No	0	–
–	–	–	–	–	–	–	–	–	–	–	4	89	143	No	1	–
★					★			–			4	97	245	No	0	–
	–	–					–	–	–		4	96	140	No	6	–
–	–	–	–	–	–	–	–	–	–	–	–[2]	–[2]	11	No	0	–
–	–	–	–	–	–	–	–	–	–	–	4	92	20	No	–	–
–	–	–		–	–		–	–	–	–	4	88	80	No	0	–
–	–	–	–	–	–	–	–	–	–	–	–[2]	–[2]	74	No	0	–
–	–	–	–	–	–	–	–	–	–	–	4	94	50	No	0	–
	–		★	–			–	–	–	–	4	91	85	No	0	–
–	–	–	–	–	–	–	–	–	–	–	–[2]	–[2]	21	No	0	–
–	–	–	–	–	–	–	–	–	–	–	4	85	23	No	0	–
								–	–		4	84	309	No	0	–
				★	★			✖	✖		–[2]	–[2]	426	No	79	–
	–	–			–	–	–	–	–	–	–[2]	–[2]	104	No	–	–
✖	–	–		–	–		–	–	–	–	4	96	103	No	1	2

***Accreditation Status:** 5=Accredited with commendation or with full standards compliance; 4=Accredited with requirements for improvement; 3=Conditional accreditation.

Detailed Ratings for All Areas

See more information on "Key Ratings for Metro Areas" table beginning on page 32

Blue is most favorable
Bold Italic is least favorable
Blank means neither better nor worse than average
"–" means insufficient data

	Death rates for all selected case types			Hospital outcomes: better (★) or worse (×) than average — Adjusted Death rates — Medical Cases											
	Number of cases	Actual death rate (%)	Adjusted death rate (%) (lower is better)	All selected cases	All selected medical cases	Heart attack	Congestive heart failure	Obstructive pulmonary disease	Pneumonia	Respiratory failure and arrest	Septicemia	Stroke	Gastrointestinal hemorrhage	Fluid, electrolyte, & acid-base disorders	Kidney failure
National Average	–	–	12.1	12.1	14.8	21.2	10.6	6.5	16.9	34.4	25.1	18.4	6.7	11.0	20.9
Louisiana *(continued)*															
Other Areas *(continued)*															
Woman's, Baton Rouge	193	–	–	–	–	–	–	–	–	–	–	–	–	–	–
Women and Children's, Lake Charles	81	9.9	12.9			–	–	–	–	–	–	–	–	–	–
Maine															
Aroostook, Presque Isle	1,306	11.8	***15.2***	✖	✖	✖		×	✖						–
Bridgton Hospital, Bridgton	799	11.4	14.0							✖	✖		–	–	–
Cary, Caribou	1,556	11.4	12.7									×	–		
Central Maine, Lewiston	3,477	10.3	12.1				×		★	✖	**★**				×
Down East, Machias	1,174	13.4	11.4												
Eastern Maine, Bangor	5,335	9.0	11.9							★				**★**	
Franklin, Farmington	1,454	13.5	13.0				✖			✖			★		✖
Henrietta D Goodall, Sanford	1,150	11.9	13.2					**★**		✖	–				✖
Houlton Regional, Houlton	1,066	9.0	11.6						★	–	–		–		–
Inland, Waterville	803	11.3	13.5							–			–		–
Maine, Portland	8,583	8.7	**10.4**	**★**	**★**	**★**			★		**★**	×			
Maine Coast, Ellsworth	1,302	12.2	12.0									✖			★
Maine General, Waterville	4,566	11.1	12.7				✖				★				
Mayo Regional, Dover-Foxcroft	995	16.5	***18.8***	✖	✖		✖		✖	–			✖	✖	–
Mercy, Portland	4,392	11.2	12.5												
Mid Coast, Brunswick	1,917	12.2	12.4				✖			★					
Miles, Damariscotta	1,121	8.4	**9.1**	**★**	**★**		**★**	**★**			–		–		–
Millinocket Regional, Millinocket	624	10.3	14.1		×					–	–		–	–	–
Northern Maine, Fort Kent	764	13.4	13.7							–	–		–		–
Parkview, Brunswick	848	9.9	10.7										–		–
Penobscot Bay, Rockport	2,474	10.9	**10.7**	**★**	★				**★**	✖			★	★	
Redington - Fairview General, Skowhegan	1,416	11.2	11.5												–
Rumford Hospital, Rumford	799	11.9	***14.5***	✖	×		✖			–	–		–	✖	–
St Joseph, Bangor	2,256	10.0	11.4			×			★	**★**				**★**	
St Mary's Regional, Lewiston	2,191	10.5	10.7	★	★					★		×			
Sebasticook Valley, Pittsfield	836	14.7	***18.2***	✖	✖			✖	×	–	–	✖	✖		–
Southern Maine, Biddeford	3,258	14.4	***14.7***	✖	✖		✖	✖	×		**★**				✖
Stephens, Norway	1,089	12.3	11.7									✖		–	
Waldo County General, Belfast[1]	1,218	12.9	13.4									✖	–	×	×
York Hospital, York	1,797	11.5	***14.4***	✖	✖					✖					

Footnotes are on page 350.

Hospital outcomes: better (★) or worse (✕) than average											Results of accreditation review on full survey		Other facts			
Adjusted Death rates			Adjusted Adverse outcome rates													
Surgical cases			Surgical cases													
All selected surgical cases	Coronary artery bypass surgery	Large bowel surgery	All selected surgical cases	Coronary artery bypass surgery	Large bowel surgery	Gall bladder removal	Total knee replacement	Total hip replacement	Simple prostatectomy	Carotid endarterectomy	Accreditation status*	Overall evaluation score (higher is better)	Number of beds	Major medical school affiliation?	Number of residents	Computerized drug order system (1 to 5 scale, higher is preferred; see page 23 for details)
2.3	3.8	6.5	7.7	10.3	11.9	7.5	6.7	6.4	5.4	8.2	–	91	161	–	–	–
–	–	–		–	–	–	–	–	–	–	4	98	220	No	0	–
–	–	–	–	–	–	–	–	–	–	–	4	89	80	No	0	–
	–	–		–		–		–	–	–	4	**87**	80	No	0	–
–	–	–		–	–	–	–	–	–	–	4	**87**	40	No	0	–
	–	–		–	✕	–	–	–			4	93	46	No	0	–
	–		✕	–			✕			★	4	91	100	No	16	–
–	–	–		–		–	–	–	–	–	3	91	36	No	0	–
	✕	★						★			5	91	304	Yes	36	–
–	–	–		–		–	–	–	–	–	4	91	50	No	0	–
	–	–		–		–	–	–	–	–	4	90	49	No	0	–
	–	–		–		–	–	–	–	–	4	93	49	No	0	–
–	–	–		–	–	–	✕	–	–	–	–[2]	–[2]	44	No	0	–
★	★			★			✕				5	**82**	560	Yes	184	–
	–	–	✕	–		–	✕	–	–	–	4	91	48	No	0	–
	–		★	–			★				4	**87**	294	No	0	–
–	–	–		–	–	–		–	–	–	4	90	46	No	0	–
★	–	★		–				★	✕	–	4	**88**	166	No	0	–
★	–	–	★	–	★	–		–	–	–	4	91	72	No	0	–
–	–	–		–	–	–	–	–	–	–	4	95	32	No	0	–
–	–	–		–	–	–	–	–	–	–	4	**84**	20	No	0	–
–	–	–	–	–	–	–	–	–	–	–	4	90	52	No	0	–
–	–	–		–	–	–	–	–	–	–	4	**84**	48	No	0	–
	–			–					–	–	–[2]	–[2]	85	No	0	–
	–	–		–		–	–	–	–	–	4	91	65	No	0	–
–	–	–		–	–	–	–	–	–	–	4	92	27	No	0	–
	–			–		–				–	4	91	84	No	0	–
	–			–			–	–	–	★	4	**81**	187	No	0	–
–	–	–	–	–	–	–	–	–	–	–	–[2]	–[2]	26	No	0	–
	–			–						–	4	**83**	121	Yes	4	–
	–	–		–		–	✕	–	–	–	4	94	50	No	0	–
–	–	–		–		–	–	–	–	–	4	**84**	45	No	0	–
	–	–		–		–		–	–	–	–[2]	–[2]	79	No	0	–

***Accreditation Status:** 5=Accredited with commendation or with full standards compliance; 4=Accredited with requirements for improvement; 3=Conditional accreditation.

Detailed Ratings for All Areas

See more information on "Key Ratings for Metro Areas" table beginning on page 32

Blue is most favorable
Bold Italic is least favorable
Blank means neither better nor worse than average
"–" means insufficient data

	Death rates for all selected case types			Hospital outcomes: better (★) or worse (×) than average — Adjusted Death rates — Medical Cases											
	Number of cases	Actual death rate (%)	Adjusted death rate (%) (lower is better)	All selected cases	All selected medical cases	Heart attack	Congestive heart failure	Obstructive pulmonary disease	Pneumonia	Respiratory failure and arrest	Septicemia	Stroke	Gastrointestinal hemorrhage	Fluid, electrolyte, & acid-base disorders	Kidney failure
National Average	–	–	12.1	12.1	14.8	21.2	10.6	6.5	16.9	34.4	25.1	18.4	6.7	11.0	20.9
Maryland															
Baltimore Area															
Bon Secours, Baltimore[1]	3,363	10.6	**9.5**	**★**	**★**		**★**		**★**						**★**
Franklin Square, Baltimore[1]	8,230	12.5	**11.2**	**★**	**★**					**★**			★		★
Good Samaritan, Baltimore	6,555	10.8	**9.2**	**★**	**★**	★	**★**		**★**	**★**		**★**	★	★	
Greater Baltimore, Baltimore	6,650	10.1	**10.3**	**★**	**★**					**★**	★	**★**		**★**	
Harbor, Baltimore	4,538	11.5	**9.4**	**★**	**★**		**★**	**★**	**★**			★			
James Lawrence Kernan, Baltimore	215	0.5	**2.3**	**★**	★	–	–	–	–	–	–	–	–	–	–
Johns Hopkins, Baltimore	4,583	7.7	**9.9**	**★**	**★**		**★**		**★**			**★**		★	
Johns Hopkins Bayview, Baltimore	4,960	13.6	11.4				★				***×***			**★**	
Maryland General, Baltimore	3,106	14.0	**10.1**	**★**	**★**		**★**		**★**			**★**		**★**	
Mercy, Baltimore	2,956	7.1	**8.8**	**★**	**★**		**★**	**★**	**★**			**★**			**★**
Northwest, Randallstown	6,226	14.7	11.4	★	★		★	***×***	★			**★**			
St Agnes, Baltimore[1]	8,313	12.6	11.8											***×***	
St Joseph, Towson	10,029	9.9	12.5		***×***	**★**	×		***×***						
Sinai, Baltimore	7,761	13.3	**10.6**	**★**	**★**	★	**★**	**★**		★	***×***	**★**			
Union, Baltimore	4,609	10.2	11.1	★			**★**				***×***				
University of Maryland, Baltimore[1]	2,475	12.0	**10.7**	**★**	**★**		**★**		**★**		×				
Washington, DC, Area															
Anne Arundel, Annapolis	6,426	12.8	11.5							**★**					×
Doctors, Lanham	4,436	11.9	**9.8**	**★**	**★**	**★**	★		**★**			**★**		★	★
Fort Washington Medical Center, Fort Washington	1,211	12.2	**10.1**	**★**	**★**				**★**						★
Holy Cross, Silver Spring	6,453	14.3	11.8									★			
Howard County General, Columbia	3,690	14.5	11.5							**★**					
Laurel Regional, Laurel	2,132	15.0	12.3												
Montgomery General, Olney	3,502	13.7	11.8									***×***	★		
North Arundel, Glen Burnie	7,555	12.2	11.7							**★**					
Prince George's, Cheverly[1]	2,828	13.5	**10.6**	**★**	**★**	★	**★**								
Shady Grove Adventist, Rockville	3,833	15.7	***13.7***	***×***	***×***	***×***	×	***×***				×	×		
Southern Maryland, Clinton[1]	4,931	14.2	**11.0**	**★**	**★**		**★**					★			★
Suburban, Bethesda[1]	6,017	12.2	**10.2**	**★**	**★**		**★**			★				**★**	
Washington Adventist, Takoma Park	4,586	10.5	**9.4**	**★**	**★**	**★**	**★**	★	**★**		★				**★**
Other Areas															
Atlantic General, Berlin[1]	1,594	13.7	11.3							**★**					
Calvert, Prince Frederick	2,478	10.2	**10.4**	**★**	**★**										

Footnotes are on page 350.

Hospital outcomes: better (★) or worse (×) than average — Adjusted Death rates — Surgical cases			Adjusted Adverse outcome rates — Surgical cases								Results of accreditation review on full survey		Other facts			
All selected surgical cases	Coronary artery bypass surgery	Large bowel surgery	All selected surgical cases	Coronary artery bypass surgery	Large bowel surgery	Gall bladder removal	Total knee replacement	Total hip replacement	Simple prostatectomy	Carotid endarterectomy	Accreditation status*	Overall evaluation score (higher is better)	Number of beds	Major medical school affiliation?	Number of residents	Computerized drug order system (1 to 5 scale, higher is preferred; see page 23 for details)
2.3	3.8	6.5	7.7	10.3	11.9	7.5	6.7	6.4	5.4	8.2	–	91	161	–	–	–
	–			–		–	–	–	–	–	4	92	106	No	4	–
	–			–							4	**96**	243	No	15	–
	–		×	–				✖			4	93	231	No	31	–
★	–	★		–			×				4	90	239	No	45	–
	–			–				–			4	***88***	156	No	32	–
–	–	–		–	–	–		–	–	–	4	91	122	No	0	–
			✖	✖	✖				✖		4	91	844	**Yes**	0	–
	–			–		–		–	–		4	92	363	**Yes**	50	–
	–			–		–	–	–		–	4	91	201	**Yes**	43	–
	–			–		–		–			4	90	200	**Yes**	10	–
	–			–				–	–	–	4	**98**	160	No	0	–
	–			–		×			★		4	92	565	No	86	–
		★						✖			4	***81***	355	No	0	–
		★				✖		✖		–	4	93	387	No	138	–
★							✖				5	**94**	318	No	76	–
		×		★		–	–	–	–		4	91	606	**Yes**	585	–
	–		★	–			★		–		4	93	308	No	0	–
	–			–						×	4	***88***	198	No	0	–
–	–	–		–	–	–	–	–	–	–	4	***88***	37	No	0	–
	–			–							5	**96**	370	**Yes**	0	–
	–			–	✖			–	–		4	**97**	163	No	0	–
	–	–		–		–	–	–	–	–	4	91	133	No	0	–
	–			–			✖	✖		–	4	**95**	153	No	0	–
	–		✖	–			×	–	✖		5	89	207	No	0	–
✖	–	✖	✖		✖	–	–	–	–		4	**94**	370	No	54	–
	–		✖	–			✖	✖		–	4	**99**	253	No	0	–
	–	★		–		×	★	–	–		4	90	330	No	0	–
	–		✖	–			✖	×			4	92	197	No	0	–
★	★				★			–	✖	✖	4	**98**	316	No	24	–
–	–	–		–	–	–	–	–	–	–	4	89	62	No	3	–
	–			–	★	–	×	–	–	–	5	**96**	109	No	0	–

***Accreditation Status:** 5=Accredited with commendation or with full standards compliance; 4=Accredited with requirements for improvement; 3=Conditional accreditation.

Detailed Ratings for All Areas

See more information on "Key Ratings for Metro Areas" table beginning on page 32

Blue is most favorable
Bold Italic is least favorable
Blank means neither better nor worse than average
"–" means insufficient data

	Death rates for all selected case types			Hospital outcomes: better (★) or worse (×) than average — Adjusted Death rates — Medical Cases											
	Number of cases	Actual death rate (%)	Adjusted death rate (%) (lower is better)	All selected cases	All selected medical cases	Heart attack	Congestive heart failure	Obstructive pulmonary disease	Pneumonia	Respiratory failure and arrest	Septicemia	Stroke	Gastrointestinal hemorrhage	Fluid, electrolyte, & acid-base disorders	Kidney failure
National Average	–	–	12.1	12.1	14.8	21.2	10.6	6.5	16.9	34.4	25.1	18.4	6.7	11.0	20.9
Maryland *(continued)*															
Other Areas *(continued)*															
Carroll County General, Westminster	4,526	12.1	11.7							★					
Civista, La Plata[1]	2,563	12.0	**10.5**	★	★		★	★							
Dorchester General, Cambridge	1,699	12.6	12.2				★	×	✖						
Edward McCready, Crisfield[1]	689	11.6	10.9			–					✖	★	–	★	
Frederick Memorial, Frederick	6,195	10.9	11.7							×	★				
Garrett County, Oakland	1,572	14.9	***15.0***	✖	✖			✖	✖	✖					×
Harford, Havre De Grace	2,837	14.1	11.9					★							★
Kent & Queen Anne's, Chestertown	1,484	11.4	11.8												
Memorial, Cumberland	5,190	11.8	**10.9**	★	★			★	★						
Memorial, Easton	4,149	11.4	12.9	×				✖			×				
Peninsula Regional, Salisbury[1]	8,591	11.0	11.8			★									
Sacred Heart, Cumberland	5,706	11.3	**9.5**	★	★		★	★	★	★	★				
St Mary's, Leonardtown	2,430	11.9	11.7												
Union, Elkton	2,683	12.9	**10.6**	★	★				★						
Washington County, Hagerstown[1]	7,114	12.2	**10.8**	★	★	★	★			★	★			✖	
Massachusetts															
Boston Area															
Addison Gilbert, Gloucester	–	–	–	–	–	–	–	–	–	–	–	–	–	–	–
Anna Jaques, Newburyport	2,684	11.0	11.1							×					
Beth Israel Deaconess, Boston	9,235	10.6	**11.1**	★	★	★		★				★			
Beverly Hospital, Beverly[1]	4,747	12.9	12.5					★							
Boston Medical Center, Boston[1]	2,993	8.2	**9.4**	★	★		★	★	★		✖			★	★
Brigham and Women's, Boston	6,717	7.3	**10.1**	★	★	★		★			✖				★
Brockton Hospital, Brockton	4,388	12.6	12.0										✖		
Cambridge Hospital, Cambridge[1]	2,386	13.9	12.0					✖							
Caritas, Norwood	4,602	14.2	12.6							✖					
Caritas Good Samaritan, Brockton	5,635	13.5	12.4												
Caritas Southwood, Norfolk	968	12.3	11.5										–		
Carney, Boston	3,417	10.4	**7.9**	★	★		★	★	★	★	★	★	★		★
Charlton - Fall River Site of Southcoast, Fall River[1]	15,293	11.7	**10.3**	★	★		★	★	★	★	★				
Children's, Boston	–	–	–	–	–	–	–	–	–	–	–	–	–	–	–
Dana-Farber Cancer Institute, Boston	65	30.8	***21.0***	✖	✖	–	–	–	–	–	–	–	–		–
Deaconess, Waltham	2,906	10.2	**9.2**	★	★		★		★			★			

Footnotes are on page 350.

Hospital outcomes: better (★) or worse (×) than average											Results of accreditation review on full survey		Other facts			
Adjusted Death rates			Adjusted Adverse outcome rates													
Surgical cases			Surgical cases													
All selected surgical cases	Coronary artery bypass surgery	Large bowel surgery	All selected surgical cases	Coronary artery bypass surgery	Large bowel surgery	Gall bladder removal	Total knee replacement	Total hip replacement	Simple prostatectomy	Carotid endarterectomy	Accreditation status*	Overall evaluation score (higher is better)	Number of beds	Major medical school affiliation?	Number of residents	Computerized drug order system (1 to 5 scale, higher is preferred; see page 23 for details)
2.3	3.8	6.5	7.7	10.3	11.9	7.5	6.7	6.4	5.4	8.2	–	91	161	–	–	–
	–			–		✖	✖	–	–		4	97	168	No	0	–
	–			–		–	–	–	–	✖	4	91	121	No	0	–
	–	–		–		–	–	–	–	–	5	95	60	No	0	–
–	–	–	–	–	–	–	–	–	–	–	4	86	45	No	0	–
	–			–					✖		5	97	155	No	0	–
	–		★	–	★	–		–	–	–	–[2]	–[2]	76	No	0	–
	–	–		–		–	–	–	–		4	96	140	No	0	–
★	–	–		–		–	–	–	–		4	85	64	No	0	–
	–	✖		–		★	✖		–		4	93	187	No	0	–
	–			–		×					4	93	133	No	2	–
				★	✖				×	★	4	82	300	No	0	–
	–	×		–						✖	4	89	199	No	0	–
	–	–		–		✖		–	–	–	5	98	100	No	0	–
	–	–		–		–		–	–	–	4	91	105	No	0	–
	–			–							4	95	287	No	0	–
–	–	–	–	–	–	–	–	–	–	–	–[2]	–[2]	–	–	–	–
	–	–	★	–			–	–	–	–	4	84	136	No	0	–
★				×	✖				★	★	4	92	541	Yes	384	–
×	–			–			✖			×	4	90	339	Yes	16	–
						–		–	–	–	5	90	337	Yes	621	–
★	★	★			★		✖	×	★		4	88	694	Yes	776	–
	–			–				–			5	95	206	Yes	0	–
	–			–	★	–	–	–	–	–	4	90	269	Yes	81	–
	–		★	–	★		★	–	–		4	82	289	Yes	14	–
	–			–				–			–[2]	–[2]	193	No	0	–
–	–	–		–	–	–	–	–	–	–	–[2]	–[2]	170	No	–	–
	–	★		–			✖	–	–	×	–[2]	–[2]	147	Yes	48	–
	–		✖	–		✖	✖	×	×	✖	4	93	790	No	0	–
–	–	–	–	–	–	–	–	–	–	–	4	94	324	–	522	–
–	–	–	–	–	–	–	–	–	–	–	4	95	30	Yes	0	5
	–			–				–		–	4	86	199	No	1	–

***Accreditation Status:** 5=Accredited with commendation or with full standards compliance; 4=Accredited with requirements for improvement; 3=Conditional accreditation.

Detailed Ratings for All Areas

See more information on "Key Ratings for Metro Areas" table beginning on page 32

Blue is most favorable
Bold Italic is least favorable
Blank means neither better nor worse than average
"–" means insufficient data

	Death rates for all selected case types				Hospital outcomes: better (★) or worse (×) than average — Adjusted Death rates — Medical Cases										
	Number of cases	Actual death rate (%)	Adjusted death rate (%) (lower is better)	All selected cases	All selected medical cases	Heart attack	Congestive heart failure	Obstructive pulmonary disease	Pneumonia	Respiratory failure and arrest	Septicemia	Stroke	Gastrointestinal hemorrhage	Fluid, electrolyte, & acid-base disorders	Kidney failure
National Average	–	–	12.1	12.1	14.8	21.2	10.6	6.5	16.9	34.4	25.1	18.4	6.7	11.0	20.9
Massachusetts *(continued)*															
Boston Area *(continued)*															
Deaconess - Glover, Needham	1,659	13.7	12.8			✖									
Deaconess - Nashoba, Ayer	1,268	12.0	11.1												
Emerson, West Concord	2,630	11.0	**10.6**	★	★							★			
Faulkner, Boston	2,842	12.0	**9.8**	★	★				★						★
Franciscan Children's, Boston	–	–	–	–	–	–	–	–	–	–	–	–	–	–	–
Hale, Haverhill	3,111	14.5	***14.9***	✖	✖			✖	✖			×			✖
Hallmark Health - Lawrence, Medford[1]	–	–	–	–	–	–	–	–	–	–	–	–	–	–	–
Hallmark Hlth - Melrose-Wakefield Campus, Melrose	3,017	10.8	**9.6**	★	★		★		★					★	
Holy Family, Methuen	4,131	12.9	12.8		×	×	★		×			✖		✖	
Jordan, Plymouth	3,474	13.0	***13.9***	✖	✖		✖	✖	✖						
Lahey Clinic, Burlington	6,453	8.0	**10.5**	★	★	★	★				★	★		✖	
Lahey Clinic Northshore, Peabody	–	–	–	–	–	–	–	–	–	–	–	–	–	–	–
Lawrence F Quigley, Chelsea[1]	193	9.8	9.7			–	–	–		–	–	–	–	–	–
Lawrence General, Lawrence	4,141	12.3	12.5									×		★	
Lemuel Shattuck, Jamaica Plain	–	–	–	–	–	–	–	–	–	–	–	–	–	–	–
Lowell General, Lowell	2,748	13.7	***13.6***	✖	✖				✖		×				
Marlborough Hospital, Marlborough	1,912	13.6	11.7					★							
Massachusetts General, Boston	10,542	8.7	**10.1**	★	★	★	★				×	★			★
Metrowest, Natick[1]	–	–	–	–	–	–	–	–	–	–	–	–	–	–	–
Metrowest, Framingham	6,271	13.1	12.3												✖
Milton Hospital, Milton	3,012	12.0	13.0		×			✖		×					
Morton, Taunton	3,465	13.2	***14.1***	✖	✖		✖		✖		×				
Mt Auburn, Cambridge	5,086	11.8	11.8			★									
New England Baptist, Boston	3,003	5.4	**8.6**	★	★				★	–		★			
New England Medical Center, Boston[1]	2,620	8.4	**9.5**	★	★	★		★					★		
Newton - Wellesley, Newton Lower Falls	4,126	12.2	**9.2**	★	★		★		★		★	★	★	★	
North Shore Children's, Salem	–	–	–	–	–	–	–	–	–	–	–	–	–	–	–
Quincy Medical Center, Quincy	4,155	14.7	***13.3***	✖	✖					✖	✖			✖	
St Anne's, Fall River[1]	2,871	11.6	**10.5**	★	★		★		★				★		
St Elizabeth's, Brighton	4,957	11.5	**9.8**	★	★	★	★		★				★		★
St Luke's, New Bedford	–	–	–	–	–	–	–	–	–	–	–	–	–	–	–
Saints, Lowell	4,407	14.2	***14.3***	✖	✖		✖		✖		✖	×			×
Salem Hospital, Salem[1]	5,190	11.1	12.5			✖									
Somerville Hospital, Somerville	–	–	–	–	–	–	–	–	–	–	–	–	–	–	–

Footnotes are on page 350.

Hospital outcomes: better (★) or worse (×) than average											Results of accreditation review on full survey		Other facts			
Adjusted Death rates			Adjusted Adverse outcome rates													
Surgical cases			Surgical cases													
All selected surgical cases	Coronary artery bypass surgery	Large bowel surgery	All selected surgical cases	Coronary artery bypass surgery	Large bowel surgery	Gall bladder removal	Total knee replacement	Total hip replacement	Simple prostatectomy	Carotid endarterectomy	Accreditation status*	Overall evaluation score (higher is better)	Number of beds	Major medical school affiliation?	Number of residents	Computerized drug order system (1 to 5 scale, higher is preferred; see page 23 for details)
2.3	3.8	6.5	7.7	10.3	11.9	7.5	6.7	6.4	5.4	8.2	–	91	161	–	–	–
	–	–	★	–	★	–	–	–	–	–	4	93	41	No	0	–
–	–	–		–		–	–	–	–	–	4	93	41	No	3	–
★	–			–					–	–	4	91	172	No	4	–
	–		★	–		★		–		–	4	92	125	No	5	–
–	–	–	–	–	–	–	–	–	–	–	4	91	–	–	–	–
	–	–		–		–		–	–	–	4	93	108	No	0	–
–	–	–	–	–	–	–	–	–	–	–	4	90	–	–	–	–
	–			–		–	–	–	–	✖	4	97	190	No	–	–
	–			–		–		–	✖		4	93	228	No	0	–
	–			–				–	×	–	4	94	94	No	0	–
★	★			★	✖		✖				4	88	234	No	114	–
–	–	–	–	–	–	–	–	–	–	–	–[2]	–[2]	–	–	–	–
–	–	–	–	–	–	–	–	–	–	–	–[2]	–[2]	159	No	8	–
	–			–		★	✖	–	–		4	83	189	Yes	0	–
–	–	–	–	–	–	–	–	–	–	–	4	88	230	–	0	–
	–	✖		–	✖	–	★	–	–		4	94	210	No	0	–
	–	–		–		–		–	–	–	4	89	66	No	0	–
★	★						×			✖	4	92	853	Yes	1,095	–
–	–	–	–	–	–	–	–	–	–	–	–[2]	–[2]	–	–	–	–
	–			–				✖			4	92	381	No	35	–
	–			–				–		–	4	96	88	No	0	–
	–			–			✖	–	✖	–	4	97	131	No	0	–
★	★					×				–	3	94	172	Yes	50	–
★	–	★	×	–		–	×	✖	–	–	4	94	130	No	0	–
					✖	–			–		4	96	323	Yes	329	–
	–			–	★			–	–	–	5	93	228	Yes	27	–
–	–	–	–	–	–	–	–	–	–	–	–[2]	–[2]	–	–	–	–
	–			–				–	×	–	4	96	134	No	0	–
	–			–		–	–	–	–	–	–[2]	–[2]	139	No	0	–
★	★			★		–	✖	–		–	–[2]	–[2]	225	Yes	158	–
–	–	–	–	–	–	–	–	–	–	–	4	90	–	–	–	–
	–			–		★				✖	4	92	150	No	0	–
	–			–	✖	★					4	89	228	No	14	–
–	–	–	–	–	–	–	–	–	–	–	–[2]	–[2]	–	–	–	–

***Accreditation Status:** 5=Accredited with commendation or with full standards compliance; 4=Accredited with requirements for improvement; 3=Conditional accreditation.

Detailed Ratings for All Areas

See more information on "Key Ratings for Metro Areas" table beginning on page 32

Blue is most favorable
Bold Italic is least favorable
Blank means neither better nor worse than average
"–" means insufficient data

	Death rates for all selected case types				Hospital outcomes: better (★) or worse (×) than average — Adjusted Death rates — Medical Cases										
	Number of cases	Actual death rate (%)	Adjusted death rate (%) (lower is better)	All selected cases	All selected medical cases	Heart attack	Congestive heart failure	Obstructive pulmonary disease	Pneumonia	Respiratory failure and arrest	Septicemia	Stroke	Gastrointestinal hemorrhage	Fluid, electrolyte, & acid-base disorders	Kidney failure
National Average	–	–	12.1	12.1	14.8	21.2	10.6	6.5	16.9	34.4	25.1	18.4	6.7	11.0	20.9
Massachusetts *(continued)*															
Boston Area *(continued)*															
South Shore, South Weymouth	6,840	13.2	12.1						×	✖					**★**
Sturdy, Attleboro	2,653	14.7	***14.3***	✖	✖		✖	✖	✖				✖		
Tobey - Southcoast, Wareham	–	–	–	–	–	–	–	–	–	–	–	–	–	–	–
Union, Lynn	4,100	13.4	***13.1***	✖	✖				✖						
Whidden, Everett	–	–	–	–	–	–	–	–	–	–	–	–	–	–	–
Winchester Hospital, Winchester	3,641	11.8	**10.8**	**★**	★					★		**★**			
Other Areas															
Athol Memorial, Athol	965	14.2	13.0							×	–		–		–
Baystate, Springfield	8,622	12.7	12.6	×	×		✖	✖							
Berkshire, Pittsfield	5,689	12.7	***13.3***	✖	✖		✖	✖	×					✖	✖
Cape Cod, Hyannis	9,078	10.6	11.4	★							**★**	**★**	✖		
Clinton Hospital, Clinton[1]	709	15.0	12.6			✖		–		–		–	–	×	
Cooley Dickinson, Northampton	3,939	11.9	***13.4***	✖	✖				✖	✖			✖		
Fairview, Great Barrington	940	12.6	11.6					–		**★**					✖
Falmouth Hospital, Falmouth	3,210	10.4	11.3					✖			★				
Franklin, Greenfield	2,651	13.5	***13.3***	✖	✖	✖	✖							★	
Harrington, Southbridge	1,761	13.1	12.7				✖								
Health Alliance, Leominster	2,021	15.9	***14.7***	✖	✖		×	✖	×			✖			✖
Heywood, Gardner	1,788	13.1	10.8	★											
Holyoke Hospital, Holyoke	4,347	14.0	***13.8***	✖	✖		✖		✖				✖	×	
Hubbard Regional, Webster	914	17.4	***14.6***	✖	✖		×	✖	×						
Martha's Vineyard, Oak Bluffs	562	10.1	12.1					–		–	–		–		–
Mary Lane, Ware[1]	762	15.5	***14.3***	✖	✖			✖					–	–	×
Mercy, Springfield	5,464	15.3	***13.6***	✖	✖		×		×	✖			×	✖	
Milford - Whitinsville Regional, Milford	2,879	13.2	11.0	★	★			**★**						**★**	
Nantucket Cottage, Nantucket	245	14.7	15.5	×	×	–		–		–	–	–	–	–	–
Noble, Westfield	1,735	14.3	13.1												
North Adams Regional, North Adams	2,528	10.7	11.9			**★**									
St Vincent, Worcester	7,290	12.8	***13.1***	✖	✖		×		✖		✖				
Soldiers' Home, Holyoke	113	23.9	***26.3***	✖	✖	–	–	–	✖	–	–	–	–	–	–
University of Massachusetts, Worcester	5,842	11.1	**11.1**	**★**	**★**			**★**						**★**	
Wing, Palmer	1,251	11.1	12.8						×						

Footnotes are on page 350.

Hospital outcomes: better (★) or worse (×) than average											Results of accreditation review on full survey		Other facts			
Adjusted Death rates			Adjusted Adverse outcome rates													
Surgical cases			Surgical cases													
All selected surgical cases	Coronary artery bypass surgery	Large bowel surgery	All selected surgical cases	Coronary artery bypass surgery	Large bowel surgery	Gall bladder removal	Total knee replacement	Total hip replacement	Simple prostatectomy	Carotid endarterectomy	Accreditation status*	Overall evaluation score (higher is better)	Number of beds	Major medical school affiliation?	Number of residents	Computerized drug order system (1 to 5 scale, higher is preferred; see page 23 for details)
2.3	3.8	6.5	7.7	10.3	11.9	7.5	6.7	6.4	5.4	8.2	–	91	161	–	–	–
★	–	★	★	–						–	4	97	219	No	0	–
	–		★	–	★		×	–	–	–	5	94	124	No	0	–
–	–	–	–	–	–	–	–	–	–	–	4	95	–	–	–	–
	–			–			★	–	×		4	85	189	No	4	–
–	–	–	–	–	–	–	–	–	–	–	4	93	–	–	–	–
★	–	★		–		–	×		–	✖	4	90	161	No	3	–
–	–	–	–	–	–	–	–	–	–	–	4	90	30	No	0	–
		✖	×		✖						5	94	564	Yes	256	–
	–			–			★		–		4	92	290	No	34	–
★	–		★	–			★		★		4	91	214	Yes	3	–
–	–	–	–	–	–	–	–	–	–	–	4	91	44	No	0	–
	–			–						–	4	81	125	No	0	–
–	–	–		–		–	–	–	–	–	–[2]	–[2]	25	No	0	–
	–	★		–	★	–	✖	–	–	–	4	90	83	No	0	–
	–			–		–		–	–	–	4	87	85	No	0	–
–	–	–		–	–	–	–	–	–	–	4	90	113	No	0	–
	–			–		–	★	–	–	–	4	88	173	No	0	–
–	–	–	★	–	★	–	–	–	–	–	4	92	126	No	0	–
	–			–		✖		–			4	88	103	No	0	–
–	–	–	–	–	–	–	–	–	–	–	4	85	26	No	0	–
–	–	–	–	–	–	–	–	–	–	–	4	90	21	No	0	–
–	–	–	–	–	–	–	–	–	–	–	–[2]	–[2]	31	No	0	–
	–			–						×	4	85	311	No	0	–
	–			–			–	–	–	–	4	92	108	Yes	0	–
–	–	–	–	–	–	–	–	–	–	–	4	84	19	No	0	–
	–	–		–		–	–	–	–	✖	4	90	97	No	0	–
	–			–			★	✖	–	–	4	93	69	No	0	–
				★							4	92	369	Yes	10	–
–	–	–	–	–	–	–	–	–	–	–	4	95	27	No	0	–
			✖			✖	✖				4	92	325	Yes	–	–
–	–	–	★	–	–	–	–	–	–	–	4	95	43	No	1	–

***Accreditation Status:** 5=Accredited with commendation or with full standards compliance; 4=Accredited with requirements for improvement; 3=Conditional accreditation.

Detailed Ratings for All Areas

See more information on "Key Ratings for Metro Areas" table beginning on page 32

Blue is most favorable
Bold Italic is least favorable
Blank means neither better nor worse than average
"–" means insufficient data

	Death rates for all selected case types			Hospital outcomes: better (★) or worse (×) than average — Adjusted Death rates	Medical Cases										
	Number of cases	Actual death rate (%)	Adjusted death rate (%) (lower is better)	All selected cases	All selected medical cases	Heart attack	Congestive heart failure	Obstructive pulmonary disease	Pneumonia	Respiratory failure and arrest	Septicemia	Stroke	Gastrointestinal hemorrhage	Fluid, electrolyte, & acid-base disorders	Kidney failure
National Average	–	–	12.1	12.1	14.8	21.2	10.6	6.5	16.9	34.4	25.1	18.4	6.7	11.0	20.9
Michigan															
Greater Detroit Area															
Bi-County, Warren	4,295	15.8	12.1			✖	★								
Bon Secours, Grosse Pointe[1]	6,869	9.5	**10.9**	★	★							★			★
Botsford General, Farmington	6,759	16.2	12.3			✖	★		★	✖		✖		×	
Chelsea Community, Chelsea	1,079	13.9	***14.4***	✖	✖		×		✖	–		✖	–		
Children's, Detroit	–	–	–	–	–	–	–	–	–	–	–	–	–	–	–
Cottage, Grosse Pointe Farms[1]	802	13.1	12.1										–	–	
Crittenton, Columbus	4,713	9.1	**10.0**	★	★				★			★			
Detroit Receiving, Detroit	3,091	15.5	**10.6**	★	★	★	★		**★**					**★**	
Garden City Osteopathic, Garden City	6,172	14.9	11.6			✖	★		**★**		★	✖		×	
Harper University, Detroit	5,269	7.2	**9.9**	★	★	★	★		**★**		★	★			★
Henry Ford, Detroit[1]	11,749	11.7	**9.4**	★	★		★		★	★		★		★	★
Henry Ford, Wyandotte	7,245	10.7	11.4			×	★					**★**			
Huron Valley - Sinai, Commerce	3,489	12.8	12.4						✖						
Hutzel, Detroit	–	–	–	–	–	–	–	–	–	–	–	–	–	–	–
Madison Community, Madison Heights	408	7.1	**8.5**	★	★	–		**★**		–	–	–	–	–	–
Mt Clemens General, Mt Clemens	5,349	13.0	***14.8***	✖	✖		✖	✖	✖			✖	✖	✖	
North Oakland, Pontiac	2,671	11.2	11.2			×	★	★						×	**★**
Oakwood, Dearborn	13,580	11.4	**10.7**	★	★	★	**★**		★						★
Oakwood Annapolis, Wayne	4,233	14.2	11.7			✖	**★**								
Oakwood Heritage, Taylor	3,494	17.1	***15.0***	✖	✖		✖	×	✖	✖	✖				
Oakwood Seaway, Trenton	1,982	17.0	***13.6***	✖	✖	✖		×						✖	
POH, Pontiac	2,267	13.3	11.3						**★**						×
Providence, Southfield	9,084	9.7	**11.1**	★	★			×	★	**★**		★			
Riverside Osteopathic, Trenton	2,946	12.7	13.2	×	×						✖				
St John, Detroit	10,884	10.9	**11.0**	★	★	★	★					★		✖	
St John Detroit Riverview, Detroit	4,288	12.7	**9.1**	★	★		★	★	★		★	★			★
St John Macomb, Warren	7,692	13.3	**10.8**	★	★		**★**	**★**	**★**	★		★			
St John Northeast, Detroit	2,730	12.8	11.6												
St John Oakland, Madison Heights[1]	3,179	14.4	11.6												
St Joseph Mercy, Ann Arbor[1]	10,046	10.6	***13.1***	✖	✖			✖			✖	×			
St Joseph Mercy Oakland, Pontiac	7,179	11.3	11.9			★				**★**				✖	
St Joseph's Mercy - East, Mt Clemens	–	–	–	–	–	–	–	–	–	–	–	–	–	–	–
St Joseph's Mercy of Macomb, Clinton Township[1]	7,471	12.7	**11.2**	★	★		**★**					★			
St Mary Mercy, Livonia	7,391	13.0	12.1					★						✖	

Footnotes are on page 350.

Hospital outcomes: better (★) or worse (×) than average											Results of accreditation review on full survey		Other facts			
Adjusted Death rates			Adjusted Adverse outcome rates													
Surgical cases			Surgical cases													
All selected surgical cases	Coronary artery bypass surgery	Large bowel surgery	All selected surgical cases	Coronary artery bypass surgery	Large bowel surgery	Gall bladder removal	Total knee replacement	Total hip replacement	Simple prostatectomy	Carotid endarterectomy	Accreditation status*	Overall evaluation score (higher is better)	Number of beds	Major medical school affiliation?	Number of residents	Computerized drug order system (1 to 5 scale, higher is preferred; see page 23 for details)
2.3	3.8	6.5	7.7	10.3	11.9	7.5	6.7	6.4	5.4	8.2	–	91	161	–	–	–
	–			–		–			–		–[2]	–[2]	164	Yes	86	–
★	–	★		–			★			✖	4	84	237	No	69	–
	–			–					–		–[2]	–[2]	325	Yes	149	–
–	–	–		–	–	–	–	–	–	–	4	97	97	No	0	–
–	–	–	–	–	–	–	–	–	–	–	4	96	218	–	0	–
–	–	–		–	–	–	–	–	–	–	–[2]	–[2]	65	No	0	–
★	–		★	–			★	★			–[2]	–[2]	227	No	8	–
✖	–	✖	✖	–	✖	–	–	–	–	–	5	98	258	Yes	0	–
	–			–			★	★	–		–[2]	–[2]	270	Yes	85	–
			✖	✖		–	–	–		✖	4	92	542	Yes	0	–
			✖		✖			✖			–[2]	–[2]	668	Yes	592	–
	–			–				★		✖	4	87	355	No	0	–
	–			–		–			–		5	98	136	No	0	–
–	–	–	–	–	–	–	–	–	–	–	–[2]	–[2]	–	–	–	–
–	–	–	–	–	–	–	–	–	–	–	3	79	50	No	0	–
								–	–	✖	–[2]	–[2]	242	Yes	83	–
	–			–			–	–	–	–	4	86	220	No	41	–
★	★	★	✖	✖	★	✖	✖			✖	4	91	585	Yes	114	4
	–	×		–			–	–		–	4	88	183	No	0	–
	–	–		–		–	–	–	–	✖	4	81	257	No	0	–
	–	–		–		–	–	–	–		4	92	82	No	0	–
	–			–		–	–	–	–	–	–[2]	–[2]	130	Yes	102	–
★		★	★		★		★	✖			4	86	379	No	144	–
	–		★	–			★		–		–[2]	–[2]	138	No	30	–
	★	×	✖		✖			✖		✖	4	95	656	Yes	183	–
	–			–		–	–	–	–	–	4	87	230	No	9	–
	–			–					×		4	87	274	No	0	–
	–	–	✖	–	✖	–	–	–	–	–	4	89	222	No	0	–
×	–			–			–	–	–	–	4	88	196	Yes	76	–
	×			✖							4	97	467	Yes	88	–
			✖			✖	✖				4	95	428	No	85	–
–	–	–	–	–	–	–	–	–	–	–	–[2]	–[2]	–	–	–	–
	–			–		×	★	★			4	83	462	No	0	–
	–			–			×				4	96	263	No	0	–

***Accreditation Status:** 5=Accredited with commendation or with full standards compliance; 4=Accredited with requirements for improvement; 3=Conditional accreditation.

Detailed Ratings for All Areas

See more information on "Key Ratings for Metro Areas" table beginning on page 32

Blue is most favorable
Bold Italic is least favorable
Blank means neither better nor worse than average
"–" means insufficient data

	Death rates for all selected case types			Hospital outcomes: better (★) or worse (×) than average — Adjusted Death rates — Medical Cases											
	Number of cases	Actual death rate (%)	Adjusted death rate (%) (lower is better)	All selected cases	All selected medical cases	Heart attack	Congestive heart failure	Obstructive pulmonary disease	Pneumonia	Respiratory failure and arrest	Septicemia	Stroke	Gastrointestinal hemorrhage	Fluid, electrolyte, & acid-base disorders	Kidney failure
National Average	–	–	12.1	12.1	14.8	21.2	10.6	6.5	16.9	34.4	25.1	18.4	6.7	11.0	20.9
Michigan *(continued)*															
Greater Detroit Area *(continued)*															
Saline Community, Saline	894	10.7	12.1										–	✖	–
Sinai - Grace, Detroit	7,474	12.3	**10.1**	**★**	**★**		**★**	★	**★**			**★**			**★**
University of Michigan, Ann Arbor	4,504	11.3	12.2										**★**	✖	
William Beaumont, Royal Oak	20,475	10.9	**10.1**	**★**	**★**	**★**	**★**	**★**	**★**		**★**		**★**	**★**	**★**
William Beaumont, Troy	6,468	10.5	**10.5**	**★**	**★**			×	**★**		**★**	★			★
Other Areas															
Allegan General, Allegan	1,029	11.1	13.2			–					–	×			–
Alpena General, Alpena	3,270	10.9	12.7												
Battle Creek Health System, Battle Creek	6,077	13.2	***13.3***	✖	✖	✖	✖	✖	×		**★**	×			
Bay Medical Center, Bay City	6,884	9.5	11.9					★							
Bell, Ishpeming	809	11.1	13.3					–		–	–		–	–	–
Bixby, Adrian	2,021	13.4	***14.5***	✖	✖		✖							×	–
Borgess, Kalamazoo	8,734	11.7	***13.6***	✖	✖		✖	✖	✖					✖	
Borgess - Lee, Dowagiac	921	11.2	12.0									**★**	–	–	–
Bronson Methodist, Kalamazoo	5,211	11.5	***13.2***	✖	✖				✖						
Caro Community, Caro	427	15.2	14.8	×			×	–		–	–		–		–
Carson City Hospital, Carson City	814	14.0	***15.5***	✖	✖		✖			–			–	–	–
Central Michigan, Mt Pleasant[1]	1,749	9.4	13.4							–					–
Charlevoix Area, Charlevoix	799	9.9	14.1			–	✖	–		–	–		–		–
Chippewa County War Memorial, Sault Sainte Marie	1,053	11.2	12.0			×				–			–		–
Clinton, St Johns	526	13.7	***17.3***	✖	✖	–	✖	–		–	–	×	–	–	–
Community, Cheboygan	1,428	11.9	12.0											★	–
Community, Watervliet	1,198	9.1	10.7					★		–			–		
Community of Branch County, Coldwater	1,907	12.2	13.2		✖	×	×	×						★	
Covenant, Saginaw	7,674	9.9	**10.9**	**★**	**★**	★					**★**				
Deckerville Community, Deckerville	190	10.5	10.4			–	–	–		–	–	–	–	–	–
Dickinson County, Iron Mountain[1]	2,267	10.9	10.8	★	★				**★**					★	✖
Doctors, Jackson	1,120	11.2	13.9	×						×			–		–
Eaton Rapids Medical Center, Eaton Rapids	403	12.2	12.7				✖	–		–	–		–	–	–
Gerber, Fremont[1]	1,400	12.9	12.5					✖						**★**	
Grand View, Ironwood	1,469	11.3	11.8					✖							–
Gratiot, Alma	2,451	12.4	11.6							×				×	
Hackley, Muskegon[1]	3,996	12.0	***14.0***	✖	✖		✖		×			✖			

Footnotes are on page 350.

Hospital outcomes: better (★) or worse (×) than average											Results of accreditation review on full survey		Other facts			
Adjusted Death rates			Adjusted Adverse outcome rates													
Surgical cases			Surgical cases													
All selected surgical cases	Coronary artery bypass surgery	Large bowel surgery	All selected surgical cases	Coronary artery bypass surgery	Large bowel surgery	Gall bladder removal	Total knee replacement	Total hip replacement	Simple prostatectomy	Carotid endarterectomy	Accreditation status*	Overall evaluation score (higher is better)	Number of beds	Major medical school affiliation?	Number of residents	Computerized drug order system (1 to 5 scale, higher is preferred; see page 23 for details)
2.3	3.8	6.5	7.7	10.3	11.9	7.5	6.7	6.4	5.4	8.2	–	91	161	–	–	–
–	–	–	–	–	–	–	–	–	–	–	4	**97**	39	No	0	–
✖	✖	✖	✖	✖	✖	★		–	✖		4	92	477	**Yes**	0	–
			✖	×	×				–		4	**95**	726	**Yes**	737	–
★			×			★	✖			✖	4	**96**	899	**Yes**	316	–
	–		✖	–			✖				4	92	189	No	18	–
	–			–		–			–	–	4	**87**	63	No	0	–
	–			–		×				★	4	90	121	No	0	–
	–			–					–		4	**99**	256	No	0	–
	–						★	★		✖	4	**94**	332	No	11	–
–	–	–	★	–		–	–	–	–	–	4	**87**	30	No	1	–
	–	–		–				–	–	–	4	**87**	77	No	0	–
	★				✖					★	4	90	383	No	0	–
–	–	–		–	–	–	–	–	–	–	4	**88**	40	No	0	–
						★			★		4	**96**	307	**Yes**	0	–
–	–	–	–	–	–	–	–	–	–	–	–[2]	–[2]	18	No	0	–
–	–	–		–		–	–	–	–	–	–[2]	–[2]	63	**Yes**	8	–
	–	–	★	–	–	–	★	–			4	**97**	118	No	0	–
–	–	–		–	–	–	–	–	–	–	4	89	33	No	0	–
–	–	–	★	–	–	–	–	–	–	–	3	**88**	35	No	0	–
–	–	–	★	–	–	–	–	–	–	–	4	91	28	No	0	–
	–	–		–		×	–	–	–	–	4	90	42	No	0	–
–	–	–	★	–	–	–	–	–	–	–	4	**87**	56	No	0	–
★	–	–		–		–		–	–	–	–[2]	–[2]	88	No	7	–
				✖			★	★		✖	–[2]	–[2]	412	No	–	–
–	–	–	–	–	–	–	–	–	–	–	4	90	17	No	0	–
	–		★	–			★	–	–	–	4	90	96	No	0	–
–	–	–		–	–	–	–	–	–	–	–[2]	–[2]	65	No	0	–
–	–	–	–	–	–	–	–	–	–	–	4	91	21	No	0	–
	–	–	★	–	★	–	★	–	–	–	4	89	73	No	0	–
	–	–		–		–	–	–	★	–	4	**94**	54	No	0	–
	–			–				–	✖		4	92	127	No	3	–
	–		★	–			★			★	4	91	181	No	0	–

***Accreditation Status:** 5=Accredited with commendation or with full standards compliance; 4=Accredited with requirements for improvement; 3=Conditional accreditation.

Detailed Ratings for All Areas

See more information on "Key Ratings for Metro Areas" table beginning on page 32

Blue is most favorable
Bold Italic is least favorable
Blank means neither better nor worse than average
"–" means insufficient data

	Death rates for all selected case types			Hospital outcomes: better (★) or worse (×) than average – Adjusted Death rates	Medical Cases										
	Number of cases	Actual death rate (%)	Adjusted death rate (%) (lower is better)	All selected cases	All selected medical cases	Heart attack	Congestive heart failure	Obstructive pulmonary disease	Pneumonia	Respiratory failure and arrest	Septicemia	Stroke	Gastrointestinal hemorrhage	Fluid, electrolyte, & acid-base disorders	Kidney failure
National Average	–	–	12.1	12.1	14.8	21.2	10.6	6.5	16.9	34.4	25.1	18.4	6.7	11.0	20.9
Michigan *(continued)*															
Other Areas *(continued)*															
Harbor Beach Community, Harbor Beach	346	8.4	11.6			–		–		–	–	–	–	–	–
Hayes Green Beach, Charlotte	635	14.3	14.3	×	×		×			–			–	–	–
Herrick, Tecumseh	1,069	10.4	12.3										–		–
Hills and Dales General, Cass City	670	13.3	***17.8***	✖	✖	–	✖	✖		–	–		–	–	–
Hillsdale Community, Hillsdale	1,466	9.2	11.1						**★**					–	
Holland Community, Holland	3,099	12.6	***14.5***	✖	✖		✖		✖			✖			
Hurley, Flint	3,900	13.4	12.0			✖									
Huron, Bad Axe	1,009	8.3	***14.7***	✖	✖	✖		–		–	–	✖	–		–
Ingham Regional, Lansing	6,750	9.4	11.2	★		★		★			**★**			✖	
Ionia County, Ionia[1]	712	11.8	14.2	×	×			–		–	–	✖	–	–	–
Iron County, Iron River	1,209	11.7	12.4				✖	**★**		–			★		✖
Kelsey, Lakeview	352	10.8	10.7					–		–	–		–	–	–
Keweenaw, Laurium	970	13.1	13.0							–					×
Lakeland, St Joseph	6,533	11.8	12.6			**★**			✖			✖		✖	
Lakeshore, Shelby	445	10.3	13.0			★		–		–	–	–	–	–	–
Lakeview, Paw Paw	945	10.6	10.9								★				–
Lapeer Regional, Lapeer	3,025	10.8	**10.4**	**★**	**★**				**★**		★	★			★
Marlette Community, Marlette	667	11.2	13.8			✖		–		–			–	–	–
Marquette General, Marquette[1]	3,737	7.9	11.7												
McKenzie, Sandusky	581	13.4	***15.5***	✖	✖		✖	–		–	–		–		–
McLaren Regional, Flint	10,393	11.2	**11.1**	**★**	**★**			**★**	**★**		**★**				
McPherson, Howell	1,744	16.3	13.3	×	×	×					✖			✖	★
Mecosta County General, Big Rapids	1,184	12.6	***15.8***	✖	✖	×	✖		×	–		✖		–	–
Memorial, Owosso	2,460	12.7	***16.1***	✖	✖	✖		✖	✖		×	×	✖		
Memorial of West Michigan, Ludington	1,965	9.5	**9.8**	**★**	**★**			★			★		**★**		
Mercy, Cadillac	2,248	11.1	12.9												
Mercy, Grayling[1]	1,787	10.1	11.8												–
Mercy, Monroe	4,068	10.6	13.0	×	✖		×								
Mercy, Port Huron	3,361	12.2	13.1	×	✖		✖							✖	
Mercy General, Muskegon	5,136	10.2	12.4												
Metropolitian, Grand Rapids	3,261	15.3	***13.2***	✖	✖						×				
MidMichigan, Clare	1,540	11.1	13.1			✖	✖							–	
MidMichigan, Gladwin	1,063	9.8	11.0			–				–			–	–	–
MidMichigan, Midland	4,957	9.9	11.0	★	★				★		**★**	✖			

Footnotes are on page 350.

Hospital outcomes: better (★) or worse (✕) than average											Results of accreditation review on full survey		Other facts			
Adjusted Death rates			Adjusted Adverse outcome rates													
Surgical cases			Surgical cases													
All selected surgical cases	Coronary artery bypass surgery	Large bowel surgery	All selected surgical cases	Coronary artery bypass surgery	Large bowel surgery	Gall bladder removal	Total knee replacement	Total hip replacement	Simple prostatectomy	Carotid endarterectomy	Accreditation status*	Overall evaluation score (higher is better)	Number of beds	Major medical school affiliation?	Number of residents	Computerized drug order system (1 to 5 scale, higher is preferred; see page 23 for details)
2.3	3.8	6.5	7.7	10.3	11.9	7.5	6.7	6.4	5.4	8.2	–	91	161	–	–	–
–	–	–	–	–	–	–	–	–	–	–	–[2]	–[2]	21	No	0	–
–	–	–	–	–	–	–	–	–	–	–	4	90	35	No	0	–
–	–	–		–	–	–		–	–	–	4	89	63	No	0	–
✖	–	–		–		–	–	–	–	–	4	94	47	No	0	–
	–	–		–		✖	✖	–	–	–	3	81	52	No	0	–
	–			–						–	–[2]	–[2]	155	No	0	–
	–			–			–	–	–	–	4	92	463	Yes	81	–
	–	–		–				–	–	–	4	83	64	No	0	–
				★	✕				–		4	90	332	No	107	–
–	–	–		–	–	–	–	–	–	–	4	96	51	No	0	–
–	–	–	★	–	–	★	–	–	–	–	4	90	18	No	0	–
–	–	–	–	–	–	–	–	–	–	–	4	87	52	No	–	–
–	–	–	★	–		–	–	–	–	–	4	89	49	No	0	–
											4	88	167	No	0	–
–	–	–	–	–	–	–	–	–	–	–	4	94	24	No	0	–
–	–	–	★	–		–	–	–	–	–	–[2]	–[2]	48	No	0	–
	–			–			★	✕	–	–	4	88	144	No	0	–
–	–	–		–	–	–	–	–	–	–	4	92	48	No	0	–
									★		4	86	282	No	18	–
–	–	–	–	–	–	–	–	–	–	–	–[2]	–[2]	25	No	0	–
			✕			✖					4	88	436	Yes	63	–
–	–	–		–	–	–		–	–	–	4	99	45	No	0	–
–	–	–		–	–	–	✕	–	–	–	4	95	50	No	0	–
	–			–			★	–	–		4	92	114	No	0	–
★	–		★	–			★	–	–		–[2]	–[2]	85	No	0	–
	–	–		–				–	–	–	4	95	89	No	0	–
	–	–		–		–		–		–	4	92	34	No	0	–
	–			–			★			✖	4	92	173	No	0	–
	–			–					–		4	91	119	No	0	–
✖	✖		✖	✖			★	✖			4	89	191	No	20	–
	–		★	–				–	★		–[2]	–[2]	214	Yes	57	–
–	–	–		–		–	–	–	–	–	4	94	64	No	0	–
–	–	–	–	–	–	–	–	–	–	–	4	93	42	No	0	–
	–			–				★			4	95	250	No	18	–

***Accreditation Status:** 5=Accredited with commendation or with full standards compliance; 4=Accredited with requirements for improvement; 3=Conditional accreditation.

Detailed Ratings for All Areas

See more information on "Key Ratings for Metro Areas" table beginning on page 32

Blue is most favorable
Bold Italic is least favorable
Blank means neither better nor worse than average
"–" means insufficient data

	Death rates for all selected case types			Hospital outcomes: better (★) or worse (×) than average — Adjusted Death rates											
					Medical Cases										
	Number of cases	Actual death rate (%)	Adjusted death rate (%) (lower is better)	All selected cases	All selected medical cases	Heart attack	Congestive heart failure	Obstructive pulmonary disease	Pneumonia	Respiratory failure and arrest	Septicemia	Stroke	Gastrointestinal hemorrhage	Fluid, electrolyte, & acid-base disorders	Kidney failure
National Average	–	–	12.1	12.1	14.8	21.2	10.6	6.5	16.9	34.4	25.1	18.4	6.7	11.0	20.9
Michigan *(continued)*															
Other Areas *(continued)*															
Munising Memorial, Munising	270	15.2	***16.5***	✖	✖	–	–	–		–	–	×	–	–	–
Munson, Traverse City	8,327	8.6	**10.6**	★	★	★							★	★	
North Ottawa, Grand Haven	1,470	13.1	***16.5***	✖	✖		×		✖	–		✖	–		
Northern Michigan Regional, Petoskey[1]	3,962	7.9	11.7												✖
Oaklawn, Marshall	956	14.5	***16.2***	✖	✖			–	✖	✖	–	×	–	–	–
OSF - St Francis, Escanaba	1,566	11.6	12.7				★			✖					–
Otsego, Gaylord	921	10.3	11.0					–					–		–
Pennock, Hastings	1,873	10.4	11.3							✖	★				–
Port Huron Hospital, Port Huron	4,302	12.6	***14.6***	✖	✖		✖		✖			✖		✖	
Portage, Hancock[1]	906	12.7	12.1					–		–	–			–	
St John River District, East China	1,393	13.1	***13.9***	✖	✖	✖	✖			×		×			–
St Joseph, Tawas City[1]	1,442	12.1	***16.9***	✖	✖		✖		✖	–	–	✖			✖
St Mary's, Saginaw	6,572	9.7	12.0												
St Mary's Mercy, Grand Rapids	5,171	13.3	11.5												
Scheurer, Pigeon[1]	490	10.2	13.3			–		–		–	–		–	–	–
Schoolcraft, Manistique	308	15.6	***17.2***	✖	✖	–	✖	–		✖	–	–	–	–	–
Sheridan Community, Sheridan	207	8.2	10.3			–	–	–		–	–	–	–	–	–
South Haven Community, South Haven	660	18.6	***18.8***	✖	✖		✖	✖			✖	×	–	–	
Sparrow, Lansing	6,030	11.8	***13.7***	✖	✖		×			✖		✖	✖		
Spectrum Health, Grand Rapids	9,367	10.3	**10.8**	★	★	★				×					
Spectrum Health, Reed City	807	9.9	10.9			×							–		–
Spectrum Health Blodgett Campus, Grand Rapids	6,932	10.1	12.6		✖				✖	✖	★				
Sturgis Hospital, Sturgis	1,354	13.2	***14.2***	✖	✖	✖	✖	×			★				
Three Rivers Area, Three Rivers	959	17.0	***17.1***	✖	✖		✖		✖		×	✖			–
Trillium, Albion	645	10.2	11.9					–			–		–		–
United, Greenville[1]	1,547	11.3	12.2								×				×
W A Foote, Jackson	6,490	10.9	11.8							★					
West Branch Regional, West Branch	2,064	9.2	12.8			✖									–
West Shore, Manistee	1,284	11.6	***13.9***	✖	×			–		–					✖
Zeeland Community, Zeeland	1,321	12.3	12.4				✖			–					–
Minnesota															
Twin Cities Area															
Abbott Northwestern, Minneapolis	10,518	8.7	**9.8**	★	★	★			★		★	★	★		★

Footnotes are on page 350.

Hospital outcomes: better (★) or worse (×) than average											Results of accreditation review on full survey		Other facts			
Adjusted Death rates			Adjusted Adverse outcome rates													
Surgical cases			Surgical cases													
All selected surgical cases	Coronary artery bypass surgery	Large bowel surgery	All selected surgical cases	Coronary artery bypass surgery	Large bowel surgery	Gall bladder removal	Total knee replacement	Total hip replacement	Simple prostatectomy	Carotid endarterectomy	Accreditation status*	Overall evaluation score (higher is better)	Number of beds	Major medical school affiliation?	Number of residents	Computerized drug order system (1 to 5 scale, higher is preferred; see page 23 for details)
2.3	3.8	6.5	7.7	10.3	11.9	7.5	6.7	6.4	5.4	8.2	–	91	161	–	–	–
–	–	–	–	–	–	–	–	–	–	–	4	89	40	No	0	–
★	★						✖	✖			4	94	368	No	15	–
	–	–	✖	–		–	✖	–	–	–	4	89	81	No	0	–
★						✖					3	90	204	No	0	–
	–	–		–		–		–	–	–	4	96	94	No	0	–
–	–	–		–	–	–	–	–	–	–	4	93	66	No	0	–
–	–	–		–		–		–	–	–	4	95	53	No	0	–
	–		★	–	★	–		–	–	–	4	92	88	No	0	–
	★								–		4	89	173	No	0	–
	–	–		–		–	–	–	–	–	4	98	44	No	0	–
	–		★	–		–	–	–	–	–	4	94	68	No	0	–
	–	–		–		–		–	–	–	4	89	49	No	0	–
	★		×				★			✖	4	83	268	No	0	–
	–		★	–			★				–[2]	–[2]	324	No	50	–
–	–	–		–	–	–	–	–	–	–	4	91	23	No	0	–
–	–	–	–	–	–	–	–	–	–	–	–[2]	–[2]	20	No	0	–
–	–	–	–	–	–	–	–	–	–	–	–[2]	–[2]	18	No	0	–
–	–	–	–	–	–	–	–	–	–	–	4	96	52	No	0	–
						★			–		–[2]	–[2]	513	Yes	106	–
★			✖							✖	4	88	857	Yes	222	–
–	–	–	★	–	–	–	–	–	–	–	4	93	31	No	0	–
★		★									–[2]	–[2]	410	Yes	61	–
–	–	–		–	–	–	–	–	–	–	4	94	67	No	0	–
–	–	–		–	–	–	–	–	–	–	4	94	60	No	0	–
–	–	–		–	★	–	–	–	–	–	4	85	56	No	0	–
–	–	–	★	–	★	–	–	–	–	–	4	94	89	No	0	–
	–			–							–[2]	–[2]	422	No	0	–
	–			–			✖	–	–		4	87	88	No	0	–
	–			–		–	–	–	–		–[2]	–[2]	54	No	0	–
–	–	–		–		–	–	–	–	–	4	97	57	No	0	–
★		★	★	★			★				4	88	642	No	42	2

***Accreditation Status:** 5=Accredited with commendation or with full standards compliance; 4=Accredited with requirements for improvement; 3=Conditional accreditation.

Detailed Ratings for All Areas

See more information on "Key Ratings for Metro Areas" table beginning on page 32

Blue is most favorable
Bold Italic is least favorable
Blank means neither better nor worse than average
"–" means insufficient data

	Death rates for all selected case types			Hospital outcomes: better (★) or worse (×) than average											
				Adjusted Death rates											
					Medical Cases										
	Number of cases	Actual death rate (%)	Adjusted death rate (%) (lower is better)	All selected cases	All selected medical cases	Heart attack	Congestive heart failure	Obstructive pulmonary disease	Pneumonia	Respiratory failure and arrest	Septicemia	Stroke	Gastrointestinal hemorrhage	Fluid, electrolyte, & acid-base disorders	Kidney failure
National Average	–	–	12.1	12.1	14.8	21.2	10.6	6.5	16.9	34.4	25.1	18.4	6.7	11.0	20.9
Minnesota *(continued)*															
Twin Cities Area *(continued)*															
Buffalo Hospital, Buffalo	997	13.4	12.6				***✖***	–		–					–
Children's, Minneapolis	–	–	–	–	–	–	–	–	–	–	–	–	–	–	–
Children's, St Paul	–	–	–	–	–	–	–	–	–	–	–	–	–	–	–
Fairview - Riverside Campus, Minneapolis	3,799	10.7	12.2						***✖***				***✖***		
Fairview - University Campus, Minneapolis[1]	–	–	–	–	–	–	–	–	–	–	–	–	–	–	–
Fairview Ridges, Burnsville	1,611	9.1	11.5								★				
Fairview Southdale, Edina	7,320	8.8	**10.2**	**★**	**★**	**★**		**★**	★		**★**			★	
Hennepin County, Minneapolis	3,000	11.7	**9.4**	**★**	**★**		**★**		★					**★**	★
Lakeview, Stillwater	1,013	10.5	***15.3***	***✖***	***✖***		×	–				***✖***	–		–
Mercy, Coon Rapids[1]	3,576	8.8	**10.3**	**★**	**★**	**★**									
Methodist, St Louis Park[1]	8,138	9.7	**10.8**	**★**	**★**	**★**		×		×	★	★	**★**		
Monticello Big Lake, Monticello[1]	345	13.3	***16.5***	***✖***	***✖***	–	***✖***	–		–	–		–	–	–
North Memorial, Robbinsdale[1]	6,329	11.2	***13.2***	***✖***	***✖***				***✖***			***✖***		×	
Regina, Hastings[1]	891	11.4	***15.5***	***✖***	***✖***			–	***✖***	–	–		–	×	–
Regions, St Paul	4,220	12.0	**10.3**	**★**	**★**	★	**★**	**★**	★						**★**
Ridgeview, Waconia	2,472	10.3	12.5			***✖***									
St Francis Regional, Shakopee	1,014	11.5	13.3							–					–
St John's, Maplewood	4,434	10.1	12.4											***✖***	
St Joseph's, St Paul	5,069	10.1	11.7					***✖***							
United, St Paul[1]	6,991	8.9	**8.9**	**★**	**★**	**★**	**★**	**★**	**★**	**★**	★		★	**★**	**★**
Unity, Fridley[1]	3,077	10.5	11.2								★				
Woodwinds, Woodbury	19	–	–	–	–	–	–	–	–	–	–	–	–	–	–
Other Areas															
Albany Area, Albany	242	12.8	14.4			–	–	–		–	–	–	–	–	–
Albert Lea - Mayo Health, Albert Lea[1]	1,906	11.9	12.9									***✖***			
Appleton Municipal, Appleton[1]	186	16.1	15.1			–	–	–	×	–	–	–	–	–	–
Arlington Municipal, Arlington	337	15.7	15.4	×	***✖***	–		–	×	–	–		–		***✖***
Arnold, Adrian	95	17.9	14.6			–	–	–		–	–	–	–	–	–
Austin Medical Center, Austin	2,170	9.7	**10.1**	**★**	**★**			**★**							
Bridges, Ada	242	8.7	8.6			–		–	★	–	–	–	–	–	–
Cambridge Medical Center, Cambridge	1,583	11.4	11.7						★						***✖***
Cannon Falls Community, Cannon Falls	280	12.1	14.8			–		–		–	–	–	–	–	–
Chippewa County - Montevideo, Montevideo	546	11.9	13.3					–		–	–	***✖***	–	–	–

Footnotes are on page 350.

Hospital outcomes: better (★) or worse (✕) than average											Results of accreditation review on full survey		Other facts			
Adjusted Death rates			Adjusted Adverse outcome rates													
Surgical cases			Surgical cases													
All selected surgical cases	Coronary artery bypass surgery	Large bowel surgery	All selected surgical cases	Coronary artery bypass surgery	Large bowel surgery	Gall bladder removal	Total knee replacement	Total hip replacement	Simple prostatectomy	Carotid endarterectomy	Accreditation status*	Overall evaluation score (higher is better)	Number of beds	Major medical school affiliation?	Number of residents	Computerized drug order system (1 to 5 scale, higher is preferred; see page 23 for details)
2.3	3.8	6.5	7.7	10.3	11.9	7.5	6.7	6.4	5.4	8.2	–	91	161	–	–	–
–	–	–		–	–	–	–	–	–	–	4	**85**	30	No	0	2
–	–	–	–	–	–	–	–	–	–	–	–[2]	–[2]	163	–	7	–
–	–	–	–	–	–	–	–	–	–	–	–[2]	–[2]	105	–	0	–
						✕		★			4	**84**	948	No	0	4
–	–	–	–	–	–	–	–	–	–	–	–[2]	–[2]	–	–	–	–
	–	–	★	–		–	★		–	–	4	**85**	127	No	0	4
	✕	★	★			★					4	**85**	348	No	0	4
	–		★	–		–	★		–	–	4	**83**	360	No	201	3
–	–	–	★	–	–	–	★	–	–	–	5	**98**	62	No	0	1
★	★		★	★		✕					4	**88**	198	No	0	4
★			★		★		★			✕	4	89	367	No	24	4
–	–	–	–	–	–	–	–	–	–	–	4	**94**	12	No	0	2
							✕				4	91	376	**Yes**	0	1
–	–	–	★	–	–	–	–	–	–	–	4	**96**	96	No	0	2
										–	4	**86**	390	**Yes**	45	2
	–	–	★	–					–	–	4	92	102	No	0	2
✕	–	✕		–	✕	–		–	–	–	4	**88**	63	No	0	2
	–		★	–			★				4	**96**	150	No	3	2
	✕										5	**97**	292	**Yes**	7	2
			★				★				4	**84**	483	No	6	2
	–			–					★		4	**88**	201	No	0	4
–	–	–	–	–	–	–	–	–	–	–	–[2]	–[2]	70	No	–	2
–	–	–	–	–	–	–	–	–	–	–	–[2]	–[2]	15	No	0	1
	–	–		–		✕	–	–		–	4	**87**	72	No	0	–
–	–	–	–	–	–	–	–	–	–	–	–[2]	–[2]	20	No	0	–
–	–	–	–	–	–	–	–	–	–	–	–[2]	–[2]	17	No	0	–
–	–	–	–	–	–	–	–	–	–	–	–[2]	–[2]	9	No	0	–
★	–	–	★	–	–	–	★	–	–	–	4	89	117	No	–	–
–	–	–	–	–	–	–	–	–	–	–	–[2]	–[2]	8	No	0	–
	–	–	★	–		–	★	–	–	–	4	**84**	81	No	7	2
–	–	–	–	–	–	–	–	–	–	–	–[2]	–[2]	14	No	0	–
–	–	–	★	–	–	–	–	–	–	–	–[2]	–[2]	29	No	0	–

***Accreditation Status:** 5=Accredited with commendation or with full standards compliance; 4=Accredited with requirements for improvement; 3=Conditional accreditation.

Detailed Ratings for All Areas

See more information on "Key Ratings for Metro Areas" table beginning on page 32

Blue is most favorable
Bold Italic is least favorable
Blank means neither better nor worse than average
"–" means insufficient data

	Death rates for all selected case types			Hospital outcomes: better (★) or worse (×) than average												
				Adjusted Death rates												
				Medical Cases												
	Number of cases	Actual death rate (%)	Adjusted death rate (%) (lower is better)	All selected cases	All selected medical cases	Heart attack	Congestive heart failure	Obstructive pulmonary disease	Pneumonia	Respiratory failure and arrest	Septicemia	Stroke	Gastrointestinal hemorrhage	Fluid, electrolyte, & acid-base disorders	Kidney failure
National Average	–	–	12.1	12.1	14.8	21.2	10.6	6.5	16.9	34.4	25.1	18.4	6.7	11.0	20.9
Minnesota *(continued)*															
Other Areas *(continued)*															
Clearwater County, Bagley[1]	416	15.1	12.5					–		–	–		–	★	–
Cloquet Community, Cloquet	744	12.2	11.9					✖		–			–	★	–
Community, Winona[1]	1,674	13.7	***14.3***	✖	✖	✖	✖		✖	–			★		
Cook Community, Cook[1]	172	10.5	12.7			–	–	–		–	–	–	–	–	–
Cook County North Shore, Grand Marais	158	13.3	15.0			–	–	–		–	–	–	–	–	–
Cuyuna Regional, Crosby	813	8.6	9.1	★	★			–			–		–	–	–
Deer River Healthcare Center, Deer River	393	9.4	10.3			–		–		–	–	–	–		–
District One, Faribault	1,206	10.4	11.2										–		
Divine Providence, Ivanhoe	148	12.8	14.2			–	–	–		–	–	–	–	–	–
Douglas County, Alexandria	2,247	9.2	12.5			✖									–
Ely - Bloomenson, Ely	348	17.0	***17.3***	✖	✖	–	✖	–	✖	–	–		–	–	–
Fairmont Community, Fairmont	1,354	11.7	11.8											×	
Fairnew University, Hibbing[1]	2,081	13.3	12.5			✖	✖	★							
Fairview Lakes Regional, Wyoming[1]	925	13.1	12.7						×				–	–	–
Fairview Northland Regional, Princeton[1]	971	14.6	***14.3***	✖	✖				×	–			–		–
Fairview Red Wing, Red Wing	1,206	12.5	***14.2***	✖	✖			–	×			×			–
Falls, International Falls[1]	499	13.8	13.3					–		–	–		–		–
First Care, Fosston	361	12.2	12.0					–		–	–		–	–	–
Glacial Ridge, Glenwood	479	18.2	***15.1***	✖	✖		×	–		–	–		–	–	–
Glencoe Regional, Glencoe[1]	775	12.0	13.8				✖	–		–	–	✖	–		–
Graceville Health Center, Graceville	159	21.4	***19.2***	✖	✖		–	–	✖	–	–	–	–	–	–
Granite Falls Municipal, Granite Falls[1]	437	11.2	10.2					–		–	–		–	–	–
Grant County, Elbow Lake	421	10.9	10.3			–		–		–			–	–	–
Hendricks Community, Hendricks	250	18.8	14.6			–		–		–	–		–	–	–
Hutchinson Area, Hutchinson[1]	980	11.1	12.5				✖	–		–			★		–
Immanuel St Joseph's, Mankato	3,050	9.7	***13.5***	✖	✖										
Itasca, Grand Rapids	1,386	12.3	12.6					★	✖						×
Jackson Medical Center, Jackson	293	14.0	13.0			–		–		–	–	–	–	–	–
Johnson, Dawson[1]	202	13.4	12.8			–	–	–		–	–	–	–	–	–
Kanabec, Mora	740	11.6	12.2				✖			–			–		–
Kittson, Hallock	119	13.4	13.8			–	–	–	–	–	–	–	–	–	–
Lake City Medical Center, Lake City[1]	422	10.7	12.5			–		–		–	–		–		–
Lake Region, Fergus Falls[1]	2,168	9.4	10.2	★	★				★						
Lake View, Two Harbors	212	15.6	16.2	×	×	–	–	–	✖	–	–	–	–	–	–

Footnotes are on page 350.

Hospital outcomes: better (★) or worse (×) than average											Results of accreditation review on full survey		Other facts			
Adjusted Death rates			Adjusted Adverse outcome rates													
Surgical cases			Surgical cases													
All selected surgical cases	Coronary artery bypass surgery	Large bowel surgery	All selected surgical cases	Coronary artery bypass surgery	Large bowel surgery	Gall bladder removal	Total knee replacement	Total hip replacement	Simple prostatectomy	Carotid endarterectomy	Accreditation status*	Overall evaluation score (higher is better)	Number of beds	Major medical school affiliation?	Number of residents	Computerized drug order system (1 to 5 scale, higher is preferred; see page 23 for details)
2.3	3.8	6.5	7.7	10.3	11.9	7.5	6.7	6.4	5.4	8.2	–	91	161	–	–	–
–	–	–	–	–	–	–	–	–	–	–	–[2]	–[2]	92	No	0	–
–	–	–		–	–	–	–	–	–	–	–[2]	–[2]	36	No	0	–
	–	–		–		–	–	–	–	–	4	90	76	No	0	–
–	–	–	–	–	–	–	–	–	–	–	–[2]	–[2]	14	No	0	1
–	–	–	–	–	–	–	–	–	–	–	–[2]	–[2]	12	No	0	–
–	–	–	★	–	–	–	–	–	–	–	–[2]	–[2]	30	No	0	–
–	–	–	–	–	–	–	–	–	–	–	–[2]	–[2]	20	No	0	–
–	–	–		–	–	–		–	–	–	4	**88**	52	No	0	–
–	–	–	–	–	–	–	–	–	–	–	–[2]	–[2]	69	No	0	–
★	–	★	★	–		★		★		–	4	**88**	99	No	0	–
–	–	–	–	–	–	–	–	–	–	–	–[2]	–[2]	26	No	0	–
–	–	–		–	–	–		–		–	4	90	52	No	0	–
	–		★	–	★		–	–	–	–	4	**84**	65	No	0	2
–	–	–		–		–	–	–	–	–	4	**86**	38	No	0	2
–	–	–		–	–	–	–	–	–	–	4	**87**	40	No	0	2
–	–	–	★	–	–	–	★	★	–	–	4	90	70	No	0	4
–	–	–	–	–	–	–	–	–	–	–	4	**94**	35	No	0	–
–	–	–	–	–	–	–	–	–	–	–	–[2]	–[2]	22	No	0	–
–	–	–	–	–	–	–	–	–	–	–	–[2]	–[2]	19	No	0	–
–	–	–		–	–	–	–	–	–	–	–[2]	–[2]	39	No	0	–
–	–	–	–	–	–	–	–	–	–	–	–[2]	–[2]	92	No	0	–
–	–	–	–	–	–	–	–	–	–	–	4	**83**	94	No	0	–
–	–	–	–	–	–	–	–	–	–	–	–[2]	–[2]	15	No	0	–
–	–	–	–	–	–	–	–	–	–	–	–[2]	–[2]	14	No	0	–
	–	–		–		–	–	–	–	–	5	92	60	No	0	–
	–	–		–			★		–	–	4	89	147	No	0	–
	–	–	★	–		–	★	–	–	–	4	91	49	No	0	–
–	–	–	–	–	–	–	–	–	–	–	–[2]	–[2]	20	No	0	–
–	–	–	–	–	–	–	–	–	–	–	–[2]	–[2]	93	No	0	–
–	–	–	–	–	–	–	–	–	–	–	4	**95**	35	No	0	–
–	–	–	–	–	–	–	–	–	–	–	–[2]	–[2]	21	No	0	–
–	–	–	–	–	–	–	–	–	–	–	4	**96**	18	No	0	–
	–	–	★	–		×	★		–	–	4	89	92	No	0	–
–	–	–	–	–	–	–	–	–	–	–	–[2]	–[2]	16	No	0	–

***Accreditation Status:** 5=Accredited with commendation or with full standards compliance; 4=Accredited with requirements for improvement; 3=Conditional accreditation.

Detailed Ratings for All Areas

See more information on "Key Ratings for Metro Areas" table beginning on page 32

Blue is most favorable
Bold Italic is least favorable
Blank means neither better nor worse than average
"–" means insufficient data

	Death rates for all selected case types			Hospital outcomes: better (★) or worse (×) than average — Adjusted Death rates — Medical Cases											
	Number of cases	Actual death rate (%)	Adjusted death rate (%) (lower is better)	All selected cases	All selected medical cases	Heart attack	Congestive heart failure	Obstructive pulmonary disease	Pneumonia	Respiratory failure and arrest	Septicemia	Stroke	Gastrointestinal hemorrhage	Fluid, electrolyte, & acid-base disorders	Kidney failure
National Average	–	–	12.1	12.1	14.8	21.2	10.6	6.5	16.9	34.4	25.1	18.4	6.7	11.0	20.9
Minnesota *(continued)*															
Other Areas *(continued)*															
Lakeside, Pine City[1]	130	20.8	***17.8***	✖	✖	–	–	–		–	–	–	–	✖	–
Lakewood, Staples	439	13.7	14.2					–	✖	–	–		–	–	–
Long Prairie Memorial, Long Prairie[1]	348	18.7	***15.8***	✖	✖		×	–		–	–				–
Luverne Community, Luverne	662	12.1	10.6					–		–	★				–
Madelia Community, Madelia	292	12.7	14.7			–		–		–	–	–	–	–	–
Madison Hospital, Madison	261	12.3	13.3			–		–		–	–	–	–	–	–
Meeker County, Litchfield	817	13.6	13.1				×	–		–				★	
Melrose Area - Centracare, Melrose	287	14.3	15.4	×	×	–	×	–		–	–	–	–	–	–
Mercy, Moose Lake[1]	461	13.4	12.2					–		–			–		–
Mille Lacs, Onamia	368	11.4	12.4			–				–	–	–	–		–
Miller Dwan, Duluth	396	7.3	10.0			–	★	–		–	–	–	–	–	
Minnesota Valley, Le Sueur	91	15.4	16.3			–	–	–		–	–	–	–	–	–
Murray County, Slayton	403	11.4	14.2			–		–		–	–	–	–	–	–
New Ulm Medical Center, New Ulm	1,065	9.2	11.1							–		★	–		–
North Country Regional, Bemidji[1]	2,196	8.6	12.1					★							–
North Valley, Warren	363	14.6	13.8			✖		–		–	–	–	–		–
Northern Itasca, Bigfork	228	7.0	7.0	★	★	–	–	–		–	–	–	–	–	–
Northfield Hospital, Northfield[1]	725	7.7	11.2							–	–		–	–	–
Northwest, Thief River Falls	1,153	12.4	***14.0***	✖	×	✖					–				
Olmsted, Rochester	717	6.3	9.0	★	★	★				–	–	–	–	–	–
Ortonville Area, Ortonville[1]	314	15.0	***17.0***	✖	✖		✖	–		–	–	✖	–	–	–
Owatonna Hospital, Owatonna	998	10.7	11.1							–					–
Paynesville Area, Paynesville[1]	373	13.9	15.3	×	×		✖	–		–	–		–	–	–
Perham Memorial, Perham[1]	405	11.4	12.6					–		–	–	–	–	–	–
PHS Indian, Cass Lake	106	6.6	9.3			–	–	–	–	–	–	–	–	–	–
PHS Indian, Redlake	113	10.6	17.1			–	–	–	–	–	–	–	–	–	–
Pine, Sandstone	171	15.2	13.5			–	–	–		–	–	–	–	–	–
Pipestone County, Pipestone	458	14.2	***16.2***	✖	✖	–		–	✖	–	–		–		–
Queen of Peace, New Prague	916	8.3	11.7					–		–	–		–	–	–
Redwood Area, Redwood Falls	501	15.8	***15.1***	✖	✖			–	×	–	–		–	–	–
Rice, Willmar	2,241	7.5	11.5				★			–				–	
Riverview, Crookston[1]	867	12.3	12.5					–					–		×
Rochester Methodist (Mayo Clinic), Rochester	4,243	1.7	9.7	★		–	–	–		–		–	–		–
Roseau Area, Roseau	499	16.2	***15.9***	✖	✖			–	✖	–	–	✖	–	–	–

Footnotes are on page 350.

Hospital outcomes: better (★) or worse (×) than average											Results of accreditation review on full survey		Other facts			
Adjusted Death rates			Adjusted Adverse outcome rates													
Surgical cases			Surgical cases													
All selected surgical cases	Coronary artery bypass surgery	Large bowel surgery	All selected surgical cases	Coronary artery bypass surgery	Large bowel surgery	Gall bladder removal	Total knee replacement	Total hip replacement	Simple prostatectomy	Carotid endarterectomy	Accreditation status*	Overall evaluation score (higher is better)	Number of beds	Major medical school affiliation?	Number of residents	Computerized drug order system (1 to 5 scale, higher is preferred; see page 23 for details)
2.3	3.8	6.5	7.7	10.3	11.9	7.5	6.7	6.4	5.4	8.2	–	91	161	–	–	–
–	–	–	–	–	–	–	–	–	–	–	–[2]	–[2]	10	No	–	–
–	–	–	–	–	–	–	–	–	–	–	–[2]	–[2]	40	No	0	–
–	–	–	–	–	–	–	–	–	–	–	–[2]	–[2]	12	No	0	–
–	–	–	★	–	–	–	–	–	–	–	–[2]	–[2]	29	No	0	–
–	–	–	–	–	–	–	–	–	–	–	4	**94**	25	No	0	–
–	–	–	–	–	–	–	–	–	–	–	–[2]	–[2]	13	No	2	–
–	–	–		–	–	–	–	–	–	–	–[2]	–[2]	38	No	0	–
–	–	–	–	–	–	–	–	–	–	–	–[2]	–[2]	12	No	0	1
–	–	–	–	–	–	–	–	–	–	–	–[2]	–[2]	118	No	5	–
–	–	–	–	–	–	–	–	–	–	–	4	89	98	No	0	–
–	–	–		–	–	–	–	–	–	–	4	***88***	152	No	0	–
–	–	–	–	–	–	–	–	–	–	–	–[2]	–[2]	17	No	0	–
–	–	–	–	–	–	–	–	–	–	–	–[2]	–[2]	25	No	0	–
	–	–		–		–		★	–	–	4	90	47	No	0	2
	–			–				×		–	4	89	85	No	0	–
–	–	–	–	–	–	–	–	–	–	–	–[2]	–[2]	20	No	0	–
–	–	–	–	–	–	–	–	–	–	–	–[2]	–[2]	56	No	0	–
–	–	–	★	–	–	–		–	–	–	–[2]	–[2]	27	No	0	–
	–	–		–			–	–	–	–	4	***77***	40	No	0	–
–	–	–		–		–		–	–	–	4	***88***	63	No	0	1
–	–	–	–	–	–	–	–	–	–	–	–[2]	–[2]	105	No	2	–
–	–	–		–	–	–	★	–	–	–	4	89	44	No	0	–
–	–	–	–	–	–	–	–	–	–	–	–[2]	–[2]	94	No	0	–
–	–	–	–	–	–	–	–	–	–	–	5	92	123	No	5	–
–	–	–	–	–	–	–	–	–	–	–	4	***78***	13	No	0	–
–	–	–	–	–	–	–	–	–	–	–	4	***87***	23	No	0	–
–	–	–	–	–	–	–	–	–	–	–	–[2]	–[2]	20	No	0	–
–	–	–	–	–	–	–	–	–	–	–	–[2]	–[2]	76	No	0	–
–	–	–	×	–	–	–	×	–	–	–	4	93	31	No	0	–
–	–	–	–	–	–	–	–	–	–	–	–[2]	–[2]	30	No	0	–
	–		★	–			★	★		–	4	91	118	No	0	–
–	–	–		–	–	–	–	–	–	–	4	92	72	No	0	–
★	–	★		–	★			×	★	–	4	**95**	335	**Yes**	19	–
–	–	–	–	–	–	–	–	–	–	–	4	**96**	37	No	0	–

***Accreditation Status:** 5=Accredited with commendation or with full standards compliance; 4=Accredited with requirements for improvement; 3=Conditional accreditation.

Detailed Ratings for All Areas

See more information on "Key Ratings for Metro Areas" table beginning on page 32

Blue is most favorable
Bold Italic is least favorable
Blank means neither better nor worse than average
"–" means insufficient data

	Death rates for all selected case types			Hospital outcomes: better (★) or worse (×) than average — Adjusted Death rates — Medical Cases											
	Number of cases	Actual death rate (%)	Adjusted death rate (%) (lower is better)	All selected cases	All selected medical cases	Heart attack	Congestive heart failure	Obstructive pulmonary disease	Pneumonia	Respiratory failure and arrest	Septicemia	Stroke	Gastrointestinal hemorrhage	Fluid, electrolyte, & acid-base disorders	Kidney failure
National Average	–	–	12.1	12.1	14.8	21.2	10.6	6.5	16.9	34.4	25.1	18.4	6.7	11.0	20.9
Minnesota *(continued)*															
Other Areas *(continued)*															
St Cloud Hospital, St Cloud	6,764	8.9	11.7												
St Elizabeth, Wabasha	443	9.3	10.2					–	★	–	–		–		–
St Francis, Breckenridge	1,038	12.7	11.4							–					
St Gabriel's, Little Falls	1,307	11.5	13.0					–		–					–
St James, St James	269	14.1	14.3					–		–	–	×	–	–	–
St Joseph's, Brainerd	3,480	8.0	9.4	★	★		★	★			★			★	
St Josephs, Park Rapids[1]	1,264	15.1	***13.9***	**×**	**×**					–					**×**
St Luke's, Duluth	3,506	9.2	12.1				×								
St Mary's, Duluth	6,965	8.7	9.6	★	★	★			★	★	★		★		★
St Mary's Regional, Detroit Lakes	1,152	10.6	10.5												–
St Marys (Mayo Clinic), Rochester	13,990	7.7	9.1	★	★	★	★	★	★			★	★		
St Michael's, Sauk Centre	332	13.6	13.7			–	★	–		–	–		–	–	–
St Peter, St Peter	295	11.9	12.7			–		–		–	–		–	–	–
Sioux Valley Canby Campus, Canby	314	13.7	***18.5***	**×**	**×**	–	–	–	**×**	–	–	–	–	–	–
Sleepy Eye Municipal, Sleepy Eye	416	9.9	12.6			–		–		–	–	–	–	–	–
Springfield Medical Center, Springfield[1]	344	13.7	15.3	×	**×**	–		–		–	–		–	–	–
Stevens, Morris	800	10.8	10.1	★	★			–		–	–		–	★	–
Swift County - Benson, Benson	339	13.9	14.8					–		–	–		–	–	–
Tri-County, Wadena	937	12.3	11.8							–			–		–
Tyler Healthcare Center, Tyler	264	10.2	10.9			–	–	–		–	–	–	–	–	–
United, Blue Earth	677	10.5	11.1					–			–		–	–	–
Virginia Regional, Virginia	1,619	13.5	***16.5***	**×**	**×**		**×**	**×**					×	**×**	**×**
Waseca - Mayo Health, Waseca[1]	320	9.4	9.8			–		–		–	–		–	–	–
Weiner, Marshall	695	12.7	13.7			**×**	×	–			–		–	–	–
Wheaton Community, Wheaton	376	14.4	14.5			×	×	–		–	–	–	–	–	–
White, Aurora	201	11.4	13.9			–	–	–		–	–	–	–	–	–
Windom Area, Windom	507	11.2	13.0					**×**		–	–		–	–	–
Worthington Regional, Worthington	1,033	10.5	13.6							–		**×**			–
Mississippi															
Aberdeen Monroe County, Aberdeen	453	19.0	***15.5***	**×**	**×**	–			**×**	–		–	–		–
Alliance, Holly Springs	516	12.4	13.1			–	★	★	**×**	–	**×**	–	–		–
Baptist, Booneville	1,532	11.9	12.4										–		
Baptist - Desoto, Southaven	2,570	14.1	***15.7***	**×**	**×**	**×**	**×**		**×**		×		**×**	×	

Footnotes are on page 350.

Hospital outcomes: better (★) or worse (✕) than average											Results of accreditation review on full survey		Other facts			
Adjusted Death rates			Adjusted Adverse outcome rates													
Surgical cases			Surgical cases													
All selected surgical cases	Coronary artery bypass surgery	Large bowel surgery	All selected surgical cases	Coronary artery bypass surgery	Large bowel surgery	Gall bladder removal	Total knee replacement	Total hip replacement	Simple prostatectomy	Carotid endarterectomy	Accreditation status*	Overall evaluation score (higher is better)	Number of beds	Major medical school affiliation?	Number of residents	Computerized drug order system (1 to 5 scale, higher is preferred; see page 23 for details)
2.3	3.8	6.5	7.7	10.3	11.9	7.5	6.7	6.4	5.4	8.2	–	91	161	–	–	–
	★		✕	★	✕						4	94	406	No	7	2
–	–	–	–	–	–	–	–	–	–	–	4	93	25	No	0	–
–	–	–		–		–	–	–	–	–	4	97	171	No	2	–
	–	–	★	–		–	★	★	–	–	4	88	49	No	0	–
–	–	–	–	–	–	–	–	–	–	–	–[2]	–[2]	24	No	0	–
	–		★	–		–	★		★	–	4	89	152	No	0	–
	–			–		✕	–	–	–	–	4	92	39	No	0	–
						✕					4	87	242	No	0	1
★		★	★		★		★			★	4	92	288	Yes	0	3
–	–	–		–	–	–	–	–	–	–	4	94	63	No	0	–
★	★	★		★	★					✕	4	93	797	Yes	76	3
–	–	–	–	–	–	–	–	–	–	–	–[2]	–[2]	78	No	1	1
–	–	–	–	–	–	–	–	–	–	–	–[2]	–[2]	118	No	5	–
–	–	–	–	–	–	–	–	–	–	–	–[2]	–[2]	19	No	0	–
–	–	–	–	–	–	–	–	–	–	–	–[2]	–[2]	18	No	0	–
–	–	–	–	–	–	–	–	–	–	–	4	95	23	No	0	–
–	–	–	–	–	–	–	–	–	–	–	4	89	39	No	0	–
–	–	–	–	–	–	–	–	–	–	–	–[2]	–[2]	17	No	0	–
–	–	–		–	–		–	–	–	–	4	89	30	No	0	–
–	–	–	–	–	–	–	–	–	–	–	–[2]	–[2]	63	No	0	–
–	–	–		–	–	–	–	–	–	–	4	84	24	No	0	–
✕	–	✕	✕	–	✕		–	–	–	–	4	94	83	No	0	1
–	–	–	–	–	–	–	–	–	–	–	4	83	26	No	0	–
–	–	–		–	–	–	–	–	–	–	4	86	49	No	0	–
–	–	–	–	–	–	–	–	–	–	–	–[2]	–[2]	25	No	0	–
–	–	–	–	–	–	–	–	–	–	–	–[2]	–[2]	85	No	0	2
–	–	–	–	–	–		–	–	–	–	–[2]	–[2]	35	No	0	–
–	–	–	✕	–	–	–	✕	–	–	–	4	92	66	No	0	–
–	–	–	–	–	–	–	–	–	–	–	–[2]	–[2]	37	No	0	–
–	–	–	–	–	–	–	–	–	–	–	–[2]	–[2]	40	No	0	–
–	–	–	–	–	–	–	–	–	–	–	4	91	99	No	0	–
	–			–				–	–	–	4	83	140	No	0	–

***Accreditation Status:** 5=Accredited with commendation or with full standards compliance; 4=Accredited with requirements for improvement; 3=Conditional accreditation.

Detailed Ratings for All Areas

See more information on "Key Ratings for Metro Areas" table beginning on page 32

Blue is most favorable
Bold Italic is least favorable
Blank means neither better nor worse than average
"–" means insufficient data

	Death rates for all selected case types			Hospital outcomes: better (★) or worse (×) than average — Adjusted Death rates — Medical Cases											
	Number of cases	Actual death rate (%)	Adjusted death rate (%) (lower is better)	All selected cases	All selected medical cases	Heart attack	Congestive heart failure	Obstructive pulmonary disease	Pneumonia	Respiratory failure and arrest	Septicemia	Stroke	Gastrointestinal hemorrhage	Fluid, electrolyte, & acid-base disorders	Kidney failure
National Average	–	–	12.1	12.1	14.8	21.2	10.6	6.5	16.9	34.4	25.1	18.4	6.7	11.0	20.9
Mississippi *(continued)*															
Baptist - Golden Triangle, Columbus	3,159	13.3	***14.9***	✖	✖		✖	×			✖		×		✖
Baptist - North Mississippi, Oxford	5,108	13.1	***17.1***	✖	✖	✖	✖	✖	✖		✖	×		×	✖
Baptist - Union County, New Albany	1,815	12.7	***17.0***	✖	✖	✖	✖		✖	–	✖	✖		×	✖
Beacham, Magnolia	800	8.0	8.2	★	★	–		★		–	–	★	–	★	
Biloxi Regional, Biloxi	3,037	11.2	11.9			×						×		★	
Bolivar, Cleveland	2,258	14.6	12.6												
Calhoun Health Services, Calhoun City	558	15.1	***16.1***	✖	✖	–				–		✖	–		–
Central Mississippi, Jackson	4,142	15.4	***15.0***	✖	✖	✖		×	✖	×	✖			✖	
Choctaw County, Ackerman	188	16.5	***17.0***	✖	✖	–	–	–	✖	–	–	–	–	–	–
Claiborne County, Port Gibson	181	16.6	15.7			–	–	–		✖	–	–	–		–
Clay County, West Point	1,299	15.5	***15.0***	✖	✖	–					✖	✖			×
Covington County, Collins	670	17.8	***21.0***	✖	✖	✖	✖		✖	–	✖	–	–		–
Delta Regional, Greenville	2,439	16.7	***17.9***	✖	✖	✖			✖	✖	✖	✖		×	✖
Field, Centreville	743	14.0	***16.1***	✖	✖		×	–		–	×		–		
Forrest General, Hattiesburg	8,215	11.9	***13.4***	✖	✖		✖				×				
Franklin County, Meadville	472	14.2	***18.6***	✖	✖	–	✖	–		–	–	✖	–	–	–
Garden Park, Gulfport	1,622	11.3	12.9						✖				–		
George County, Lucedale	1,271	10.1	12.2					★		✖	✖			★	–
Gilmore, Amory	1,432	13.5	12.5			✖	★				×				–
Greenwood Leflore, Greenwood	3,131	12.6	***16.2***	✖	✖	✖	✖		✖		✖	×		✖	✖
Grenada Lake, Grenada	2,288	13.3	***13.4***	✖	✖	✖		×		–				★	✖
Gulf Coast, Biloxi	1,708	11.2	13.5	×	×	✖	✖								★
H C Watkins, Quitman	750	12.9	10.7			–		–		–			–	★	–
Hancock, Bay St Louis	1,751	12.9	11.0												
Hardy Wilson, Hazlehurst	798	15.8	***16.4***	✖	✖			–	✖	–	–	×	–		✖
Humphreys County, Belzoni	356	13.2	15.0	×	×	–		–		–	–	–	–	–	–
Iuka Hospital, Iuka[1]	1,286	13.2	***14.7***	✖	✖	✖				–		✖	–		
Jasper General, Bay Springs	123	23.6	***23.2***	✖	✖	–	–	–	✖	–	–	–	–	–	–
Jeff Anderson Regional, Meridian	5,068	11.1	10.9	★	★				★	×				★	
Jefferson County, Fayette	74	0.0	0.0	★	★	–	★	–	–	–	–	–	–	–	–
Kilmichael Hospital, Kilmichael	422	11.8	15.1	×	×	–			✖	–	–	✖	–		–
King's Daughters, Brookhaven	2,204	14.2	***14.0***	✖	✖	✖		✖	✖		×				
King's Daughters, Greenville	1,031	10.0	13.9			–			★	–			–		
King's Daughters, Yazoo City[1]	1,085	16.2	***15.3***	✖	✖	✖		–				×	–	×	✖
Laird, Union	843	6.5	7.1	★	★		★	★	★	★			–		–

Footnotes are on page 350.

Hospital outcomes: better (★) or worse (×) than average											Results of accreditation review on full survey		Other facts			
Adjusted Death rates			Adjusted Adverse outcome rates													
Surgical cases			Surgical cases													
All selected surgical cases	Coronary artery bypass surgery	Large bowel surgery	All selected surgical cases	Coronary artery bypass surgery	Large bowel surgery	Gall bladder removal	Total knee replacement	Total hip replacement	Simple prostatectomy	Carotid endarterectomy	Accreditation status*	Overall evaluation score (higher is better)	Number of beds	Major medical school affiliation?	Number of residents	Computerized drug order system (1 to 5 scale, higher is preferred; see page 23 for details)
2.3	3.8	6.5	7.7	10.3	11.9	7.5	6.7	6.4	5.4	8.2	–	91	161	–	–	–
	–			–						–	4	***87***	328	No	0	–
✖		✖	×		✖		★		–	✖	4	92	204	No	0	–
–	–	–		–	–	–	–	–	–	–	4	**96**	153	No	0	–
–	–	–	–	–	–	–	–	–	–	–	–[2]	–[2]	37	No	0	–
	–	–		–			–	–	–		4	**95**	153	No	0	–
–	–	–		–	–	–	–	–	–	–	4	***78***	113	No	0	–
–	–	–	–	–	–	–	–	–	–	–	–[2]	–[2]	30	No	0	–
✖		×	✖					–	–	–	4	**95**	317	No	0	–
–	–	–	–	–	–	–	–	–	–	–	–[2]	–[2]	13	No	0	–
–	–	–	–	–	–	–	–	–	–	–	–[2]	–[2]	32	No	0	–
–	–	–	–	–	–	–	–	–	–	–	4	92	60	**Yes**	0	–
–	–	–	–	–	–	–	–	–	–	–	4	***84***	82	No	0	–
✖	–	✖		–		–	–	–	–	–	4	***72***	160	No	0	–
–	–	–	–	–	–	–	–	–	–	–	4	89	66	No	0	–
✖		✖	✖		✖				✖		4	**97**	537	No	0	–
–	–	–	–	–	–	–	–	–	–	–	–[2]	–[2]	43	No	0	–
–	–	–		–			–	–	–	–	4	91	97	No	0	–
–	–	–	–	–	–	–	–	–	–	–	–[2]	–[2]	47	No	0	–
–	–	–		–	–	–	–	–	–	–	4	89	95	No	0	–
	–			–	×			–		✖	5	93	204	No	0	–
–	–	–		–	–	–	–	–	–	–	4	***81***	114	No	0	–
	–	–		–		–		–	–	–	4	***88***	189	No	0	–
–	–	–	–	–	–	–	–	–	–	–	–[2]	–[2]	32	No	0	–
	–	–		–			–	–	–	–	4	90	104	No	0	–
–	–	–	–	–	–	–	–	–	–	–	–[2]	–[2]	49	No	0	–
–	–	–	–	–	–	–	–	–	–	–	–[2]	–[2]	28	No	0	–
–	–	–	–	–	–	–	–	–	–	–	4	93	48	No	0	–
–	–	–	–	–	–	–	–	–	–	–	–[2]	–[2]	20	No	0	–
		–						–			4	***86***	260	No	0	–
–	–	–	–	–	–	–	–	–	–	–	–[2]	–[2]	27	No	0	–
–	–	–	–	–	–	–	–	–	–	–	–[2]	–[2]	19	No	0	–
	–	–		–			–	–	–	–	4	90	109	No	0	–
✖	–	–	✖	–	✖	–	–	–	–	–	4	***87***	103	No	0	–
–	–	–	–	–	–	–	–	–	–	–	–[2]	–[2]	54	No	0	–
–	–	–	–	–	–	–	–	–	–	–	–[2]	–[2]	50	No	0	–

***Accreditation Status:** 5=Accredited with commendation or with full standards compliance; 4=Accredited with requirements for improvement; 3=Conditional accreditation.

Detailed Ratings for All Areas

See more information on "Key Ratings for Metro Areas" table beginning on page 32

Blue is most favorable
Bold Italic is least favorable
Blank means neither better nor worse than average
"–" means insufficient data

	Death rates for all selected case types			Hospital outcomes: better (★) or worse (×) than average — Adjusted Death rates											
					Medical Cases										
	Number of cases	Actual death rate (%)	Adjusted death rate (%) (lower is better)	All selected cases	All selected medical cases	Heart attack	Congestive heart failure	Obstructive pulmonary disease	Pneumonia	Respiratory failure and arrest	Septicemia	Stroke	Gastrointestinal hemorrhage	Fluid, electrolyte, & acid-base disorders	Kidney failure
National Average	–	–	12.1	12.1	14.8	21.2	10.6	6.5	16.9	34.4	25.1	18.4	6.7	11.0	20.9
Mississippi *(continued)*															
Lawrence County, Monticello	631	10.1	10.7			–				–	–		–	★	–
Leake, Carthage	793	19.4	***17.1***	✖	✖		✖	–		–	–	✖	–	×	×
Lucius Olen Crosby, Picayune	1,604	15.5	***16.2***	✖	✖				✖	✖	✖		–		×
Madison County, Canton	562	11.6	13.4			–		–		–	–	★	–		–
Magee General, Magee	1,385	13.1	***15.0***	✖	✖		✖			–	✖		–	✖	
Magnolia Regional, Corinth	3,381	12.5	12.2												×
Marion General, Columbia	1,400	16.7	***18.7***	✖	✖		✖	✖	✖	–	✖	✖		✖	✖
Memorial, Gulfport	5,258	11.5	11.8									★			★
Mississippi Baptist, Jackson[1]	8,241	9.9	12.3					×							
Mississippi State, Whitfield	206	25.2	***17.8***	✖	✖	–	–	–	✖	–		–	–		–
Montfort Jones, Kosciusko	1,106	14.8	12.2								×				–
Natchez Community, Natchez	2,128	13.7	***15.9***	✖	✖	✖	✖	✖	✖		✖				
Natchez Regional, Natchez	1,838	14.6	***18.0***	✖	✖		✖	✖	✖	×	✖	✖	✖	×	
Neshoba County General, Philadelphia	926	10.6	12.6			–				–			–		–
Newton Regional, Newton	632	15.8	***15.9***	✖	✖	–				–		✖	–		✖
North Mississippi, Tupelo	10,746	12.0	***13.7***	✖	✖		✖		✖	×	✖		✖	✖	
North Oak Regional, Senatobia	598	16.1	***18.2***	✖	✖	–	✖	–		–	–	–	–	✖	–
North Sunflower County, Ruleville	491	17.9	***15.3***	✖	✖	–		★	✖	–		✖	–		
Northwest Mississippi Regional, Clarksdale	3,082	11.1	12.1			✖						★		★	
Noxubee General, Macon	430	13.5	12.5			–		–		–	✖		–		–
Oktibbeha County, Starkville	1,170	16.7	***16.6***	✖	✖				✖	×	✖				
Parkview Regional, Vicksburg[1]	2,157	14.9	12.7								×				
Pearl River County, Poplarville	347	11.2	13.6			–		–		–	–	–	–	–	–
Perry County General, Richton	238	15.5	13.5			–		–		–	–		–	–	–
Pontotoc Health Services, Pontotoc[1]	465	15.9	12.9			–		–		–	–	–	–	–	–
Prentiss Regional, Prentiss[1]	409	13.7	15.0	×	×	–		–		–	–	–	–		✖
Quitman County, Marks	501	10.2	10.0			–		–			–	–	–		–
Rankin, Brandon	1,783	14.9	***15.4***	✖	✖	×	✖				✖	✖			✖
Riley, Meridian	3,437	10.6	10.1	★	★				★	★			★	★	
River Oaks, Jackson[1]	1,782	7.9	13.0							–			–		
River Region, Vicksburg[1]	2,319	11.1	10.4	★	★		★								
Rush Foundation, Meridian	4,100	11.0	9.8	★	★				★		★		★	★	★
St Dominic - Jackson, Jackson	7,920	10.6	12.5												
Scott Regional, Morton	830	9.4	10.3			–	✖	–	★	–	–	★	–		
Sharkey Isaquena, Rolling Fork	236	11.0	14.1			–	–	–		–	–	–	–		–

Footnotes are on page 350.

Hospital outcomes: better (★) or worse (×) than average											Results of accreditation review on full survey		Other facts			
Adjusted Death rates			Adjusted Adverse outcome rates													
Surgical cases			Surgical cases													
All selected surgical cases	Coronary artery bypass surgery	Large bowel surgery	All selected surgical cases	Coronary artery bypass surgery	Large bowel surgery	Gall bladder removal	Total knee replacement	Total hip replacement	Simple prostatectomy	Carotid endarterectomy	Accreditation status*	Overall evaluation score (higher is better)	Number of beds	Major medical school affiliation?	Number of residents	Computerized drug order system (1 to 5 scale, higher is preferred; see page 23 for details)
2.3	3.8	6.5	7.7	10.3	11.9	7.5	6.7	6.4	5.4	8.2	–	91	161	–	–	–
–	–	–	–	–	–	–	–	–	–	–	–[2]	–[2]	53	No	0	–
–	–	–	–	–	–	–	–	–	–	–	–[2]	–[2]	32	No	0	–
–	–	–	–	–	–	–	–	–	–	–	–[2]	–[2]	71	No	0	–
–	–	–	–	–	–	–	–	–	–	–	–[2]	–[2]	67	No	0	–
–	–	–	–	–	–	–	–	–	–	–	–[2]	–[2]	64	No	0	–
✖	–	–	✖	–			✖	–	–	–	4	92	163	No	1	–
–	–	–	–	–	–	–	–	–	–	–	–[2]	–[2]	79	No	0	–
								–		✖	4	***88***	335	No	0	–
	✖		✖	✖							4	***81***	639	No	0	–
–	–	–	–	–	–	–	–	–	–	–	4	***86***	818	No	0	–
–	–	–	–	–	–	–	–	–	–	–	–[2]	–[2]	72	No	0	–
–	–	–		–	★	–	✖	–	–	–	4	**94**	101	No	0	–
–	–	–		–		–	–	–	–	–	4	***75***	112	No	0	–
–	–	–	–	–	–	–	–	–	–	–	–[2]	–[2]	48	No	0	–
–	–	–	–	–	–	–	–	–	–	–	–[2]	–[2]	49	No	–	–
×		✖	✖		✖	×			✖	✖	4	89	624	No	0	–
–	–	–	–	–	–	–	–	–	–	–	4	***87***	52	No	0	–
–	–	–	–	–	–	–	–	–	–	–	–[2]	–[2]	44	No	0	–
	–			–			–	–		–	4	**94**	175	No	0	–
–	–	–	–	–	–	–	–	–	–	–	–[2]	–[2]	49	No	0	–
	–	–		–		–	–	–	–	–	4	**95**	96	No	0	–
×	–			–			–	–		–	–[2]	–[2]	197	No	1	–
–	–	–	–	–	–	–	–	–	–	–	–[2]	–[2]	24	No	0	–
–	–	–	–	–	–	–	–	–	–	–	–[2]	–[2]	22	No	0	–
–	–	–	–	–	–	–	–	–	–	–	4	93	27	No	0	–
–	–	–	–	–	–	–	–	–	–	–	–[2]	–[2]	41	No	0	–
–	–	–	–	–	–	–	–	–	–	–	–[2]	–[2]	36	No	0	–
	–	–		–		–	–	–	–	–	5	**99**	90	No	0	–
	–	–		–			–	–	–	–	4	**97**	180	No	0	–
	–	–		–	–	–		–	–	–	4	89	109	No	0	–
	–	–		–	–	–	–	–	–	–	–[2]	–[2]	348	No	0	–
	–			–				–		–	–[2]	–[2]	195	No	0	–
×	✖			✖		✖	★	★			4	90	571	No	0	–
–	–	–	–	–	–	–	–	–	–	–	–[2]	–[2]	30	No	–	–
–	–	–	–	–	–	–	–	–	–	–	–[2]	–[2]	29	No	0	–

***Accreditation Status:** 5=Accredited with commendation or with full standards compliance; 4=Accredited with requirements for improvement; 3=Conditional accreditation.

Detailed Ratings for All Areas

See more information on "Key Ratings for Metro Areas" table beginning on page 32

Blue is most favorable
Bold Italic is least favorable
Blank means neither better nor worse than average
"–" means insufficient data

	Death rates for all selected case types				Hospital outcomes: better (★) or worse (×) than average — Adjusted Death rates — Medical Cases										
	Number of cases	Actual death rate (%)	Adjusted death rate (%) (lower is better)	All selected cases	All selected medical cases	Heart attack	Congestive heart failure	Obstructive pulmonary disease	Pneumonia	Respiratory failure and arrest	Septicemia	Stroke	Gastrointestinal hemorrhage	Fluid, electrolyte, & acid-base disorders	Kidney failure
National Average	–	–	12.1	12.1	14.8	21.2	10.6	6.5	16.9	34.4	25.1	18.4	6.7	11.0	20.9
Mississippi *(continued)*															
Simpson General, Mendenhall	474	14.3	***15.3***	✖	✖	–				–	–		–		–
Singing River, Pascagoula[1]	6,418	9.9	**11.1**	**★**	★							★	★		
South Central Regional, Laurel	3,661	11.8	12.9	×	×		×			✖					
South Panola, Batesville	792	16.7	***17.3***	✖	✖	–	✖		✖	–		✖	–		–
South Sunflower County, Indianola	814	12.3	***14.6***	✖	✖	–		–		–		×	–		–
Southwest Mississippi Regional, McComb	3,241	12.3	11.9			✖			★						
Tallahatchie General, Charleston	209	16.7	14.8			–	–	–		–	–	–	–	–	–
Tippah County, Ripley	1,172	19.7	***16.0***	✖	✖		✖	★	✖	✖				×	–
Trace Regional, Houston[1]	969	10.7	10.6					–		★			–		
Tyler Holmes, Winona	640	15.0	***14.8***	✖	✖	–	✖			–	–		–	×	–
University Hospital - Holmes County, Lexington	756	9.1	11.7			–				–			–	**★**	–
University Hosp - University of Mississippi, Jackson[1]	2,043	14.9	***14.0***	✖	✖						✖	✖			
Walthall County General, Tylertown	832	12.7	13.3			–				–			–	★	
Wayne General, Waynesboro	1,483	13.9	***14.6***	✖	✖	×		✖	✖	–					✖
Webster, Eupora[1]	1,072	14.3	13.6	×	×	✖	✖	–			✖		–		–
Wesley, Hattiesburg	3,669	9.9	***14.4***	✖	✖	✖	✖		✖		×				
Winston, Louisville[1]	599	16.9	***17.8***	✖	✖	✖		–		–		✖	–	✖	–
Woman's Hospital at River Oaks, Jackson	66	–	–	–	–	–	–	–	–	–	–	–	–	–	–
Yalobusha General, Water Valley	300	13.0	15.3	×	×	–	✖	–	★	–	–		–	–	–
Missouri															
Kansas City Area															
Baptist, Kansas City	3,439	14.0	12.5								✖				
Children's Mercy, Kansas City	–	–	–	–	–	–	–	–	–	–	–	–	–	–	–
Independence Regional, Independence	4,406	11.5	12.9	×	×	×		×							
Lee's Summit Hospital, Lee's Summit	2,331	16.0	***16.4***	✖	✖	✖	✖		✖	✖	✖	✖			
Medical Center, Independence	1,744	14.0	***14.1***	✖	✖				✖						×
Research, Kansas City	7,471	10.4	11.6			**★**									
St Joseph, Kansas City[1]	4,991	11.8	11.1	★	**★**	**★**			**★**						
St Luke's, Kansas City	7,310	8.1	**10.7**	**★**	**★**	**★**						**★**		★	
St Luke's Northland, Kansas City	–	–	–	–	–	–	–	–	–	–	–	–	–	–	–
St Mary's, Blue Springs	1,639	13.8	***14.5***	✖	✖				✖					×	✖
Trinity Lutheran, Kansas City	3,180	10.8	**10.7**	**★**	**★**										
Truman, Kansas City	1,478	9.7	**8.7**	**★**	**★**	★		**★**	**★**		★				**★**
Truman - Lakewood, Kansas City	470	17.2	***16.9***	✖	✖	–		✖		–	–	–	–	✖	–

Footnotes are on page 350.

Hospital outcomes: better (★) or worse (×) than average											Results of accreditation review on full survey		Other facts			
Adjusted Death rates			Adjusted Adverse outcome rates													
Surgical cases			Surgical cases													
All selected surgical cases	Coronary artery bypass surgery	Large bowel surgery	All selected surgical cases	Coronary artery bypass surgery	Large bowel surgery	Gall bladder removal	Total knee replacement	Total hip replacement	Simple prostatectomy	Carotid endarterectomy	Accreditation status*	Overall evaluation score (higher is better)	Number of beds	Major medical school affiliation?	Number of residents	Computerized drug order system (1 to 5 scale, higher is preferred; see page 23 for details)
2.3	3.8	6.5	7.7	10.3	11.9	7.5	6.7	6.4	5.4	8.2	–	91	161	–	–	–
–	–	–	–	–	–	–	–	–	–	–	–²	–²	49	No	0	–
			✖						✖	✖	5	**98**	273	No	0	–
	–			–			★	–		–	4	92	201	No	0	–
–	–	–	–	–	–	–	–	–	–	–	–²	–²	70	No	0	–
–	–	–	–	–	–	–	–	–	–	–	4	92	69	No	0	–
✕	–			–			–	–		–	4	93	120	No	0	–
–	–	–	–	–	–	–	–	–	–	–	–²	–²	16	No	0	–
–	–	–	–	–	–	–	–	–	–	–	4	**97**	70	No	0	–
–	–	–	–	–	–	–	–	–	–	–	4	**94**	84	No	0	–
–	–	–	–	–	–	–	–	–	–	–	–²	–²	49	No	0	–
–	–	–	–	–	–	–	–	–	–	–	4	91	80	No	0	–
✖	–	–		✖		–		–	–	–	4	**86**	613	**Yes**	336	–
–	–	–	–	–	–	–	–	–	–	–	–²	–²	49	No	0	–
–	–	–	–	–	–	–	–	–	–	–	4	**88**	80	No	0	–
–	–	–	–	–	–	–	–	–	–	–	4	90	43	No	0	–
✕	–		✖	–			✖	✖		✖	4	**88**	211	No	0	–
–	–	–	–	–	–	–	–	–	–	–	–²	–²	65	No	0	–
–	–	–	–	–	–	–	–	–	–	–	4	**94**	76	No	0	–
–	–	–	–	–	–	–	–	–	–	–	–²	–²	26	No	0	–
	–					–				–	4	92	242	No	22	–
–	–	–	–	–	–	–	–	–	–	–	4	92	177	–	83	–
			★	★			★		–		–²	–²	259	No	0	–
	–			–		–		–	–	–	5	91	83	No	0	–
	–	–		–		–		–	–	–	4	**88**	99	**Yes**	0	–
		★	✖		✖						4	89	448	No	0	–
			★		★		★				4	**86**	267	No	0	–
★			★	★				★		✕	4	92	480	**Yes**	47	–
–	–	–	–	–	–	–	–	–	–	–	4	92	63	–	0	–
	–	–		–		–		–	–	–	4	**94**	115	No	0	–
						–	✖	–	–	–	4	**87**	304	No	15	–
–	–	–		–	–	–	–	–	–	–	–²	–²	227	**Yes**	0	–
–	–	–	–	–	–	–	–	–	–	–	–²	–²	90	**Yes**	1	–

***Accreditation Status:** 5=Accredited with commendation or with full standards compliance; 4=Accredited with requirements for improvement; 3=Conditional accreditation.

Detailed Ratings for All Areas

See more information on "Key Ratings for Metro Areas" table beginning on page 32

Blue is most favorable
Bold Italic is least favorable
Blank means neither better nor worse than average
"–" means insufficient data

	Death rates for all selected case types			Hospital outcomes: better (★) or worse (×) than average — Adjusted Death rates											
				Medical Cases											
	Number of cases	Actual death rate (%)	Adjusted death rate (%) (lower is better)	All selected cases	All selected medical cases	Heart attack	Congestive heart failure	Obstructive pulmonary disease	Pneumonia	Respiratory failure and arrest	Septicemia	Stroke	Gastrointestinal hemorrhage	Fluid, electrolyte, & acid-base disorders	Kidney failure
National Average	–	–	12.1	12.1	14.8	21.2	10.6	6.5	16.9	34.4	25.1	18.4	6.7	11.0	20.9
Missouri *(continued)*															
St. Louis Area															
Barnes - Jewish, St Louis	15,048	9.9	10.2	★	★	★	★			★		★			★
Barnes - Jewish West County, St Louis	1,625	3.4	9.7	★		–		–	★	–	–		–		–
Cardinal Glennon Children's, St Louis	–	–	–	–	–	–	–	–	–	–	–	–	–	–	–
Christian Northeast, St Louis[1]	9,256	14.5	11.2	★	★		★			★					
Christian Northwest, Florissant[1]	96	9.4	12.6			–	–	–	–	–	–	–	–	–	–
DePaul, Bridgeton	5,293	14.3	11.5					★		★					
Des Peres, St Louis	1,471	14.8	13.5	×	×										×
Forest Park, St Louis	4,811	15.6	12.8	×	×			×					✖		
Missouri Baptist, St Louis	7,146	9.5	11.6												
St Alexius, St Louis	1,810	14.8	11.3												
St Anthony's, St Louis	9,687	12.9	11.8												
St John's Mercy, Creve Coeur	6,609	11.1	11.9											×	
St Louis Children's, St Louis	–	–	–	–	–	–	–	–	–	–	–	–	–	–	–
St Louis ConnectCare, St Louis	159	7.5	6.2	★	★	–	–	–	–	–		–	–	–	–
St Louis University, St Louis	3,199	11.7	10.0	★	★		★		★	★				★	
St Luke's, Chesterfield	8,792	9.9	9.4	★	★	★	★		★	★				★	★
St Mary's, Richmond Heights	6,402	11.4	10.2	★	★		★			★	★	★	★	★	
Southpointe, St Louis	1,545	16.2	11.5					–	★						
SSM St Joseph, Kirkwood	4,042	12.9	11.1	★	★	★				★					
Other Areas															
Audrain, Mexico	3,033	11.9	9.7	★	★		★	★	★	★	★				
Aurora Community, Aurora	856	13.9	9.5	★	★			–	★				–		
Barnes - Jewish St Peters, St Peters	1,411	10.8	12.2					✖							
Barton County, Lamar	661	12.7	11.9					–		–			–		–
Bates County, Butler	1,245	10.8	12.7					–		–	–	✖	–		–
Boone, Columbia	6,048	8.1	10.0	★	★	★			★		★	★			
Bothwell Regional, Sedalia	3,988	10.3	12.0			✖								★	
Breech Regional, Lebanon	983	15.9	***16.1***	✖	✖			✖	×	✖		×	✖		–
Callaway, Fulton	599	16.4	***16.8***	✖	✖	–	✖	–	✖	–			–	–	–
Cameron Community, Cameron	1,101	18.1	***17.3***	✖	✖	✖	✖		✖		–		×		–
Capital Region, Jefferson City[1]	3,959	13.1	10.9	★	★				★					★	
Carroll County, Carrollton	349	16.6	***20.3***	✖	✖	–		✖	✖	–	–	–	–	–	–
Cass, Harrisonville	748	12.2	***16.8***	✖	✖	–			✖	–	–	✖	–		–

Footnotes are on page 350.

Hospital outcomes: better (★) or worse (×) than average											Results of accreditation review on full survey		Other facts			
Adjusted Death rates			Adjusted Adverse outcome rates													
Surgical cases			Surgical cases													
All selected surgical cases	Coronary artery bypass surgery	Large bowel surgery	All selected surgical cases	Coronary artery bypass surgery	Large bowel surgery	Gall bladder removal	Total knee replacement	Total hip replacement	Simple prostatectomy	Carotid endarterectomy	Accreditation status*	Overall evaluation score (higher is better)	Number of beds	Major medical school affiliation?	Number of residents	Computerized drug order system (1 to 5 scale, higher is preferred; see page 23 for details)
2.3	3.8	6.5	7.7	10.3	11.9	7.5	6.7	6.4	5.4	8.2	–	91	161	–	–	–
			✖			✖			✖	✖	3	89	941	**Yes**	761	1
★	–	–	✖	–	–	–	✖	✖	–	–	4	90	81	No	0	1
–	–	–	–	–	–	–	–	–	–	–	4	91	172	–	0	–
✖							★			★	4	**95**	510	No	96	1
–	–	–	–	–	–	–	–	–	–	–	4	**95**	223	No	–	1
✖											4	91	291	No	3	1
	–	–				–	–	–	–	–	–[2]	–[2]	93	**Yes**	4	1
×	–					–			–	–	4	93	268	No	72	1
											4	**87**	370	No	0	1
	–	–		–	★	–	–	–	–	–	5	**94**	163	No	0	1
×			✖	✖	×		✖	✖	★	✖	4	91	588	No	0	1
		★									4	92	876	No	83	4
–	–	–	–	–	–	–	–	–	–	–	4	**94**	235	–	74	–
–	–	–	–	–	–	–	–	–	–	–	–[2]	–[2]	24	No	0	–
						–	–	✖	–		4	**95**	303	**Yes**	478	1
				✖							4	**95**	369	No	39	1
											–[2]	–[2]	410	**Yes**	26	1
–	–	–		–	–	–	–	–	–	–	4	**86**	219	No	2	1
			×			–	✖				4	**94**	169	No	0	1
✖	–	–		–				★	–	–	4	**88**	114	No	0	–
–	–	–	–	–	–	–	–	–	–	–	–[2]	–[2]	27	No	0	–
	–	–		–		–		–	–	–	4	**86**	76	No	0	1
–	–	–	–	–	–	–	–	–	–	–	–[2]	–[2]	42	No	0	–
–	–	–		–	–	–	–	–	–	–	–[2]	–[2]	40	No	0	–
			★	★					★		4	90	316	No	0	–
	–			–			✖		–	★	4	**78**	167	No	0	–
–	–	–		–	–	–	–	–	–	–	3	**82**	41	No	0	–
–	–	–	–	–	–	–	–	–	–	–	4	**98**	31	No	0	–
–	–	–		–	–	–	–	–	–	–	–[2]	–[2]	48	No	0	–
	×					×	★		–	–	4	92	114	**Yes**	8	–
–	–	–	–	–	–	–	–	–	–	–	–[2]	–[2]	50	No	0	–
–	–	–	★	–	–	–	–	–	–	–	4	**85**	37	No	0	–

***Accreditation Status:** 5=Accredited with commendation or with full standards compliance; 4=Accredited with requirements for improvement; 3=Conditional accreditation.

Detailed Ratings for All Areas

See more information on "Key Ratings for Metro Areas" table beginning on page 32

Blue is most favorable
Bold Italic is least favorable
Blank means neither better nor worse than average
"–" means insufficient data

	Death rates for all selected case types			Hospital outcomes: better (★) or worse (×) than average — Adjusted Death rates											
					Medical Cases										
	Number of cases	Actual death rate (%)	Adjusted death rate (%) (lower is better)	All selected cases	All selected medical cases	Heart attack	Congestive heart failure	Obstructive pulmonary disease	Pneumonia	Respiratory failure and arrest	Septicemia	Stroke	Gastrointestinal hemorrhage	Fluid, electrolyte, & acid-base disorders	Kidney failure
National Average	–	–	12.1	12.1	14.8	21.2	10.6	6.5	16.9	34.4	25.1	18.4	6.7	11.0	20.9
Missouri *(continued)*															
Other Areas (continued)															
Cedar County, El Dorado Springs	578	12.5	12.7			–					–		–		×
Citizens, Bolivar	1,752	15.5	***15.8***	✖	✖	✖	×	×	✖		×				×
Columbia Regional, Columbia	2,287	7.8	11.4					✖						**★**	
Cooper County, Boonville	624	16.5	***16.6***	✖	✖			–	✖	–	–	✖	–	×	–
Cox, Springfield[1]	11,580	12.3	12.1			×								★	
Cox-Monett Hospital, Monett	662	11.9	11.5								–		–		–
Crossroads Regional, Wentzville	744	15.2	11.9										–		
Doctor's, Springfield	121	8.3	9.1			–	–	–		–	–	–	–	–	–
Doctors Regional, Poplar Bluff[1]	2,347	12.1	12.1							×					
Excelsior Springs Medical Center, Excelsior Springs	542	15.7	***16.4***	✖	✖	–		–		–	–		–	–	–
Freeman, Joplin[1]	3,879	11.1	***13.4***	✖	✖				✖	×			✖		★
Freeman, Neosho	1,184	15.5	***16.1***	✖	✖		✖	–	✖						–
Gentry County, Albany	565	11.9	13.2					×		–	–		–	–	–
Golden Valley, Clinton	2,282	12.8	***14.5***	✖	✖	✖	✖		✖	–					
Hannibal Regional, Hannibal	3,165	12.7	12.8										✖		×
Harrison County, Bethany	635	11.7	10.1						★		–		–	–	
Heartland Regional, St Joseph	9,609	10.9	**11.1**	**★**	**★**							**★**			
Hedrick, Chillicothe	1,106	12.0	11.7			✖				–				★	✖
Hermann Area, Hermann	259	15.8	***16.1***	✖	✖	–		–		–	–	–	–	–	–
Jefferson, Crystal City	4,285	11.3	**9.6**	**★**	**★**		**★**	★	**★**	**★**				**★**	
John Fitzgibbon, Marshall	1,228	11.2	***14.4***	✖	✖		✖	×			–				
Lafayette Regional, Lexington	1,108	14.2	***15.8***	✖	✖	✖				–		✖			×
Lake Regional, Osage Beach	2,577	12.1	12.7				✖					×	**★**		✖
Liberty Hospital, Liberty	4,104	11.5	12.2				★	✖					★		
Lincoln County, Troy	1,068	11.1	12.6					★			–				–
McCune - Brooks, Carthage	1,165	11.3	11.6												–
Mineral Area Regional, Farmington	1,810	14.8	***14.5***	✖	✖	✖	✖	**★**		✖	✖				✖
Missouri Baptist, Sullivan	964	17.0	***15.1***	✖	✖	✖					✖		–		✖
Missouri Delta, Sikeston	2,427	14.6	***14.6***	✖	✖				✖	✖		×			✖
Missouri Southern, Dexter	720	18.9	***19.8***	✖	✖		✖	✖	✖	–	–	✖	–	✖	–
Moberly Regional, Moberly	1,807	14.4	11.1					×			**★**				
Nevada Regional, Nevada	1,046	14.2	***16.3***	✖	✖		✖		✖	–					✖
North Kansas City Hospital, North Kansas City	5,451	10.4	11.9												
Northeast Regional, Kirksville[1]	2,561	12.1	13.0			✖									

Footnotes are on page 350.

Hospital outcomes: better (★) or worse (×) than average											Results of accreditation review on full survey		Other facts			
Adjusted Death rates – Surgical cases			Adjusted Adverse outcome rates – Surgical cases													
All selected surgical cases	Coronary artery bypass surgery	Large bowel surgery	All selected surgical cases	Coronary artery bypass surgery	Large bowel surgery	Gall bladder removal	Total knee replacement	Total hip replacement	Simple prostatectomy	Carotid endarterectomy	Accreditation status*	Overall evaluation score (higher is better)	Number of beds	Major medical school affiliation?	Number of residents	Computerized drug order system (1 to 5 scale, higher is preferred; see page 23 for details)
2.3	3.8	6.5	7.7	10.3	11.9	7.5	6.7	6.4	5.4	8.2	–	91	161	–	–	–
–	–	–	–	–	–	–	–	–	–	–	–[2]	–[2]	34	No	0	–
	–	–	×	–		–	✖	–	–	–	4	90	74	No	0	–
	–	–		–		–		×	–	–	4	91	265	No	1	–
–	–	–	–	–	–	–	–	–	–	–	4	***86***	25	No	0	–
✖	✖			✖			★		★		–[2]	–[2]	521	**Yes**	172	–
–	–	–	–	–	–	–	–	–	–	–	–[2]	–[2]	53	No	0	–
–	–	–	–	–	–	–	–	–	–	–	4	***87***	67	No	0	1
–	–	–	–	–	–	–	–	–	–	–	–[2]	–[2]	45	No	–	–
	–	–		–				–		–	4	***86***	155	No	0	–
–	–	–	–	–	–	–	–	–	–	–	4	92	24	No	0	–
									–		–[2]	–[2]	237	No	12	–
–	–	–		–	–	–	–	–	–	–	–[2]	–[2]	54	No	0	–
–	–	–	–	–	–	–	–	–	–	–	–[2]	–[2]	25	No	0	–
	–			–	×			–	–	–	4	***95***	94	No	0	–
	–			–			★		✖		4	89	105	No	0	–
–	–	–	–	–	–	–	–	–	–	–	–[2]	–[2]	21	No	0	–
×											4	***83***	292	No	0	–
–	–	–	–	–	–	–	–	–	–	–	4	***88***	80	No	0	–
–	–	–	–	–	–	–	–	–	–	–	–[2]	–[2]	41	No	0	–
	–				★		–	–	–		3	***81***	208	No	0	1
–	–	–		–	–	–	–	–	–	–	–[2]	–[2]	43	No	0	–
–	–	–	–	–	–	–	–	–	–	–	4	92	37	No	0	–
	–	–	★		★	–	★		–	–	4	***96***	84	No	0	–
	–			–				★		×	4	***88***	168	No	0	–
–	–	–		–		–	–	–	–	–	4	91	20	No	0	–
–	–	–		–	–	–	–	–	–	–	–[2]	–[2]	54	No	0	–
–	–	–	★	–	–	–	–	–	–	–	–[2]	–[2]	110	No	9	–
–	–	–	–	–	–	–	–	–	–	–	–[2]	–[2]	40	No	0	–
	–	–		–			–	–	✖	–	4	***83***	140	No	0	–
–	–	–	–	–	–	–	–	–	–	–	–[2]	–[2]	48	No	0	–
	–	–		–	★	–		–	–	–	4	90	92	No	0	–
✖	–	–		–		–	–	–	–	–	5	***98***	71	No	0	–
✖		✖	✖	×						✖	4	***94***	311	No	0	–
	–			–		★		–		✖	–[2]	–[2]	150	**Yes**	23	–

***Accreditation Status:** 5=Accredited with commendation or with full standards compliance; 4=Accredited with requirements for improvement; 3=Conditional accreditation.

Detailed Ratings for All Areas

See more information on "Key Ratings for Metro Areas" table beginning on page 32

Blue is most favorable
Bold Italic is least favorable
Blank means neither better nor worse than average
"–" means insufficient data

	Death rates for all selected case types			Hospital outcomes: better (★) or worse (×) than average — Adjusted Death rates											
					Medical Cases										
	Number of cases	Actual death rate (%)	Adjusted death rate (%) (lower is better)	All selected cases	All selected medical cases	Heart attack	Congestive heart failure	Obstructive pulmonary disease	Pneumonia	Respiratory failure and arrest	Septicemia	Stroke	Gastrointestinal hemorrhage	Fluid, electrolyte, & acid-base disorders	Kidney failure
National Average	–	–	12.1	12.1	14.8	21.2	10.6	6.5	16.9	34.4	25.1	18.4	6.7	11.0	20.9
Missouri *(continued)*															
Other Areas *(continued)*															
Ozarks, West Plains	2,477	14.9	***15.0***	✖	✖	✖	✖	✖	×		✖	×			–
Parkland, Farmington	2,348	15.5	***13.4***	✖	✖	×	×					✖			
Pemiscot, Hayti[1]	1,209	11.2	11.9			✖							–	★	–
Perry County, Perryville	679	13.8	11.6			–		–		–			–	✖	–
Pershing, Brookfield	834	16.5	13.9	×	×		✖			–					–
Phelps County Regional, Rolla	3,271	12.3	12.4			✖				✖			★		
Pike County, Louisiana	683	17.1	***15.3***	✖	✖		✖	–	✖			×	–		–
Ray County, Richmond	991	10.5	9.3	★	★			★	★		✖				–
Ripley County, Doniphan	532	11.7	11.7			–				–	–	–	–	–	–
Sac-Osage, Osceola	850	9.9	11.2							–			–	–	–
St Francis, Cape Girardeau	5,069	11.3	***13.9***	✖	✖		✖		✖						
St Francis, Maryville[1]	1,014	13.3	12.8					–		–			×		
St Francis, Mountain View	391	15.3	***16.8***	✖	✖	–	✖	–		–	–		–	✖	–
St John's Regional, Joplin	8,599	10.4	12.6				×	×							
St John's Regional, Springfield	13,479	11.0	***12.7***	✖	×		✖						✖		
St Johns Mercy, Washington	2,372	12.8	12.7			✖			×	★					
St Joseph, St Charles	3,690	12.7	11.1	★						★	✖		★		
St Joseph West, Lake St Louis	1,242	13.8	12.6					✖					–		
St Luke's Northland, Smithville	1,209	12.9	13.1			✖				✖	✖				–
St Marys, Jefferson City	4,344	11.7	11.9						✖					★	
Salem Memorial, Salem[1]	672	12.4	13.8					–		–	–		–	–	–
Samaritan, Macon	470	14.5	***16.9***	✖	✖	–		–		✖	–	–	–	–	–
Scotland County, Memphis	263	15.2	12.8			–		–		–	–		–	–	–
Skaggs, Branson	2,856	10.7	12.1									×			
South Barry County, Cassville	599	16.4	14.1	×		–				–			–	–	–
Southeast Missouri, Cape Girardeau	4,157	11.0	12.3												✖
Ste Genevieve County, Ste Genevieve	844	10.4	12.2										–		–
Texas County, Houston	1,394	13.1	13.4									×			–
Three Rivers - North Campus, Poplar Bluff	3,099	12.6	***14.7***	✖	✖	✖	✖		✖						✖
Twin Rivers Regional, Kennett	1,186	18.6	***18.4***	✖	✖	✖	✖		✖		✖	✖			×
University of Missouri, Columbia	3,096	10.9	***13.3***	✖	✖			×	✖						
Western Missouri, Warrensburg	1,192	16.2	***16.1***	✖	✖				✖	×	★				✖
Wright, Trenton	646	13.9	***15.2***	✖	✖		✖			–	–		–	✖	–

Footnotes are on page 350.

Hospital outcomes: better (★) or worse (×) than average											Results of accreditation review on full survey		Other facts			
Adjusted Death rates			Adjusted Adverse outcome rates													
Surgical cases			Surgical cases													
All selected surgical cases	Coronary artery bypass surgery	Large bowel surgery	All selected surgical cases	Coronary artery bypass surgery	Large bowel surgery	Gall bladder removal	Total knee replacement	Total hip replacement	Simple prostatectomy	Carotid endarterectomy	Accreditation status*	Overall evaluation score (higher is better)	Number of beds	Major medical school affiliation?	Number of residents	Computerized drug order system (1 to 5 scale, higher is preferred; see page 23 for details)
2.3	3.8	6.5	7.7	10.3	11.9	7.5	6.7	6.4	5.4	8.2	–	91	161	–	–	–
	–		★	–		★	–		–	–	–[2]	–[2]	104	No	0	–
	–	–		–		–	–	–		–	4	92	94	No	0	–
–	–	–	–	–	–	–	–	–	–	–	–[2]	–[2]	109	No	0	–
–	–	–		–	–	–	–	–	–	–	4	93	47	No	0	–
–	–	–	–	–	–	–	–	–	–	–	–[2]	–[2]	29	No	0	–
	–			–		–	✖	–		–	4	93	176	No	0	–
–	–	–	–	–	–	–	–	–	–	–	–[2]	–[2]	31	No	0	–
–	–	–		–		–	–	–	–	–	–[2]	–[2]	39	No	0	–
–	–	–	–	–	–	–	–	–	–	–	–[2]	–[2]	26	No	0	–
–	–	–	–	–	–	–	–	–	–	–	4	92	47	No	0	–
						✖			✖		4	89	238	No	0	–
–	–	–	–	–	–	–	–	–	–	–	4	92	53	No	0	–
–	–	–	–	–	–	–	–	–	–	–	4	97	17	No	0	–
			★	★					★	★	4	87	357	No	0	–
✖					×		★	★		×	4	92	681	No	0	–
	–		★	–		–		–	–		5	96	185	No	–	1
			★	★				–	–		4	92	294	Yes	0	1
–	–	–	★	–	–	–	–	–	–	–	–[2]	–[2]	47	No	0	1
	–	–		–		–	–	–	–	–	–[2]	–[2]	43	Yes	0	–
			★	★		✖	★	–			4	97	157	No	0	–
–	–	–	–	–	–	–	–	–	–	–	–[2]	–[2]	33	No	0	–
–	–	–	–	–	–	–	–	–	–	–	–[2]	–[2]	28	No	0	–
–	–	–	–	–	–	–	–	–	–	–	–[2]	–[2]	32	No	0	–
	–			–				–	–	–	3	79	76	No	0	–
–	–	–	–	–	–	–	–	–	–	–	–[2]	–[2]	18	No	0	–
★			★			★					4	96	220	No	0	–
–	–	–	–	–	–	–	–	–	–	–	–[2]	–[2]	34	No	0	–
–	–	–		–	–	–	–	–	–	–	–[2]	–[2]	66	No	0	–
✖	–			–				–	–	–	4	83	149	No	0	–
–	–	–		–	–	–	–	–	–	–	4	93	116	No	0	–
			✖	✖			✖	–	–	✖	–[2]	–[2]	378	Yes	330	–
✖	–	–		–		–	–	–	–	–	4	94	56	No	0	–
–	–	–	–	–	–	–	–	–	–	–	4	93	34	No	0	–

***Accreditation Status:** 5=Accredited with commendation or with full standards compliance; 4=Accredited with requirements for improvement; 3=Conditional accreditation.

Detailed Ratings for All Areas

See more information on "Key Ratings for Metro Areas" table beginning on page 32

Blue is most favorable
Bold Italic is least favorable
Blank means neither better nor worse than average
"–" means insufficient data

	Death rates for all selected case types			Hospital outcomes: better (★) or worse (×) than average — Adjusted Death rates												
					Medical Cases											
	Number of cases	Actual death rate (%)	Adjusted death rate (%) (lower is better)	All selected cases	All selected medical cases	Heart attack	Congestive heart failure	Obstructive pulmonary disease	Pneumonia	Respiratory failure and arrest	Septicemia	Stroke	Gastrointestinal hemorrhage	Fluid, electrolyte, & acid-base disorders	Kidney failure
National Average	–	–	12.1	12.1	14.8	21.2	10.6	6.5	16.9	34.4	25.1	18.4	6.7	11.0	20.9
Montana															
Barrett, Dillon	574	9.6	10.9			–		–		–			–	–	–
Beartooth, Red Lodge	228	17.1	12.6			–	–	–			–	–	–	–	–
Benefis, Great Falls	5,101	9.0	11.1	★	★				★		★	★			
Big Horn County, Hardin	230	14.3	14.6			✖	–	–		–	–	–	–	–	–
Bozeman Deaconess, Bozeman	1,656	7.4	9.9	★	★				★		★		–		–
Broadwater, Townsend	78	9.0	10.1			–	–	–	–	–	–	–	–	–	–
Central Montana, Lewistown	680	12.6	14.2	×			✖			–	–		–		–
Clark Fork Valley, Plains	356	9.0	11.9			–	★	–		–	–	–	–	–	–
Community, Anaconda	543	10.7	14.3		×	×				–	–	–	–	–	–
Community, Missoula	1,418	10.2	13.3						✖			×			–
Daniels, Scobey	119	12.6	14.8			–	–	–	–	–	–	–	–	–	–
Deaconess Billings Clinic, Billings	5,084	8.8	10.2	★	★	★			★		★	★			
Fallon, Baker[1]	168	12.5	9.1			–	–	–		–	–	–	–	–	–
Glacier County, Cut Bank	205	11.7	15.2			–	–	–		–	–	–	–	–	–
Glendive Medical Center, Glendive	427	14.3	***15.5***	✖	✖	–	–	–		–	✖		–	–	–
Holy Rosary, Miles City	725	13.1	13.8			✖		–						–	–
Kalispell Regional, Kalispell	2,525	8.6	11.7											★	✖
Liberty County, Chester	193	13.0	11.8			–	–	–		–	–	–	–	–	–
Livingston Memorial, Livingston	713	10.8	10.9					–		–			–	–	
Madison Valley, Ennis	151	14.6	10.5			–	–	–	–	–	–		–	–	
Marcus Daly, Hamilton	808	11.9	13.8					✖			–	×	–		–
Marias, Shelby	387	10.1	14.8			–	–	–		–	–	–	–	–	–
Mineral, Superior	162	10.5	11.1			–	–	–		–	–	–	–	–	–
North Valley, Whitefish	634	11.8	13.5							–				–	–
Northern Montana, Havre	1,090	10.4	9.4	★	★	–			★				★		
PHS Indian, Bighorn	85	2.4	3.8	★	★	–	–	–	–	–	–	–	–	–	–
Pondera, Conrad	383	7.8	8.2	★	★	–		–	★	–	–		–	–	–
Rosebud, Forsyth	142	13.4	14.5			–	–	–		–	–	–	–	–	–
Roundup Memorial, Roundup	247	16.2	14.6			–		–		–	–	–	–	✖	–
Ruby Valley, Sheridan	101	17.8	***23.2***	✖	✖	–	–	–	✖	–	–	–	–	–	–
St James, Butte[1]	1,974	13.0	***15.3***	✖	✖		×	✖				✖	★		–
St John's Lutheran, Libby	531	13.2	***16.9***	✖	✖	–				✖	–		✖	–	–
St Joseph, Polson	303	11.6	15.2			–		–		–	–	✖	–	–	–
St Luke, Ronan	245	11.0	12.7			–		–		–	–	–	–	–	–
St Patrick, Missoula[1]	4,008	9.2	11.0	★		★	✖								

Footnotes are on page 350.

Hospital outcomes: better (★) or worse (✕) than average											Results of accreditation review on full survey		Other facts			
Adjusted Death rates			Adjusted Adverse outcome rates													
Surgical cases			Surgical cases													
All selected surgical cases	Coronary artery bypass surgery	Large bowel surgery	All selected surgical cases	Coronary artery bypass surgery	Large bowel surgery	Gall bladder removal	Total knee replacement	Total hip replacement	Simple prostatectomy	Carotid endarterectomy	Accreditation status*	Overall evaluation score (higher is better)	Number of beds	Major medical school affiliation?	Number of residents	Computerized drug order system (1 to 5 scale, higher is preferred; see page 23 for details)
2.3	3.8	6.5	7.7	10.3	11.9	7.5	6.7	6.4	5.4	8.2	–	91	161	–	–	–
–	–	–		–	–	–	–	–	–	–	–[2]	–[2]	23	No	0	–
–	–	–	–	–	–	–	–	–	–	–	–[2]	–[2]	22	No	0	–
	✖			✕				★	✖		4	***81***	330	No	0	–
–	–	–	–	–	–	–	–	–	–	–	–[2]	–[2]	16	No	0	–
	–	–		–		–			–	–	–[2]	–[2]	70	No	0	–
–	–	–	–	–	–	–	–	–	–	–	–[2]	–[2]	44	No	0	–
–	–	–	–	–	–	–	–	–	–	–	–[2]	–[2]	39	No	0	–
–	–	–	–	–	–	–	–	–	–	–	–[2]	–[2]	16	No	0	–
–	–	–	–	–	–	–	–	–	–	–	–[2]	–[2]	25	No	0	–
	–	–		–		–		★	–		4	***88***	117	No	0	–
–	–	–	–	–	–	–	–	–	–	–	–[2]	–[2]	6	No	0	–
★		★	★	★					★	★	4	89	216	No	0	–
–	–	–	–	–	–	–	–	–	–	–	–[2]	–[2]	12	No	0	–
–	–	–	–	–	–	–	–	–	–	–	–[2]	–[2]	59	No	0	–
–	–	–	–	–	–	–	–	–	–	–	4	***86***	26	No	0	–
–	–	–		–	–	–		–	–	–	4	91	44	No	0	–
	–		★	–						★	4	92	150	No	0	–
–	–	–	–	–	–	–	–	–	–	–	–[2]	–[2]	11	No	0	–
–	–	–	★	–		–	–	–	–	–	–[2]	–[2]	32	No	0	–
–	–	–	–	–	–	–	–	–	–	–	–[2]	–[2]	9	No	0	–
–	–	–		–	–	–	–	–	–	–	–[2]	–[2]	48	No	0	–
–	–	–	–	–	–	–	–	–	–	–	–[2]	–[2]	16	No	0	–
–	–	–	–	–	–	–	–	–	–	–	–[2]	–[2]	30	No	0	–
–	–	–	★	–	–	–	–	–	–	–	–[2]	–[2]	43	No	0	–
–	–	–	★	–	★	–	–	–	–	–	–[2]	–[2]	92	No	0	–
–	–	–	–	–	–	–	–	–	–	–	–[2]	–[2]	24	No	0	–
–	–	–	–	–	–	–	–	–	–	–	–[2]	–[2]	20	No	0	–
–	–	–	–	–	–	–	–	–	–	–	–[2]	–[2]	20	No	0	–
–	–	–	–	–	–	–	–	–	–	–	–[2]	–[2]	11	No	0	–
–	–	–	–	–	–	–	–	–	–	–	–[2]	–[2]	8	No	0	–
✖	–	✖	✖	–	✖		–	–		–	4	***85***	100	No	0	–
–	–	–	–	–	–	–	–	–	–	–	–[2]	–[2]	26	No	0	–
–	–	–	–	–	–	–	–	–	–	–	4	**94**	22	No	0	–
–	–	–	–	–	–	–	–	–	–	–	–[2]	–[2]	24	No	0	–
★	★		★	★			★		★	★	4	89	177	No	0	–

***Accreditation Status:** 5=Accredited with commendation or with full standards compliance; 4=Accredited with requirements for improvement; 3=Conditional accreditation.

Detailed Ratings for All Areas

See more information on "Key Ratings for Metro Areas" table beginning on page 32

Blue is most favorable
Bold Italic is least favorable
Blank means neither better nor worse than average
"–" means insufficient data

	Death rates for all selected case types			Hospital outcomes: better (★) or worse (×) than average											
				Adjusted Death rates											
					Medical Cases										
Hospital	Number of cases	Actual death rate (%)	Adjusted death rate (%) (lower is better)	All selected cases	All selected medical cases	Heart attack	Congestive heart failure	Obstructive pulmonary disease	Pneumonia	Respiratory failure and arrest	Septicemia	Stroke	Gastrointestinal hemorrhage	Fluid, electrolyte, & acid-base disorders	Kidney failure
National Average	–	–	12.1	12.1	14.8	21.2	10.6	6.5	16.9	34.4	25.1	18.4	6.7	11.0	20.9
Montana *(continued)*															
St Peter's, Helena	1,990	11.9	***13.8***	✖	✖			✖				×			
St Vincent, Billings[1]	4,590	7.9	10.5 (blue)	★ (blue)	★ (blue)				★ (blue)	★ (blue)	★			★ (blue)	
Sheridan, Plentywood	284	13.0	15.2			–		–	✖	–	–	–	–	–	–
Sidney Health Center, Sidney	798	9.0	9.3 (blue)	★ (blue)	★ (blue)			–	★ (blue)	–			–	★	
Stillwater, Columbus	136	12.5	10.5			–	–	–		–	–	–	–	–	–
USPHS - IHS Blackfeet, Browning	271	6.3	9.8			–	–	–		–	–	–	–	–	–
Wheatland, Harlowton	103	15.5	18.1	×	×	–	–	–	–	–	–	–	–	–	–
Nebraska															
Alegent Health - Bergan Mercy, Omaha[1]	6,612	8.1	9.6 (blue)	★ (blue)	★ (blue)	★			★ (blue)	★ (blue)	★ (blue)	★ (blue)		★ (blue)	
Alegent Health - Immanuel, Omaha	4,543	10.2	***13.1***	✖	✖		✖								✖
Alegent Health - Midlands, Papillion	1,294	15.1	***16.1***	✖	✖	✖	✖						✖		✖
Beatrice Community, Beatrice	722	14.5	***14.9***	✖	✖			–		–	–		–	–	–
Box Butte General, Alliance	388	8.5	10.0			–		–	★	–	–	–	–	–	–
BryanLGH East, Lincoln[1]	8,629	6.9	11.9			★ (blue)	✖				★ (blue)				
Chase County, Imperial	286	12.9	15.5	×	×	–	–	–		–	–	–	–	–	–
Cherry County, Valentine	243	10.3	11.9			–	–	–		–	–	–	–	–	–
Columbus Community, Columbus	1,244	12.9	***15.6***	✖	✖			✖	✖	–		×	✖	–	–
Community, Falls City	607	18.3	***15.9***	✖	✖		×	–		–	–	✖		–	–
Community, McCook	1,057	10.6	***14.5***	✖	✖			–	×	–	–		–		–
Crete Municipal, Crete	289	14.5	***16.4***	✖	✖	–	✖	–	×	–	–	–	–	–	–
Faith Regional, Norfolk	2,553	10.2	***14.4***	✖	✖		✖		✖						✖
Fremont Area, Fremont	2,001	9.4	12.3						×						
Good Samaritan, Kearney[1]	3,813	8.2	10.9	★	★ (blue)										★
Gordon Memorial, Gordon[1]	340	17.1	***17.7***	✖	✖		✖	–		–	–	–	–	–	–
Great Plains Regional, North Platte	1,954	9.8	11.9				×	✖							
Jennie M Melham, Broken Bow	609	14.3	***16.0***	✖	✖	–		✖			–	✖	–	–	–
Johnson County, Tecumseh	205	18.0	***18.7***	✖	✖	–	–	–		–	–	–	–	–	–
Mary Lanning, Hastings	2,269	10.5	13.3	×	✖	✖			×				✖		
Memorial, Blair[1]	601	18.8	***17.8***	✖	✖		×	–	×	–	–		✖	–	✖
Memorial, Sidney	578	13.0	***15.8***	✖	✖			–	✖	–	–		–	–	–
Nebraska Methodist, Omaha	4,695	9.6	***14.5***	✖	✖	×	✖		×				×		
NHS University, Omaha	4,473	11.9	***14.2***	✖	✖		✖	✖	✖	✖					
Ogallala Community, Ogallala	320	15.6	***17.3***	✖	✖	–		–	✖	–	–	×	–	–	–
Osmond General, Osmond	396	14.4	13.1			–	×	–		–	–		–	–	–
Pender Community, Pender	531	13.4	***16.8***	✖	✖	–	×	–	✖	–	–		–		–

Footnotes are on page 350.

Hospital outcomes: better (★) or worse (×) than average											Results of accreditation review on full survey		Other facts			
Adjusted Death rates			Adjusted Adverse outcome rates													
Surgical cases			Surgical cases													
All selected surgical cases	Coronary artery bypass surgery	Large bowel surgery	All selected surgical cases	Coronary artery bypass surgery	Large bowel surgery	Gall bladder removal	Total knee replacement	Total hip replacement	Simple prostatectomy	Carotid endarterectomy	Accreditation status*	Overall evaluation score (higher is better)	Number of beds	Major medical school affiliation?	Number of residents	Computerized drug order system (1 to 5 scale, higher is preferred; see page 23 for details)
2.3	3.8	6.5	7.7	10.3	11.9	7.5	6.7	6.4	5.4	8.2	–	91	161	–	–	–
	–	–	★	–		–			–	–	–²	–²	55	No	0	–
★	★		★	★						★	4	**84**	221	No	0	–
–	–	–	–	–	–	–	–	–	–	–	–²	–²	93	No	0	–
–	–	–	★	–	–	–	–	–	–	–	–²	–²	42	No	0	–
–	–	–	–	–	–	–	–	–	–	–	–²	–²	13	No	0	–
–	–	–	–	–	–	–	–	–	–	–	4	92	25	No	0	–
–	–	–	–	–	–	–	–	–	–	–	–²	–²	18	No	1	–
							×				4	**87**	308	No	0	–
	★								–		4	92	334	No	0	–
–	–	–		–		–	–	–	–	–	4	**88**	151	No	0	–
–	–	–		–	–	–	–		–	–	4	91	48	**Yes**	0	–
–	–	–	–	–	–	–	–	–	–	–	4	**82**	44	No	0	–
						✖				★	4	91	488	No	0	–
–	–	–	–	–	–	–	–	–	–	–	–²	–²	25	No	0	–
–	–	–	–	–	–	–	–	–	–	–	–²	–²	27	No	0	–
	–	–	★	–		–		–	–	–	4	91	52	No	0	–
–	–	–	–	–	–	–	–	–	–	–	–²	–²	35	No	0	–
–	–	–		–	–	–		–	–	–	4	**88**	44	No	0	–
–	–	–	–	–	–	–	–	–	–	–	–²	–²	35	No	0	–
	–			–					★		3	**82**	126	No	0	–
	–	–	★	–		–	★	★		–	4	**88**	97	No	0	–
				★		✖					4	**88**	247	No	1	–
–	–	–	–	–	–	–	–	–	–	–	–²	–²	40	No	0	–
	–	–		–		–			–	–	4	90	99	No	0	–
–	–	–	–	–	–	–	–	–	–	–	–²	–²	39	No	0	–
–	–	–	–	–	–	–	–	–	–	–	–²	–²	30	No	0	–
★	–	–	★	–		–				–	4	92	137	No	0	–
–	–	–	–	–	–		–	–	–	–	3	**83**	33	No	0	–
–	–	–		–	–	–	–	–	–	–	–²	–²	102	No	1	–
×	✖			✖	★		★				–²	–²	359	**Yes**	0	–
		×			✖				✖		4	**96**	352	**Yes**	350	–
–	–	–	–	–	–	–	–	–	–	–	–²	–²	29	No	0	–
–	–	–	–	–	–	–	–	–	–	–	–²	–²	30	No	0	–
–	–	–	–	–	–	–	–	–	–	–	–²	–²	30	No	0	–

***Accreditation Status:** 5=Accredited with commendation or with full standards compliance; 4=Accredited with requirements for improvement; 3=Conditional accreditation.

Detailed Ratings for All Areas

See more information on "Key Ratings for Metro Areas" table beginning on page 32

Blue is most favorable
Bold Italic is least favorable
Blank means neither better nor worse than average
"–" means insufficient data

	Death rates for all selected case types			Hospital outcomes: better (★) or worse (×) than average — Adjusted Death rates											
					Medical Cases										
	Number of cases	Actual death rate (%)	Adjusted death rate (%) (lower is better)	All selected cases	All selected medical cases	Heart attack	Congestive heart failure	Obstructive pulmonary disease	Pneumonia	Respiratory failure and arrest	Septicemia	Stroke	Gastrointestinal hemorrhage	Fluid, electrolyte, & acid-base disorders	Kidney failure
National Average	–	–	12.1	12.1	14.8	21.2	10.6	6.5	16.9	34.4	25.1	18.4	6.7	11.0	20.9
Nebraska *(continued)*															
Perkins County, Grant	345	8.4	11.2			–		–		–	–	–	–	–	–
Phelps, Holdrege	835	13.4	14.1	×	×						–	✖	–		–
Plainview Public, Plainview	284	7.7	9.2			–		–		–	–	–	–	–	–
Providence, Wayne	496	12.5	13.7					×		–	–	×	–	–	–
Regional West, Scottsbluff	2,659	11.2	***18.0***	✖	✖	✖	✖	✖	✖				✖		
St Elizabeth Regional, Lincoln	2,690	10.1	***13.8***	✖	✖		✖								✖
St Francis, Grand Island	3,468	11.9	***13.9***	✖	✖	×	✖		✖						×
St Joseph, Omaha	3,202	12.1	12.1			★									
Tri-County Area, Lexington[1]	651	16.4	***15.4***	✖	✖	★		–		–			✖	–	
Tri-Valley, Cambridge[1]	368	12.2	13.3			–		–		–	–	–	–	–	–
Valley County, Ord	425	14.1	14.6	×	×	–		–		–	–		–		–
Nevada															
Las Vegas Area															
Boulder City Hospital, Boulder City	639	13.1	13.2			–	✖				–		–	–	–
Desert Springs, Las Vegas	6,059	12.6	12.6			★		✖				✖	✖		
Lake Mead, North Las Vegas	2,077	15.1	13.0					★				✖			
Mountainview, Las Vegas	3,110	13.3	***13.3***	✖	✖		✖								
St Rose Dominican, Henderson	2,995	15.3	***15.5***	✖	✖		✖	✖	✖	✖					
Summerlin, Las Vegas	1,311	15.7	12.1			×									
Sunrise, Las Vegas	10,100	11.7	12.4			★					×				
University, Las Vegas	3,694	10.7	9.2	★	★		★	★	★	★		★		★	★
Valley, Las Vegas	8,015	14.0	***14.7***	✖	✖			✖	✖		✖	✖	✖	✖	✖
Other Areas															
Carson - Tahoe, Carson City	3,547	12.9	***13.3***	✖	✖	×				×		✖			
Churchill, Fallon	1,025	15.6	***14.8***	✖	✖			×				✖	–		–
Grover C Dils, Caliente	130	11.5	14.0			–	–	–	–	–	–	–	–	–	–
Humboldt General, Winnemucca	182	14.3	15.0			–	–	–		–	–	–	–	–	–
Northeastern Nevada Regional, Elko	720	11.4	12.4					–			✖				–
Northern Nevada, Sparks	1,408	12.7	12.3			×		✖							
Nye Regional, Tonopah	116	6.9	7.9			–	–	–		–	–	–	–	–	–
St Marys Regional, Reno	4,287	10.9	10.1	★	★	★		★	★						
South Lyon, Yerington	178	14.0	16.9	×	×	–	–	–		–	–	–	–	–	–
Washoe, Reno[1]	5,382	14.2	***14.2***	✖	✖	★	✖		✖	✖		✖		✖	

Footnotes are on page 350.

Hospital outcomes: better (★) or worse (×) than average											Results of accreditation review on full survey		Other facts			
Adjusted Death rates			Adjusted Adverse outcome rates													
Surgical cases			Surgical cases													
All selected surgical cases	Coronary artery bypass surgery	Large bowel surgery	All selected surgical cases	Coronary artery bypass surgery	Large bowel surgery	Gall bladder removal	Total knee replacement	Total hip replacement	Simple prostatectomy	Carotid endarterectomy	Accreditation status*	Overall evaluation score (higher is better)	Number of beds	Major medical school affiliation?	Number of residents	Computerized drug order system (1 to 5 scale, higher is preferred; see page 23 for details)
2.3	3.8	6.5	7.7	10.3	11.9	7.5	6.7	6.4	5.4	8.2	–	91	161	–	–	–
–	–	–	–	–	–	–	–	–	–	–	–[2]	–[2]	20	No	0	–
–	–	–		–	–	–	–	–	–	–	4	**87**	31	No	0	–
–	–	–	–	–	–	–	–	–	–	–	–[2]	–[2]	19	No	0	–
–	–	–	–	–	–	–	–	–	–	–	–[2]	–[2]	32	No	0	–
	–			–				★			4	90	178	No	0	–
×	✖			✖					–		4	**95**	197	No	0	–
	–		✖	–				✖	✖	–	4	**83**	162	No	0	–
		–					–	–	–		4	**94**	278	**Yes**	0	–
–	–	–	–	–	–	–	–	–	–	–	4	89	25	No	0	–
–	–	–	–	–	–	–	–	–	–	–	–[2]	–[2]	29	No	0	–
–	–	–	–	–	–	–	–	–	–	–	–[2]	–[2]	26	No	0	–
–	–	–	–	–	–	–	–	–	–	–	–[2]	–[2]	20	No	0	–
×										✖	4	**85**	238	No	8	–
✖	–			–		–			–	–	–[2]	–[2]	184	No	0	–
	–			–				–			5	**96**	120	No	0	2
×	–	✖	✖	–					–		4	**96**	143	No	0	–
–	–	–		–	–	–	✖	–	–	–	4	**96**	148	No	1	–
	×										4	**94**	675	No	0	–
								–	–	–	4	**86**	504	**Yes**	0	–
✖	✖								×	✖	4	**94**	365	No	8	–
★	–		★	–		★			–		4	90	124	No	0	–
–	–	–		–		–	–	–	–	–	4	91	40	No	1	–
–	–	–	–	–	–	–	–	–	–	–	–[2]	–[2]	4	No	0	–
–	–	–	–	–	–	–	–	–	–	–	–[2]	–[2]	22	No	0	–
–	–	–		–	–	–	–	–	–	–	4	93	50	No	0	–
	–	–		–		–		–	–		5	**95**	100	No	0	–
–	–	–	–	–	–	–	–	–	–	–	–[2]	–[2]	45	No	0	–
									–		5	**96**	257	No	0	–
–	–	–	–	–	–	–	–	–	–	–	–[2]	–[2]	14	No	0	–
✖		✖	✖			✖	✖		–		4	92	436	**Yes**	46	–

***Accreditation Status:** 5=Accredited with commendation or with full standards compliance; 4=Accredited with requirements for improvement; 3=Conditional accreditation.

Detailed Ratings for All Areas

See more information on "Key Ratings for Metro Areas" table beginning on page 32

Blue is most favorable
Bold Italic is least favorable
Blank means neither better nor worse than average
"–" means insufficient data

	Death rates for all selected case types			Hospital outcomes: better (★) or worse (×) than average											
				Adjusted Death rates											
				Medical Cases											
	Number of cases	Actual death rate (%)	Adjusted death rate (%) (lower is better)	All selected cases	All selected medical cases	Heart attack	Congestive heart failure	Obstructive pulmonary disease	Pneumonia	Respiratory failure and arrest	Septicemia	Stroke	Gastrointestinal hemorrhage	Fluid, electrolyte, & acid-base disorders	Kidney failure
National Average	–	–	12.1	12.1	14.8	21.2	10.6	6.5	16.9	34.4	25.1	18.4	6.7	11.0	20.9
New Hampshire															
Alice Peck Day, Lebanon	265	7.9	12.9			–	–	–	★	–	–	–	–	–	–
Androscoggin Valley, Berlin	996	12.3	11.3						★				★		–
Catholic, Manchester	4,145	11.3	***14.1***	✖	✖	★	✖	✖	×			✖	×		✖
Cheshire, Keene	2,445	13.0	***15.6***	✖	✖		✖	✖	✖					×	✖
Concord Hospital, Concord	4,460	11.1	***13.0***	✖	✖	★	✖		×						
Cottage, Woodsville	679	13.5	12.8					–		–		✖		–	–
Elliot, Manchester	3,070	11.2	***14.6***	✖	✖		✖	✖			✖				
Exeter Hospital, Exeter	2,152	12.2	12.9		×			✖				×			✖
Franklin Regional, Franklin	1,258	14.2	12.6			×	✖	★					–	–	–
Frisbie, Rochester	1,434	12.6	***15.2***	✖	✖			✖			✖	✖			
Huggins, Wolfeboro	918	12.6	12.6							–				–	–
Lakes Region General, Laconia	2,253	10.4	12.9			✖			★	–			★		✖
Littleton Regional, Littleton	687	11.8	14.1		×	✖		–	×	–			–		–
Mary Hitchcock, Lebanon	4,233	9.1	10.1	★	★	★						★		★	
Memorial, North Conway	530	11.9	***15.8***	✖	✖			–		–	–		–	–	–
Monadnock, Peterborough	662	15.4	***17.6***	✖	✖		✖		✖	–	–		–	–	–
New London Hospital, New London[1]	663	11.0	11.7					–		–				–	–
Parkland, Derry	1,172	10.8	10.6								★				
Portsmouth Regional, Portsmouth[1]	2,546	10.3	12.6				×					×			
St Joseph, Nashua	1,977	11.2	11.0												
Southern New Hampshire, Nashua	2,171	13.3	12.6											✖	
Speare, Plymouth	514	17.1	***16.3***	✖	✖	✖	✖	×		–			–	–	–
Valley Regional, Claremont	778	12.2	10.6												–
Weeks, Lancaster[1]	550	12.7	12.7					–		–	–		–		–
Wentworth - Douglass, Dover	2,308	10.7	12.0					×		✖	★				
New Jersey															
Delaware Valley Area															
Cooper, Camden[1]	3,235	11.7	12.6								✖				
Deborah Heart and Lung, Browns Mills	1,682	5.1	9.4	★	★	★			–		–	–	–	–	–
Kennedy - University Medical Center, Cherry Hill	–	–	–	–	–	–	–	–	–	–	–	–	–	–	–
Kennedy - University Medical Center, Stratford	8,989	15.9	12.3					★		✖	×	×			
Kennedy - University Medical Center, Turnersville	–	–	–	–	–	–	–	–	–	–	–	–	–	–	–
Our Lady of Lourdes, Camden	4,955	12.0	12.4				★				×				
Rancocas, Willingboro	3,634	14.9	***13.5***	✖	✖					✖					

Footnotes are on page 350.

Hospital outcomes: better (★) or worse (×) than average											Results of accreditation review on full survey		Other facts			
Adjusted Death rates			Adjusted Adverse outcome rates													
Surgical cases			Surgical cases													
All selected surgical cases	Coronary artery bypass surgery	Large bowel surgery	All selected surgical cases	Coronary artery bypass surgery	Large bowel surgery	Gall bladder removal	Total knee replacement	Total hip replacement	Simple prostatectomy	Carotid endarterectomy	Accreditation status*	Overall evaluation score (higher is better)	Number of beds	Major medical school affiliation?	Number of residents	Computerized drug order system (1 to 5 scale, higher is preferred; see page 23 for details)
2.3	3.8	6.5	7.7	10.3	11.9	7.5	6.7	6.4	5.4	8.2	–	91	161	–	–	–
–	–	–	–	–	–	–	–	–	–	–	–[2]	–[2]	22	No	0	–
–	–	–		–	–	–	–	–	–	–	–[2]	–[2]	64	No	0	–
×		✖	✖		✖	✖	–	–	–		4	***86***	204	No	0	–
	–			–		–		–	–	–	4	92	141	No	0	–
	–		★	★							4	90	179	No	18	–
–	–	–		–	–	–	–	–	–	–	–[2]	–[2]	34	No	0	–
	–			–			×		✖		4	***88***	225	No	0	–
	–			–				–	–	–	5	**96**	80	No	0	–
–	–	–		–	–	–	–	–	–	–	4	**95**	49	No	0	–
	–	–		–		–	–	–	–	–	–[2]	–[2]	70	No	0	–
	–	–		–		–	–	–	–	–	–[2]	–[2]	55	No	0	–
	–			–		–			–		–[2]	–[2]	117	No	0	–
–	–	–	★	–	–	–	–	–	–	–	–[2]	–[2]	49	No	0	–
										★	4	91	315	**Yes**	275	–
–	–	–		–	–	–	–	–	–	–	–[2]	–[2]	35	No	0	–
–	–	–		–	–	–	–	–	–	–	4	92	62	No	0	–
–	–	–		–	–	–	–	–	–	–	4	**99**	35	No	0	–
	–	–		–		–	–	–	–		4	***88***	79	No	0	–
		–				–	★	✖	–	–	4	93	179	No	0	4
	–		★	–		–		–	–		4	92	208	No	0	–
	–	–		–			✖	–	–	–	4	**95**	175	No	3	–
–	–	–	–	–	–	–	–	–	–	–	–[2]	–[2]	28	No	0	–
–	–	–	★	–	–	–	–	–	–	–	–[2]	–[2]	59	No	0	–
–	–	–	–	–	–	–	–	–	–	–	–[2]	–[2]	31	No	0	–
	–			–		–		–	–		–[2]	–[2]	115	No	0	–
					✖	–	–	–	–		4	92	370	**Yes**	44	–
		–	✖	✖	–	–	–	–	–		4	93	161	No	7	–
–	–	–	–	–	–	–	–	–	–	–	–[2]	–[2]	458	–	5	–
	–		✖	–			✖			×	–[2]	–[2]	607	**Yes**	–	–
–	–	–	–	–	–	–	–	–	–	–	–[2]	–[2]	–	–	–	–
✖	✖		✖	✖	×		–	–	✖		4	**96**	349	**Yes**	30	–
	–	✖		–	✖		–	–	✖	–	4	93	237	No	0	–

***Accreditation Status:** 5=Accredited with commendation or with full standards compliance; 4=Accredited with requirements for improvement; 3=Conditional accreditation.

Detailed Ratings for All Areas

See more information on "Key Ratings for Metro Areas" table beginning on page 32

Blue is most favorable
Bold Italic is least favorable
Blank means neither better nor worse than average
"–" means insufficient data

	Death rates for all selected case types				Hospital outcomes: better (★) or worse (×) than average — Adjusted Death rates — Medical Cases											
	Number of cases	Actual death rate (%)	Adjusted death rate (%) (lower is better)	All selected cases	All selected medical cases	Heart attack	Congestive heart failure	Obstructive pulmonary disease	Pneumonia	Respiratory failure and arrest	Septicemia	Stroke	Gastrointestinal hemorrhage	Fluid, electrolyte, & acid-base disorders	Kidney failure
National Average	–	–	12.1	12.1	14.8	21.2	10.6	6.5	16.9	34.4	25.1	18.4	6.7	11.0	20.9
New Jersey *(continued)*															
Delaware Valley Area *(continued)*															
Underwood - Memorial, Woodbury	5,262	13.0	11.6												✖
Virtua, Marlton[1]	–	–	–	–	–	–	–	–	–	–	–	–	–	–	–
Virtua, Mt Holly	5,701	14.5	12.5			✖								★	
Virtua, Voorhees	–	–	–	–	–	–	–	–	–	–	–	–	–	–	–
Virtua West Jersey, Berlin	–	–	–	–	–	–	–	–	–	–	–	–	–	–	–
Northern and Central New Jersey															
Barnert, Paterson	1,230	10.4	**9.2**	**★**	**★**			★	★	**★**	★				
Bayonne Hospital, Bayonne	4,538	10.0	**9.5**	**★**	**★**		**★**	**★**	**★**	**★**	**★**				
Bayshore, Holmdel	5,037	13.8	**11.0**	**★**	**★**		★								**★**
Centrastate, Freehold[1]	4,856	13.4	**10.4**	**★**	**★**		**★**		**★**					★	
Chilton, Pompton Plains	4,412	16.2	12.4						×						
Christ, Jersey City	3,794	11.7	**10.2**	**★**	**★**		**★**					★		**★**	
Christian, Wyckoff	–	–	–	–	–	–	–	–	–	–	–	–	–	–	–
Clara Maass, Belleville[1]	4,742	12.1	**10.1**	**★**	**★**	×	**★**	★	**★**	**★**	★	**★**			
Columbus, Newark	2,469	9.2	**8.8**	**★**	**★**	✖	**★**	**★**	**★**			**★**		★	**★**
East Orange General, East Orange	2,654	11.7	**8.5**	**★**	**★**		**★**		**★**		**★**	**★**	★	**★**	
Englewood Hospital, Englewood	6,298	11.5	**9.7**	**★**	**★**		**★**		**★**		**★**	**★**			**★**
General, Passaic	5,449	10.2	**11.1**	**★**	★	**★**								✖	
Greenville, Jersey City	910	12.0	**9.0**	**★**	**★**		**★**		**★**						–
Hackensack University, Hackensack	12,165	11.0	**10.7**	**★**	**★**	**★**	★					**★**			
Hackettstown Community, Hackettstown	2,348	14.2	11.3			×	✖		**★**	★					
Holy Name, Teaneck	6,402	11.2	**10.4**	**★**	**★**			★	**★**		★	**★**		**★**	
Hospital Center, Orange	3,260	9.7	**8.1**	**★**	**★**		**★**		**★**		**★**	**★**	★		**★**
Hunterdon, Flemington[1]	3,007	12.6	11.5						★						
Irvington General, Irvington	2,399	10.4	**7.7**	**★**	**★**		**★**	★	**★**		**★**	★			★
Jersey City Medical Center, Jersey City	1,360	15.7	**9.7**	**★**	**★**				**★**	**★**					
Jersey Shore, Neptune[1]	7,294	13.8	***13.0***	✖	✖		✖							✖	
JFK, Edison	8,123	11.9	**9.7**	**★**	**★**				**★**		★	**★**			
Meadowlands, Secaucus	1,900	12.1	11.7					★		**★**					
Monmouth, Long Branch	4,614	12.8	**10.8**	**★**	**★**		**★**								
Morristown Memorial, Morristown	8,451	11.4	12.7	×	✖		✖						✖	×	
Mountainside, Montclair	6,842	13.4	11.6							★					
Muhlenberg Regional, Plainfield	5,068	12.8	11.7			×	★	**★**							

Footnotes are on page 350.

Hospital outcomes: better (★) or worse (×) than average											Results of accreditation review on full survey		Other facts			
Adjusted Death rates			Adjusted Adverse outcome rates													
Surgical cases			Surgical cases													
All selected surgical cases	Coronary artery bypass surgery	Large bowel surgery	All selected surgical cases	Coronary artery bypass surgery	Large bowel surgery	Gall bladder removal	Total knee replacement	Total hip replacement	Simple prostatectomy	Carotid endarterectomy	Accreditation status*	Overall evaluation score (higher is better)	Number of beds	Major medical school affiliation?	Number of residents	Computerized drug order system (1 to 5 scale, higher is preferred; see page 23 for details)
2.3	3.8	6.5	7.7	10.3	11.9	7.5	6.7	6.4	5.4	8.2	–	91	161	–	–	–
	–		✖	–		✖	✖	✖			5	94	242	No	12	–
–	–	–	–	–	–	–	–	–	–	–	–[2]	–[2]	157	–	5	–
	–			–				✖			–[2]	–[2]	348	Yes	24	–
–	–	–	–	–	–	–	–	–	–	–	–[2]	–[2]	271	–	12	–
–	–	–	–	–	–	–	–	–	–	–	–[2]	–[2]	104	–	2	–
–	–	–		–		–	–	–	–	–	4	96	182	No	0	–
	–			–		★	–	–	✖	–	4	88	278	No	10	–
	–			–			–	–	✖	–	4	86	155	No	0	–
✖	–	✖		–	✖		–	–			4	93	241	No	0	–
	–			–			✖	–	✖		5	96	256	No	0	–
	–			–			–	–		–	4	86	382	No	0	–
–	–	–	–	–	–	–	–	–	–	–	4	94	–	–	–	–
	–		✖	–		★		–	✖	✖	4	91	644	No	59	–
	–	–		–			–	–		–	–[2]	–[2]	206	No	6	–
×	–	–		–		–	–	–	–	–	4	91	209	No	0	–
	–		✖	–	✖			✖	✖		5	93	318	Yes	28	–
			✖				✖	✖	✖	✖	4	94	303	No	–	2
–	–	–		–		–	–	–	–	–	4	94	86	No	0	–
	★	★	✖			×	✖	✖		✖	5	96	556	Yes	129	–
	–	–		–	✖	–	–		–	–	4	94	106	No	0	–
	–			–				–			4	97	341	No	21	–
	–			–		–	✖	–	–	–	4	91	205	No	0	–
	–			–				–	–		4	94	176	No	18	–
★	–	–		–		–	–	–	–	–	4	92	157	No	3	–
–	–	–		–		–	–	–	–	–	5	91	487	Yes	52	–
				★			×	✖			4	91	1,084	Yes	78	–
★	–	★	✖	–	★		✖		✖	✖	4	97	380	No	35	–
✖	–	–	✖	–				–	–	–	5	96	143	No	1	–
	–		✖	–			✖	✖			5	94	435	Yes	46	–
	★		✖	★	✖	✖				✖	4	99	483	Yes	122	2
	–		✖	–	✖		✖	×	✖	✖	5	99	396	No	–	2
	–		✖	–	×	×		×			–[2]	–[2]	303	No	30	–

***Accreditation Status:** 5=Accredited with commendation or with full standards compliance; 4=Accredited with requirements for improvement; 3=Conditional accreditation.

Detailed Ratings for All Areas

See more information on "Key Ratings for Metro Areas" table beginning on page 32

Blue is most favorable
Bold Italic is least favorable
Blank means neither better nor worse than average
"–" means insufficient data

	Death rates for all selected case types				Hospital outcomes: better (★) or worse (×) than average — Adjusted Death rates — Medical Cases										
	Number of cases	Actual death rate (%)	Adjusted death rate (%) (lower is better)	All selected cases	All selected medical cases	Heart attack	Congestive heart failure	Obstructive pulmonary disease	Pneumonia	Respiratory failure and arrest	Septicemia	Stroke	Gastrointestinal hemorrhage	Fluid, electrolyte, & acid-base disorders	Kidney failure
National Average	–	–	12.1	12.1	14.8	21.2	10.6	6.5	16.9	34.4	25.1	18.4	6.7	11.0	20.9
New Jersey *(continued)*															
Northern and Central New Jersey *(continued)*															
Newark Beth Israel, Newark	3,409	8.9	**8.8**	**★**	**★**		**★**		**★**		**★**	**★**			
Newton Memorial, Newton	3,006	13.8	11.2						**★**	**★**					
Overlook, Summit	6,912	11.9	**10.8**	**★**	**★**				**★**			**★**			
Palisades of New York Presbyterian, North Bergen	3,893	14.2	**10.8**	**★**	**★**		**★**			★			**★**		
Pascack Valley, Westwood	5,279	14.1	12.1												
Passaic Beth Israel, Passaic	2,750	15.1	12.1												✖
Rahway Hospital, Rahway	5,406	13.7	12.7	×	×	✖								✖	
Raritan Bay, Perth Amboy	6,474	14.0	**10.5**	**★**	**★**	✖	**★**		**★**	**★**					**★**
Raritan Bay - Old Bridge Division, Old Bridge	–	–	–	–	–	–	–	–	–	–	–	–	–	–	–
Riverview, Red Bank	5,724	12.6	11.8										✖		
Robert Wood Johnson University, New Brunswick	5,706	10.6	11.4												
St Barnabas, Livingston	7,900	11.7	**10.1**	**★**	**★**		**★**		**★**	★			★		
St Claire's, Sussex[1]	998	12.0	13.5		×								–	✖	–
St Clare's, Dover	3,467	12.5	12.1					×							
St Clares, Denville	4,479	13.0	11.7			✖			**★**		✖	**★**	**★**		
St Francis, Jersey City	2,000	14.2	12.6			✖						**★**		✖	
St James, Newark	1,291	11.4	11.7			✖								×	✖
St Joseph's, Wayne	3,983	16.7	12.8	×	×	✖			✖			★			
St Joseph's Regional, Paterson	6,111	13.7	12.3								×				
St Mary, Hoboken	3,081	10.7	**10.5**	**★**	**★**			**★**	★						
St Mary's, Passaic	1,958	13.4	11.3						★		**★**				
St Michaels, Newark	2,299	9.7	**9.9**	**★**	**★**				**★**		★				
St Peter's University, New Brunswick	5,493	12.5	**11.0**	**★**	**★**		**★**		★				★	×	★
Somerset, Somerville	5,516	13.5	12.3												
Trinitas (East Jersey St), Elizabeth[1]	2,429	13.6	11.3			×	**★**						**★**		
Trinitas (Williamson St), Elizabeth	4,170	11.5	**8.8**	**★**	**★**		**★**	**★**	**★**				**★**		**★**
Union Hospital, Union	4,245	16.6	11.7												
University, Newark	1,348	11.3	**10.1**	**★**	**★**		**★**	**★**		★	✖				**★**
Valley, Ridgewood	10,583	10.5	**10.8**	**★**	**★**	**★**			**★**						
Warren, Phillipsburg	3,304	12.1	12.0				**★**	✖					★		
West Hudson, Kearny	2,244	11.6	**10.5**	**★**	**★**			**★**	★						
Other Areas															
Atlantic City Medical Center, Atlantic City	6,598	13.4	**9.7**	**★**	**★**		**★**	**★**	**★**	**★**	**★**			**★**	

Footnotes are on page 350.

Hospital outcomes: better (★) or worse (×) than average											Results of accreditation review on full survey		Other facts			
Adjusted Death rates			Adjusted Adverse outcome rates													
Surgical cases			Surgical cases													
All selected surgical cases	Coronary artery bypass surgery	Large bowel surgery	All selected surgical cases	Coronary artery bypass surgery	Large bowel surgery	Gall bladder removal	Total knee replacement	Total hip replacement	Simple prostatectomy	Carotid endarterectomy	Accreditation status*	Overall evaluation score (higher is better)	Number of beds	Major medical school affiliation?	Number of residents	Computerized drug order system (1 to 5 scale, higher is preferred; see page 23 for details)
2.3	3.8	6.5	7.7	10.3	11.9	7.5	6.7	6.4	5.4	8.2	–	91	161	–	–	–
		–				–	–	–	–	–	5	94	532	Yes	148	–
	–			–			–	–	–	–	4	90	162	No	0	–
★	–	★		–	★		✖	✖		✖	5	97	490	Yes	83	2
	–			–			–		–	–	4	94	202	No	0	–
	–		✖	–				✖			5	98	214	No	4	–
	–			–		–	–	–	✖	–	4	96	210	No	2	–
	–		✖	–			–	–	×	✖	4	94	236	No	0	–
★	–			–		×	–	–			5	93	365	No	27	–
–	–	–	–	–	–	–	–	–	–	–	–[2]	–[2]	–	–	–	–
	–	★		–							4	96	479	No	–	–
	★		✖		✖			✖	–	✖	5	97	445	Yes	5	–
★	–	★								✖	4	94	581	Yes	147	–
–	–	–	★	–	–	–	–	–	–	–	–[2]	–[2]	106	No	–	–
	–			–			–	–	✖		4	97	512	No	0	–
	–		×	–		✖					4	97	512	Yes	0	–
	–			–		–	–	–	–	–	4	97	161	No	0	–
–	–	–		–	–	–	–	–	–	–	4	93	189	No	3	–
	–			–	×		–	–		–	4	95	146	No	0	–
×	×		✖	✖				–	–		4	95	621	No	141	–
	–			–		★	–	–		–	4	93	223	No	6	–
	–			–			–	–		–	4	93	229	No	0	–
		–				–	–	–	–	✖	4	88	270	No	96	–
	–	★	✖	–		✖		✖	✖		5	96	396	Yes	0	–
	–			–			★			✖	4	92	261	No	20	–
	–		×	–			–	–	–	–	4	93	265	No	0	–
	–			–	×		–	–	–		4	87	284	No	8	4
	–		✖	–			–	✖	✖	–	5	99	148	Yes	49	–
✖	–	–			✖	–	–	–	–	–	5	97	500	Yes	281	–
★	★		✖	★	×	✖	✖	✖			4	93	427	No	0	–
	–			–			–	–	✖		4	91	193	No	5	–
	–			–			–	–		–	4	93	171	No	0	–
	–		✖	–			✖	✖		✖	4	95	399	No	28	–

***Accreditation Status:** 5=Accredited with commendation or with full standards compliance; 4=Accredited with requirements for improvement; 3=Conditional accreditation.

Detailed Ratings for All Areas

See more information on "Key Ratings for Metro Areas" table beginning on page 32

Blue is most favorable
Bold Italic is least favorable
Blank means neither better nor worse than average
"–" means insufficient data

	Death rates for all selected case types			Hospital outcomes: better (★) or worse (×) than average — Adjusted Death rates											
					Medical Cases										
	Number of cases	Actual death rate (%)	Adjusted death rate (%) (lower is better)	All selected cases	All selected medical cases	Heart attack	Congestive heart failure	Obstructive pulmonary disease	Pneumonia	Respiratory failure and arrest	Septicemia	Stroke	Gastrointestinal hemorrhage	Fluid, electrolyte, & acid-base disorders	Kidney failure
National Average	–	–	12.1	12.1	14.8	21.2	10.6	6.5	16.9	34.4	25.1	18.4	6.7	11.0	20.9
New Jersey *(continued)*															
Other Areas *(continued)*															
Burdette Tomlin, Cape May Court House	5,682	14.6	11.5			✖			★ (blue)						
Capital, Trenton	3,146	12.0	9.9 (blue)	★ (blue)	★ (blue)		★ (blue)	★ (blue)	★ (blue)						
Capital - Mercer, Trenton	3,212	12.3	***13.6***	✖	✖	✖			✖						
Community, Toms River	18,206	14.9	10.6 (blue)	★ (blue)	★ (blue)		★ (blue)		★ (blue)	★ (blue)			★ (blue)		★
Elmer Hospital, Elmer	1,448	11.5	10.5	★	★ (blue)		★ (blue)		★		×				
Kimball, Lakewood	7,581	18.5	11.7				★			★ (blue)	×		★ (blue)		
Medical Center, Princeton	4,801	12.2	10.9 (blue)	★ (blue)	★ (blue)				★ (blue)				★		
Memorial Hospital of Salem County, Salem	2,795	14.9	***13.4***	✖	✖					✖		×	★		
Robert Wood Johnson University, Hamilton	3,881	15.1	***13.9***	✖	✖	✖					✖				×
St Francis, Trenton	3,305	12.8	11.2			★ (blue)					×				
Shore, Somers Point	4,503	13.7	12.1							×					
South Jersey, Bridgeton[1]	3,999	13.6	11.9				★						×		
South Jersey - Newcomb, Vineland	2,048	17.2	***14.5***	✖	✖				✖		✖			×	
Southern Ocean County, Manahawkin	4,384	14.5	12.8	×	×				✖						
William B Kessler, Hammonton	1,796	14.1	10.4 (blue)	★ (blue)	★ (blue)				★ (blue)						
New Mexico															
Acoma-Canoncito-Laguna, USPHS, IHS, San Fidel	176	10.8	12.1			–	–	–		–	–	–	–	–	–
Artesia General, Artesia	434	10.8	12.5					–		–	–		–		–
Carlsbad Medical Center, Carlsbad	1,696	14.2	***14.4***	✖	✖		×			×					
Cibola General, Grants	293	12.3	13.9			–	–	–		–	–	–	–	–	–
Eastern New Mexico, Roswell	2,536	13.2	***14.7***	✖	✖				✖			✖			
Espanola Hospital, Espanola	911	11.7	12.6							–				–	–
Gallup Indian, Gallup	705	8.7	12.2			–		–		–	–	–	–		–
Gerald Champion Regional, Alamogordo	1,851	12.5	***13.8***	✖	✖	✖									
Gila Regional, Silver City	1,457	11.1	12.0						★					✖	
Guadalupe County, Santa Rosa	92	5.4	7.7			–	–	–	–	–	–	–	–	–	–
Heart Hospital of New Mexico, Albuquerque	526	4.6	6.9 (blue)	★ (blue)	★ (blue)	★ (blue)		–	–	–	–	–	–	–	–
Holy Cross, Taos	978	9.7	10.7					–		–				–	–
Lea Regional, Hobbs	1,634	11.9	9.9 (blue)	★ (blue)	★ (blue)			★ (blue)				★			
Lincoln County, Ruidoso	324	16.4	14.7			–	–	–		–	–		–	–	–
Los Alamos Medical Center, Los Alamos	463	14.5	***15.7***	✖	✖		–	–	×	–			–	–	–
Lovelace, Albuquerque[1]	3,070	11.8	***13.8***	✖	✖	★		✖	✖					✖	
Memorial, Las Cruces	4,599	12.2	***14.4***	✖	✖		×	×	✖				×	✖	

Footnotes are on page 350.

Hospital outcomes: better (★) or worse (×) than average											Results of accreditation review on full survey		Other facts			
Adjusted Death rates			Adjusted Adverse outcome rates													
Surgical cases			Surgical cases													
All selected surgical cases	Coronary artery bypass surgery	Large bowel surgery	All selected surgical cases	Coronary artery bypass surgery	Large bowel surgery	Gall bladder removal	Total knee replacement	Total hip replacement	Simple prostatectomy	Carotid endarterectomy	Accreditation status*	Overall evaluation score (higher is better)	Number of beds	Major medical school affiliation?	Number of residents	Computerized drug order system (1 to 5 scale, higher is preferred; see page 23 for details)
2.3	3.8	6.5	7.7	10.3	11.9	7.5	6.7	6.4	5.4	8.2	–	91	161	–	–	–
	–		✖	–				–	✖	–	4	92	206	No	0	–
	–	–	×	–			–	–	✖	–	4	93	375	No	–	–
	–		✖	–	✖		✖		✖		–[2]	–[2]	344	No	–	–
	–		✖	–							4	91	465	No	0	–
	–	–		–			–	–	–	–	–[2]	–[2]	91	No	–	–
	–			–			✖		–	–	4	96	300	No	0	–
	–			–							5	97	299	Yes	0	–
	–			–		✖	–	–	–	–	4	94	122	No	0	2
	–		✖	–	✖		–	–	✖	–	4	96	160	No	0	–
★	★			★		★	✖	–			–[2]	–[2]	158	No	17	–
	–		×	–				–		×	4	92	179	No	0	–
	–			–				–	–	✖	4	89	340	No	0	–
	–	–		–		–	–	–	–	–	–[2]	–[2]	139	No	4	–
	–			–		★	–	–			5	98	120	No	0	–
	–	–		–			–	–	–	–	4	98	93	No	2	–
–	–	–	–	–	–	–	–	–	–	–	4	95	15	No	0	–
–	–	–	–	–	–	–	–	–	–	–	–[2]	–[2]	20	No	0	–
	–	–					★	–	–	–	4	82	73	No	0	–
–	–	–	–	–	–	–	–	–	–	–	4	84	22	No	0	–
×	–		★	–			★	–			4	92	168	No	6	–
–	–	–		–	–	–	–	–	–	–	4	95	80	No	0	–
–	–	–		–	–	–	–	–	–	–	4	85	79	No	5	–
×	–	–		–					–	–	4	81	73	No	0	–
	–	–		–		–	–	–		–	4	88	67	No	0	–
–	–	–	–	–	–	–	–	–	–	–	–[2]	–[2]	12	No	0	–
	–	–			–	–	–	–	–	–	4	90	55	No	–	–
–	–	–		–	–	–	–	–	–	–	4	88	34	No	0	–
	–	–		–		–	–	–	–	–	4	83	141	No	1	–
–	–	–	–	–	–	–	–	–	–	–	4	85	27	No	0	–
–	–	–	–	–	–	–	–	–	–	–	4	89	47	No	1	–
	★			★	✖				–	–	4	94	119	No	0	–
✖			✖							✖	4	96	243	No	7	–

***Accreditation Status:** 5=Accredited with commendation or with full standards compliance; 4=Accredited with requirements for improvement; 3=Conditional accreditation.

Detailed Ratings for All Areas

See more information on "Key Ratings for Metro Areas" table beginning on page 32

Blue is most favorable
Bold Italic is least favorable
Blank means neither better nor worse than average
"–" means insufficient data

	Death rates for all selected case types				Hospital outcomes: better (★) or worse (×) than average — Adjusted Death rates — Medical Cases											
	Number of cases	Actual death rate (%)	Adjusted death rate (%) (lower is better)	All selected cases	All selected medical cases	Heart attack	Congestive heart failure	Obstructive pulmonary disease	Pneumonia	Respiratory failure and arrest	Septicemia	Stroke	Gastrointestinal hemorrhage	Fluid, electrolyte, & acid-base disorders	Kidney failure
National Average	–	–	12.1	12.1	14.8	21.2	10.6	6.5	16.9	34.4	25.1	18.4	6.7	11.0	20.9
New Mexico *(continued)*															
Mimbres, Deming	937	13.1	13.6										✖	×	–
Miners' Colfax, Raton	576	13.5	13.6							–			–		–
Nor-Lea General, Lovington	221	10.9	12.9			–	–	–		–	–	–	–	–	–
Northeastern Regional, Las Vegas	1,228	13.3	13.1												–
Northern Navajo, Shiprock	640	8.8	11.4			–		–		–	–	–	–		–
PHS Indian, Crownpoint	132	6.8	9.4			–	–	–		–	–	–	–	–	–
PHS Santa Fe Indian, Santa Fe	162	9.9	11.7			–	–	–		–	–	–	–	–	–
Plains Regional, Clovis	2,448	12.7	***17.2***	✖	✖		✖		✖	✖	✖	✖	✖		×
Presbyterian, Albuquerque[1]	6,615	9.3	10.9	★	★	★	✖	★					★	★	
Presbyterian Kaseman, Albuquerque	1,637	10.8	11.5												–
Rehoboth McKinley Christian, Gallup[1]	841	7.8	8.9	★	★				★	–			–		
St Joseph, Albuquerque[1]	4,132	11.9	12.2			★									
St Joseph Northeast Heights, Albuquerque	1,140	9.3	10.3	★	★				★						–
St Joseph West Mesa, Albuquerque	654	12.1	14.6	×	×			–		–	×		–	–	–
St Vincent, Santa Fe	2,358	12.0	***14.7***	✖	✖				✖	×			✖		
San Juan Regional, Farmington	2,952	11.7	12.1												
Union County General, Clayton	277	13.4	12.8			–	★	–		–	–	–	–	–	–
University, Albuquerque	1,578	14.3	***15.1***	✖	✖			×		–			✖		
Zuni PHS Indian, Zuni	136	8.8	9.1			–	–	–		–	–	–	–	–	–
New York															
Buffalo Area															
Bertrand Chaffee, Springville	939	13.6	10.7				★			–					–
Children's, Buffalo	–	–	–	–	–	–	–	–	–	–	–	–	–	–	–
Erie County, Buffalo	2,868	17.6	***14.8***	✖	✖	✖			✖	✖				×	
Kaleida Health - Buffalo General, Buffalo[1]	13,538	10.4	***12.7***	✖	✖				✖		✖				
Kaleida Hlth - Millard Filmore Suburban, Williamsville	–	–	–	–	–	–	–	–	–	–	–	–	–	–	–
Kalieda Hlth - Millard Filmore - Gates Circle, Buffalo[1]	–	–	–	–	–	–	–	–	–	–	–	–	–	–	–
Kenmore Mercy, Kenmore	5,013	12.1	***13.5***	✖	✖	✖						✖		✖	
Mercy, Buffalo	6,849	13.8	***13.2***	✖	✖	✖	✖				✖			✖	
Our Lady of Victory, Lackawanna	3,038	13.4	12.6				★		✖	×		★		✖	
Roswell Park Cancer Institute, Buffalo	454	13.0	14.9	×	×	–	–	–		–	–	–	–		–
St Joseph, Cheektowaga	4,245	13.6	11.5			★								✖	×
Sheehan, Buffalo	438	7.1	8.2	★	★			–	–	★	–	★	–	–	–
Sisters of Charity, Buffalo	4,478	12.2	11.9												

Footnotes are on page 350.

Hospital outcomes: better (★) or worse (×) than average											Results of accreditation review on full survey		Other facts			
Adjusted Death rates			Adjusted Adverse outcome rates													
Surgical cases			Surgical cases													
All selected surgical cases	Coronary artery bypass surgery	Large bowel surgery	All selected surgical cases	Coronary artery bypass surgery	Large bowel surgery	Gall bladder removal	Total knee replacement	Total hip replacement	Simple prostatectomy	Carotid endarterectomy	Accreditation status*	Overall evaluation score (higher is better)	Number of beds	Major medical school affiliation?	Number of residents	Computerized drug order system (1 to 5 scale, higher is preferred; see page 23 for details)
2.3	3.8	6.5	7.7	10.3	11.9	7.5	6.7	6.4	5.4	8.2	–	91	161	–	–	–
–	–	–		–	–	–	–	–	–	–	–[2]	–[2]	119	No	1	–
–	–	–	–	–	–	–	–	–	–	–	–[2]	–[2]	68	No	0	–
–	–	–	–	–	–	–	–	–	–	–	–[2]	–[2]	28	No	0	–
–	–	–		–	–		–	–	–	–	4	89	54	No	0	–
–	–	–	–	–	–	–	–	–	–	–	4	92	59	No	0	–
–	–	–	–	–	–	–	–	–	–	–	–[2]	–[2]	32	No	0	–
–	–	–	–	–	–	–	–	–	–	–	4	93	39	No	0	–
✖	–	–		–			★	–	✖	–	–[2]	–[2]	74	No	0	–
			★	★							4	***77***	383	No	0	–
–	–	–	★	–	–	–	★		–	–	–[2]	–[2]	138	No	0	–
–	–	–	★	–	–	–	–	–	–	–	4	***87***	118	No	0	–
			★								4	91	179	No	0	–
–	–	–	★	–	–	–	–	–	–	–	–[2]	–[2]	78	No	0	–
–	–	–		–	–	–	–	–	–	–	–[2]	–[2]	52	No	0	–
	–			–			★	×	✖	–	4	89	198	No	6	–
	–			–				–	–	–	4	91	130	No	0	–
–	–	–	–	–	–	–	–	–	–	–	–[2]	–[2]	25	No	0	–
✖	–	✖	✖	–	✖	✖	–	–	–	–	4	91	261	**Yes**	0	–
–	–	–	–	–	–	–	–	–	–	–	4	92	25	No	0	–
–	–	–	–	–	–	–	–	–	–	–	–[2]	–[2]	49	No	1	–
–	–	–	–	–	–	–	–	–	–	–	–[2]	–[2]	313	–	26	–
		–					–	–	–	–	4	***85***	417	**Yes**	0	–
			✖	×			★		✖		4	89	1,310	**Yes**	22	–
–	–	–	–	–	–	–	–	–	–	–	–[2]	–[2]	–	–	–	–
–	–	–	–	–	–	–	–	–	–	–	–[2]	–[2]	588	–	138	–
	–		✖	–				✖			4	91	184	No	5	–
	–		✖	–				✖			4	91	276	No	21	–
	–		✖	–		–		✖	–		–[2]	–[2]	232	No	6	–
–	–	–		–		–	–	–	–	–	4	**96**	119	No	48	–
	–			–							4	**96**	208	No	0	–
–	–	–	–	–	–	–	–	–	–	–	4	***84***	109	No	2	–
	–		✖	–	✖	×		✖		✖	4	***87***	215	No	14	–

***Accreditation Status:** 5=Accredited with commendation or with full standards compliance; 4=Accredited with requirements for improvement; 3=Conditional accreditation.

Detailed Ratings for All Areas

See more information on "Key Ratings for Metro Areas" table beginning on page 32

Blue is most favorable
Bold Italic is least favorable
Blank means neither better nor worse than average
"–" means insufficient data

	Death rates for all selected case types				Hospital outcomes: better (★) or worse (×) than average — Adjusted Death rates — Medical Cases										
	Number of cases	Actual death rate (%)	Adjusted death rate (%) (lower is better)	All selected cases	All selected medical cases	Heart attack	Congestive heart failure	Obstructive pulmonary disease	Pneumonia	Respiratory failure and arrest	Septicemia	Stroke	Gastrointestinal hemorrhage	Fluid, electrolyte, & acid-base disorders	Kidney failure
National Average	–	–	12.1	12.1	14.8	21.2	10.6	6.5	16.9	34.4	25.1	18.4	6.7	11.0	20.9
New York *(continued)*															
New York City, Long Island, and Westchester County															
Allen Pavilion (New York Presbyterian), New York	–	–	–	–	–	–	–	–	–	–	–	–	–	–	–
Bellevue, New York	1,461	9.7	**9.7**	**★**	**★**		**★**								
Beth Israel - Kings Highway Division, Brooklyn	–	–	–	–	–	–	–	–	–	–	–	–	–	–	–
Beth Israel - Petrie Division, New York	13,221	10.6	**8.9**	**★**	**★**	**★**	**★**		**★**	★	**★**	**★**	**★**	**★**	**★**
Beth Israel - Singer Division, New York[1]	–	–	–	–	–	–	–	–	–	–	–	–	–	–	–
Bronx - Lebanon, Bronx	2,565	13.5	**10.4**	**★**	**★**		**★**		★	–					
Brookdale, Brooklyn	4,082	12.3	**10.4**	**★**	**★**						**★**	**★**			
Brookhaven, Patchogue	4,859	16.5	***13.5***	✖	✖	✖		✖	✖					✖	**★**
Brooklyn - Caledonian Campus, Brooklyn	–	–	–	–	–	–	–	–	–	–	–	–	–	–	–
Brooklyn Hospital Center, Brooklyn[1]	5,531	16.4	**10.7**	**★**	**★**	✖	★	★	**★**			**★**			
Brunswick General, Amityville	2,815	15.0	11.4							★					
Cabrini, New York	3,536	9.5	**8.4**	**★**	**★**	**★**	**★**	★	**★**			**★**	★		
Calvary, Bronx	–	–	–	–	–	–	–	–	–	–	–	–	–	–	–
Central Suffolk, Riverhead	2,331	13.9	12.9												
Community, Dobbs Ferry	705	13.9	13.2					★		–	✖		–	✖	–
Coney Island, Brooklyn	2,999	20.0	12.1			✖	★								
Doctors', Staten Island	982	8.9	11.0							–	–		–		–
Eastern Long Island, Greenport	886	12.1	11.8				×						–	–	–
Elmhurst Hospital, Elmhurst[1]	1,817	15.8	13.2	×		✖					✖				
Flushing Hospital, Flushing	4,428	19.9	***12.8***	✖	✖			★	✖						
Franklin, Valley Stream[1]	4,392	15.6	***14.5***	✖	✖		✖	✖				×	✖	✖	
Good Samaritan, West Islip	6,913	14.0	***13.2***	✖	✖	✖	✖	✖					✖	✖	
Harlem, New York	1,624	10.7	**9.5**	**★**	**★**		**★**							★	
Hospital for Joint Diseases, New York	916	0.7	7.2			–	–	–	–	–	–	–	–	–	–
Hospital for Special Surgery, New York	4,002	0.2	**4.0**	**★**	–	–	–	–	–	–	–	–	–	–	–
Hudson Valley, Peekskill	2,409	12.4	12.9						✖						
Huntington Hospital, Huntington	5,269	13.0	**10.8**	**★**	**★**			**★**	★						
Interfaith, Brooklyn	1,277	14.3	**8.7**	**★**	**★**		**★**		**★**		**★**				★
Interfaith - Brooklyn Jewish Division, Brooklyn	–	–	–	–	–	–	–	–	–	–	–	–	–	–	–
Island, Hempstead	1,443	19.4	***15.1***	✖	✖		✖	×	✖					✖	
Jacobi, Bronx	2,097	16.4	11.3				**★**				✖				★
Jamaica Hospital, Jamaica	3,794	16.3	**10.8**	**★**	**★**	**★**	**★**	**★**		★				✖	
John T Mather, Port Jefferson	4,152	14.7	12.5			✖				×			★		
Kings County, Brooklyn	1,395	13.5	12.4			✖	★								

Footnotes are on page 350.

Hospital outcomes: better (★) or worse (×) than average											Results of accreditation review on full survey		Other facts			
Adjusted Death rates			Adjusted Adverse outcome rates													
Surgical cases			Surgical cases													
All selected surgical cases	Coronary artery bypass surgery	Large bowel surgery	All selected surgical cases	Coronary artery bypass surgery	Large bowel surgery	Gall bladder removal	Total knee replacement	Total hip replacement	Simple prostatectomy	Carotid endarterectomy	Accreditation status*	Overall evaluation score (higher is better)	Number of beds	Major medical school affiliation?	Number of residents	Computerized drug order system (1 to 5 scale, higher is preferred; see page 23 for details)
2.3	3.8	6.5	7.7	10.3	11.9	7.5	6.7	6.4	5.4	8.2	–	91	161	–	–	–
–	–	–	–	–	–	–	–	–	–	–	–[2]	–[2]	–	–	–	–
	–	–		–	★	–	–	–	–	–	4	93	771	Yes	320	4
–	–	–	–	–	–	–	–	–	–	–	–[2]	–[2]	–	–	–	–
★		★					★			✖	4	94	1,245	Yes	396	–
–	–	–	–	–	–	–	–	–	–	–	–[2]	–[2]	–	–	–	–
	–	–	✖	–		–	–	–	✖	–	4	93	509	Yes	300	–
×	–	✖	✖	–			–	–	✖	–	4	96	525	Yes	167	–
	–			–		✖	–	–	–		4	93	321	No	0	–
–	–	–	–	–	–	–	–	–	–	–	–[2]	–[2]	–	–	–	–
	–		×	–	✖	–	–	–		–	5	96	653	Yes	242	–
	–		✖	–	✖		✖	–	–	–	4	81	380	No	0	–
	–		✖	–			✖			–	4	90	349	Yes	123	–
–	–	–	–	–	–	–	–	–	–	–	5	99	–	–	–	–
	–		✖	–			✖	–	–	✖	–[2]	–[2]	136	No	7	–
–	–	–		–	–	–	–	–	–	–	5	98	50	No	0	–
	–	–		–		–	–	–	–	–	5	96	406	Yes	114	2
–	–	–		–	–	–	–	–	–	–	4	87	117	No	1	–
–	–	–		–	–	–	–	–	–	–	4	90	80	No	0	–
–	–	–	×	–	–	–	–	–	–	–	–[2]	–[2]	506	Yes	0	4
	–		×	–			–	–		–	–[2]	–[2]	250	Yes	110	–
	–			–			–	–	✖	–	5	96	190	No	17	–
	–		✖	–			–	✖	×	✖	4	94	525	Yes	86	–
–	–	–	✖	–	–	–	–	–	–	–	4	93	297	Yes	163	5
–	–	–		–	–	–			–	–	4	97	163	No	17	5
★	–	–		–	–	–			–	–	4	98	138	Yes	35	–
	–			–		–	–	–	–	–	–[2]	–[2]	92	No	0	–
	–		×	–				✖		–	–[2]	–[2]	263	No	0	–
–	–	–	–	–	–	–	–	–	–	–	–[2]	–[2]	886	No	134	–
–	–	–	–	–	–	–	–	–	–	–	4	89	375	–	106	–
–	–	–	–	–	–	–	–	–	–	–	4	77	213	No	5	–
–	–	–		–		–	–	–	–	–	4	93	545	Yes	225	5
	–	–		–		–	–	–	–	–	4	95	384	No	91	–
	–			–		–	–	–	–	×	4	92	248	No	0	–
–	–	–	–	–	–	–	–	–	–	–	4	93	686	No	395	5

***Accreditation Status:** 5=Accredited with commendation or with full standards compliance; 4=Accredited with requirements for improvement; 3=Conditional accreditation.

Detailed Ratings for All Areas

See more information on "Key Ratings for Metro Areas" table beginning on page 32

Blue is most favorable
Bold Italic is least favorable
Blank means neither better nor worse than average
"–" means insufficient data

	Death rates for all selected case types			Hospital outcomes: better (★) or worse (×) than average — Adjusted Death rates — Medical Cases											
	Number of cases	Actual death rate (%)	Adjusted death rate (%) (lower is better)	All selected cases	All selected medical cases	Heart attack	Congestive heart failure	Obstructive pulmonary disease	Pneumonia	Respiratory failure and arrest	Septicemia	Stroke	Gastrointestinal hemorrhage	Fluid, electrolyte, & acid-base disorders	Kidney failure
National Average	–	–	12.1	12.1	14.8	21.2	10.6	6.5	16.9	34.4	25.1	18.4	6.7	11.0	20.9
New York *(continued)*															
New York City, Long Island, and Westchester County *(continued)*															
Kingsbrook Jewish, Brooklyn	3,055	16.4	**10.1**	★	★			★	★		★	★			
Lawrence, Bronxville	4,376	12.5	**10.7**	★	★				★		★				★
Lenox Hill, New York	7,441	7.6	**8.8**	★	★		★	★	★		★	★	★	★	★
Lincoln Medical and Mental Health, Bronx	2,083	9.6	**9.7**	★	★		★	★		–					
Long Beach Medical Center, Long Beach	3,425	17.7	12.7												
Long Island College, Brooklyn	4,297	12.2	**9.1**	★	★		★	★	★	★		★	★		
Long Island Jewish, New Hyde Park	8,163	12.4	11.5			★	★		✖			★			
Lutheran, Brooklyn	4,411	13.3	**9.9**	★	★		★	★		★		★			
Maimonides, Brooklyn	10,914	11.8	**8.8**	★	★	★	★	★	★		★	★			
Mary Immaculate (St Vincent Catholic), Jamaica	–	–	–	–	–	–	–	–	–	–	–	–	–	–	–
Massapequa General, Seaford	1,889	13.9	12.3			×								★	
Memorial Sloan - Kettering Cancer, New York	2,554	12.1	**10.6**	★		✖	✖			★	★				
Mercy, Rockville Centre	5,242	13.2	**10.8**	★	★								★		★
Metropolitan, New York	1,332	8.8	**8.0**	★	★		★	★					–		★
Montefiore, Bronx	13,092	13.9	11.6												★
Montefiore - Jackie Weiler, Bronx	–	–	–	–	–	–	–	–	–	–	–	–	–	–	–
Mt Sinai, New York[1]	9,945	10.9	**11.2**	★		★					×	★		×	★
Mt Sinai of Queens, Long Island City[1]	–	–	–	–	–	–	–	–	–	–	–	–	–	–	–
Mt Vernon Hospital, Mt Vernon	1,800	10.2	**7.6**	★	★	★	★	★	★		★			★	
Nassau University, East Meadow[1]	2,121	23.6	***15.3***	✖	✖	✖		★	✖			✖		✖	✖
New Island, Bethpage	2,553	11.2	11.0		★		★								
New York, Brooklyn	2,838	13.7	11.4							★					★
New York Hospital of Queens, Flushing	8,434	15.0	***14.6***	✖	✖		×	×	✖		✖	✖			
New York Methodist, Brooklyn	8,056	13.0	**9.6**	★	★		★	★	★		★	★	★		★
New York Presbyterian, New York	4,322	11.3	11.5							★	✖	★			
New York United, Port Chester	2,737	11.5	**10.2**	★	★		★	★				★			
New York Weill Cornell of NY Presbyterian, New York[1]	12,187	9.6	**10.4**	★	★	★				★		★			
New York Westchester Square, Bronx	4,142	12.8	11.9						✖		×	★			
North Central Bronx, Bronx	500	9.4	**8.1**	★	★			–	★	–		★	–	–	–
North General, New York	1,470	18.0	***14.9***	✖	✖	✖				✖					
North Shore University, Forest Hills	2,955	15.0	11.9												
North Shore University, Glen Cove	3,974	14.4	12.1											✖	
North Shore University, Manhasset	10,507	10.2	**10.3**	★	★	★				★		★		★	
North Shore University, Plainview	3,979	14.6	12.6			✖									

Footnotes are on page 350.

Hospital outcomes: better (★) or worse (×) than average											Results of accreditation review on full survey		Other facts			
Adjusted Death rates			Adjusted Adverse outcome rates													
Surgical cases			Surgical cases													
All selected surgical cases	Coronary artery bypass surgery	Large bowel surgery	All selected surgical cases	Coronary artery bypass surgery	Large bowel surgery	Gall bladder removal	Total knee replacement	Total hip replacement	Simple prostatectomy	Carotid endarterectomy	Accreditation status*	Overall evaluation score (higher is better)	Number of beds	Major medical school affiliation?	Number of residents	Computerized drug order system (1 to 5 scale, higher is preferred; see page 23 for details)
2.3	3.8	6.5	7.7	10.3	11.9	7.5	6.7	6.4	5.4	8.2	–	91	161	–	–	–
	–			–		–	–	–		–	4	92	864	No	93	–
	–			–							5	96	198	No	0	–
★			✖	×	✖			✖	✖	✖	–[2]	–[2]	600	Yes	191	–
–	–	–		–	–	–	–	–	–	–	4	95	438	Yes	226	5
	–	–		–		–	–	–	–	–	4	92	134	No	32	–
	–		✖	–			✖	–		–	4	96	388	Yes	262	–
		★	✖	×							–[2]	–[2]	802	Yes	500	–
	–		✖	–	✖				–	✖	5	92	415	Yes	138	–
★	★	★	×	✖		★		✖			4	90	626	Yes	352	5
–	–	–	–	–	–	–	–	–	–	–	–[2]	–[2]	–	–	–	–
	–			–		–	–	–	–	–	–[2]	–[2]	122	No	1	–
★	–	★		–		–	–	–	–	–	5	98	437	Yes	252	3
★	–			–			★			–	5	96	327	No	0	–
–	–	–		–		–	–	–	–	–	–[2]	–[2]	325	Yes	178	5
	★			★					✖		4	94	967	Yes	826	5
–	–	–	–	–	–	–	–	–	–	–	–[2]	–[2]	–	–	–	–
★	★	★		×						✖	4	*88*	1,173	Yes	560	2
–	–	–	–	–	–	–	–	–	–	–	4	*88*	208	–	7	–
	–	–		–		–	–	–	–	–	4	*88*	206	No	6	–
–	–	–	×	–	✖	–	–	–	–	–	4	96	1,384	Yes	292	–
	–			–			–	–	–	–	4	90	125	No	0	–
	–			–		–	–	–		–	4	*87*	125	No	0	–
			✖	×			✖	✖	✖	✖	5	96	439	Yes	67	–
	–		✖	–	✖	✖	–	–		✖	4	95	560	No	226	–
	★				✖						–[2]	–[2]	1,346	Yes	537	–
	–		★	–	★		–	–		–	4	*84*	161	No	0	–
★	★		✖						✖	✖	4	91	2,346	Yes	1,114	–
	–			–				–			4	94	205	No	0	–
–	–	–	–	–	–	–	–	–	–	–	5	97	255	No	23	5
✖	–	✖	✖	–	✖	–	–	–	–	–	4	93	160	Yes	47	–
×	–		✖	–		–	✖	–	✖	–	–[2]	–[2]	231	No	8	–
	–			–				★		–	5	97	246	No	21	–
★	★	★							✖		5	98	731	Yes	350	–
	–			–						–	5	99	279	No	7	–

***Accreditation Status:** 5=Accredited with commendation or with full standards compliance; 4=Accredited with requirements for improvement; 3=Conditional accreditation.

Detailed Ratings for All Areas

See more information on "Key Ratings for Metro Areas" table beginning on page 32

Blue is most favorable
Bold Italic is least favorable
Blank means neither better nor worse than average
"–" means insufficient data

	Death rates for all selected case types				Hospital outcomes: better (★) or worse (×) than average — Adjusted Death rates — Medical Cases										
	Number of cases	Actual death rate (%)	Adjusted death rate (%) (lower is better)	All selected cases	All selected medical cases	Heart attack	Congestive heart failure	Obstructive pulmonary disease	Pneumonia	Respiratory failure and arrest	Septicemia	Stroke	Gastrointestinal hemorrhage	Fluid, electrolyte, & acid-base disorders	Kidney failure
National Average	–	–	12.1	12.1	14.8	21.2	10.6	6.5	16.9	34.4	25.1	18.4	6.7	11.0	20.9
New York *(continued)*															
New York City, Long Island, and Westchester County *(continued)*															
North Shore University, Syosset	–	–	–	–	–	–	–	–	–	–	–	–	–	–	–
Northern Westchester, Mt Kisco	2,983	9.9	10.1	★	★			★				★	★		
NYU Downtown, New York	1,954	13.1	9.5	★	★		★	★	★	–					★
NYU Hospital Center, New York	7,889	6.0	7.3	★	★	★	★	★	★		★	★	★		★
Our Lady of Mercy, Bronx[1]	5,596	15.2	9.5	★	★		★	★	★	★		★		★	
Our Lady of Mercy - D'Urso Pavilion, Bronx	–	–	–	–	–	–	–	–	–	–	–	–	–	–	–
Parkway, Forest Hills	5,769	15.3	11.3	★	★								★		★
Peninsula, Far Rockaway	2,885	19.9	***14.0***	✖	✖				✖						
Phelps, North Tarrytown	2,955	11.6	11.6												
Queens, Jamaica	737	12.2	10.7			–				–			–		
St Agnes, White Plains[1]	962	9.6	9.6	★	★	–				–			–		–
St Barnabas, Bronx	2,393	14.3	9.2	★	★		★		★		★			★	
St Catherine of Siena, Smithtown	773	11.0	10.0	★	★		★	–				★	–		
St Charles, Port Jefferson[1]	1,600	12.5	***15.7***	✖	✖		✖		✖	✖				✖	
St Clare's, New York	991	13.9	8.6	★	★		★	–	★	–				★	
St Francis, Roslyn	7,907	5.9	8.3	★	★	★	★	★	★			★	★		
St John's Episcopal - South Shore, Far Rockaway	–	–	–	–	–	–	–	–	–	–	–	–	–	–	–
St John's Queens (St Vincent Catholic), Flushing	–	–	–	–	–	–	–	–	–	–	–	–	–	–	–
St John's Riverside, Yonkers	3,912	9.8	9.0	★	★		★	★	★	★		★			
St Joseph's, Flushing[1]	–	–	–	–	–	–	–	–	–	–	–	–	–	–	–
St Joseph's, Yonkers	2,792	17.1	12.3			✖			✖	★					
St Luke's - Roosevelt - Roosevelt Division, New York	–	–	–	–	–	–	–	–	–	–	–	–	–	–	–
St Luke's - Roosevelt - St Luke's Division, New York	7,536	11.3	9.7	★	★	★	★	★		★		★		★	
St Mary's (St Vincent Catholic), Brooklyn	–	–	–	–	–	–	–	–	–	–	–	–	–	–	–
St Vincent Catholic, Jamaica[1]	12,696	18.0	***13.1***	✖	✖	✖			✖		✖			✖	
St Vincent Catholic of New York, Staten Island	–	–	–	–	–	–	–	–	–	–	–	–	–	–	–
St Vincents, New York	4,585	12.0	11.2	★			★			×	✖				
St Vincents of New York - Bayley Seton, Staten Island	800	15.5	10.0	★	★		★								
Sound Shore of Westchester, New Rochelle	4,055	15.8	11.9			✖							★		
South Nassau, Oceanside	6,517	13.5	12.5			✖			✖						
Southampton Hospital, Southampton	2,252	10.5	11.8				✖			★					
Southside, Bay Shore	3,094	14.0	***13.2***	✖	✖	✖								✖	
Staten Island University - North, Staten Island	7,672	15.9	***13.8***	✖	✖	✖			✖	×	×		×	×	
Staten Island University - South, Staten Island	7,672	15.9	***13.8***	✖	✖	✖			✖	×	×		×	×	

Footnotes are on page 350.

Hospital outcomes: better (★) or worse (×) than average											Results of accreditation review on full survey		Other facts			
Adjusted Death rates			Adjusted Adverse outcome rates													
Surgical cases			Surgical cases													
All selected surgical cases	Coronary artery bypass surgery	Large bowel surgery	All selected surgical cases	Coronary artery bypass surgery	Large bowel surgery	Gall bladder removal	Total knee replacement	Total hip replacement	Simple prostatectomy	Carotid endarterectomy	Accreditation status*	Overall evaluation score (higher is better)	Number of beds	Major medical school affiliation?	Number of residents	Computerized drug order system (1 to 5 scale, higher is preferred; see page 23 for details)
2.3	3.8	6.5	7.7	10.3	11.9	7.5	6.7	6.4	5.4	8.2	–	91	161	–	–	–
–	–	–	–	–	–	–	–	–	–	–	5	**100**	186	–	6	–
★	–	★		–				×		–	4	93	239	No	0	–
	–	–		–		–	–	–	✖	–	4	91	149	**Yes**	61	**5**
★	★		✖	×			★				5	92	718	**Yes**	998	**5**
	–			–			–	–	✖	–	4	***88***	489	**Yes**	153	–
–	–	–	–	–	–	–	–	–	–	–	–[2]	–[2]	–	–	–	–
	–		✖	–		✖	–	–	✖	–	4	***84***	251	No	3	–
	–			–		–	–	–	–	–	4	91	196	No	7	–
★	–	★	×	–					✖	×	5	**96**	235	No	0	–
–	–	–	–	–	–	–	–	–	–	–	4	**94**	266	**Yes**	0	–
–	–	–		–	–	–	–	–	–	–	4	91	142	**Yes**	4	–
–	–	–		–	–	–	–	–	–	–	4	92	458	No	50	–
–	–	–	–	–	–	–	–	–	–	–	–[2]	–[2]	366	No	17	–
	–	–	✖	–		–	✖		–	–	4	92	291	No	11	–
–	–	–	–	–	–	–	–	–	–	–	4	***87***	236	No	9	–
★	★	★		★			–	–	✖	✖	5	**97**	279	No	0	–
–	–	–	–	–	–	–	–	–	–	–	4	93	314	–	22	–
–	–	–	–	–	–	–	–	–	–	–	–[2]	–[2]	–	–	–	–
	–			–			–	–			4	93	237	No	0	–
–	–	–	–	–	–	–	–	–	–	–	–[2]	–[2]	–	–	–	–
	–	–		–			–	–		–	4	91	194	No	32	–
–	–	–	–	–	–	–	–	–	–	–	–[2]	–[2]	–	–	–	–
★			✖	✖					✖		4	***87***	724	**Yes**	242	4
–	–	–	–	–	–	–	–	–	–	–	–[2]	–[2]	–	–	–	–
✖	–			–				–		–	4	89	981	**Yes**	284	–
–	–	–	–	–	–	–	–	–	–	–	4	93	449	–	137	–
★			✖	×	✖	✖		–	✖		4	90	590	**Yes**	143	–
–	–	–		–	–	–	–	–	–	–	–[2]	–[2]	198	**Yes**	3	–
	–		★	–			–			–	4	**95**	257	**Yes**	64	2
	–		✖	–			×		✖	✖	5	**94**	321	No	24	–
	–			–				–	–		4	90	127	No	0	–
	–			–	✖		–	–	–	–	4	**96**	439	No	27	–
	–		✖	–			★		✖		–[2]	–[2]	617	**Yes**	114	2
	–		✖	–			★		✖		–[2]	–[2]	451	**Yes**	99	2

***Accreditation Status:** 5=Accredited with commendation or with full standards compliance; 4=Accredited with requirements for improvement; 3=Conditional accreditation.

Detailed Ratings for All Areas

See more information on "Key Ratings for Metro Areas" table beginning on page 32

Blue is most favorable
Bold Italic is least favorable
Blank means neither better nor worse than average
"–" means insufficient data

	Death rates for all selected case types			Hospital outcomes: better (★) or worse (×) than average											
					Adjusted Death rates										
					Medical Cases										
	Number of cases	Actual death rate (%)	Adjusted death rate (%) (lower is better)	All selected cases	All selected medical cases	Heart attack	Congestive heart failure	Obstructive pulmonary disease	Pneumonia	Respiratory failure and arrest	Septicemia	Stroke	Gastrointestinal hemorrhage	Fluid, electrolyte, & acid-base disorders	Kidney failure
National Average	–	–	12.1	12.1	14.8	21.2	10.6	6.5	16.9	34.4	25.1	18.4	6.7	11.0	20.9
New York *(continued)*															
New York City, Long Island, and Westchester County *(continued)*															
SUNY Downstate, Brooklyn	939	9.4	10.8								–		–		
Union, Bronx	–	–	–	–	–	–	–	–	–	–	–	–	–	–	–
University, Stony Brook	4,440	10.7	**10.9**	**★**	**★**	**★**				***✖***		★			
Victory, Brooklyn	3,653	17.2	***14.0***	***✖***	***✖***				×					***✖***	
Westchester, Valhalla[1]	2,088	9.2	12.0								×		–		
White Plains Hospital, White Plains	4,482	11.2	**10.7**	**★**	**★**							**★**			
Winthrop - University, Mineola	8,933	10.0	**10.4**	**★**	**★**			**★**				★			**★**
Woodhull, Brooklyn	1,719	10.0	**8.9**	**★**	**★**	×	**★**		**★**	**★**					
Wyckoff Heights, Brooklyn	3,198	11.4	**9.3**	**★**	**★**		**★**	**★**	**★**						**★**
Rochester Area															
Genesee, Rochester	4,283	10.4	**10.8**	**★**	**★**						★				**★**
Highland, Rochester	2,953	13.9	***14.3***	***✖***	***✖***	***✖***			***✖***			***✖***			
Lakeside, Brockport	1,476	11.9	12.5			***✖***									
Park Ridge, Rochester	4,858	10.0	11.4									**★**			
Rochester General, Rochester	9,710	8.4	**11.0**	**★**	**★**	**★**				★					
Strong, Rochester	6,293	10.1	11.6				***✖***								
Other Areas															
A O Fox, Oneonta	2,239	11.8	12.8												
Adirondack, Saranac Lake	1,724	9.4	10.7		★										
Albany Medical Center, Albany	4,592	7.8	11.2												★
Albany Memorial, Albany	3,983	12.1	12.0							★					
Albert Lindley Lee, Fulton	1,695	10.9	12.9			×									–
Alice Hyde, Malone	1,582	10.5	13.6	×					***✖***	–		★			–
Amsterdam Memorial, Amsterdam	1,549	12.3	10.8								★				
Arden Hill, Goshen	2,498	14.8	12.3							***✖***			×	★	
Arnot Ogden, Elmira	3,225	11.1	***14.0***	***✖***	***✖***		***✖***		***✖***	***✖***					***✖***
Auburn Memorial, Auburn	4,512	10.5	11.7			**★**		***✖***							
Bassett Hospital of Schoharie County, Cobleskill	802	16.2	***16.0***	***✖***	***✖***	–		***✖***	***✖***	***✖***	–		–		–
Bellevue Woman's, Schenectady	52	–	–	–	–	–	–	–	–	–	–	–	–	–	–
Benedictine, Kingston	2,344	12.2	12.5												
Brooks, Dunkirk	1,527	13.8	***15.1***	***✖***	***✖***		***✖***				–	***✖***		***✖***	×
Canton - Potsdam Hospital, Potsdam	1,610	11.8	13.5	×	×		***✖***								–
Carthage Area, Carthage	823	7.0	**8.2**	**★**	**★**				**★**	–	–		–	–	–

Footnotes are on page 350.

Hospital outcomes: better (★) or worse (×) than average											Results of accreditation review on full survey		Other facts			
Adjusted Death rates – Surgical cases			Adjusted Adverse outcome rates – Surgical cases													
All selected surgical cases	Coronary artery bypass surgery	Large bowel surgery	All selected surgical cases	Coronary artery bypass surgery	Large bowel surgery	Gall bladder removal	Total knee replacement	Total hip replacement	Simple prostatectomy	Carotid endarterectomy	Accreditation status*	Overall evaluation score (higher is better)	Number of beds	Major medical school affiliation?	Number of residents	Computerized drug order system (1 to 5 scale, higher is preferred; see page 23 for details)
2.3	3.8	6.5	7.7	10.3	11.9	7.5	6.7	6.4	5.4	8.2	–	91	161	–	–	–
	–	–			–	–	–	–	–	–	5	**96**	376	**Yes**	133	–
–	–	–	–	–	–	–	–	–	–	–	–[2]	–[2]	197	–	4	–
					✖		–	–	✖		4	89	490	**Yes**	324	–
	–			–			–	–		–	–[2]	–[2]	410	No	33	–
★	★	–				–	–	–	–		3	**94**	641	**Yes**	238	–
★	–	★		–							5	91	307	No	0	–
★	★	★		★				×	✖	✖	5	**97**	502	**Yes**	200	–
–	–	–	–	–	–	–	–	–	–	–	4	**94**	382	No	93	3
	–			–			–	–	–	–	5	**96**	324	No	148	–
	–			–		✖		×			–[2]	–[2]	229	**Yes**	48	–
	–			–							–[2]	–[2]	200	**Yes**	52	–
×	–	–		–		–	–	–	–	–	4	90	72	No	0	–
★	–			–					×	✖	4	***84***	340	No	37	2
	×		✖	×		×		✖	✖	✖	5	**95**	488	No	24	–
		★	✖	✖			★			✖	4	92	651	**Yes**	751	–
	–	–		–				✖	–	×	4	***84***	115	No	0	–
	–			–	×		★		–	–	4	**95**	78	No	0	–
	★		✖	✖	✖				–	★	–[2]	–[2]	558	**Yes**	382	–
	–		★	–					–		4	92	90	No	0	–
✖	–	–		–		–	–		–	–	4	89	67	No	0	–
✖	–	–		–		–	–	–		–	4	89	80	No	0	–
	–	–		–		–	★	–	–	–	4	**94**	82	No	0	**5**
	–	–		–			–	–	–	–	4	91	174	No	4	–
	–			✖		–					4	***87***	207	No	0	–
	–			–				✖	–		4	***88***	164	**Yes**	0	–
–	–	–	–	–	–	–	–	–	–	–	3	***86***	40	No	0	2
–	–	–	–	–	–	–	–	–	–	–	4	93	55	No	0	–
	–			–		–	–	–	–	×	4	***86***	222	**Yes**	2	2
	–			–			★		–	–	4	91	60	No	0	–
	–	–		–			–	–	–	–	4	***83***	94	No	0	–
–	–	–	–	–	–	–	–	–	–	–	4	92	48	No	0	–

***Accreditation Status:** 5=Accredited with commendation or with full standards compliance; 4=Accredited with requirements for improvement; 3=Conditional accreditation.

Detailed Ratings for All Areas

See more information on "Key Ratings for Metro Areas" table beginning on page 32

Blue is most favorable
Bold Italic is least favorable
Blank means neither better nor worse than average
"–" means insufficient data

	Death rates for all selected case types				Hospital outcomes: better (★) or worse (×) than average — Adjusted Death rates — Medical Cases										
	Number of cases	Actual death rate (%)	Adjusted death rate (%) (lower is better)	All selected cases	All selected medical cases	Heart attack	Congestive heart failure	Obstructive pulmonary disease	Pneumonia	Respiratory failure and arrest	Septicemia	Stroke	Gastrointestinal hemorrhage	Fluid, electrolyte, & acid-base disorders	Kidney failure
National Average	–	–	12.1	12.1	14.8	21.2	10.6	6.5	16.9	34.4	25.1	18.4	6.7	11.0	20.9
New York *(continued)*															
Other Areas *(continued)*															
Catskill Regional, Harris	2,206	13.2	10.6	★	★								★		
Cayuga, Ithaca	2,765	12.8	***13.6***	✖	✖		✖	★		✖	★			×	
Champlain Valley Physicians, Plattsburgh	4,507	10.2	11.0	★											★
Chenango, Norwich	1,267	12.2	12.0							✖	–	×	★		
Claxton - Hepburn, Ogdensburg	1,865	12.1	***15.5***	✖	✖	✖			✖		–	×	–		
Clifton Fine, Star Lake	250	3.6	6.2	★	★	–	–	–	–	–	–	–	–	–	–
Clifton Springs Hospital, Clifton Springs	1,522	8.6	10.6												
Columbia, Hudson	3,237	14.0	***13.3***	✖	✖			×				✖			
Community, Hamilton	1,171	10.2	***15.2***	✖	✖		✖			–	–		–		–
Community General, Syracuse	5,620	11.1	12.4					✖							✖
Corning Hospital, Corning	2,745	9.2	10.5	★	★			★	★					★	
Cornwall Hospital, Cornwall	2,135	9.9	8.2	★	★		★	★	★	★	★	★			
Cortland Memorial, Cortland	2,588	12.7	***14.8***	✖	✖	✖	✖	✖	×	–					✖
Crouse, Syracuse	7,208	10.6	***12.9***	✖	✖				✖						
Delaware Valley, Walton	580	8.6	9.2	★	★					–	–	–	–		–
E J Noble - Samaritan, Alexandria Bay	307	12.1	12.5					–		–	–	–	–	–	–
Edward John Noble, Gouverneur	588	8.0	8.9	★	★	–	★				–		–	★	–
Ellenville Community, Ellenville	387	12.9	12.2			✖		–		–	–		–	–	–
Ellis, Schenectady	6,359	9.8	10.7	★	★	★					★				
F F Thompson, Canandaigua[1]	2,317	10.3	11.7				✖								
Faxton - St Luke's - Faxton Campus, Utica[1]	2,612	11.7	11.2						★						
Faxton - St Luke's - St Luke's Campus, Utica[1]	6,068	11.1	10.9	★	★		★	★		★		★			
Geneva General, Geneva	2,418	10.5	10.3	★	★			★		★	★				
Glens Falls Hospital, Glens Falls	5,826	10.7	11.4									✖			
Good Samaritan, Suffern	3,937	13.7	10.3	★	★				★		★	★		×	
Horton, Middletown	3,653	12.9	***13.6***	✖	✖	✖		×							
The Hospital, Sidney	956	10.8	13.3							–	–		–	–	–
Inter Community, Newfane	1,216	14.4	***15.9***	✖	✖	×				×		✖			✖
Ira Davenport, Bath	827	13.8	***16.4***	✖	✖			×		–		×	✖		–
Jones, Wellsville	1,794	10.8	11.2					★			★				
Kingston Hospital, Kingston	2,987	12.2	***13.8***	✖	✖			✖	✖						
Lake Shore, Irving	847	14.5	***17.3***	✖	✖	✖	✖			–			–		–
Lewis County General, Lowville	894	8.8	10.6			✖				–				–	–
Little Falls Hospital, Little Falls	2,300	15.8	***15.9***	✖	✖	✖	×		✖	–			×	✖	–

Footnotes are on page 350.

Hospital outcomes: better (★) or worse (✕) than average											Results of accreditation review on full survey		Other facts			
Adjusted Death rates			Adjusted Adverse outcome rates													
Surgical cases			Surgical cases													
All selected surgical cases	Coronary artery bypass surgery	Large bowel surgery	All selected surgical cases	Coronary artery bypass surgery	Large bowel surgery	Gall bladder removal	Total knee replacement	Total hip replacement	Simple prostatectomy	Carotid endarterectomy	Accreditation status*	Overall evaluation score (higher is better)	Number of beds	Major medical school affiliation?	Number of residents	Computerized drug order system (1 to 5 scale, higher is preferred; see page 23 for details)
2.3	3.8	6.5	7.7	10.3	11.9	7.5	6.7	6.4	5.4	8.2	–	91	161	–	–	–
	–			–			–	–	✕	–	4	93	204	No	0	–
	–			–				–		–	4	**95**	145	No	0	–
	–		★	–		★	★		–	★	4	92	329	No	0	–
	–	–		–		–		–	–	–	4	89	58	No	0	–
★	–	–		–			–	–	–	–	4	**84**	120	No	0	–
–	–	–	–	–	–	–	–	–	–	–	–[2]	–[2]	20	No	0	–
★	–		★	–		–			–		4	**78**	100	No	0	–
	–			–			–	–		–	4	89	131	No	0	–
–	–	–		–	–	✖			–	–	4	90	84	No	0	–
	–			–				★		✖	–[2]	–[2]	219	No	0	–
	–			–				–	–	–	–[2]	–[2]	144	No	5	–
	–	–		–			–	–	–	–	4	**94**	125	No	0	–
	–	–	✕	–	✖		–	–	–	–	4	93	115	No	0	–
	–			–							4	93	455	**Yes**	12	–
–	–	–	–	–	–	–	–	–	–	–	4	89	38	No	1	–
–	–	–	–	–	–	–	–	–	–	–	–[2]	–[2]	54	No	0	–
–	–	–	–	–	–	–	–	–	–	–	4	**86**	47	No	0	–
–	–	–	–	–	–	–	–	–	–	–	–[2]	–[2]	31	No	0	–
★	★				✖						4	92	269	No	0	–
	–		✕	–	✕	–		✖	–	★	4	**85**	113	No	0	–
	–		★	–		–	★	★	–		–[2]	–[2]	166	No	–	–
	–		✕	–							–[2]	–[2]	432	No	5	–
	–		★	–		–	★		–		4	**95**	136	No	0	–
	–			–							4	**87**	410	No	41	–
	–			–				✖	–		–[2]	–[2]	308	No	20	–
	–		✕	–			★			✖	4	93	169	No	0	–
–	–	–	–	–	–	–	–	–	–	–	4	89	47	No	0	–
✖	–	–		–	–	–	–	–	–	–	–[2]	–[2]	71	No	0	–
–	–	–	–	–	–	–	–	–	–	–	4	**87**	186	No	2	–
	–	–	✖	–		–	✖	–	–	–	4	93	70	No	0	–
	–			–						–	4	**94**	152	No	0	–
–	–	–		–	–	–	–	–	–	–	–[2]	–[2]	62	No	0	–
–	–	–	★	–	–	–	–	–	–	–	4	93	54	No	0	–
–	–	–		–		–	–	–	–	–	4	90	100	No	2	–

***Accreditation Status:** 5=Accredited with commendation or with full standards compliance; 4=Accredited with requirements for improvement; 3=Conditional accreditation.

Detailed Ratings for All Areas

See more information on "Key Ratings for Metro Areas" table beginning on page 32

Blue is most favorable
Bold Italic is least favorable
Blank means neither better nor worse than average
"–" means insufficient data

	Death rates for all selected case types				Hospital outcomes: better (★) or worse (×) than average — Adjusted Death rates — Medical Cases											
	Number of cases	Actual death rate (%)	Adjusted death rate (%) (lower is better)	All selected cases	All selected medical cases	Heart attack	Congestive heart failure	Obstructive pulmonary disease	Pneumonia	Respiratory failure and arrest	Septicemia	Stroke	Gastrointestinal hemorrhage	Fluid, electrolyte, & acid-base disorders	Kidney failure
National Average	–	–	12.1	12.1	14.8	21.2	10.6	6.5	16.9	34.4	25.1	18.4	6.7	11.0	20.9
New York *(continued)*															
Other Areas *(continued)*															
Lockport Memorial, Lockport	2,376	12.1	12.8			✖							×		
Mary Imogene Bassett, Cooperstown	3,528	10.2	11.7					×		×				★	
Mary McClellan, Cambridge[1]	720	14.4	***14.9***	✖	✖		✖			–	–	✖		–	–
Massena Memorial, Massena	1,546	14.7	***17.1***	✖	✖	✖			✖		✖	✖	–		–
Medina Memorial, Medina[1]	1,219	14.9	***16.7***	✖	✖	✖	✖	–		✖				–	
Mercy, Port Jervis	1,688	10.7	12.4				×								–
Moses Ludington, Ticonderoga	279	10.0	11.3			–		–		–	–	–	–	–	–
Mt St Mary's, Lewiston	3,028	13.3	***14.6***	✖	✖	✖	✖					✖			
Nathan Littauer, Gloversville[1]	2,388	10.2	12.3												–
Niagara Falls Memorial, Niagara Falls	2,148	13.5	***13.5***	✖	✖	✖		✖			★				
Nicholas Noyes, Dansville	1,553	11.7	12.8							✖				×	
Northern Dutchess, Rhinebeck	1,127	13.5	***14.1***	✖	×	✖					×		–		–
Nyack Hospital, Nyack	4,585	14.2	11.1	★	★						★				
Oneida Healthcare Center, Oneida[1]	1,641	10.0	13.3			✖									–
Oswego Hospital, Oswego	1,845	12.0	13.5	×	✖	✖			×					✖	–
Our Lady of Lourdes, Binghamton	6,045	10.7	10.6	★	★			★	★	★					
Putnam, Carmel	2,508	12.9	11.1						★					✖	
Rome Memorial, Rome	2,715	12.9	***14.7***	✖	✖	✖	×		✖			✖			
St Anthony, Warwick	1,017	13.0	11.6								✖				–
St Clares, Schenectady	4,111	11.7	11.9												
St Elizabeth, Utica	4,244	10.4	11.2				★								
St Francis, Poughkeepsie	3,592	12.8	***13.8***	✖	✖	×			✖					✖	
St James Mercy, Hornell	1,501	10.5	11.2										–		
St Joseph's, Elmira	2,219	10.9	11.1												
St Joseph's, Syracuse	10,544	8.2	10.7	★	★	★					★				
St Luke's, Newburgh	3,186	10.9	10.0	★	★		★			★		★			
St Mary's, Amsterdam	2,459	12.1	10.4	★	★		★				★				
St Peter's, Albany	8,918	11.2	***13.0***	✖	✖		✖	✖					×	✖	★
Samaritan, Troy	3,159	14.5	***14.6***	✖	✖	✖	×				✖	✖		✖	
Samaritan, Watertown	3,684	10.4	12.5							–					
Saratoga Hospital, Saratoga Springs	2,739	11.8	9.9	★	★		★	★	★		★				
Schuyler, Montour Falls	871	11.3	10.6								★		–		–
Seton, Troy[1]	4,605	13.0	***13.4***	✖	✖				×	–		✖		✖	
Soldiers and Sailors, Penn Yan	990	13.1	12.5							×					–

Footnotes are on page 350.

Hospital outcomes: better (★) or worse (✕) than average — Adjusted Death rates, Surgical cases: All selected surgical cases	Adjusted Death rates, Surgical cases: Coronary artery bypass surgery	Adjusted Death rates, Surgical cases: Large bowel surgery	Adjusted Adverse outcome rates, Surgical cases: All selected surgical cases	Adjusted Adverse outcome rates: Coronary artery bypass surgery	Adjusted Adverse outcome rates: Large bowel surgery	Adjusted Adverse outcome rates: Gall bladder removal	Adjusted Adverse outcome rates: Total knee replacement	Adjusted Adverse outcome rates: Total hip replacement	Adjusted Adverse outcome rates: Simple prostatectomy	Adjusted Adverse outcome rates: Carotid endarterectomy	Results of accreditation review on full survey: Accreditation status*	Results of accreditation review on full survey: Overall evaluation score (higher is better)	Other facts: Number of beds	Other facts: Major medical school affiliation?	Other facts: Number of residents	Other facts: Computerized drug order system (1 to 5 scale, higher is preferred; see page 23 for details)
2.3	3.8	6.5	7.7	10.3	11.9	7.5	6.7	6.4	5.4	8.2	–	91	161	–	–	–
	–	–		–			–	–	–		–[2]	–[2]	134	No	3	–
	–			–					–	★	4	89	180	**Yes**	50	–
–	–	–	–	–	–	–	–	–	–	–	4	**80**	114	No	0	–
–	–	–		–	–	–	–	–	–	–	4	93	50	No	0	–
×	–	–		–	✖	–	–	–	–	–	4	**95**	71	No	0	–
	–	–		–		★	–	–	–	–	4	92	141	No	0	–
–	–	–	–	–	–	–	–	–	–	–	4	**82**	39	No	0	–
	–			–				×			4	**87**	179	No	0	–
	–	×		–	✖				×	–	4	90	124	No	0	–
	–			–		–	–	✖		–	–[2]	–[2]	288	No	9	–
	–	–		–		–	–	–		–	4	**80**	49	No	0	–
×	–	–		–	–	–	–	–	–	–	4	91	68	No	0	2
★	–		✖	–			–	–		✖	5	**98**	317	No	0	–
	–	–		–		–	–	–	–	–	4	**94**	101	No	0	–
	–			–	★	–	–	–	–	–	4	**87**	55	No	0	–
	–			–							4	93	184	No	3	–
	–		★	–		–			–	–	4	89	164	No	3	4
	–		✖	–	✖		–	–	–	✖	4	**85**	129	No	0	–
–	–	–		–	–	–	–	–	–	–	4	**97**	73	No	0	–
	–		×	–	✖				✖	–	4	92	200	No	8	2
								–	✖		4	89	172	No	25	–
	–			–	✖				✖	–	4	93	314	No	19	–
–	–	–		–	–	–	–	–	–	–	4	91	136	No	0	–
	–			–		–			–	–	4	**88**	169	No	0	–
★	★		✖				✖	✖			4	**87**	431	**Yes**	59	–
	–			–			–	–	–	✖	4	90	175	No	0	–
	–			–				–		–	–[2]	–[2]	143	No	0	–
							★				4	**97**	442	**Yes**	70	–
	–			–				–		–	4	92	135	No	0	–
	–			–				×	✖	×	4	**79**	178	No	7	–
	–			–				–	–		4	**95**	132	No	0	–
–	–	–		–	–	–	–	–	–	–	–[2]	–[2]	35	No	0	–
	–		✖	–				✖	✖	–	4	91	187	No	6	–
–	–	–		–	–	–	–	–	–	–	4	92	51	No	0	–

***Accreditation Status:** 5=Accredited with commendation or with full standards compliance; 4=Accredited with requirements for improvement; 3=Conditional accreditation.

Detailed Ratings for All Areas

See more information on "Key Ratings for Metro Areas" table beginning on page 32

Blue is most favorable
Bold Italic is least favorable
Blank means neither better nor worse than average
"–" means insufficient data

	Death rates for all selected case types			Hospital outcomes: better (★) or worse (×) than average — Adjusted Death rates — Medical Cases											
	Number of cases	Actual death rate (%)	Adjusted death rate (%) (lower is better)	All selected cases	All selected medical cases	Heart attack	Congestive heart failure	Obstructive pulmonary disease	Pneumonia	Respiratory failure and arrest	Septicemia	Stroke	Gastrointestinal hemorrhage	Fluid, electrolyte, & acid-base disorders	Kidney failure
National Average	–	–	12.1	12.1	14.8	21.2	10.6	6.5	16.9	34.4	25.1	18.4	6.7	11.0	20.9
New York *(continued)*															
Other Areas *(continued)*															
Tri-County, Gowanda	709	15.1	***14.7***	✖	✖			×		–					–
United, Batavia	2,135	13.0	12.6												×
United Health Services, Johnson City[1]	8,602	11.8	***13.1***	✖	✖	★	✖					✖		✖	✖
Upstate Medical University, Syracuse	3,180	10.0	11.5				✖	×				★			
Vassar Brothers, Poughkeepsie	5,353	14.5	12.5					✖							✖
ViaHealth of Wayne, Newark	1,323	13.6	12.7									×			–
Westfield Memorial, Westfield	516	13.4	13.0			–	✖			–	–		–		–
Woman's Christian, Jamestown	4,931	11.5	11.0	★	★	✖	★	★				★			
Wyoming County, Warsaw	1,507	12.3	11.8												
North Carolina															
Charlotte Area															
Carolinas, Charlotte[1]	8,797	10.0	11.7			★	✖					★			
Mercy, Charlotte	4,340	10.1	10.1	★	★	★			★	★				★	
Mercy South, Charlotte	–	–	–	–	–	–	–	–	–	–	–	–	–	–	–
Presbyterian, Charlotte	11,844	13.0	11.8			★			×				★		
Presbyterian, Matthews	1,872	10.1	10.7												★
Presbyterian - Orthopaedic, Charlotte	1,286	0.3	8.3		–	–	–	–	–	–	–	–	–	–	–
University, Charlotte	1,535	13.0	12.1			✖		★							–
Forsyth and Guilford Counties															
Forsyth, Winston-Salem	13,491	13.0	***12.8***	✖	✖		×		✖						
High Point Regional, High Point[1]	7,366	11.1	11.6			★									
Medical Park, Winston-Salem	788	0.3	2.5	★	–	–	–	–	–	–	–	–	–	–	–
Moses H Cone, Greensboro[1]	12,591	11.2	12.0			★		✖	✖						
North Carolina Baptist, Winston-Salem	7,415	14.3	11.2	★	★		★	★						✖	
Wesley Long, Greensboro	2,954	9.8	12.9		✖			✖	×		✖				
Triangle Area															
Duke University, Durham	7,539	11.3	12.0								✖			★	
Durham Regional, Durham	6,376	12.4	***15.1***	✖	✖		✖		✖		✖	×	✖	✖	
Raleigh Community, Raleigh	2,995	11.4	10.4	★	★				★				★		
Rex, Raleigh[1]	9,347	10.1	10.2	★	★	★			★			★		★	★
University of North Carolina, Chapel Hill	5,631	11.0	10.4	★	★				★					★	
Wakemed, Raleigh	8,374	10.6	10.5	★	★		★					★			★
Western Wake, Cary	1,772	11.9	10.2	★	★						★				

Footnotes are on page 350.

Hospital outcomes: better (★) or worse (×) than average											Results of accreditation review on full survey		Other facts			
Adjusted Death rates			Adjusted Adverse outcome rates													
Surgical cases			Surgical cases													
All selected surgical cases	Coronary artery bypass surgery	Large bowel surgery	All selected surgical cases	Coronary artery bypass surgery	Large bowel surgery	Gall bladder removal	Total knee replacement	Total hip replacement	Simple prostatectomy	Carotid endarterectomy	Accreditation status*	Overall evaluation score (higher is better)	Number of beds	Major medical school affiliation?	Number of residents	Computerized drug order system (1 to 5 scale, higher is preferred; see page 23 for details)
2.3	3.8	6.5	7.7	10.3	11.9	7.5	6.7	6.4	5.4	8.2	–	91	161	–	–	–
–	–	–		–	–	–	–	–	–	–	4	84	65	No	0	–
	–	–		–		–		–	–	–	4	84	119	No	0	–
							★			✖	–[2]	–[2]	516	Yes	62	–
		–	✖	✖	×	–	✖		–	✖	4	90	356	Yes	243	–
	–		✖	–			–	–	×	✖	4	91	249	No	0	4
	–	–		–		–	–	–	–	–	4	94	75	No	0	–
–	–	–	–	–	–	–	–	–	–	–	–[2]	–[2]	32	No	0	–
	–	–		–		★				–	4	93	291	No	0	–
	–	–		–		✖	–	–	–	–	4	88	81	No	0	–
✖	✖		✖	✖	✖		★	★		✖	4	95	761	Yes	197	–
						✖		–	–		4	94	224	No	0	–
–	–	–	–	–	–	–	–	–	–	–	–[2]	–[2]	–	–	–	–
							–	–			4	97	551	No	0	–
	–	–		–		–	–	–	–	–	–[2]	–[2]	82	No	0	–
	–	–	★	–	–	–	★	★	–	–	–[2]	–[2]	140	No	3	–
	–	–		–		–	×	–	–	–	4	95	122	No	0	–
			✖		✖	✖				✖	4	95	692	Yes	10	–
											5	97	311	No	0	–
★	–	★	★	–		★	–	–		–	5	97	51	No	8	–
★	★						★		✖	×	4	91	805	No	52	–
		✖	✖	×	✖		✖				4	87	765	Yes	487	–
	–		★	–			★	★	–	★	–[2]	–[2]	309	No	–	–
	★			★					★	✖	4	95	852	Yes	420	–
		×			✖					✖	4	87	213	No	0	–
	–			–					–	–	4	90	164	No	0	–
★					✖						4	92	296	No	0	–
							✖				5	95	677	Yes	474	–
★	★			★		✖			–		5	98	661	Yes	0	–
–	–	–		–		–	–	–	–	–	4	99	92	No	–	–

***Accreditation Status:** 5=Accredited with commendation or with full standards compliance; 4=Accredited with requirements for improvement; 3=Conditional accreditation.

Detailed Ratings for All Areas

See more information on "Key Ratings for Metro Areas" table beginning on page 32

Blue is most favorable
Bold Italic is least favorable
Blank means neither better nor worse than average
"–" means insufficient data

	Death rates for all selected case types				Hospital outcomes: better (★) or worse (×) than average — Adjusted Death rates — Medical Cases											
	Number of cases	Actual death rate (%)	Adjusted death rate (%) (lower is better)	All selected cases	All selected medical cases	Heart attack	Congestive heart failure	Obstructive pulmonary disease	Pneumonia	Respiratory failure and arrest	Septicemia	Stroke	Gastrointestinal hemorrhage	Fluid, electrolyte, & acid-base disorders	Kidney failure
National Average	–	–	12.1	12.1	14.8	21.2	10.6	6.5	16.9	34.4	25.1	18.4	6.7	11.0	20.9
North Carolina *(continued)*															
Other Areas															
Alamance Regional, Burlington	4,959	12.9	***14.6***	✖	✖	✖	✖		✖			✖	★		
Albemarle, Elizabeth City	4,393	11.5	11.4												
Alexander, Taylorsville	561	9.8	8.8	★	★	–		–	★			★	–	★	
Alleghany, Sparta	1,064	12.2	10.2	★	★			★		★			–	★	–
Angel, Franklin	1,751	14.6	***13.6***	✖	✖										
Annie Penn, Reidsville	2,101	11.5	12.7			✖						×			
Anson, Wadesboro	1,125	10.3	8.2	★	★		★		★						–
Ashe, Jefferson[1]	1,343	16.9	***15.8***	✖	✖	✖	✖				✖	✖	✖		✖
Beaufort County, Washington[1]	2,010	11.8	***15.4***	✖	✖	✖		✖			✖	✖			✖
Betsy Johnson Regional, Dunn	1,954	10.6	10.8	★											
Bladen County, Elizabethtown	960	15.7	***14.0***	✖	×				×						–
Blowing Rock Hospital, Blowing Rock[1]	242	15.3	13.0			–	–	–		–	–	–	–	–	–
Brunswick, Supply	1,275	12.6	***14.1***	✖	✖				✖	×					–
Caldwell, Lenoir	2,137	12.4	11.7												
Cape Fear Valley, Fayetteville[1]	6,933	13.2	12.3			★								×	✖
Carteret General, Morehead City	2,934	12.9	***13.7***	✖	✖	✖		✖							
Catawba, Hickory	3,281	11.4	11.0	★	★					★					
Central Carolina, Sanford	2,891	15.3	***14.3***	✖	✖	✖			✖	✖	×				
Charles A Cannon Jr, Linville	1,114	9.1	10.3			–			★		–			★	–
Chatham, Siler City	910	11.3	11.1					–					–		–
Chowan, Edenton	1,282	14.7	***14.4***	✖	✖			–	✖				✖		✖
Cleveland Regional, Shelby	4,724	13.2	***13.8***	✖	✖	✖	×				✖				
Columbus County, Whiteville	3,347	10.8	10.5	★	★					★					
Craven Regional, New Bern[1]	6,522	10.5	12.4												
Davie County, Mocksville	412	13.8	13.5			–		–			–	–	–	–	–
Davis Regional, Statesville	1,976	8.0	8.5	★	★		★	★	★	★					
Duplin General, Kenansville	1,074	15.7	***14.7***	✖	✖				✖	–		✖			
FirstHealth Moore Regional, Pinehurst	9,078	8.5	9.5	★	★	★	★			★		★	★		
FirstHealth Richmond, Rockingham	1,854	10.0	11.0							✖					★
Franklin Regional, Louisburg	1,750	16.1	10.7	★	★		★	★				✖			
Frye Regional, Hickory	5,269	11.7	12.0												
Gaston Memorial, Gastonia	8,458	13.0	***13.9***	✖	✖	×	✖		✖		✖	✖			✖
Good Hope, Erwin	1,595	14.5	***13.7***	✖	✖				✖	–		★			–
Grace, Morganton	2,281	18.1	***16.4***	✖	✖	✖	✖		✖		×			×	✖

Footnotes are on page 350.

Hospital outcomes: better (★) or worse (×) than average											Results of accreditation review on full survey		Other facts			
Adjusted Death rates			Adjusted Adverse outcome rates													
Surgical cases			Surgical cases													
All selected surgical cases	Coronary artery bypass surgery	Large bowel surgery	All selected surgical cases	Coronary artery bypass surgery	Large bowel surgery	Gall bladder removal	Total knee replacement	Total hip replacement	Simple prostatectomy	Carotid endarterectomy	Accreditation status*	Overall evaluation score (higher is better)	Number of beds	Major medical school affiliation?	Number of residents	Computerized drug order system (1 to 5 scale, higher is preferred; see page 23 for details)
2.3	3.8	6.5	7.7	10.3	11.9	7.5	6.7	6.4	5.4	8.2	–	91	161	–	–	–
	–			–					–		4	89	238	No	0	–
	–			–			–	–		–	4	95	150	No	0	–
–	–	–	–	–	–	–	–	–	–	–	4	85	39	No	0	–
–	–	–	–	–	–	–	–	–	–	–	4	86	46	No	0	–
	–	–		–		–		–	–	–	4	90	59	No	0	–
	–	–		–			–	–	–	–	4	89	87	No	0	–
–	–	–	–	–	–	–	–	–	–	–	4	97	30	No	0	–
–	–	–		–	–	–	–	–	–	–	4	84	55	No	0	–
	–			–		–		–	–	–	4	91	103	No	0	–
–	–	–		–	–	✖	–	–	–	–	4	88	62	No	0	–
–	–	–	–	–	–	–	–	–	–	–	4	98	58	No	0	–
–	–	–	–	–	–	–	–	–	–	–	4	93	28	No	0	–
–	–	–		–	–	–	–	–	–	–	4	97	56	No	0	–
	–			–		–	–	–	–	–	4	90	63	No	0	–
×			✖							✖	4	94	619	Yes	0	–
	–			–				–	–	×	4	87	117	No	0	–
	–			–			★				4	92	187	No	0	–
	–	×		–			–	–	–	–	4	92	137	No	0	–
–	–	–		–	–	–	–	–	–	–	4	93	69	No	–	–
–	–	–		–	–	–	–	–	–	–	4	88	35	No	0	–
–	–	–		–		–	✖	–	–	–	4	93	71	No	0	–
×	–	✖		–	×			–			4	94	214	No	0	–
★	–		★	–			★	★	–		4	89	117	No	0	–
			★			✖	★	★	–		4	96	255	No	0	–
–	–	–	–	–	–	–	–	–	–	–	5	99	30	No	0	–
	–	–		–	–			–	–	–	4	92	132	No	1	–
–	–	–		–	–	–	–	–	–	–	4	86	70	No	0	–
★	★		★	★							4	96	371	No	0	–
–	–	–		–	–	–	–	–	–	–	4	94	90	No	0	–
–	–	–		–	–	–	–	–	–	–	–[2]	–[2]	85	No	0	–
			✖			✖		★			–[2]	–[2]	338	No	9	–
	–	✖	✖				✖			✖	5	93	348	No	0	–
–	–	–	–	–	–	–	–	–	–	–	4	89	72	No	0	–
×	–	–		–			–	–		–	4	84	149	No	0	2

***Accreditation Status:** 5=Accredited with commendation or with full standards compliance; 4=Accredited with requirements for improvement; 3=Conditional accreditation.

Detailed Ratings for All Areas

See more information on "Key Ratings for Metro Areas" table beginning on page 32

Blue is most favorable
Bold Italic is least favorable
Blank means neither better nor worse than average
"–" means insufficient data

	Death rates for all selected case types				Hospital outcomes: better (★) or worse (×) than average — Adjusted Death rates — Medical Cases										
	Number of cases	Actual death rate (%)	Adjusted death rate (%) (lower is better)	All selected cases	All selected medical cases	Heart attack	Congestive heart failure	Obstructive pulmonary disease	Pneumonia	Respiratory failure and arrest	Septicemia	Stroke	Gastrointestinal hemorrhage	Fluid, electrolyte, & acid-base disorders	Kidney failure
National Average	–	–	12.1	12.1	14.8	21.2	10.6	6.5	16.9	34.4	25.1	18.4	6.7	11.0	20.9
North Carolina *(continued)*															
Other Areas *(continued)*															
Granville, Oxford	1,207	14.6	13.4		×					–	×				–
Halifax Regional, Roanoke Rapids	3,713	14.7	12.9	×		✖		**★**	×			✖			
Harris Regional, Sylva	2,006	11.7	13.2					**★**	×					✖	–
Haywood Regional, Clyde	2,952	13.2	13.1	×	✖	✖									
Heritage, Tarboro	1,977	12.8	13.1											✖	–
Highlands - Cashiers, Highlands	416	14.2	13.1					–		**★**	–	✖	–	–	–
Hoots, Yadkinville	375	17.9	14.4			✖		–		–		–	–	✖	–
Hugh Chatham, Elkin	1,713	10.3	12.8							–					–
Iredell, Statesville	4,247	11.0	12.7			✖						✖			
J Arthur Dosher, Southport	841	9.3	12.6			–				–			–		–
Johnston, Smithfield	2,355	15.6	***15.5***	✖	✖	✖			✖		×		✖		
Kings Mountain Hospital, Kings Mountain	995	12.1	11.0			✖		**★**		✖	**★**		×		
Lake Norman Regional, Mooresville	2,283	10.7	11.6			✖		★		★	×				
Lenoir, Kinston	4,830	12.4	11.7					★					✖	✖	
Lexington Memorial, Lexington	1,870	13.0	12.6			✖				×				**★**	
Lincoln Medical Center, Lincolnton	1,695	15.8	12.2								**★**				×
Margaret R Pardee, Hendersonville	4,168	11.3	***13.1***	✖	×					✖		✖			✖
Maria Parham, Henderson	2,153	13.4	***13.8***	✖	✖				✖		×				
Martin General, Williamston	1,415	12.4	12.0				★							✖	
McDowell, Marion	1,479	14.9	***15.7***	✖	✖		✖		✖	✖					✖
Memorial Mission, Asheville	11,109	10.3	12.2			**★**			×						
Morehead, Eden	2,806	11.3	13.2	×											
Murphy Medical Center, Murphy	1,405	10.0	10.6						**★**		**★**				×
Nash, Rocky Mount[1]	5,951	12.6	12.5						✖					✖	
New Hanover Regional, Wilmington	10,615	11.5	***13.7***	✖	✖				✖		✖	✖		★	
Northeast, Concord	8,909	11.3	12.1					**★**			✖				**★**
Northern Hospital of Surry County, Mt Airy	2,574	12.5	11.2										★		
Onslow, Jacksonville	2,658	13.4	***13.9***	✖	✖			✖	✖						
Park Ridge, Fletcher	1,773	17.9	11.2												
Pender, Burgaw	896	13.8	***15.8***	✖	✖	–			✖		–	✖	–		–
Person, Roxboro	1,195	12.2	13.3			×		–			–		✖		–
Pitt County, Greenville	8,992	10.4	12.4					✖							
Pungo, Belhaven	972	12.1	11.2					★							–
Randolph, Asheboro	3,141	12.5	12.9							**★**				×	

Footnotes are on page 350.

Hospital outcomes: better (★) or worse (×) than average											Results of accreditation review on full survey		Other facts			
Adjusted Death rates			Adjusted Adverse outcome rates													
Surgical cases			Surgical cases													
All selected surgical cases	Coronary artery bypass surgery	Large bowel surgery	All selected surgical cases	Coronary artery bypass surgery	Large bowel surgery	Gall bladder removal	Total knee replacement	Total hip replacement	Simple prostatectomy	Carotid endarterectomy	Accreditation status*	Overall evaluation score (higher is better)	Number of beds	Major medical school affiliation?	Number of residents	Computerized drug order system (1 to 5 scale, higher is preferred; see page 23 for details)
2.3	3.8	6.5	7.7	10.3	11.9	7.5	6.7	6.4	5.4	8.2	–	91	161	–	–	–
–	–	–		–	–	–		–	–	–	4	91	128	No	3	–
×	–	×		–			–	–	–	–	4	90	143	No	0	–
	–	–		–	×	–		–	–	–	4	92	75	No	0	–
	–	–		–			–	–	–		4	91	130	No	0	–
	–	–	★	–		–	–	–	★	–	4	91	117	No	0	–
–	–	–	–	–	–	–	–	–	–	–	4	**98**	24	No	0	–
–	–	–	–	–	–	–	–	–	–	–	4	92	22	No	0	–
–	–	–		–	–	–	✖	–	–	–	5	**95**	81	No	0	–
	–	–		–			✖		–	–	5	**97**	154	No	0	–
–	–	–		–	–	–	–	–	–	–	4	91	40	No	0	–
	–	–		–		–	–	–	–	–	4	91	127	No	0	–
–	–	–	–	–	–	–	–	–	–	–	4	93	72	No	0	–
✖	–	–		–		–	★	–		–	4	92	105	No	0	–
	–	–		–		★		–	–	✖	–[2]	–[2]	170	No	0	–
–	–	–		–	–	–		–	–	–	4	***87***	87	No	0	–
✖	–	–		–		×	–	–	–	–	4	93	75	No	0	–
	–			–		×			–		4	93	175	No	0	–
	–	–	★	–		–	–	–		–	4	93	102	No	0	–
–	–	–	–	–	–	–	–	–	–	–	4	91	49	No	0	–
–	–	–		–	–	–	–	–	–	–	4	**94**	65	No	0	–
					✖	×			–		–[2]	–[2]	628	No	0	–
×	–	–		–		★	–	–	–	–	4	***87***	108	No	0	–
–	–	–		–	–	–	–	–	–	–	4	**94**	50	No	0	–
	–		×	–							5	**98**	245	No	0	–
				★					✖	✖	4	90	622	No	52	–
					×		★	★		✖	4	**97**	353	No	25	–
	–	–		–			–	–	–	–	5	**94**	90	No	0	–
	–			–	✖	★	–	–	✖	–	4	90	133	No	5	–
	–	–		–		–	–	–	–	–	4	***86***	96	No	0	–
–	–	–	–	–	–	–	–	–	–	–	4	91	43	No	0	–
–	–	–		–	–	–		–	–	–	4	**99**	50	No	0	–
					✖	✖		★		★	5	**98**	695	No	184	2
–	–	–	–	–	–	–	–	–	–	–	–[2]	–[2]	49	No	0	–
	–	–		–	★	✖		–	–	–	4	92	105	No	0	–

***Accreditation Status:** 5=Accredited with commendation or with full standards compliance; 4=Accredited with requirements for improvement; 3=Conditional accreditation.

Detailed Ratings for All Areas

See more information on "Key Ratings for Metro Areas" table beginning on page 32

Blue is most favorable
Bold Italic is least favorable
Blank means neither better nor worse than average
"–" means insufficient data

	Death rates for all selected case types			Hospital outcomes: better (★) or worse (×) than average											
				Adjusted Death rates											
					Medical Cases										
	Number of cases	Actual death rate (%)	Adjusted death rate (%) (lower is better)	All selected cases	All selected medical cases	Heart attack	Congestive heart failure	Obstructive pulmonary disease	Pneumonia	Respiratory failure and arrest	Septicemia	Stroke	Gastrointestinal hemorrhage	Fluid, electrolyte, & acid-base disorders	Kidney failure
National Average	–	–	12.1	12.1	14.8	21.2	10.6	6.5	16.9	34.4	25.1	18.4	6.7	11.0	20.9
North Carolina *(continued)*															
Other Areas *(continued)*															
Roanoke - Chowan, Ahoskie	2,106	13.0	***13.4***	✖	✖									✖	
Rowan Regional, Salisbury	5,206	12.7	***13.3***	✖	✖				✖	×	✖				
Rutherford Hospital, Rutherfordton	2,993	14.9	***13.5***	✖	✖	×						✖			
St Josephs, Asheville	4,152	10.3	***14.0***	✖	✖	×			✖			✖	×		
St Luke's, Columbus	1,079	13.6	***17.0***	✖	✖	✖	✖	–		–			✖		✖
Sampson Regional, Clinton	2,470	12.1	11.7			×		★							
Sandhills Regional, Hamlet	1,591	12.6	***14.9***	✖	✖	✖			✖		✖				
Scotland, Laurinburg	1,461	13.0	***17.3***	✖	✖	×		✖	✖			✖			–
Southeastern Regional, Lumberton	4,507	14.1	***14.4***	✖	✖	✖			✖	✖	✖				
Spruce Pine Community, Spruce Pine	1,459	16.2	11.2						★						
Stanly, Albemarle	2,666	13.5	12.8							×					
Stokes - Reynolds, Danbury	677	10.2	**8.2**	★	★		★	–		–	–	★	–		–
Thomasville Medical Center, Thomasville	1,535	12.7	***14.7***	✖	✖				✖		✖	✖			–
Transylvania, Brevard	1,094	12.1	12.2					–							–
Union Regional, Monroe	2,957	12.8	***13.3***	✖	✖				✖		×		✖	✖	★
US PHS Indian, Cherokee	158	12.0	17.1	×	×	–	–	–		–	–	–	–	–	–
Valdese General, Valdese	1,810	11.7	12.2							×					
Washington County, Plymouth	552	13.9	***15.5***	✖	✖	–		–		–	×		–	✖	–
Watauga, Boone	2,643	10.0	11.6												–
Wayne, Goldsboro	5,014	12.6	12.7									✖			
Wilkes Regional, North Wilkesboro	2,501	12.8	***14.9***	✖	✖	×			✖	✖		✖			
Wilson Memorial, Wilson	3,955	14.3	12.2												
North Dakota															
Altru, Grand Forks[1]	3,712	8.0	11.7								★				
Ashley Medical Center, Ashley	213	14.6	12.6			–	–	–		–	–		–	–	–
Carrington Health Center, Carrington	403	12.7	14.9	×	×	–		–		–	–		–	–	–
Cavalier County, Langdon	288	11.1	11.7			–		–		–	–		–	–	–
Dakota Heartland, Fargo	4,401	7.5	**10.6**	★	★	★				★		✖			
First Care, Park River	451	12.2	11.8					–	★	–	–		–		–
Heart of America, Rugby	674	11.7	11.4							–	–		–		–
Hillsboro Medical Center, Hillsboro	310	9.4	9.1			–		–		–	–	–	–	–	–
Jacobson, Elgin	236	13.6	15.1			–		–		–	–	–	–		–
Jamestown Hospital, Jamestown	948	13.5	***14.1***	✖	✖	✖		–						–	–

Footnotes are on page 350.

Hospital outcomes: better (★) or worse (×) than average											Results of accreditation review on full survey		Other facts			
Adjusted Death rates			Adjusted Adverse outcome rates													
Surgical cases			Surgical cases													
All selected surgical cases	Coronary artery bypass surgery	Large bowel surgery	All selected surgical cases	Coronary artery bypass surgery	Large bowel surgery	Gall bladder removal	Total knee replacement	Total hip replacement	Simple prostatectomy	Carotid endarterectomy	Accreditation status*	Overall evaluation score (higher is better)	Number of beds	Major medical school affiliation?	Number of residents	Computerized drug order system (1 to 5 scale, higher is preferred; see page 23 for details)
2.3	3.8	6.5	7.7	10.3	11.9	7.5	6.7	6.4	5.4	8.2	–	91	161	–	–	–
	–			–		–	–	–	–	–	4	93	118	No	2	–
✖	–	×	✖	–		✖	✖	✖	–		4	94	222	No	0	–
	–			–		×	–	–	–	–	4	89	111	No	0	–
	–			–	★				✖	–	–[2]	–[2]	301	No	–	–
–	–	–		–	–	–	–	–	–	–	4	94	73	No	0	–
	–	–		–			–		–	–	4	94	116	No	0	–
–	–	–		–	–	–	–	–	–	–	4	91	64	No	0	–
✖	–	✖		–	✖	–	–	–	–	–	4	90	124	No	0	–
	–	✖		–	✖			–	–	✖	4	89	166	No	0	–
–	–	–	★	–	–	–	–	–	–	–	4	86	42	No	0	–
	–	–	★	–		–	–	–	–	–	4	91	119	No	0	–
–	–	–	–	–	–	–	–	–	–	–	4	96	53	No	0	–
	–	–		–		–	–	–	–	–	4	98	89	No	0	–
	–	–		–	★		–	–	–	–	4	94	77	No	0	–
×	–	–		–				–	–	–	–[2]	–[2]	157	Yes	0	–
–	–	–	–	–	–	–	–	–	–	–	4	90	30	No	0	–
	–	–		–			–	–	–	–	–[2]	–[2]	79	No	0	–
–	–	–	–	–	–	–	–	–	–	–	4	90	33	No	0	–
	–	–		–				–	–	–	4	88	95	No	0	–
✖	–	✖	✖	–	✖						4	91	272	No	0	–
	–	–		–			–	–	✖	★	4	80	130	No	6	–
	–			–	✖			–	–		4	90	220	No	0	–
★	★									★	4	81	262	No	0	–
–	–	–	–	–	–	–	–	–	–	–	–[2]	–[2]	26	No	0	–
–	–	–	–	–	–	–	–	–	–	–	–[2]	–[2]	70	No	0	–
–	–	–	–	–	–	–	–	–	–	–	–[2]	–[2]	28	No	0	–
			★		★		★				4	82	203	Yes	5	1
–	–	–	–	–	–	–	–	–	–	–	–[2]	–[2]	20	No	0	–
–	–	–	–	–	–	–	–	–	–	–	–[2]	–[2]	20	No	0	–
–	–	–	–	–	–	–	–	–	–	–	–[2]	–[2]	74	No	0	–
–	–	–	–	–	–	–	–	–	–	–	–[2]	–[2]	50	No	0	–
–	–	–		–		–	–	–	–	–	4	93	56	No	0	–

***Accreditation Status:** 5=Accredited with commendation or with full standards compliance; 4=Accredited with requirements for improvement; 3=Conditional accreditation.

Detailed Ratings for All Areas

See more information on "Key Ratings for Metro Areas" table beginning on page 32

Blue is most favorable
Bold Italic is least favorable
Blank means neither better nor worse than average
"–" means insufficient data

	Death rates for all selected case types				Hospital outcomes: better (★) or worse (×) than average — Adjusted Death rates — Medical Cases											
	Number of cases	Actual death rate (%)	Adjusted death rate (%) (lower is better)	All selected cases	All selected medical cases	Heart attack	Congestive heart failure	Obstructive pulmonary disease	Pneumonia	Respiratory failure and arrest	Septicemia	Stroke	Gastrointestinal hemorrhage	Fluid, electrolyte, & acid-base disorders	Kidney failure
National Average	–	–	12.1	12.1	14.8	21.2	10.6	6.5	16.9	34.4	25.1	18.4	6.7	11.0	20.9
North Dakota *(continued)*															
Linton Hospital, Linton	273	16.1	***16.8***	✖	✖	–	×	–	×	–	–	–	–	–	–
Medcenter One, Bismarck	3,514	9.1	11.9				×								
Mercy, Devils Lake	980	13.7	12.5							–					–
Mercy, Williston	1,078	10.7	12.1							–	–		–	×	–
Meritcare, Fargo[1]	5,997	10.0	**11.0**	**★**	**★**	**★**							★		
Oakes Community, Oakes	594	12.3	13.1					–		–	–		–		–
Pembina County, Cavalier	353	12.5	10.8			–		–		–	–		–	–	
PHS Indian, Belcourt	206	4.4	7.1	★	★	–	–	–		–	–	–	–	–	–
Presentation, Rolla	452	6.4	**7.5**	**★**	**★**	–				–	–	–	–	–	–
St Alexius, Bismarck	3,915	6.3	**8.5**	**★**	**★**	**★**		**★**	**★**		**★**				★
St Aloisius, Harvey	502	11.4	10.0			–		–		–	–		–	★	–
St Joseph's, Dickinson	1,567	10.5	**10.4**	**★**	★										–
St Luke's, Crosby	338	14.5	15.0	×	×	–		–		–	–	–	–	–	–
Towner County, Cando	328	14.9	12.4					–	★	–	–	✖	–	–	–
Trinity, Minot[1]	3,065	8.5	**10.2**	**★**	**★**	**★**	★				★				**★**
Trinity - St Joseph's, Minot[1]	1,726	8.7	**10.2**	**★**	**★**				★					★	–
Unity, Grafton	261	12.6	9.5			–	–	–		–	–	–	–		×
West River Regional, Hettinger	1,216	9.0	**9.0**	**★**	**★**				★	–				**★**	
Wishek Community, Wishek[1]	367	12.5	12.0					–		–	–	–	–	–	–
Ohio															
Cincinnati Area															
Bethesda North, Cincinnati[1]	7,928	13.5	***14.1***	✖	✖	✖		✖	✖					✖	
Children's, Cincinnati	–	–	–	–	–	–	–	–	–	–	–	–	–	–	–
Christ, Cincinnati	6,846	9.7	**10.6**	**★**	**★**	**★**	**★**		★		★				
Deaconess, Cincinnati	4,319	15.9	11.9										**★**		
Good Samaritan, Cincinnati	6,258	11.6	12.1												
Jewish, Cincinnati	6,705	12.8	11.3	★	**★**		★							✖	**★**
Mercy - Anderson, Cincinnati	4,376	13.0	12.3			✖	✖				**★**				
Mercy Franciscan - Mt Airy, Cincinnati[1]	5,083	12.7	11.9			★		✖							
Mercy Franciscan - Western Hills, Cincinnati[1]	6,002	12.8	11.5					✖							
University, Cincinnati	3,589	13.0	**10.2**	**★**	**★**				**★**						
Cleveland Area															
Cleveland Clinic Foundation, Cleveland	10,431	6.6	**9.3**	**★**	**★**	**★**						**★**	**★**	★	**★**
Deaconess, Cleveland	2,555	12.3	12.0												

Footnotes are on page 350.

Hospital outcomes: better (★) or worse (×) than average											Results of accreditation review on full survey		Other facts			
Adjusted Death rates			Adjusted Adverse outcome rates													
Surgical cases			Surgical cases													
All selected surgical cases	Coronary artery bypass surgery	Large bowel surgery	All selected surgical cases	Coronary artery bypass surgery	Large bowel surgery	Gall bladder removal	Total knee replacement	Total hip replacement	Simple prostatectomy	Carotid endarterectomy	Accreditation status*	Overall evaluation score (higher is better)	Number of beds	Major medical school affiliation?	Number of residents	Computerized drug order system (1 to 5 scale, higher is preferred; see page 23 for details)
2.3	3.8	6.5	7.7	10.3	11.9	7.5	6.7	6.4	5.4	8.2	–	91	161	–	–	–
–	–	–	–	–	–	–	–	–	–	–	–[2]	–[2]	25	No	0	–
			★				★	–			–[2]	–[2]	186	**Yes**	0	–
–	–	–	–	–	–	–	–	–	–	–	4	**94**	35	No	0	–
	–	–		–		–	–	–	–	–	4	93	93	No	0	–
				★		×				★	4	**94**	352	**Yes**	56	1
–	–	–		–	–	–	–	–	–	–	–[2]	–[2]	25	No	0	–
–	–	–	–	–	–	–	–	–	–	–	–[2]	–[2]	29	No	0	–
–	–	–	–	–	–	–	–	–	–	–	–[2]	–[2]	42	No	0	–
–	–	–	–	–	–	–	–	–	–	–	–[2]	–[2]	54	No	0	–
★		★		★	★		★	×		★	4	89	249	No	0	–
–	–	–	–	–	–	–	–	–	–	–	–[2]	–[2]	25	No	0	–
★	–	–	★	–	★	–		–	–	–	4	***88***	90	No	0	–
–	–	–	–	–	–	–	–	–	–	–	–[2]	–[2]	29	No	0	–
–	–	–	–	–	–	–	–	–	–	–	–[2]	–[2]	32	No	0	–
	–		★		★		★				4	93	178	No	6	–
	–	–				–	–	–	–	–	4	***85***	160	No	0	–
–	–	–	–	–	–	–	–	–	–	–	–[2]	–[2]	17	No	0	–
–	–	–	–	–	–	–	–	–	–	–	4	**94**	46	No	–	–
–	–	–	–	–	–	–	–	–	–	–	–[2]	–[2]	22	No	0	–
×	×										4	**97**	261	No	9	–
–	–	–	–	–	–	–	–	–	–	–	4	92	307	–	109	–
							★		★	★	4	92	411	No	55	–
			★	★	×	★			–		4	90	155	No	5	–
											4	93	404	**Yes**	68	–
					×			★			4	89	169	No	45	–
	–			–			×	×			4	**95**	151	**Yes**	0	–
	–			–							5	**99**	226	No	0	–
	–			–	★			–	×		5	**99**	189	No	0	–
						–	–	–	–		4	92	429	**Yes**	585	–
★	★	★					×	×	★		–[2]	–[2]	942	No	762	–
	–	–	★	–		–	–	–	–	★	4	90	143	No	0	–

***Accreditation Status:** 5=Accredited with commendation or with full standards compliance; 4=Accredited with requirements for improvement; 3=Conditional accreditation.

Detailed Ratings for All Areas

See more information on "Key Ratings for Metro Areas" table beginning on page 32

Blue is most favorable
Bold Italic is least favorable
Blank means neither better nor worse than average
"–" means insufficient data

	Death rates for all selected case types			Hospital outcomes: better (★) or worse (✕) than average — Adjusted Death rates											
				Medical Cases											
	Number of cases	Actual death rate (%)	Adjusted death rate (%) (lower is better)	All selected cases	All selected medical cases	Heart attack	Congestive heart failure	Obstructive pulmonary disease	Pneumonia	Respiratory failure and arrest	Septicemia	Stroke	Gastrointestinal hemorrhage	Fluid, electrolyte, & acid-base disorders	Kidney failure
National Average	–	–	12.1	12.1	14.8	21.2	10.6	6.5	16.9	34.4	25.1	18.4	6.7	11.0	20.9
Ohio *(continued)*															
Cleveland Area *(continued)*															
Euclid Hospital, Euclid	3,559	14.1	11.6				**★**		✖	**★**					
Fairview, Cleveland	7,060	11.0	**10.8**	**★**	**★**	**★**	★		**★**	✖	✖	**★**			
Grace, Cleveland	–	–	–	–	–	–	–	–	–	–	–	–	–	–	–
Hillcrest, Mayfield Heights	8,657	9.6	**9.2**	**★**	**★**	**★**	**★**	**★**	**★**		**★**				★
Huron - Cleveland Clinic, Cleveland	1,844	12.6	**8.9**	**★**	**★**	**★**	**★**	**★**	**★**			★			
Lakewood Hospital, Lakewood[1]	5,086	10.5	**10.4**	**★**	**★**							**★**			
Lutheran, Cleveland	1,782	12.2	12.1					✕							
Marymount, Garfield Heights	5,755	9.9	**9.8**	**★**	**★**		**★**	**★**	★	**★**		**★**			
Metrohealth, Cleveland	3,188	11.6	11.6								✖				
Parma Community General, Parma	8,191	13.5	12.7	✕	✕				✖						
St John West Shore, Cleveland	4,235	13.2	***13.2***	✖	✖							✖			
St Vincent Charity, Cleveland[1]	3,436	8.7	**9.5**	**★**	**★**				**★**			★			
South Pointe - Cleveland Clinic, Warrensville Heights[1]	4,741	13.1	**10.2**	**★**	**★**		**★**				**★**	**★**			
Southwest General, Middleburg Heights	7,262	10.4	**10.7**	**★**	**★**			**★**				**★**			
UHHS, Richmond Heights	4,581	11.4	**10.4**	**★**	**★**		**★**						**★**		
University, Bedford[1]	2,592	16.5	13.0	✕	✕						✕	★	✖		
University, Cleveland	7,285	10.2	**9.5**	**★**	**★**	**★**	★		**★**		**★**	★			
University St Michael, Cleveland	1,590	9.6	**8.7**	**★**	**★**	★	**★**	★						**★**	
Columbus Area															
Arthur G James Cancer/Richard J Solove, Columbus	607	10.4	11.6			–	–	–		–		–	–		–
Children's, Columbus	–	–	–	–	–	–	–	–	–	–	–	–	–	–	–
Columbus Community, Columbus	1,391	9.8	**9.6**	**★**	**★**		**★**	**★**		**★**			–		–
Doctors - Ohio Health, Columbus	4,359	10.8	**10.4**	**★**	**★**		**★**	★	**★**		**★**				
Doctors West, Columbus	–	–	–	–	–	–	–	–	–	–	–	–	–	–	–
Grant, Columbus	5,398	9.3	***13.1***	✖	✕						✖				
Mount Carmel East, Columbus	–	–	–	–	–	–	–	–	–	–	–	–	–	–	–
Mount Carmel St Ann's, Westerville	3,272	16.0	***15.1***	✖	✖			✖	✖				✕	✖	
Mount Carmel West, Columbus[1]	15,173	12.4	***14.4***	✖	✖	✕	✖		✖			✖	✖	✖	
Ohio State University East Hospital, Columbus	2,802	14.7	**10.3**	**★**	**★**				**★**		**★**				
Ohio State University Medical Center, Columbus[1]	3,535	8.4	**9.8**	**★**	**★**	**★**			**★**						
Riverside Methodist, Columbus	13,404	10.3	12.6	✕	✖			✖	✖						✖
Other Areas															
Adams County, West Union	966	14.1	13.6			✕				–	✖				–

Footnotes are on page 350.

Hospital outcomes: better (★) or worse (×) than average											Results of accreditation review on full survey		Other facts			
Adjusted Death rates			Adjusted Adverse outcome rates													
Surgical cases			Surgical cases													
All selected surgical cases	Coronary artery bypass surgery	Large bowel surgery	All selected surgical cases	Coronary artery bypass surgery	Large bowel surgery	Gall bladder removal	Total knee replacement	Total hip replacement	Simple prostatectomy	Carotid endarterectomy	Accreditation status*	Overall evaluation score (higher is better)	Number of beds	Major medical school affiliation?	Number of residents	Computerized drug order system (1 to 5 scale, higher is preferred; see page 23 for details)
2.3	3.8	6.5	7.7	10.3	11.9	7.5	6.7	6.4	5.4	8.2	–	91	161	–	–	–
	–			–	★				–		4	**96**	147	No	0	–
			★			★	★				4	89	402	No	70	–
–	–	–	–	–	–	–	–	–	–	–	4	92	57	–	0	–
★		★									4	91	305	No	0	–
–	–	–		–		–	–	–	–	–	4	**94**	143	No	72	–
					✖			✖			4	***87***	283	No	0	–
	–			–		–				–	3	***81***	184	No	0	–
	–			–			✖				4	**94**	220	No	8	–
	–					–		–	–	–	4	90	490	**Yes**	316	2
	–		×	★			✖	✖			4	91	256	No	0	–
	–			–					–		4	**95**	183	**Yes**	5	–
					★	–			–		4	91	222	No	56	–
	–			–		★	–	–			4	***85***	198	**Yes**	59	–
				★						★	4	92	293	No	2	–
	–							–			–[2]	–[2]	98	**Yes**	0	–
	–			–			–	–	–	–	4	93	99	No	0	–
★		★			★			×			4	89	702	**Yes**	630	–
	–	–		–		–	–	–	–	–	4	***87***	199	No	1	–
	–	★		–		–	–	–	–	–	4	***87***	120	**Yes**	321	–
–	–	–	–	–	–	–	–	–	–	–	4	93	281	–	8	–
–	–	–		–	–	–	–	–	–	–	4	**94**	130	No	1	–
								✖	–	✖	4	**99**	349	No	52	–
–	–	–	–	–	–	–	–	–	–	–	–[2]	–[2]	–	–	–	–
✖		✖			×						–[2]	–[2]	408	No	54	–
–	–	–	–	–	–	–	–	–	–	–	–[2]	–[2]	–	–	–	–
	–	✖		–			–	–	–	–	4	**96**	161	No	–	–
		×									–[2]	–[2]	929	No	76	–
✖	–	×	✖	–		–	✖	✖	–	–	4	93	130	No	0	–
		–		×				–	–		4	***83***	550	**Yes**	485	–
★								★			4	91	810	**Yes**	212	–
–	–	–	–	–	–	–	–	–	–	–	4	92	31	No	0	–

***Accreditation Status:** 5=Accredited with commendation or with full standards compliance; 4=Accredited with requirements for improvement; 3=Conditional accreditation.

Detailed Ratings for All Areas

See more information on "Key Ratings for Metro Areas" table beginning on page 32

Blue is most favorable
Bold Italic is least favorable
Blank means neither better nor worse than average
"–" means insufficient data

	Death rates for all selected case types				Hospital outcomes: better (★) or worse (×) than average — Adjusted Death rates — Medical Cases											
	Number of cases	Actual death rate (%)	Adjusted death rate (%) (lower is better)	All selected cases	All selected medical cases	Heart attack	Congestive heart failure	Obstructive pulmonary disease	Pneumonia	Respiratory failure and arrest	Septicemia	Stroke	Gastrointestinal hemorrhage	Fluid, electrolyte, & acid-base disorders	Kidney failure
National Average	–	–	12.1	12.1	14.8	21.2	10.6	6.5	16.9	34.4	25.1	18.4	6.7	11.0	20.9
Ohio *(continued)*															
Other Areas *(continued)*															
Adena Regional, Chillicothe[1]	4,173	11.4	12.9	×	×				✖						
Akron General, Akron	11,072	10.9	**11.0**	**★**	**★**				**★**		**★**		★		
Alliance Community, Alliance	2,694	13.1	***14.1***	✖	✖				✖		✖				×
Amherst Hospital, Amherst	504	7.1	**8.5**	**★**	**★**	–	★	–	**★**	–	–		–		–
Ashtabula County, Ashtabula	2,625	11.7	***13.7***	✖	✖		✖								
Aultman, Canton	10,938	11.5	**11.3**	**★**	★	**★**					★				
Barberton Citizens, Barberton	4,679	12.0	11.5					**★**	**★**		✖	★	×	×	
Barnesville Hospital Association, Barnesville	1,585	10.4	11.8			×	**★**			–	–				–
Bellevue Hospital, Bellevue	957	10.7	11.2												–
Belmont, Bellaire	1,333	14.4	12.6			✖	✖	**★**	★			×			–
Berger, Circleville[1]	1,372	16.3	***15.1***	✖	✖				✖			×			
Blanchard Valley Regional, Findlay[1]	4,020	9.6	12.9	×	×					✖				★	
Brown County General, Georgetown	883	11.3	10.1	★	★		★				×		–		–
Bucyrus Community, Bucyrus	726	17.4	13.3					–					–		×
Clinton, Wilmington	2,283	11.9	12.9						✖						
Community, Hicksville	277	8.3	9.0			–	–	–	★	–	–		–	–	–
Community, Springfield	3,788	11.6	12.3			✖				✖		**★**			
Community Health Partners - West, Lorain	5,438	9.4	**10.4**	**★**	**★**			**★**	**★**		**★**	**★**			
Community Health Partners - East, Lorain[1]	690	10.4	10.5				★				–		–	–	–
Community of Williams County, Bryan[1]	2,162	9.7	12.5							✖					
Coshocton County, Coshocton	2,136	14.4	***16.3***	✖	✖		✖		✖			✖			×
Cuyahoga Falls General, Cuyahoga Falls	2,078	14.5	***14.4***	✖	✖	✖						✖	×		
Dayton Heart, Dayton	297	6.1	11.5				–	–	–	–	–	–	–	–	–
Defiance Hospital, Defiance	1,419	13.2	13.3		×	✖									–
Doctors, Nelsonville	708	11.9	14.3	×	×	✖	✖				–		–		–
Doctors of Stark County, Massillon	2,150	11.7	10.8	★	★	✖		**★**	**★**						
Dunlap, Orrville	427	15.0	14.3			✖	✖	–					–	–	–
East Liverpool City, East Liverpool	3,611	11.2	11.2						★						
East Ohio Regional, Martins Ferry	2,618	14.6	***15.0***	✖	✖	✖			✖				✖	✖	
EMH Regional, Elyria	5,229	9.9	**10.6**	**★**	**★**				★	★	★				
Fairfield, Lancaster	4,322	12.5	12.4												
Fayette County, Washington Court House	1,009	20.2	***15.2***	✖	✖		✖				✖				
Firelands Community, Sandusky	2,378	11.0	12.2						×			**★**			
Firelands Regional - South Campus, Sandusky	2,649	13.7	***14.0***	✖	✖	✖	✖		✖						

Footnotes are on page 350.

Hospital outcomes: better (★) or worse (×) than average											Results of accreditation review on full survey		Other facts			
Adjusted Death rates			Adjusted Adverse outcome rates													
Surgical cases			Surgical cases													
All selected surgical cases	Coronary artery bypass surgery	Large bowel surgery	All selected surgical cases	Coronary artery bypass surgery	Large bowel surgery	Gall bladder removal	Total knee replacement	Total hip replacement	Simple prostatectomy	Carotid endarterectomy	Accreditation status*	Overall evaluation score (higher is better)	Number of beds	Major medical school affiliation?	Number of residents	Computerized drug order system (1 to 5 scale, higher is preferred; see page 23 for details)
2.3	3.8	6.5	7.7	10.3	11.9	7.5	6.7	6.4	5.4	8.2	–	91	161	–	–	–
	–			–				–	–		4	88	187	No	0	–
						★	✖			×	4	89	473	No	139	–
	–			–				–	–	–	4	91	128	No	2	–
–	–	–	–	–	–	–	–	–	–	–	4	94	29	No	0	–
	–	–		–		–	×	–		–	4	95	137	No	0	–
	★			★				✖		×	5	96	736	Yes	92	–
	–	★		–	★					✖	4	91	205	Yes	18	–
–	–	–		–	–	–	–	–	–	–	4	92	56	No	0	–
	–	–		–		–	–	–	–	–	–[2]	–[2]	48	No	0	–
–	–	–	–	–	–	–	–	–	–	–	4	91	81	No	0	–
×	–	✖		–		–	–	–	–		4	95	75	No	0	–
	–		★	–			★			–	4	90	133	No	0	–
–	–	–	–	–	–	–	–	–	–	–	4	92	53	No	0	–
–	–	–	★	–		–	–	–	–	–	4	93	25	No	0	–
	–	–		–		–		–		–	4	96	81	No	12	–
–	–	–	–	–	–	–	–	–	–	–	4	84	22	No	0	–
	–				✖	★		–	–		4	99	160	No	0	–
★	–			–						×	4	91	282	No	0	–
–	–	–	–	–	–	–	–	–	–	–	–[2]	–[2]	358	No	–	–
	–			–		×			–	–	4	83	121	No	3	–
	–	–		–		–	–	–	–	–	4	83	151	No	3	–
	–			–				–	–		–[2]	–[2]	135	Yes	40	–
		–			–	–	–	–	–	–	4	90	47	No	–	–
★	–	–	★	–	★	–	–	–	–	–	4	94	80	No	0	–
–	–	–	–	–	–	–	–	–	–	–	–[2]	–[2]	65	Yes	0	–
	–		★	–		–			–	–	–[2]	–[2]	110	Yes	36	–
–	–	–	–	–	–	–	–	–	–	–	4	98	38	No	2	–
	–			–			–	–		–	4	93	140	No	0	–
	–			–		–	–	–	–	–	4	96	71	No	0	–
			★		★		★				4	90	266	No	0	–
✖	–			–					×		4	87	172	No	0	–
	–	–		–		–	–	–	–	–	4	89	35	No	0	–
	–	–		–	★	–		–			4	92	200	No	10	–
★	–	–		–	–	–		–	–		4	88	124	No	0	–

***Accreditation Status:** 5=Accredited with commendation or with full standards compliance; 4=Accredited with requirements for improvement; 3=Conditional accreditation.

Detailed Ratings for All Areas

See more information on "Key Ratings for Metro Areas" table beginning on page 32

Blue is most favorable
Bold Italic is least favorable
Blank means neither better nor worse than average
"–" means insufficient data

	Death rates for all selected case types			Hospital outcomes: better (★) or worse (×) than average — Adjusted Death rates — Medical Cases											
	Number of cases	Actual death rate (%)	Adjusted death rate (%) (lower is better)	All selected cases	All selected medical cases	Heart attack	Congestive heart failure	Obstructive pulmonary disease	Pneumonia	Respiratory failure and arrest	Septicemia	Stroke	Gastrointestinal hemorrhage	Fluid, electrolyte, & acid-base disorders	Kidney failure
National Average	–	–	12.1	12.1	14.8	21.2	10.6	6.5	16.9	34.4	25.1	18.4	6.7	11.0	20.9
Ohio *(continued)*															
Other Areas *(continued)*															
Fisher - Titus, Norwalk	1,733	10.6	12.7			✖									
Flower, Sylvania	3,641	13.8	***13.4***	✖	✖					✖				×	
Fort Hamilton Hospital, Hamilton	3,253	12.3	10.6	★	★					★					
Fostoria Community, Fostoria	791	11.9	13.8			✖	×				–		–		–
Fulton County, Wauseon	1,164	10.6	13.7		×		×			–	–	✖	–		
Galion Community, Galion	730	12.2	12.5							–	–				–
Genesis, Zanesville	6,874	12.3	***14.1***	✖	✖	✖	✖	✖				✖		✖	
Good Samaritan, Dayton	7,736	10.5	11.7												
Grady, Delaware	1,436	16.2	***16.5***	✖	✖		✖	×	×			×	✖		✖
Grandview, Dayton	4,611	12.3	10.2	★	★		★		★	★		×	✖		★
Greene, Xenia	2,231	14.7	12.3			✖					★				
Greenfield Area, Greenfield	475	13.5	12.5			–		–		–	–		–	–	
H B Magruder, Port Clinton	1,111	10.7	12.9							✖		✖			–
Hardin, Kenton	1,241	13.7	***15.0***	✖	✖		✖		✖	✖				✖	
Harrison, Cadiz	748	17.6	***15.6***	✖	✖	–	✖		✖	–					–
Henry County, Napoleon	525	10.5	12.4					–		–			–	–	–
Highland, Hillsboro	1,345	12.5	12.4							×					–
Hocking Valley, Logan	1,001	14.2	13.5										–		–
Holzer, Gallipolis	3,730	13.3	12.8			×							✖		✖
Joel Pomerene, Millersburg	674	15.4	***15.4***	✖	✖			–			–		–	–	–
Joint Township, St Marys	1,929	8.5	8.9	★	★		★		★		★				★
Kettering Medical Center, Kettering[1]	8,281	10.1	11.8												
Kettering Youth Services, Dayton[1]	2,468	17.7	***14.4***	✖	✖	✖	✖					✖			×
Knox, Mt Vernon	2,452	12.9	12.4			×							×		
Lake, Painesville	7,731	13.0	***13.1***	✖	✖		×	✖				✖			
Licking, Newark	3,765	13.3	***15.1***	✖	✖		✖	✖		✖	✖	✖			
Lima Memorial, Lima	4,119	9.6	12.3									★			
Lodi Community, Lodi[1]	285	8.1	13.2			–		–	–	–	–	–	–	–	–
Madison County, London	841	15.1	***16.3***	✖	✖				✖		–		–		–
Marietta Memorial, Marietta	2,735	13.1	***17.7***	✖	✖	✖	✖	✖	✖					✖	
Marion General, Marion	3,645	10.5	11.3						★			★			
Mary Rutan, Bellefontaine	1,679	12.5	***15.1***	✖	✖		✖	✖		✖	✖				
Massillon Community, Massillon	2,511	13.0	***13.8***	✖	✖						✖	×	×		
McCullough - Hyde, Oxford	1,242	13.9	***16.8***	✖	✖	×		✖	✖		–			–	✖

Footnotes are on page 350.

Hospital outcomes: better (★) or worse (×) than average											Results of accreditation review on full survey		Other facts			
Adjusted Death rates			Adjusted Adverse outcome rates													
Surgical cases			Surgical cases													
All selected surgical cases	Coronary artery bypass surgery	Large bowel surgery	All selected surgical cases	Coronary artery bypass surgery	Large bowel surgery	Gall bladder removal	Total knee replacement	Total hip replacement	Simple prostatectomy	Carotid endarterectomy	Accreditation status*	Overall evaluation score (higher is better)	Number of beds	Major medical school affiliation?	Number of residents	Computerized drug order system (1 to 5 scale, higher is preferred; see page 23 for details)
2.3	3.8	6.5	7.7	10.3	11.9	7.5	6.7	6.4	5.4	8.2	–	91	161	–	–	–
	–			–		–	×	–	–	–	5	98	65	No	0	–
×	–	×		–	×				–		5	97	224	No	18	–
	–			–				–	–		5	96	181	No	0	–
–	–	–	–	–	–	–	–	–	–	–	4	96	39	No	0	–
–	–	–		–	–	–		–	–	–	4	96	86	No	0	–
–	–	–		–	–	–	–	–	–	–	4	92	75	No	0	–
	–			–	★	✖	★				4	89	389	No	0	–
			✖							✖	4	94	496	Yes	74	–
–	–	–		–		–	–	–	–	–	4	93	70	No	0	–
						✖		–	–		–[2]	–[2]	427	Yes	–	–
✖	–	×		–		–	✖	–	–	–	4	86	138	No	0	–
–	–	–	–	–	–	–	–	–	–	–	4	83	36	No	0	–
–	–	–	★	–	–	–	–	–	–	–	4	93	33	No	0	–
–	–	–		–	–	–	–	–	–	–	4	91	51	No	0	–
–	–	–	–	–	–	–	–	–	–	–	4	87	48	No	0	–
–	–	–		–	–	–	–	–	–	–	4	91	39	No	0	–
–	–	–	–	–	–	–	–	–	–	–	4	96	51	No	0	–
–	–	–		–	–	–	–	–	–	–	4	96	62	No	0	–
	–	✖		–				–		–	4	91	149	No	0	–
–	–	–	–	–	–	–	–	–	–	–	4	92	38	No	0	–
	–	–		–		–	✖	–	–	–	5	98	83	No	2	–
						★					4	88	626	No	279	–
✖	–	✖		–			–	–	–	–	–[2]	–[2]	120	No	–	–
	–			–			–	–	–	–	4	89	75	No	0	–
	–						✖				4	91	374	No	0	–
	–			–	★			–	–		4	86	165	No	0	–
			×			✖			–	×	4	91	162	No	0	–
–	–	–	–	–	–	–	–	–	–	–	4	89	14	No	0	–
–	–	–	–	–	–	–	–	–	–	–	4	90	35	No	0	–
	–	✖		–				–			4	91	135	No	0	–
	–			–		✖	✖				4	94	188	No	0	–
	–			–				–	–	–	4	96	72	No	0	–
	–			–		–		–	–	–	4	91	139	No	0	–
✖	–	✖		–	✖	–	–	–	–	–	4	96	44	No	0	–

***Accreditation Status:** 5=Accredited with commendation or with full standards compliance; 4=Accredited with requirements for improvement; 3=Conditional accreditation.

Detailed Ratings for All Areas

See more information on "Key Ratings for Metro Areas" table beginning on page 32

Blue is most favorable
Bold Italic is least favorable
Blank means neither better nor worse than average
"–" means insufficient data

	Death rates for all selected case types			Hospital outcomes: better (★) or worse (×) than average — Adjusted Death rates — Medical Cases											
	Number of cases	Actual death rate (%)	Adjusted death rate (%) (lower is better)	All selected cases	All selected medical cases	Heart attack	Congestive heart failure	Obstructive pulmonary disease	Pneumonia	Respiratory failure and arrest	Septicemia	Stroke	Gastrointestinal hemorrhage	Fluid, electrolyte, & acid-base disorders	Kidney failure
National Average	–	–	12.1	12.1	14.8	21.2	10.6	6.5	16.9	34.4	25.1	18.4	6.7	11.0	20.9
Ohio *(continued)*															
Other Areas *(continued)*															
Medcentral, Mansfield	6,404	12.3	***15.0***	✖	✖		✖	✖	✖			×	✖	✖	
Medical College, Toledo	2,411	11.9	10.8	★	★	★						★			
Medina General, Medina	2,758	11.6	11.9					★							×
Memorial, Fremont	1,620	11.7	***14.5***	✖	✖						★	✖			✖
Memorial of Union County, Marysville	1,175	10.6	13.0							×	–		–	–	
Mercer County, Coldwater	1,249	11.6	13.7	×			✖				×		–		–
Mercy, Canton	6,168	11.8	10.8	★	★		★		★	★					
Mercy, Springfield[1]	4,286	12.7	11.0	★	★		★								
Mercy, Tiffin	1,600	9.2	10.8												★
Mercy, Urbana	1,040	11.8	11.6										–	–	–
Mercy, Willard	474	12.2	***16.3***	✖	✖	–		–	✖	–	–		–	–	–
Mercy - Clermont, Batavia	2,467	14.5	13.0												
Miami Valley, Dayton	8,696	10.0	10.4	★	★		★		★	★		★	×	×	
Middletown Regional, Middletown	3,875	13.5	***13.5***	✖	✖				✖			✖			
Morrow County, Mt Gilead[1]	709	10.0	11.0				★			–	–		–	–	–
O'Bleness, Athens	1,408	14.4	12.8			✖	✖				★				
Oak Hill Community, Oak Hill	519	17.9	***17.0***	✖	✖				✖			–	–	–	–
Pike, Waverly	813	17.3	***15.9***	✖	✖	×	✖		✖					–	
Riverside Mercy, Toledo	1,934	11.2	11.4					★							
Robinson, Ravenna	4,104	11.4	12.7						✖	–				✖	
St Charles Mercy, Oregon	4,585	11.5	11.7						★						
St Elizabeth, Youngstown	10,323	13.2	11.0	★	★	★		★	★	★				✖	★
St Joseph, Warren	3,698	11.5	10.8	★	★	★		★							
St Luke's, Maumee	5,366	13.1	***14.2***	✖	✖	×			✖	✖			★	✖	✖
St Rita's, Lima	4,988	9.7	11.3				★								
St Vincent Mercy, Toledo	7,221	11.1	12.4										✖		
Salem Community, Salem	3,734	12.6	12.3			×									
Samaritan Regional, Ashland	2,006	11.8	11.5												
Selby General, Marietta	979	12.5	12.6										✖		
Southeastern Ohio Regional, Cambridge	2,714	12.6	13.1	×	×										✖
Southern Ohio, Portsmouth	5,950	12.4	12.4						✖						
Summa, Akron[1]	15,084	12.2	10.7	★	★	★	★		★		★	★			
Toledo Hospital, Toledo	7,832	9.9	11.5			★							×		
Trinity, Steubenville	6,517	11.8	***12.8***	✖	✖	✖				★					✖

Footnotes are on page 350.

Hospital outcomes: better (★) or worse (×) than average											Results of accreditation review on full survey		Other facts			
Adjusted Death rates			Adjusted Adverse outcome rates													
Surgical cases			Surgical cases													
All selected surgical cases	Coronary artery bypass surgery	Large bowel surgery	All selected surgical cases	Coronary artery bypass surgery	Large bowel surgery	Gall bladder removal	Total knee replacement	Total hip replacement	Simple prostatectomy	Carotid endarterectomy	Accreditation status*	Overall evaluation score (higher is better)	Number of beds	Major medical school affiliation?	Number of residents	Computerized drug order system (1 to 5 scale, higher is preferred; see page 23 for details)
2.3	3.8	6.5	7.7	10.3	11.9	7.5	6.7	6.4	5.4	8.2	–	91	161	–	–	–
×	✖					✖					4	93	350	No	0	–
×			✖	✖		–			–		4	**87**	191	**Yes**	247	–
	–			–					★	–	4	**94**	118	No	0	–
	–			–		–		–	–	–	4	**94**	121	No	0	–
–	–	–	★	–	–	–	–	–	–	–	4	**94**	50	No	0	–
–	–	–		–		–	–	–	–	–	4	**97**	59	No	0	–
			×				✖				4	89	374	No	0	–
	–			–	★				–		4	**87**	218	No	8	–
	–	–	★	–		–		–	–	–	4	**97**	66	No	0	–
–	–	–	★	–	–	–	–	–	–	–	–[2]	–[2]	20	No	0	–
–	–	–	–	–	–	–	–	–	–	–	4	92	72	No	–	–
	–			–		–	–	–	–	–	4	91	85	No	0	–
			✖			✖					5	**96**	603	**Yes**	111	–
	–			–					–		–[2]	–[2]	183	No	0	–
–	–	–	–	–	–	–	–	–	–	–	4	93	37	No	0	–
–	–	–		–		–	–	–	–	–	4	92	75	No	0	–
–	–	–	–	–	–	–	–	–	–	–	–[2]	–[2]	34	No	0	–
–	–	–	–	–	–	–	–	–	–	–	4	**87**	35	No	0	–
	–	–		–		–	–	–	–	–	5	**96**	162	No	5	–
	–			–	×			–	–		4	**88**	131	No	0	–
	–			–			✖		–		4	90	289	No	0	–
			✖	✖			✖	✖			4	91	309	**Yes**	67	4
	–			–			✖		–		4	93	476	No	6	–
	–			–	✖	★				✖	–[2]	–[2]	144	No	0	–
						✖		★			4	92	351	No	0	–
			✖	✖			✖			✖	4	**95**	483	No	102	–
	–		★	–	★	★		–	–		4	90	108	No	0	–
	–	–	★	–		–		–	–	–	4	**96**	70	No	0	–
–	–	–		–	–	–		–	–	–	–[2]	–[2]	54	No	2	–
	–	–		–			–	–	–		4	**97**	93	No	0	4
	–	✖	★	–			★	–			5	**96**	205	No	0	–
★	★						★		★		5	93	536	No	161	–
★	★			★			✖	✖			4	**95**	648	No	12	–
	–			–				–		×	4	**86**	355	No	0	–

***Accreditation Status:** 5=Accredited with commendation or with full standards compliance; 4=Accredited with requirements for improvement; 3=Conditional accreditation.

Detailed Ratings for All Areas

See more information on "Key Ratings for Metro Areas" table beginning on page 32

Blue is most favorable
Bold Italic is least favorable
Blank means neither better nor worse than average
"–" means insufficient data

	Death rates for all selected case types			Hospital outcomes: better (★) or worse (×) than average — Adjusted Death rates — Medical Cases											
	Number of cases	Actual death rate (%)	Adjusted death rate (%) (lower is better)	All selected cases	All selected medical cases	Heart attack	Congestive heart failure	Obstructive pulmonary disease	Pneumonia	Respiratory failure and arrest	Septicemia	Stroke	Gastrointestinal hemorrhage	Fluid, electrolyte, & acid-base disorders	Kidney failure
National Average	–	–	12.1	12.1	14.8	21.2	10.6	6.5	16.9	34.4	25.1	18.4	6.7	11.0	20.9
Ohio *(continued)*															
Other Areas *(continued)*															
Trumbull, Warren	7,012	12.9	11.4						★			★			
UHHS Memorial, Geneva	1,066	11.8	11.5				★			–					–
Union, Dover[1]	2,775	12.6	***13.9***	✖	✖	✖		✖	×						
University - Brown, Conneaut	896	11.6	12.7					✖		–			–		–
University - Geauga Regional, Chardon	2,585	13.2	12.3				✖	★					×		
Upper Valley, Troy	3,495	14.0	***13.9***	✖	✖										
Van Wert County, Van Wert[1]	1,209	14.8	***18.6***	✖	✖			✖	✖	✖	✖	✖	–		
Wadsworth - Rittman, Wadsworth	1,479	12.5	12.7											✖	–
Wayne, Greenville	1,558	11.5	***13.8***	✖	✖	×			×			×			
Western Reserve, Youngstown	8,414	11.4	12.1				✖				★				★
Wilson, Sidney	1,740	9.8	11.5							★		×			
Wood County, Bowling Green	1,397	12.5	***15.3***	✖	✖		✖		×			✖		✖	
Wooster Community, Wooster	2,886	10.0	10.1	★	★				★		★				
Wyandot, Upper Sandusky	655	14.7	***15.2***	✖	✖	×		–		–	–	✖	–	–	
Oklahoma															
Arbuckle, Sulphur	508	14.0	13.5			–		–		–	–		–	–	–
Beaver County, Beaver	90	15.6	16.4			–	–	–	–	–	–	–	–	–	–
Bone and Joint, Oklahoma City	1,897	0.2	5.2	★	–	–	–	–	–	–	–	–	–	–	–
Bristow Memorial, Bristow	257	17.9	***17.2***	✖	✖	–	–	–		✖	–	–	–	–	–
Cancer Treatment Centers, Tulsa	168	22.0	11.2			–	–	–		–	–	–	–	–	–
Carnegie Tri-County Municipal, Carnegie	429	15.4	***15.1***	✖	✖	–		–		–	–	–	–	–	–
Chickasaw Nation, Ada[1]	318	8.5	11.3			–		–		–	–	–	–	–	–
Choctaw, Hugo	922	10.8	10.7			–				–			–		–
Choctaw Nation, Talihina[1]	100	3.0	3.7	★	★	–	–	–	–	–	–	–	–	–	–
Cimarron, Boise City	126	8.7	8.1			–	–	–	★	–	–	–	–	–	–
Claremore Regional, Claremore	1,639	12.4	10.7	★			★								✖
Cleveland Area, Cleveland[1]	358	14.8	14.9	×		–		–		–	–	–	–	–	–
Comanche County, Lawton	3,974	12.1	***14.8***	✖	✖		✖	✖			×				
Community - Lakeview, Eufaula	452	11.9	13.4					–		–	–	–	–	–	–
Cordell Memorial, Cordell	473	9.5	9.0	★	★			–	★	–	–		–		★
Craig General, Vinita	689	17.1	***16.5***	✖	✖			–	✖	–	–	✖	–		–
Creek Nation, Okemah	256	15.6	***19.4***	✖	✖	–	✖	–		–	–	–	–	–	–
Cushing Regional, Cushing	1,043	11.6	12.7							★					–

Footnotes are on page 350.

Hospital outcomes: better (★) or worse (×) than average											Results of accreditation review on full survey		Other facts			
Adjusted Death rates			Adjusted Adverse outcome rates													
Surgical cases			Surgical cases													
All selected surgical cases	Coronary artery bypass surgery	Large bowel surgery	All selected surgical cases	Coronary artery bypass surgery	Large bowel surgery	Gall bladder removal	Total knee replacement	Total hip replacement	Simple prostatectomy	Carotid endarterectomy	Accreditation status*	Overall evaluation score (higher is better)	Number of beds	Major medical school affiliation?	Number of residents	Computerized drug order system (1 to 5 scale, higher is preferred; see page 23 for details)
2.3	3.8	6.5	7.7	10.3	11.9	7.5	6.7	6.4	5.4	8.2	–	91	161	–	–	–
	–	★		–				✖		✖	4	***83***	284	No	0	–
–	–	–	–	–	–	–	–	–	–	–	4	***87***	40	No	0	–
	–			–			✖	–	–	–	4	89	104	No	0	–
–	–	–		–	–	–	–	–	–	–	4	92	51	No	0	–
	–	–		–			×		–	–	5	**96**	121	No	0	–
	–			–				–		–	4	**97**	392	No	24	–
✖	–	–		–		–		–	–	–	4	***88***	99	No	0	–
	–	–	★	–			–	–	–	–	4	89	67	No	0	–
	–			–		–	–	–	–	–	4	***85***	92	No	0	–
								✖	–		4	***79***	335	**Yes**	107	–
	–	–		–			–	–	–	–	4	***88***	81	No	0	–
–	–	–		–		–	–	–	–	–	5	**94**	80	No	0	–
	–		★	–		–		–	–	–	4	***84***	90	No	0	–
–	–	–	–	–	–	–	–	–	–	–	–[2]	–[2]	31	No	0	–
–	–	–	–	–	–	–	–	–	–	–	–[2]	–[2]	35	No	0	–
–	–	–	–	–	–	–	–	–	–	–	–[2]	–[2]	24	No	0	–
★	–	–	★	–	–	–	★	★	–	–	4	**95**	89	**Yes**	0	–
–	–	–	–	–	–	–	–	–	–	–	–[2]	–[2]	16	No	0	–
–	–	–	–	–	–	–	–	–	–	–	4	**95**	40	No	0	–
–	–	–	–	–	–	–	–	–	–	–	–[2]	–[2]	28	No	0	–
–	–	–	–	–	–	–	–	–	–	–	4	***88***	28	No	1	–
–	–	–	–	–	–	–	–	–	–	–	–[2]	–[2]	34	No	0	–
–	–	–	–	–	–	–	–	–	–	–	4	***84***	37	No	0	–
–	–	–	–	–	–	–	–	–	–	–	–[2]	–[2]	20	No	0	–
	–	–	★	–	★	–	–	–	–	–	5	**97**	68	No	0	–
–	–	–	–	–	–	–	–	–	–	–	–[2]	–[2]	19	No	0	–
✖	✖		✖	✖			★	–	–		4	***83***	283	No	0	–
–	–	–	–	–	–	–	–	–	–	–	–[2]	–[2]	33	No	0	–
–	–	–	–	–	–	–	–	–	–	–	–[2]	–[2]	28	No	0	–
–	–	–	–	–	–	–	–	–	–	–	–[2]	–[2]	29	No	0	–
–	–	–	–	–	–	–	–	–	–	–	–[2]	–[2]	34	No	0	–
–	–	–	–	–	–	–	–	–	–	–	4	92	75	No	0	–

***Accreditation Status:** 5=Accredited with commendation or with full standards compliance; 4=Accredited with requirements for improvement; 3=Conditional accreditation.

Detailed Ratings for All Areas

See more information on "Key Ratings for Metro Areas" table beginning on page 32

Blue is most favorable
Bold Italic is least favorable
Blank means neither better nor worse than average
"–" means insufficient data

	Death rates for all selected case types			Hospital outcomes: better (★) or worse (×) than average — Adjusted Death rates — Medical Cases											
	Number of cases	Actual death rate (%)	Adjusted death rate (%) (lower is better)	All selected cases	All selected medical cases	Heart attack	Congestive heart failure	Obstructive pulmonary disease	Pneumonia	Respiratory failure and arrest	Septicemia	Stroke	Gastrointestinal hemorrhage	Fluid, electrolyte, & acid-base disorders	Kidney failure
National Average	–	–	12.1	12.1	14.8	21.2	10.6	6.5	16.9	34.4	25.1	18.4	6.7	11.0	20.9
Oklahoma *(continued)*															
Deaconess, Oklahoma City	4,986	13.0	11.7						★						
Doctors, Tulsa	1,211	17.8	***14.9***	✖	✖		×	–	✖		★				
Duncan Regional, Duncan	2,567	14.7	***13.6***	✖	✖		×				✖				
Eastern Oklahoma, Poteau	1,804	13.9	***14.6***	✖	✖	×			✖	✖	✖				
Edmond Medical Center, Edmond	1,331	17.0	11.3											★	
Elkview General, Hobart	813	13.8	***14.6***	✖	✖	✖		–			×		–		–
Fairfax Memorial, Fairfax	252	13.5	11.0			–	–	–		–		–	–	–	–
Fairview Hospital, Fairview	232	21.1	***20.5***	✖	✖	–	✖	–		–	–	✖	–	–	–
Grady, Chickasha	2,588	12.8	11.9												
Great Plains Regional, Elk City	1,405	11.6	***14.7***	✖	✖		✖					✖	–		–
Harmon, Hollis	330	10.0	5.9	★	★	–	–	–	★	–		–	–	★	–
Harper County, Buffalo	199	16.1	13.7			–	–	–		–	–	–	–	–	–
Haskell County, Stigler[1]	846	13.6	14.2	×	×			✖	✖	–	×		–		–
Henryetta Medical Center, Henryetta	657	17.7	***20.4***	✖	✖	–	✖	–	✖	×	–	–	✖		–
Hillcrest, Tulsa	3,946	13.3	12.1			★						×			
Holdenville General, Holdenville	605	17.5	***21.1***	✖	✖	–	✖	–	✖	–		✖	–		–
Hurley, Coalgate	339	11.2	12.6			–		–		–	–	–	–	★	–
Integris Baptist, Oklahoma City	7,450	10.3	11.7			★									
Integris Baptist Regional, Miami	2,605	11.4	10.3	★	★			★		★	★			★	
Integris Bass Baptist, Enid	2,513	13.8	***13.8***	✖	✖		✖		✖						
Integris Blackwell Regional, Blackwell	912	14.1	10.6					–							–
Integris Clinton Regional, Clinton	1,029	13.5	10.8									×		★	–
Integris Grove General, Grove	2,118	13.5	***14.5***	✖	✖				✖		✖				✖
Integris Marshall, Madill	597	17.4	***16.2***	✖	✖	✖	×	–		–		✖	–	–	×
Integris Mayes County, Pryor	892	13.9	11.9									✖		–	
Integris Pawnee Municipal, Pawnee	370	13.2	13.2			–		–		–		–	–	–	–
Integris Southwest, Oklahoma City	4,842	14.8	***14.0***	✖	✖		✖								✖
Jackson County, Altus	2,553	10.0	12.0			✖	✖		★				★		
Jane Phillips, Bartlesville	3,495	13.8	***14.9***	✖	✖		✖	✖		✖	✖				✖
Latimer County General, Wilburton	420	11.4	11.7			–				–	–	–	–		–
Logan, Guthrie	751	16.5	***14.4***	✖	✖	✖		–		–	–		–	✖	–
Mangum City, Mangum	360	16.1	15.1	×	×	–		–		–	–		–	–	–
McAlester Regional, McAlester	3,208	14.3	***15.0***	✖	✖		✖		✖					✖	✖
McCurtain, Idabel	1,196	21.2	***17.4***	✖	✖	✖	✖		✖		✖	✖			
Medical Center of Southeastern Oklahoma, Durant	3,107	13.2	12.5								✖	★	✖	★	✖

Footnotes are on page 350.

Hospital outcomes: better (★) or worse (×) than average											Results of accreditation review on full survey		Other facts			
Adjusted Death rates			Adjusted Adverse outcome rates													
Surgical cases			Surgical cases													
All selected surgical cases	Coronary artery bypass surgery	Large bowel surgery	All selected surgical cases	Coronary artery bypass surgery	Large bowel surgery	Gall bladder removal	Total knee replacement	Total hip replacement	Simple prostatectomy	Carotid endarterectomy	Accreditation status*	Overall evaluation score (higher is better)	Number of beds	Major medical school affiliation?	Number of residents	Computerized drug order system (1 to 5 scale, higher is preferred; see page 23 for details)
2.3	3.8	6.5	7.7	10.3	11.9	7.5	6.7	6.4	5.4	8.2	–	91	161	–	–	–
✖			✖	×			✖	✖			4	**95**	219	No	9	–
✖	–	✖		–		–	–	–	–	–	–[2]	–[2]	121	No	0	–
	–	–		–			–	–	–	–	4	93	82	No	0	–
–	–	–		–	–	–	–	–	–	–	4	***87***	72	No	0	–
–	–	–		–	–	–	×	–	–	–	5	**98**	84	No	0	–
–	–	–	–	–	–	–	–	–	–	–	–[2]	–[2]	30	No	0	–
–	–	–	–	–	–	–	–	–	–	–	–[2]	–[2]	15	No	0	–
–	–	–	–	–	–	–	–	–	–	–	–[2]	–[2]	31	No	0	–
	–			–	★		×	–	–		4	93	123	No	0	–
	–	–	★	–			–	–			4	93	76	No	0	–
–	–	–	–	–	–	–	–	–	–	–	–[2]	–[2]	16	No	0	–
–	–	–	–	–	–	–	–	–	–	–	–[2]	–[2]	25	No	0	–
–	–	–	–	–	–	–	–	–	–	–	–[2]	–[2]	31	No	0	–
–	–	–	–	–	–	–	–	–	–	–	4	**94**	42	No	0	–
×						★		–			4	***85***	421	**Yes**	0	–
–	–	–	–	–	–	–	–	–	–	–	–[2]	–[2]	22	No	0	–
–	–	–	–	–	–	–	–	–	–	–	–[2]	–[2]	20	No	0	–
			✖		✖		✖				4	93	503	No	16	–
–	–	–	★	–	–	–	–	–	–	–	4	**98**	113	No	0	–
	–			–		–	★	–	–	–	4	93	207	No	0	–
–	–	–	–	–	–	–	–	–	–	–	4	**95**	34	No	0	–
–	–	–	–	–	–	–	–	–	–	–	4	90	49	No	0	–
	–	–		–		–		–	–	–	4	**99**	72	No	0	–
–	–	–	–	–	–	–	–	–	–	–	4	***83***	25	No	0	–
–	–	–	–	–	–	–	–	–	–	–	4	**96**	38	No	0	–
–	–	–	–	–	–	–	–	–	–	–	–[2]	–[2]	32	No	0	–
✖											4	***87***	325	No	0	–
✖	–			–		✖					–[2]	–[2]	76	No	0	–
	–		✖	–	★	✖	✖		–		4	***87***	158	No	0	–
–	–	–	–	–	–	–	–	–	–	–	–[2]	–[2]	33	No	0	–
–	–	–	–	–	–	–	–	–	–	–	4	93	32	No	0	–
–	–	–	–	–	–	–	–	–	–	–	–[2]	–[2]	22	No	0	–
	–	–		–				–	–	–	4	***88***	197	No	0	–
–	–	–	–	–	–	–	–	–	–	–	–[2]	–[2]	81	No	0	–
	–	–	★	–		–	–	–	–	–	4	**100**	103	**Yes**	5	–

***Accreditation Status:** 5=Accredited with commendation or with full standards compliance; 4=Accredited with requirements for improvement; 3=Conditional accreditation.

Detailed Ratings for All Areas

See more information on "Key Ratings for Metro Areas" table beginning on page 32

Blue is most favorable
Bold Italic is least favorable
Blank means neither better nor worse than average
"–" means insufficient data

	Death rates for all selected case types			Hospital outcomes: better (★) or worse (×) than average											
				Adjusted Death rates											
					Medical Cases										
	Number of cases	Actual death rate (%)	Adjusted death rate (%) (lower is better)	All selected cases	All selected medical cases	Heart attack	Congestive heart failure	Obstructive pulmonary disease	Pneumonia	Respiratory failure and arrest	Septicemia	Stroke	Gastrointestinal hemorrhage	Fluid, electrolyte, & acid-base disorders	Kidney failure
National Average	–	–	12.1	12.1	14.8	21.2	10.6	6.5	16.9	34.4	25.1	18.4	6.7	11.0	20.9
Oklahoma *(continued)*															
Memorial, Frederick[1]	684	11.0	10.5			–		***✖***	★	–	–	–	–		–
Memorial, Stilwell	731	11.9	12.2					–		–			–		–
Memorial of Texas County, Guymon	733	10.0	**8.9**	**★**	**★**			**★**	**★**				–	–	–
Mercy, Ardmore	3,932	14.8	***13.7***	***✖***	***✖***	***✖***		***✖***	×				×		
Mercy, Oklahoma City	5,246	10.6	11.4		★					**★**					
Midwest Regional, Midwest City	5,636	11.1	11.5					***✖***				**★**		**★**	**★**
Mission Hill, Shawnee	1,039	20.6	***15.9***	***✖***	***✖***		***✖***	–	***✖***						–
Muskogee Regional, Muskogee	6,589	12.5	11.3	★	★		**★**			***✖***	**★**	**★**	**★**	★	
Newman, Shattuck	546	11.2	11.9			–		–		–	–		–		–
Norman Regional, Norman	5,741	12.7	***13.1***	***✖***			×								
Okeene Municipal, Okeene	241	18.3	***18.1***	***✖***	***✖***		–	–		–	–	–	–	–	–
Okmulgee Memorial, Okmulgee	1,340	13.3	***14.6***	***✖***	***✖***			***✖***		–					
OU Medical Center, Oklahoma City	3,891	11.1	11.9							**★**			***✖***		
Park View, El Reno	1,011	12.8	***14.9***	***✖***	***✖***				***✖***		–		–		–
Pauls Valley General, Pauls Valley	1,027	15.9	12.0						×	–			**★**		–
Perry Memorial, Perry	516	14.0	13.0					–		–			–	–	–
PHS Indian Health, Claremore	239	9.2	11.9			–		–		–	–	–	–	–	–
Physicians of Oklahoma, Oklahoma City	93	5.4	10.1			–	–	–	–	–	–	–	–	–	–
Purcell Municipal, Purcell	1,034	15.0	13.1			***✖***									***✖***
Pushmataha City - Town of Antlers, Antlers	1,081	18.4	***16.4***	***✖***	***✖***	***✖***	×	***✖***	***✖***	–					×
St Anthony, Oklahoma City	3,962	10.2	**10.8**	**★**	**★**				**★**					★	
St Francis, Broken Arrow[1]	1,025	14.3	***14.9***	***✖***	***✖***			***✖***	***✖***						–
St Francis, Tulsa[1]	10,389	11.7	***12.8***	***✖***	***✖***		***✖***	***✖***		***✖***					
St John, Tulsa	9,711	11.6	***13.5***	***✖***	***✖***	×		***✖***		***✖***				***✖***	×
St Mary's Regional, Enid	3,019	13.0	**10.9**	**★**	**★**			★	**★**						
St Michael, Oklahoma City[1]	1,158	14.2	13.6	×				***✖***					–		***✖***
Sayre Memorial, Sayre	522	16.7	***15.0***	***✖***	***✖***			–		–			–		–
Seiling Municipal, Seiling	312	17.3	***15.8***	***✖***	***✖***	–		–		–	–		–	–	–
Seminole Medical Center, Seminole	257	19.8	***20.9***	***✖***	***✖***	–	***✖***	–	***✖***	–	***✖***	–	–	–	–
Sequoyah, Sallisaw	587	15.3	13.3				***✖***	–					–	×	–
Share, Alva	710	16.1	***16.9***	***✖***	***✖***	***✖***	***✖***		×	–	–		–		–
Shawnee Regional, Shawnee	2,099	17.2	***17.2***	***✖***	***✖***	***✖***	***✖***	***✖***	***✖***		***✖***				***✖***
Southcrest, Tulsa	415	8.9	10.9					–	★	–	–		–	–	–
Southwestern, Lawton	1,615	11.1	12.4							***✖***					
Southwestern, Weatherford	577	22.4	***18.7***	***✖***	***✖***	–		–	***✖***	–	***✖***	×	–		***✖***

Footnotes are on page 350.

Hospital outcomes: better (★) or worse (×) than average											Results of accreditation review on full survey		Other facts			
Adjusted Death rates			**Adjusted Adverse outcome rates**													
Surgical cases			Surgical cases													
All selected surgical cases	Coronary artery bypass surgery	Large bowel surgery	All selected surgical cases	Coronary artery bypass surgery	Large bowel surgery	Gall bladder removal	Total knee replacement	Total hip replacement	Simple prostatectomy	Carotid endarterectomy	Accreditation status*	Overall evaluation score (higher is better)	Number of beds	Major medical school affiliation?	Number of residents	Computerized drug order system (1 to 5 scale, higher is preferred; see page 23 for details)
2.3	3.8	6.5	7.7	10.3	11.9	7.5	6.7	6.4	5.4	8.2	–	91	161	–	–	–
–	–	–	–	–	–	–	–	–	–	–	–[2]	–[2]	30	No	0	–
–	–	–	–	–	–	–	–	–	–	–	–[2]	–[2]	50	No	–	–
–	–	–	–	–	–	–	–	–	–	–	–[2]	–[2]	40	No	0	–
	–		★	–				★			4	**87**	199	No	0	–
								–	×		4	91	350	No	0	–
				×			★	★	–		4	**97**	227	No	0	–
–	–	–		–	–	–	–	–	–	–	4	89	49	No	0	–
	–			–			★	✖	–	–	4	**88**	225	No	0	–
–	–	–	–	–	–	–	–	–	–	–	–[2]	–[2]	27	No	0	–
✖	✖		✖			✖	✖		✖	✖	4	**94**	271	No	0	–
–	–	–	–	–	–	–	–	–	–	–	–[2]	–[2]	50	No	0	–
–	–	–		–	–	–	–	–		–	4	**82**	66	No	–	–
			×				✖	–	–		4	**82**	941	**Yes**	445	–
–	–	–	–	–	–	–	–	–	–	–	–[2]	–[2]	54	No	0	–
–	–	–		–		–	–	–	–	–	–[2]	–[2]	42	No	0	–
–	–	–	–	–	–	–	–	–	–	–	–[2]	–[2]	28	No	0	–
–	–	–	–	–	–	–	–	–	–	–	4	**99**	46	No	0	–
–	–	–	–	–	–	–	–	–	–	–	4	91	51	No	–	–
–	–	–	–	–	–	–	–	–	–	–	–[2]	–[2]	22	No	0	–
–	–	–	–	–	–	–	–	–	–	–	–[2]	–[2]	46	No	0	–
	×		★				–	–			4	**100**	342	No	23	–
–	–	–		–	–	–	–	–	–	–	–[2]	–[2]	62	No	0	–
✖	✖	✖				×		★			5	**96**	584	**Yes**	0	–
											4	91	556	No	0	–
	–			–		★	★	–	×	–	4	**95**	123	No	0	–
–	–	–		–	–	–	–	–	–	–	4	93	128	No	36	–
–	–	–	–	–	–	–	–	–	–	–	–[2]	–[2]	46	No	0	–
–	–	–	–	–	–	–	–	–	–	–	–[2]	–[2]	18	No	0	–
–	–	–	–	–	–	–	–	–	–	–	–[2]	–[2]	32	No	0	–
–	–	–	–	–	–	–	–	–	–	–	–[2]	–[2]	41	**Yes**	0	–
–	–	–	–	–	–	–	–	–	–	–	–[2]	–[2]	37	No	0	–
	–	–		–			–	–	–	–	4	90	126	No	0	–
–	–	–		–	–	–	–	–	–	–	4	**96**	119	No	–	–
	–		★	–		–	–	–	–	★	4	**96**	158	No	0	–
–	–	–	–	–	–	–	–	–	–	–	–[2]	–[2]	46	No	0	–

***Accreditation Status:** 5=Accredited with commendation or with full standards compliance; 4=Accredited with requirements for improvement; 3=Conditional accreditation.

Detailed Ratings for All Areas

See more information on "Key Ratings for Metro Areas" table beginning on page 32

Blue is most favorable
Bold Italic is least favorable
Blank means neither better nor worse than average
"–" means insufficient data

	Death rates for all selected case types			Hospital outcomes: better (★) or worse (×) than average — Adjusted Death rates — Medical Cases											
	Number of cases	Actual death rate (%)	Adjusted death rate (%) (lower is better)	All selected cases	All selected medical cases	Heart attack	Congestive heart failure	Obstructive pulmonary disease	Pneumonia	Respiratory failure and arrest	Septicemia	Stroke	Gastrointestinal hemorrhage	Fluid, electrolyte, & acid-base disorders	Kidney failure
National Average	–	–	12.1	12.1	14.8	21.2	10.6	6.5	16.9	34.4	25.1	18.4	6.7	11.0	20.9
Oklahoma *(continued)*															
Stillwater Medical Center, Stillwater	2,046	13.4	***13.5***	✖	✖	✖									
Tahlequah City, Tahlequah	1,404	14.6	13.4	×											–
Tulsa Regional, Tulsa	3,042	15.4	12.9	×		✖			★				✖		
USPHS Lawton Indian, Lawton	81	7.4	9.1			–	–	–	–	–	–	–	–	–	–
Valley View Regional, Ada	3,267	12.7	***14.2***	✖	✖	✖	×	✖	✖	–				×	✖
Via Christi Oklahoma Regional, Ponca City	1,717	17.0	***19.4***	✖	✖	✖	✖	×	✖			✖		✖	
W W Hastings Indian, Tahlequah	569	9.1	13.9			–			✖	–	–		–	–	–
Wagoner Community, Wagoner	922	9.5	9.6	★	★	–			★						
Woodward Regional, Woodward	919	13.8	***15.5***	✖	✖	✖			✖		×				×
Oregon															
Portland Area															
Adventist, Portland	2,499	13.4	***14.2***	✖	✖		×								
Eastmoreland, Portland	526	16.9	14.0			✖		–		–	–		–	–	–
Kaiser Sunnyside, Clackamas	3,038	11.8	***15.7***	✖	✖	×	✖	✖	✖					✖	
Legacy Emanuel, Portland[1]	1,891	11.5	13.5	×											
Legacy Good Samaritan, Portland	2,947	11.1	12.3			★	✖	✖				✖			
Legacy Meridian Park, Tualatin	3,199	12.2	***14.9***	✖	✖	✖	✖			–		✖			✖
Legacy Mount Hood, Gresham	1,067	18.2	***15.5***	✖	✖	✖				×			✖		
OHSU, Portland[1]	1,537	11.0	12.1										–		
Providence, Milwaukie	1,217	15.8	***19.3***	✖	✖		✖	✖	✖	–	–	✖	✖	–	–
Providence, Portland	6,802	12.0	***13.5***	✖	✖		✖			✖	×	✖		✖	×
Providence St Vincent, Portland	7,834	10.5	***13.9***	✖	✖		✖	✖	✖		✖	✖		✖	
Tuality, Forest Grove	–	–	–	–	–	–	–	–	–	–	–	–	–	–	–
Tuality, Hillsboro	1,782	14.6	***16.2***	✖	✖		✖	✖		✖		✖	✖		
Willamette Falls, Oregon City	1,396	14.3	***16.1***	✖	✖		✖		✖			✖			–
Woodland Park, Portland	554	22.4	***15.5***	✖	✖			–	✖	×		✖	–		–
Other Areas															
Albany General, Albany	1,599	15.4	***16.0***	✖	✖		✖		✖			✖			
Ashland Community, Ashland	747	10.0	10.3								★		–		–
Bay Area, Coos Bay	3,924	10.0	***14.2***	✖	✖				✖	✖		✖			
Central Oregon, Redmond	894	11.2	***15.1***	✖	✖			✖		–			–	–	–
Columbia, Astoria	1,069	12.3	***14.2***	✖	✖	✖					–				–
Coquille Valley, Coquille	277	15.2	***18.5***	✖	✖	–	–	–	×	–	–		–	–	–
Curry General, Gold Beach	347	15.9	***18.9***	✖	✖	–	✖	–	✖	–	–	×	–	–	–

Footnotes are on page 350.

Hospital outcomes: better (★) or worse (×) than average — Adjusted Death rates — Surgical cases: All selected surgical cases	Coronary artery bypass surgery	Large bowel surgery	Adjusted Adverse outcome rates — Surgical cases: All selected surgical cases	Coronary artery bypass surgery	Large bowel surgery	Gall bladder removal	Total knee replacement	Total hip replacement	Simple prostatectomy	Carotid endarterectomy	Results of accreditation review on full survey: Accreditation status*	Overall evaluation score (higher is better)	Other facts: Number of beds	Major medical school affiliation?	Number of residents	Computerized drug order system (1 to 5 scale, higher is preferred; see page 23 for details)
2.3	3.8	6.5	7.7	10.3	11.9	7.5	6.7	6.4	5.4	8.2	–	91	161	–	–	–
	–	–		–				–	–	–	5	98	89	No	0	–
–	–	–		–		–	–	–	–	–	4	99	75	No	0	–
							★	–	–	★	–[2]	–[2]	255	Yes	108	–
–	–	–	–	–	–	–	–	–	–	–	4	85	44	No	0	–
	–		★	–			★	–		–	4	93	153	No	0	–
✖	–	×		–		–	–	–	–		4	95	90	No	0	–
–	–	–	–	–	–	–	–	–	–	–	4	98	60	No	2	–
–	–	–	–	–	–	–	–	–	–	–	–[2]	–[2]	100	No	0	–
	–	–	★	–		–	–	–	–	–	4	94	68	No	0	–
	–			–							4	95	214	No	0	–
–	–	–	★	–	–	–	–	–	–	–	–[2]	–[2]	77	Yes	0	–
×	–			–			★		–		4	89	178	No	0	–
✖	–	–				✖			–		–[2]	–[2]	329	Yes	35	–
★			★			–					–[2]	–[2]	239	Yes	39	–
	–		★	–					–	★	4	93	117	No	0	–
	–	–		–		–	–	–	–	–	4	95	58	No	0	–
	–	–				–	–	–	–		4	89	373	Yes	312	–
	–	–	★	–			★	–	–	–	4	90	27	No	0	–
			★		★		★	★		★	4	93	380	No	31	–
			★							★	4	83	389	Yes	41	–
–	–	–	–	–	–	–	–	–	–	–	–[2]	–[2]	–	–	–	–
	–	×		–	×	–	★	–	–	–	4	93	129	No	0	–
	–	–		–		–		–	–	–	4	86	91	No	0	–
–	–	–	–	–	–	–	–	–	–	–	4	83	121	No	0	–
	–	–		–	✖	–	–	–	–	–	4	89	71	No	4	–
–	–	–	★	–	–	–	–	–	–	–	4	96	49	No	0	–
	–		★	–		★				★	4	88	114	No	5	–
	–	–		–		–	–	–	–	–	4	92	48	No	0	–
–	–	–		–			–	–	–	–	4	89	37	No	0	–
–	–	–	–	–	–	–	–	–	–	–	–[2]	–[2]	20	No	0	–
–	–	–	–	–	–	–	–	–	–	–	–[2]	–[2]	24	No	0	–

***Accreditation Status:** 5=Accredited with commendation or with full standards compliance; 4=Accredited with requirements for improvement; 3=Conditional accreditation.

Detailed Ratings for All Areas

See more information on "Key Ratings for Metro Areas" table beginning on page 32

Blue is most favorable
Bold Italic is least favorable
Blank means neither better nor worse than average
"–" means insufficient data

	Death rates for all selected case types				Hospital outcomes: better (★) or worse (×) than average — Adjusted Death rates — Medical Cases											
	Number of cases	Actual death rate (%)	Adjusted death rate (%) (lower is better)	All selected cases	All selected medical cases	Heart attack	Congestive heart failure	Obstructive pulmonary disease	Pneumonia	Respiratory failure and arrest	Septicemia	Stroke	Gastrointestinal hemorrhage	Fluid, electrolyte, & acid-base disorders	Kidney failure
National Average	–	–	12.1	12.1	14.8	21.2	10.6	6.5	16.9	34.4	25.1	18.4	6.7	11.0	20.9
Oregon *(continued)*															
Other Areas (continued)															
Good Samaritan, Corvallis	2,693	8.6	**10.4**	**★**	**★**	**★**									**★**
Good Shepherd, Hermiston[1]	880	13.9	***14.7***	✖	✖		✖			–	–		–	✖	–
Grande Ronde, La Grande	1,172	12.3	12.0									✖			
Harney, Burns	234	12.8	14.1			–	✖	–		–	–	–	–	–	–
Holy Rosary, Ontario	2,065	11.1	11.5				×			**★**					
Lake District, Lakeview	201	14.4	***17.5***	✖	✖	–	–	–		–	–	–	–	–	–
Lebanon Community, Lebanon[1]	1,673	10.8	12.8				✖								–
Lower Umpqua, Reedsport[1]	371	13.5	15.2	×	✖	–	–	–	✖	–	–		–	–	–
McKenzie - Willamette, Springfield	2,512	11.3	12.4					×							
Mercy, Roseburg[1]	3,920	10.1	**10.2**	**★**	**★**				**★**		**★**				
Merle West, Klamath Falls	3,161	11.9	12.5					×							
Mid-Columbia, The Dalles	1,568	10.2	10.5	★	★					**★**	**★**	✖			
Mountain View, Madras[1]	347	12.7	***16.4***	✖	✖	–	–	–		–	–	×	–	–	–
Peace Harbor, Florence	843	12.7	***14.6***	✖	✖	×				–	–		–	–	–
Pioneer, Heppner	67	9.0	7.2			–	–	–	–	–	–	–	–	–	–
Pioneer, Prineville	480	18.8	***16.9***	✖	✖			–	×	×	–	✖	–	–	–
Providence, Hood River	660	12.3	13.9					–		–	–		–	–	–
Providence, Medford	2,761	11.8	***13.4***	✖	×				×						
Providence, Newberg	548	15.7	***15.0***	✖	✖			–			–	✖	–	–	–
Rogue Valley, Medford	4,756	9.8	12.9	×	✖		✖	✖				✖			
Sacred Heart, Eugene	8,464	11.1	***13.6***	✖	✖	★	✖		✖		×		✖	✖	
St Anthony, Pendleton	750	13.9	***15.5***	✖	✖			✖	✖	–				–	–
St Charles, Bend	4,059	8.1	12.2			**★**	✖	✖				×			
St Elizabeth, Baker City	858	12.9	***15.4***	✖	✖		✖				–		×		–
Salem Hospital, Salem	6,963	14.0	***15.9***	✖	✖		✖	✖	✖	×		✖	✖	✖	×
Samaritan Pacific, Newport[1]	1,100	13.9	13.2								×	✖		–	–
Santiam, Stayton	424	19.6	***23.2***	✖	✖	–	✖	–	✖	–	–	✖	–	✖	–
Silverton Hospital, Silverton	963	14.4	***14.0***	✖	✖		✖	–		–		✖			
Three Rivers, Grants Pass[1]	3,463	11.9	***13.6***	✖	✖		×				**★**	✖			
Tillamook County General, Tillamook	928	13.4	***14.3***	✖	✖			–				✖	✖	–	
Valley, Dallas	590	12.5	12.3					–	✖	–	–			–	
Wallowa, Enterprise	329	15.5	***16.4***	✖	✖	✖	✖	–		–	–	✖	–	–	–
Willamette Valley, McMinnville	1,661	13.1	12.4												×

Footnotes are on page 350.

Hospital outcomes: better (★) or worse (×) than average											Results of accreditation review on full survey		Other facts			
Adjusted Death rates			Adjusted Adverse outcome rates													
Surgical cases			Surgical cases													
All selected surgical cases	Coronary artery bypass surgery	Large bowel surgery	All selected surgical cases	Coronary artery bypass surgery	Large bowel surgery	Gall bladder removal	Total knee replacement	Total hip replacement	Simple prostatectomy	Carotid endarterectomy	Accreditation status*	Overall evaluation score (higher is better)	Number of beds	Major medical school affiliation?	Number of residents	Computerized drug order system (1 to 5 scale, higher is preferred; see page 23 for details)
2.3	3.8	6.5	7.7	10.3	11.9	7.5	6.7	6.4	5.4	8.2	–	91	161	–	–	–
	★		★					★	★		4	89	134	No	3	–
–	–	–	★	–	–	–	–	–	–	–	4	**84**	45	No	0	–
	–			–		–		–	–	–	4	92	49	No	0	–
–	–	–	–	–	–	–	–	–	–	–	–[2]	–[2]	44	No	0	–
	–		★	–				–	–	–	4	92	74	No	0	–
–	–	–	–	–	–	–	–	–	–	–	–[2]	–[2]	21	No	0	–
	–	–		–		–	–	–	–	–	4	91	49	No	0	–
–	–	–		–	–	–	–	–	–	–	–[2]	–[2]	21	No	0	–
	–			–					–		4	**83**	106	No	0	–
	–			–						–	4	**82**	114	No	0	–
×	–	×		–	×				–		4	92	136	No	0	–
	–	–		–		–	×	–	–		4	**97**	49	No	0	–
–	–	–	–	–	–	–	–	–	–	–	–[2]	–[2]	34	No	0	–
–	–	–	★	–	–	–	–	–	–	–	4	**86**	21	No	0	–
–	–	–	–	–	–	–	–	–	–	–	–[2]	–[2]	12	No	0	–
–	–	–		–	–	–	–	–	–	–	–[2]	–[2]	30	No	0	–
–	–	–		–	–	–	–	–	–	–	4	89	31	No	0	–
×	–		★	–		×			★	★	4	**98**	121	No	0	–
–	–	–	–	–	–	–	–	–	–	–	4	**94**	35	No	0	–
	★		★	★							4	**87**	264	No	0	–
	×						★				4	90	404	No	0	–
	–	–		–		–	–	–	–	–	4	**88**	49	No	0	–
★			★	★	★		★			★	4	89	181	No	5	–
–	–	–		–	–	–	–	–	–	–	4	**86**	36	No	1	–
				×			★			★	4	93	402	No	0	–
–	–	–		–		–	–	–	–	–	4	92	42	No	0	–
–	–	–	–	–	–	–	–	–	–	–	4	**86**	40	No	0	–
–	–	–		–		–	–	–	–	–	–[2]	–[2]	38	No	0	–
	–			–		×	★				4	93	71	No	0	–
–	–	–		–	–	–	–	–	–	–	4	**97**	30	No	1	–
–	–	–	★	–	–	–	–	–	–	–	4	**83**	36	No	0	–
–	–	–	–	–	–	–	–	–	–	–	–[2]	–[2]	24	No	0	–
	–	–		–		–		–	–	–	4	**99**	67	No	0	–

***Accreditation Status:** 5=Accredited with commendation or with full standards compliance; 4=Accredited with requirements for improvement; 3=Conditional accreditation.

Detailed Ratings for All Areas

See more information on "Key Ratings for Metro Areas" table beginning on page 32

Blue is most favorable
Bold Italic is least favorable
Blank means neither better nor worse than average
"–" means insufficient data

	Death rates for all selected case types				Hospital outcomes: better (★) or worse (×) than average — Adjusted Death rates — Medical Cases										
	Number of cases	Actual death rate (%)	Adjusted death rate (%) (lower is better)	All selected cases	All selected medical cases	Heart attack	Congestive heart failure	Obstructive pulmonary disease	Pneumonia	Respiratory failure and arrest	Septicemia	Stroke	Gastrointestinal hemorrhage	Fluid, electrolyte, & acid-base disorders	Kidney failure
National Average	–	–	12.1	12.1	14.8	21.2	10.6	6.5	16.9	34.4	25.1	18.4	6.7	11.0	20.9
Pennsylvania															
Delaware Valley Area															
Abington Memorial, Abington	7,386	13.3	11.4		★							★			
Albert Einstein, Philadelphia	5,783	13.7	11.6				**★**		★		✖				
Brandywine, Coatesville[1]	2,926	14.5	12.1						★			✖		✖	
Bryn Mawr Hospital, Bryn Mawr[1]	5,922	9.7	**10.0**	**★**	**★**	**★**			**★**	**★**					
Chester County, West Chester	4,046	12.0	11.3		★						★	★			
Chestnut Hill, Philadelphia	3,818	17.3	12.5			**★**			×		✖			✖	
Children's, Philadelphia	–	–	–	–	–	–	–	–	–	–	–	–	–	–	–
Crozer - Chester, Upland	6,864	13.8	12.0					✖		✖			✖		
Delaware County, Drexel Hill	3,722	10.8	11.5				**★**								
Doylestown Hospital, Doylestown	3,495	12.2	11.3												
Elkins Park Hospital, Elkins Park	429	11.2	**8.4**	**★**	**★**	–		–		–		–	–	–	–
Episcopal, Philadelphia	1,054	9.2	**9.7**	**★**	**★**		**★**				✖		–		–
Fox Chase Cancer Center, Philadelphia	377	18.8	***17.4***	✖	✖	–	–	–		–	–	–	–	✖	–
Frankford - Bucks County Campus, Langhorne	–	–	–	–	–	–	–	–	–	–	–	–	–	–	–
Frankford - Frankford Campus, Philadelphia	–	–	–	–	–	–	–	–	–	–	–	–	–	–	–
Frankford - Torresdale, Philadelphia	6,851	14.2	12.5			✖							✖		
Germantown, Philadelphia	–	–	–	–	–	–	–	–	–	–	–	–	–	–	–
Graduate, Philadelphia	548	6.8	**7.2**	**★**	**★**			–		–			–		–
Grand View, Sellersville	3,049	10.7	12.2					×	×	★					
Hahnemann University, Philadelphia	887	9.7	**9.1**	**★**	**★**	★	**★**	–	**★**		–		–		
Holy Redeemer, Meadowbrook[1]	4,744	11.3	11.2	★	★		**★**	★							
Jeanes, Philadelphia	5,098	12.3	**10.9**	**★**	**★**	×			**★**						
Lankenau, Wynnewood	6,486	9.7	**8.6**	**★**	**★**	**★**	**★**	**★**	**★**		**★**	**★**			★
Medical College of Pennsylvania, Philadelphia	789	9.5	**8.8**	**★**	**★**					–	–				–
Mercy, Havertown	2,207	17.5	***14.8***	✖	✖	×		✖	✖		✖	×			
Mercy, Philadelphia	–	–	–	–	–	–	–	–	–	–	–	–	–	–	–
Mercy Fitzgerald, Darby[1]	7,544	14.1	11.9			✖		★		✖				★	
Mercy Suburban, Norristown	1,920	19.4	***16.0***	✖	✖	✖	✖				×	✖		✖	
Methodist, Philadelphia	0	–	–	–	–	–	–	–	–	–	–	–	–	–	–
Montgomery, Norristown	3,902	12.9	***13.9***	✖	✖		★	✖	✖					✖	
Nazareth, Philadelphia	6,361	14.2	**10.9**	**★**	**★**		**★**		**★**						
North Penn, Lansdale	1,913	14.9	***13.9***	✖	✖			✖	✖						
Northeastern, Philadelphia	–	–	–	–	–	–	–	–	–	–	–	–	–	–	–
Paoli Memorial, Paoli	2,571	12.1	12.8								★	✖			

Footnotes are on page 350.

Hospital outcomes: better (★) or worse (×) than average											Results of accreditation review on full survey		Other facts			
Adjusted Death rates			Adjusted Adverse outcome rates													
Surgical cases			Surgical cases													
All selected surgical cases	Coronary artery bypass surgery	Large bowel surgery	All selected surgical cases	Coronary artery bypass surgery	Large bowel surgery	Gall bladder removal	Total knee replacement	Total hip replacement	Simple prostatectomy	Carotid endarterectomy	Accreditation status*	Overall evaluation score (higher is better)	Number of beds	Major medical school affiliation?	Number of residents	Computerized drug order system (1 to 5 scale, higher is preferred; see page 23 for details)
2.3	3.8	6.5	7.7	10.3	11.9	7.5	6.7	6.4	5.4	8.2	–	91	161	–	–	–
					✖		✖	✖	★		4	93	424	No	98	–
✖			✖			✖		–		–	4	90	379	Yes	71	–
	–			–		–	–	–	–	–	4	**95**	164	No	0	–
						★					4	**96**	260	No	30	–
×	–	×		–					–		4	92	195	No	0	–
★	–	★	★	–		★	–	–	–	–	5	**97**	140	No	26	–
–	–	–	–	–	–	–	–	–	–	–	–[2]	–[2]	387	–	178	–
			★	★			★		–		4	90	574	Yes	82	–
	–			–				✖	✖		4	93	231	No	16	–
	–			–				–	–	–	4	**94**	178	No	0	–
–	–	–	–	–	–	–	–	–	–	–	4	**97**	158	No	3	–
×	–	–			–	–	–	–	–	–	–[2]	–[2]	218	Yes	11	–
–	–	–		–		–	–	–	–	–	4	**94**	76	No	4	–
–	–	–	–	–	–	–	–	–	–	–	–[2]	–[2]	–	–	–	–
–	–	–	–	–	–	–	–	–	–	–	–[2]	–[2]	–	–	–	–
	–			★		★			–	✖	4	***85***	537	Yes	86	–
–	–	–	–	–	–	–	–	–	–	–	4	92	110	–	4	–
–	–	–		–	–	–	–	–	–	–	4	93	198	No	9	–
	–		★	–	★				–	–	–[2]	–[2]	174	No	0	–
	×	–			–	–	–	–	–	–	4	92	540	Yes	128	–
	–		✖	–			✖	×		✖	4	***88***	210	No	0	–
	–			–				–	–		4	**94**	182	No	0	–
★						✖					–[2]	–[2]	287	Yes	91	–
–	–	–	–	–	–	–	–	–	–	–	4	90	369	Yes	38	–
–	–	–		–	–	–	–	–	–	–	4	**94**	97	No	0	–
–	–	–	–	–	–	–	–	–	–	–	–[2]	–[2]	–	–	–	–
	–		×	–	✖	★		–			4	89	499	Yes	114	–
×	–	–		–	–	–	–	–	–	–	3	***87***	115	Yes	3	–
–	–	–	–	–	–	–	–	–	–	–	–[2]	–[2]	271	Yes	15	–
	–	✖	✖	–	✖		✖	✖			4	91	182	No	18	–
	–			–				–	–	–	4	89	199	No	0	–
	–	–		–			–	–	–	–	–[2]	–[2]	107	No	3	–
–	–	–	–	–	–	–	–	–	–	–	–[2]	–[2]	166	–	4	–
	–			–					–		–[2]	–[2]	138	No	0	–

***Accreditation Status:** 5=Accredited with commendation or with full standards compliance; 4=Accredited with requirements for improvement; 3=Conditional accreditation.

Detailed Ratings for All Areas

See more information on "Key Ratings for Metro Areas" table beginning on page 32

Blue is most favorable
Bold Italic is least favorable
Blank means neither better nor worse than average
"–" means insufficient data

	Death rates for all selected case types			Hospital outcomes: better (★) or worse (×) than average											
				Adjusted Death rates											
					Medical Cases										
	Number of cases	Actual death rate (%)	Adjusted death rate (%) (lower is better)	All selected cases	All selected medical cases	Heart attack	Congestive heart failure	Obstructive pulmonary disease	Pneumonia	Respiratory failure and arrest	Septicemia	Stroke	Gastrointestinal hemorrhage	Fluid, electrolyte, & acid-base disorders	Kidney failure
National Average	–	–	12.1	12.1	14.8	21.2	10.6	6.5	16.9	34.4	25.1	18.4	6.7	11.0	20.9
Pennsylvania *(continued)*															
Delaware Valley Area *(continued)*															
Pennsylvania, Philadelphia	5,286	5.2	8.4	★	★		★		★			★			
Phoenixville Hospital, Phoenixville[1]	2,367	13.8	13.0		×			×							✖
Pottstown Memorial, Pottstown	3,393	16.4	***16.0***	✖	✖	✖	✖	✖	✖				×	✖	
Presbyterian, Philadelphia	3,259	12.3	9.3	★	★	★	★	★	★				★	★	★
Riddle, Media	4,561	15.0	***12.9***	✖	✖			✖		✖					
Roxborough, Philadelphia	2,749	12.7	10.6	★	★				★						
St Agnes, Philadelphia	2,749	12.1	9.5	★	★		★		★	★	★			★	★
St Christophers for Children, Philadelphia	–	–	–	–	–	–	–	–	–	–	–	–	–	–	–
St Joseph's, Philadelphia[1]	1,312	11.8	9.2	★	★	–	★		★						
St Lukes, Quakertown	1,149	15.9	13.2			✖									
St Mary, Langhorne	4,692	15.4	***14.1***	✖	✖			✖	✖	✖			✖		
Southern Chester County, West Grove	1,769	12.2	11.6			✖			★						
Springfield Hospital, Springfield	–	–	–	–	–	–	–	–	–	–	–	–	–	–	–
Taylor, Ridley Park	–	–	–	–	–	–	–	–	–	–	–	–	–	–	–
Temple - Lower Bucks, Bristol	2,944	13.9	12.8						×						
Temple University, Philadelphia	3,730	10.3	9.8	★	★		★	★	★	★			★		★
Thomas Jefferson University, Philadelphia	8,251	7.5	9.4	★	★		★		★			★	★		★
University of Pennsylvania, Philadelphia	4,265	8.2	10.1	★	★	★			★		×	★			
Warminster Hospital, Warminster	443	14.7	10.9					–		–	–	–	–		–
Wills Eye, Philadelphia	183	3.3	7.9			–	–	–	–	–	–	–	–	–	–
Pittsburgh Area															
Alle-Kiski, Natrona Heights	5,644	12.8	***12.9***	✖	✖	✖									✖
Allegheny General, Pittsburgh	6,828	9.1	10.0	★	★	★	★				★			★	★
Children's, Pittsburgh	–	–	–	–	–	–	–	–	–	–	–	–	–	–	–
Forbes Regional, Monroeville	6,336	13.0	12.4			✖		✖	×						
Jefferson, Pittsburgh[1]	9,099	11.4	12.4			✖			✖	✖	★			★	
Magee - Womens, Pittsburgh[1]	295	1.4	10.2		–	–	–	–	–	–	–	–	–	–	–
Mercy, Pittsburgh	7,141	10.4	11.0	★	★	★									★
Mercy Providence, Pittsburgh	1,527	9.9	10.7				★	★							
Pittsburgh's Ohio Valley General, McKees Rocks	2,371	10.7	12.9			×					✖				
St Clair, Pittsburgh	6,495	13.5	***14.8***	✖	✖	✖	✖	✖	✖	✖	✖	✖	✖		
St Francis Central Hospital, Pittsburgh	1,243	8.5	11.8							✖	–		–		
St Francis Medical Center, Pittsburgh	4,974	9.5	9.9	★	★				★				★		

Footnotes are on page 350.

Hospital outcomes: better (★) or worse (×) than average											Results of accreditation review on full survey		Other facts			
Adjusted Death rates			Adjusted Adverse outcome rates													
Surgical cases			Surgical cases													
All selected surgical cases	Coronary artery bypass surgery	Large bowel surgery	All selected surgical cases	Coronary artery bypass surgery	Large bowel surgery	Gall bladder removal	Total knee replacement	Total hip replacement	Simple prostatectomy	Carotid endarterectomy	Accreditation status*	Overall evaluation score (higher is better)	Number of beds	Major medical school affiliation?	Number of residents	Computerized drug order system (1 to 5 scale, higher is preferred; see page 23 for details)
2.3	3.8	6.5	7.7	10.3	11.9	7.5	6.7	6.4	5.4	8.2	–	91	161	–	–	–
★			✖				✖				4	98	346	Yes	44	–
	–			–		–	–	–	–	–	4	85	106	No	0	–
×	–		✖	–		✖	✖	–	–	–	–[2]	–[2]	201	No	0	–
						–	–	–	–	–	4	92	240	No	40	–
	–			–						–	–[2]	–[2]	175	No	0	–
×	–	✖		–		–	–	–	–	–	4	91	129	No	4	–
	–	–		–		–	–	–	–	–	4	87	153	No	4	–
–	–	–	–	–	–	–	–	–	–	–	5	97	130	–	7	–
–	–	–	–	–	–	–	–	–	–	–	4	94	315	Yes	22	–
–	–	–		–	–	–	–	–	–	–	4	86	89	No	–	–
			★	★			★			–	4	92	257	No	0	–
	–	–		–		–	–	–	–	–	4	91	31	No	0	–
–	–	–	–	–	–	–	–	–	–	–	–[2]	–[2]	–	–	–	–
–	–	–	–	–	–	–	–	–	–	–	–[2]	–[2]	–	–	–	–
	–					✖			–	✖	4	92	163	Yes	4	–
						–			–	–	4	91	423	Yes	403	–
★		★	✖		×		✖	✖			4	81	771	Yes	549	–
							✖	✖	–		4	95	659	Yes	855	–
–	–	–	–	–	–	–	–	–	–	–	5	96	132	No	3	–
–	–	–	★	–	–	–	–	–	–	–	4	93	115	Yes	24	–
	–		★	–				★			4	96	237	No	0	–
											4	97	443	Yes	279	–
–	–	–	–	–	–	–	–	–	–	–	5	92	235	–	14	–
	–			–	★		✖				4	97	310	No	18	–
	–			–			★				4	86	466	No	38	–
–	–	–	★	–	–	–	–	–	–	–	4	84	204	Yes	14	2
	★	✖			×	×			–		4	92	369	No	136	–
	–	–		–		–	–	–	–	–	4	89	146	No	0	–
	–		★	–	★			–	–		5	97	118	No	0	–
	–					★		★		✖	–[2]	–[2]	266	No	10	–
		–				–	–	–	–	–	–[2]	–[2]	117	Yes	9	–
	★			★	★			–	–		4	84	495	Yes	97	2

***Accreditation Status:** 5=Accredited with commendation or with full standards compliance; 4=Accredited with requirements for improvement; 3=Conditional accreditation.

Detailed Ratings for All Areas

See more information on "Key Ratings for Metro Areas" table beginning on page 32

Blue is most favorable
Bold Italic is least favorable
Blank means neither better nor worse than average
"–" means insufficient data

	Death rates for all selected case types			Hospital outcomes: better (★) or worse (×) than average											
				Adjusted Death rates											
					Medical Cases										
	Number of cases	Actual death rate (%)	Adjusted death rate (%) (lower is better)	All selected cases	All selected medical cases	Heart attack	Congestive heart failure	Obstructive pulmonary disease	Pneumonia	Respiratory failure and arrest	Septicemia	Stroke	Gastrointestinal hemorrhage	Fluid, electrolyte, & acid-base disorders	Kidney failure
National Average	–	–	12.1	12.1	14.8	21.2	10.6	6.5	16.9	34.4	25.1	18.4	6.7	11.0	20.9
Pennsylvania *(continued)*															
Pittsburgh Area *(continued)*															
Sewickley Valley, Sewickley	4,180	10.0	12.7												
Suburban General, Pittsburgh	2,644	10.9	11.4				**★**	×				★			★
UPMC Braddock, Braddock	3,135	12.7	11.8			×		✖							
UPMC McKeesport, McKeesport	6,834	11.8	**9.9**	**★**	**★**		**★**	**★**	**★**	**★**				★	★
UPMC Passavant, Pittsburgh	6,495	12.4	12.6			**★**			×						
UPMC Presbyterian, Pittsburgh	7,709	9.8	**10.5**	**★**	**★**	**★**		**★**		**★**				**★**	
UPMC St Margaret, Pittsburgh	5,384	11.9	12.6												
UPMC Shadyside, Pittsburgh	10,715	9.7	**10.7**	**★**	**★**	**★**	**★**					**★**			
UPMC South Side, Pittsburgh	3,374	11.9	11.5							✖		★			
Western Pennsylvania, Pittsburgh	5,885	11.8	11.2	★	★		**★**							**★**	
Other Areas															
Aliquippa Community, Aliquippa	1,964	11.6	11.8			✖	**★**							✖	
Altoona Hospital, Altoona	6,337	12.8	***15.0***	✖	✖	✖	✖	✖	✖	✖	×		✖		✖
Armstrong County, Kittanning	3,160	13.0	***13.4***	✖	✖		×		×						
Ashland Regional, Ashland	2,342	14.4	11.9				**★**	**★**							✖
Barnes - Kasson County, Susquehanna	612	10.9	12.4			–				–	–		–	×	–
Berwick Hospital, Berwick	1,663	12.0	***14.4***	✖	✖	✖	×	**★**	✖						–
Bloomsburg Hospital, Bloomsburg	1,335	17.2	***16.8***	✖	✖			–	✖	–		✖		–	✖
Bon Secours Holy Family, Altoona	2,913	16.0	***14.8***	✖	✖		✖	×		✖		✖			
Bradford Regional, Bradford	2,284	13.0	***15.1***	✖	✖			✖	✖	×					
Brookville Hospital, Brookville	1,376	9.5	11.5					★							
Brownsville General, Brownsville	1,975	10.4	**9.9**	**★**	**★**		**★**				**★**				
Bucktail, Renovo	124	16.1	***20.9***	✖	✖	–	–	–	–	–	–	–	–	–	–
Butler Memorial, Butler[1]	4,614	11.6	11.9				×								
Canonsburg General, Canonsburg	2,515	13.4	12.9			✖	★								
Carlisle Hospital, Carlisle[1]	3,470	13.4	***16.4***	✖	✖	×	✖		✖	×		✖	✖	✖	
Centre, State College	3,587	11.3	12.6				✖						×	★	×
Chambersburg Hospital, Chambersburg	5,237	10.6	12.3						✖						
Charles Cole, Coudersport	1,612	10.7	12.5												
Citizens General, New Kensington	3,424	8.8	**8.7**	**★**	**★**		★		**★**	**★**	**★**			**★**	
Clarion Hospital, Clarion	2,262	12.7	***15.3***	✖	✖			✖		×				✖	×
Clearfield Hospital, Clearfield	2,452	12.1	13.0			✖									
Community, Lancaster	1,776	11.8	13.3			×									

Footnotes are on page 350.

Hospital outcomes: better (★) or worse (×) than average											Results of accreditation review on full survey		Other facts			
Adjusted Death rates			Adjusted Adverse outcome rates													
Surgical cases			Surgical cases													
All selected surgical cases	Coronary artery bypass surgery	Large bowel surgery	All selected surgical cases	Coronary artery bypass surgery	Large bowel surgery	Gall bladder removal	Total knee replacement	Total hip replacement	Simple prostatectomy	Carotid endarterectomy	Accreditation status*	Overall evaluation score (higher is better)	Number of beds	Major medical school affiliation?	Number of residents	Computerized drug order system (1 to 5 scale, higher is preferred; see page 23 for details)
2.3	3.8	6.5	7.7	10.3	11.9	7.5	6.7	6.4	5.4	8.2	–	91	161	–	–	–
	–	✖	✖	–	✖						4	**95**	168	No	0	–
	–			–		–		–	–		4	91	118	No	4	–
	–			–	★			–	–	✖	4	92	128	No	0	–
	–			–	★			–			5	92	202	No	50	–
			✖	✖						✖	4	**97**	175	No	0	–
★	★										–[2]	–[2]	722	**Yes**	447	–
	–			–					–	–	4	**96**	201	**Yes**	40	3
★	★			★					✖	✖	–[2]	–[2]	357	No	26	–
✖	–	×	✖	–			✖	–	–		4	**94**	113	No	0	–
			✖	✖			–	–	✖	✖	4	**86**	512	No	108	–
	–			–		–	–	–	–	–	4	**96**	96	No	0	–
									✖	✖	4	93	189	No	17	–
	–			–				–	–	✖	4	**94**	185	No	0	–
	–			–		–	–	–	–	–	4	**88**	76	No	2	–
–	–	–	–	–	–	–	–	–	–	–	–[2]	–[2]	49	No	0	–
–	–	–	★	–	–	–	–	–	–	–	4	**95**	100	No	0	–
	–	–		–		–		–	–	–	–[2]	–[2]	266	No	0	–
	–	✖		–	✖			–	–		4	89	136	No	0	–
	–		×	–	✖	–	✖	–			–[2]	–[2]	105	No	0	–
	–	–		–		–	–	–	–	–	4	90	63	No	0	–
	–	–	★	–	★		–	–	–	–	4	92	94	No	0	–
–	–	–	–	–	–	–	–	–	–	–	–[2]	–[2]	50	No	0	–
	–					×	✖	–		–	4	**94**	217	No	0	–
	–			–			✖	–	–	–	4	**88**	120	No	2	–
	–		✖	–		✖	✖	✖			–[2]	–[2]	110	No	0	–
	–		✖	–		–	✖	✖	–		5	91	170	No	0	–
	–			–							4	**86**	205	No	0	–
✖	–	✖		–	×	–		–	–	–	4	91	70	No	0	–
	–			–		✖	–	–		–	–[2]	–[2]	180	No	0	–
✖	–	–		–				–		–	–[2]	–[2]	77	No	9	–
	–			–				–	–	–	4	93	81	No	0	–
	–	×		–				–	–	–	–[2]	–[2]	116	No	4	–

***Accreditation Status:** 5=Accredited with commendation or with full standards compliance; 4=Accredited with requirements for improvement; 3=Conditional accreditation.

Detailed Ratings for All Areas

See more information on "Key Ratings for Metro Areas" table beginning on page 32

Blue is most favorable
Bold Italic is least favorable
Blank means neither better nor worse than average
"–" means insufficient data

	Death rates for all selected case types			Hospital outcomes: better (★) or worse (×) than average — Adjusted Death rates											
				Medical Cases											
	Number of cases	Actual death rate (%)	Adjusted death rate (%) (lower is better)	All selected cases	All selected medical cases	Heart attack	Congestive heart failure	Obstructive pulmonary disease	Pneumonia	Respiratory failure and arrest	Septicemia	Stroke	Gastrointestinal hemorrhage	Fluid, electrolyte, & acid-base disorders	Kidney failure
National Average	–	–	12.1	12.1	14.8	21.2	10.6	6.5	16.9	34.4	25.1	18.4	6.7	11.0	20.9
Pennsylvania *(continued)*															
Other Areas *(continued)*															
Community, Scranton[1]	4,009	11.6	12.4				×	✖							
Conemaugh, Johnstown	7,287	10.6	**10.4**	**★**	**★**	**★**	**★**	**★**							**★**
Corry Memorial, Corry	852	12.0	13.1							–		✖	–		–
Divine Providence, Williamsport[1]	1,111	10.3	11.6												
Dubois Regional, Dubois	3,424	10.7	***13.2***	✖	✖		✖		✖	×	×				
Easton Hospital, Easton	7,580	11.6	**10.0**	**★**	**★**	★	**★**		**★**						
Elk Regional, St Marys	2,357	10.5	11.5												
Ellwood City Hospital, Ellwood City	1,663	10.8	***13.8***	✖	✖		✖								✖
Endless Mountain, Montrose	664	12.5	13.6				×			–	–		–		–
Ephrata Community, Ephrata	2,696	10.5	11.4			×				×		★			
Evangelical, Lewisburg	3,476	12.4	12.6									✖			
Frick, Mt Pleasant	3,723	9.8	**10.5**	**★**	**★**			★	★						
Geisinger, Danville	5,067	11.1	11.3			**★**	✖					**★**			
Geisinger Wyoming Valley, Wilkes-Barre	2,387	11.6	***14.9***	✖	✖	✖	✖	×	×						
Gettysburg Hospital, Gettysburg	2,545	10.5	11.7												✖
Gnaden Huetten, Lehighton[1]	1,622	9.6	11.7							✖					
Good Samaritan, Lebanon	5,388	10.4	11.4									**★**			
Good Samaritan Regional, Pottsville	5,036	11.4	**11.1**	**★**	**★**			**★**			**★**				
Greene County, Waynesburg	1,681	12.5	***14.6***	✖	✖	✖			×	–		×		×	
Hamot, Erie[1]	5,338	10.4	**11.0**	**★**	★							**★**		×	
Hanover Hospital, Hanover	3,931	10.2	11.9												✖
Hazleton - St Joseph, Hazleton	2,322	14.9	***14.2***	✖	✖	✖			✖		×				✖
Hazleton General, Hazleton	3,848	13.8	***13.8***	✖	✖	✖						✖		✖	
Highlands, Connellsville	1,316	11.1	12.7												
Holy Spirit, Camp Hill[1]	7,444	12.2	**10.5**	**★**	**★**		★		★		**★**		**★**	★	
Indiana Hospital, Indiana	3,987	13.4	***13.9***	✖	✖	✖			✖		✖	×			
J C Blair, Huntingdon	1,862	10.3	10.8								**★**				
Jameson, New Castle	3,763	11.7	***13.1***	✖	×	×	✖							×	✖
Jeannette District, Jeannette	3,221	12.8	11.5			✖	×			**★**		★			
Jersey Shore Hospital, Jersey Shore	775	8.1	**9.2**	**★**	**★**		**★**			–	–		–	–	–
Kane Community, Kane	954	12.6	12.3			×		★							
Lancaster General, Lancaster	10,342	11.0	11.8			**★**			✖	×					
Lancaster General - Susquehanna Division, Columbia	633	13.7	12.8					–			–				–
Lancaster Regional, Lancaster[1]	3,857	12.2	12.0			**★**	✖			★					

Footnotes are on page 350.

Hospital outcomes: better (★) or worse (×) than average											Results of accreditation review on full survey		Other facts			
Adjusted Death rates			Adjusted Adverse outcome rates													
Surgical cases			Surgical cases													
All selected surgical cases	Coronary artery bypass surgery	Large bowel surgery	All selected surgical cases	Coronary artery bypass surgery	Large bowel surgery	Gall bladder removal	Total knee replacement	Total hip replacement	Simple prostatectomy	Carotid endarterectomy	Accreditation status*	Overall evaluation score (higher is better)	Number of beds	Major medical school affiliation?	Number of residents	Computerized drug order system (1 to 5 scale, higher is preferred; see page 23 for details)
2.3	3.8	6.5	7.7	10.3	11.9	7.5	6.7	6.4	5.4	8.2	–	91	161	–	–	–
★	★			★					–	✖	4	**94**	258	No	17	–
	★			★					×	✖	4	91	400	No	68	–
–	–	–	–	–	–	–	–	–	–	–	4	89	55	No	0	–
	–			–			–	–		–	4	**97**	285	No	19	–
★	–			–			✖	–	★	–	4	**86**	189	No	0	–
							×				4	89	233	**Yes**	36	–
	–	–		–	–	–		–	–		4	91	66	No	0	–
	–	–		–		–		–	–	–	–[2]	–[2]	118	No	3	–
–	–	–	–	–	–	–	–	–	–	–	–[2]	–[2]	32	No	0	–
	–		★	–	★		★	–	–	–	–[2]	–[2]	134	No	–	–
	–			–					–	–	–[2]	–[2]	115	No	5	–
	–			–		★		–		✖	4	**99**	153	No	0	–
★	★		★	★		★				★	4	**84**	333	No	187	–
	–			–	★	–	✖		–		4	**88**	132	No	0	–
	–			–			–	–		–	4	**94**	76	No	0	–
	–	–		–		–	–	–	–	–	4	92	111	No	0	–
	–			–	×	★					4	89	159	No	0	–
	–			–		×		–		✖	4	89	153	No	0	–
	–	–	✖	–		–	✖	–	–	–	4	92	45	No	0	–
		★									4	**95**	309	**Yes**	36	4
★	–	★		–						–	4	**85**	101	No	0	–
	–			–			–	–	–	–	4	92	109	No	0	–
✖	–			–				–	–	–	4	**85**	152	No	4	–
–	–	–		–	✖	–	–	–	–	–	4	**96**	92	No	–	–
★	–			–			✖				5	**98**	263	No	0	–
	–			–				–		–	4	91	130	No	0	–
	–			–			–	–	–	–	4	**87**	104	No	0	–
	–			–					–	–	–[2]	–[2]	175	No	0	–
	–	×		–				–	–	–	4	91	126	No	0	–
–	–	–		–	–	–	–	–	–	–	4	**94**	49	No	0	–
–	–	–	–	–	–	–	–	–	–	–	–[2]	–[2]	39	No	0	–
★	★			★				★	✖	×	5	**96**	463	No	53	–
–	–	–	–	–	–	–	–	–	–	–	–[2]	–[2]	62	No	0	–
								–			4	**94**	187	No	0	–

***Accreditation Status:** 5=Accredited with commendation or with full standards compliance; 4=Accredited with requirements for improvement; 3=Conditional accreditation.

Detailed Ratings for All Areas

See more information on "Key Ratings for Metro Areas" table beginning on page 32

Blue is most favorable
Bold Italic is least favorable
Blank means neither better nor worse than average
"–" means insufficient data

	Death rates for all selected case types			Hospital outcomes: better (★) or worse (×) than average — Adjusted Death rates											
				Medical Cases											
	Number of cases	Actual death rate (%)	Adjusted death rate (%) (lower is better)	All selected cases	All selected medical cases	Heart attack	Congestive heart failure	Obstructive pulmonary disease	Pneumonia	Respiratory failure and arrest	Septicemia	Stroke	Gastrointestinal hemorrhage	Fluid, electrolyte, & acid-base disorders	Kidney failure
National Average	–	–	12.1	12.1	14.8	21.2	10.6	6.5	16.9	34.4	25.1	18.4	6.7	11.0	20.9
Pennsylvania *(continued)*															
Other Areas *(continued)*															
Latrobe Area, Latrobe	5,909	12.9	***14.0***	✖	✖	✖			✖			✖			
Lehigh Valley, Allentown[1]	11,893	10.1	11.2	★											★
Lehigh Valley - Muhlenberg Campus, Bethlehem	3,374	11.3	10.8	★	★		★	×	★						
Lewistown Hospital, Lewistown	3,828	11.7	12.9	×											
Lock Haven Hospital, Lock Haven[1]	1,137	12.9	***14.9***	✖	✖		✖					✖			–
Marian, Carbondale	2,617	14.2	***13.4***	✖	✖		✖				×				
Meadville Medical Center, Meadville	3,742	10.7	11.6							★					
The Medical Center, Beaver	7,691	12.5	***13.0***	✖	✖				×	✖		✖			
Memorial, Towanda[1]	1,010	14.8	***15.8***	✖	✖		✖		✖	✖				✖	–
Memorial, York	2,725	10.9	12.8					✖							
Mercy, Scranton	7,066	12.1	10.1	★	★	★	★		★	★			★		
Mercy, Wilkes-Barre	4,554	12.3	12.2					★							
Metro, Erie	1,073	9.8	13.5		×					–			–		–
Meyersdale Community, Meyersdale	469	16.0	11.2			–		–					–	–	–
Mid-Valley, Peckville[1]	1,068	14.0	11.7				★				★		–	–	
Millcreek, Erie	1,240	11.7	11.9												
Miners, Hastings	1,161	14.7	***15.9***	✖	✖						✖	✖	★	✖	✖
Monongahela Valley, Monongahela	5,797	10.8	12.7			✖				×					
Monsour, Jeannette	889	10.0	9.0	★	★	–		★		–			–		–
Moses Taylor, Scranton	4,706	12.8	11.6												
Muncy Valley, Muncy	713	12.3	11.2							–	–			–	–
Nason, Roaring Spring	803	14.9	***18.1***	✖	✖			–	✖			✖	–	–	–
Northwest, Franklin	4,446	10.4	12.3									★			
Palmerton Hospital, Palmerton	1,865	11.7	13.0												
Penn State Milton S Hershey, Hershey	3,792	12.2	12.4				×					★			
Philipsburg Area, Philipsburg	868	11.3	13.1							–			–	–	–
Pinnacle Health, Harrisburg[1]	12,633	11.2	11.6			★						★			
Pocono, East Stroudsburg	4,567	11.2	10.9	★	★		★				★	★	×		×
Pottsville Hospital, Pottsville	3,392	13.6	***15.2***	✖	✖	✖	×	✖	✖	✖	✖				×
Punxsutawney Area, Punxsutawney	1,401	11.6	10.6	★											
Reading Hospital, Reading	11,856	10.8	12.3			★		✖		✖					
Robert Packer, Sayre	4,546	9.9	12.7				×			★					
Sacred Heart, Allentown	3,789	9.5	11.9												
St Francis, Cranberry Township	114	13.2	12.8			–	–	–		–	–	–	–	–	–

Footnotes are on page 350.

Hospital outcomes: better (★) or worse (×) than average											Results of accreditation review on full survey		Other facts			
Adjusted Death rates			Adjusted Adverse outcome rates													
Surgical cases			Surgical cases													
All selected surgical cases	Coronary artery bypass surgery	Large bowel surgery	All selected surgical cases	Coronary artery bypass surgery	Large bowel surgery	Gall bladder removal	Total knee replacement	Total hip replacement	Simple prostatectomy	Carotid endarterectomy	Accreditation status*	Overall evaluation score (higher is better)	Number of beds	Major medical school affiliation?	Number of residents	Computerized drug order system (1 to 5 scale, higher is preferred; see page 23 for details)
2.3	3.8	6.5	7.7	10.3	11.9	7.5	6.7	6.4	5.4	8.2	–	91	161	–	–	–
	–			–							4	90	195	No	17	–
★	★		×					✖			4	97	498	Yes	108	4
	–			–		✖		–	–		–[2]	–[2]	148	No	3	–
✖	–		×	–	✖		✖	–	–	–	4	90	158	No	0	–
	–	–		–		–	–	–	–	–	4	91	75	No	0	–
	–			–			✖	–	–	–	4	92	104	No	0	–
	–		✖	–	×	×	✖	✖	–	–	4	89	208	No	8	–
								★	✖		4	96	434	No	18	–
–	–	–		–	–	–	–	–	–	–	4	93	49	No	0	–
✖	–	✖	✖	–	✖			–	–	✖	–[2]	–[2]	119	No	35	–
★			★					–	–		4	86	243	No	0	–
	–	×					–	–	–		4	85	195	No	30	–
–	–	–		–	–	–		–	–	–	–[2]	–[2]	111	No	12	–
–	–	–	–	–	–	–	–	–	–	–	4	87	20	No	0	–
–	–	–		–	★	–	–	–	–	–	–[2]	–[2]	40	No	0	–
–	–	–	×	–	×	–	–	–	–	–	–[2]	–[2]	101	No	45	–
✖	–	–		–	–	–	–	–	–	–	–[2]	–[2]	40	No	0	–
✖	–			–			★	–	–		4	92	240	No	0	–
–	–	–	–	–	–	–	–	–	–	–	4	83	149	No	0	–
	–			–					–		4	91	144	No	0	–
–	–	–		–	–	–	–	–	–	–	4	93	45	No	–	–
×	–	–	✖	–		–	–	–	–	–	4	94	40	No	0	–
	–			–					–		4	86	198	No	0	–
	–	–		–		–	–	–	–	–	4	96	70	No	0	–
			✖						–	✖	4	85	415	No	355	–
–	–	–		–	–	–	–	–	–	–	–[2]	–[2]	94	No	–	–
			✖		★		✖	✖	✖		4	91	659	No	113	–
	–			–			–	–			4	88	192	No	7	–
	–			–				–		×	4	88	197	No	0	–
–	–	–	★	–	★	–	–	–	–	–	4	91	51	No	0	–
	✖	★	✖	✖		✖	✖	✖	✖		4	91	594	No	60	–
						–		✖	–		4	92	238	Yes	58	–
	–								–		4	88	138	No	24	–
–	–	–	–	–	–	–	–	–	–	–	4	79	32	No	6	–

***Accreditation Status:** 5=Accredited with commendation or with full standards compliance; 4=Accredited with requirements for improvement; 3=Conditional accreditation.

Detailed Ratings for All Areas

See more information on "Key Ratings for Metro Areas" table beginning on page 32

Blue is most favorable
Bold Italic is least favorable
Blank means neither better nor worse than average
"–" means insufficient data

	Death rates for all selected case types			Hospital outcomes: better (★) or worse (×) than average — Adjusted Death rates											
					Medical Cases										
	Number of cases	Actual death rate (%)	Adjusted death rate (%) (lower is better)	All selected cases	All selected medical cases	Heart attack	Congestive heart failure	Obstructive pulmonary disease	Pneumonia	Respiratory failure and arrest	Septicemia	Stroke	Gastrointestinal hemorrhage	Fluid, electrolyte, & acid-base disorders	Kidney failure
National Average	–	–	12.1	12.1	14.8	21.2	10.6	6.5	16.9	34.4	25.1	18.4	6.7	11.0	20.9
Pennsylvania *(continued)*															
Other Areas *(continued)*															
St Francis, New Castle	1,577	14.1	***14.4***	✖	✖					✖		×			
St Joseph, Reading	4,327	14.2	***14.5***	✖	✖				✖			✖	×		✖
St Luke's, Bethlehem	10,252	9.7	9.5 (blue)	★ (blue)	★ (blue)	★ (blue)	★ (blue)		★ (blue)		★ (blue)		★	★ (blue)	★ (blue)
St Luke's Miners, Coaldale	1,793	12.4	10.6	★	★			★ (blue)	★						
St Vincent, Erie	6,294	10.5	12.0			★ (blue)	×							✖	
Shamokin Area, Coal Township	1,540	15.2	***14.4***	✖	✖		×	✖	×				–	×	
Sharon Regional, Sharon	4,575	9.8	10.7 (blue)	★ (blue)	★ (blue)					★ (blue)				★ (blue)	
Soldiers and Sailors, Wellsboro	2,145	11.8	12.6			×	★ (blue)		✖						
Somerset Hospital, Somerset	2,171	12.7	12.8							✖					
Sunbury Community, Sunbury	2,228	16.2	12.1										★		
Titusville Area, Titusville	1,499	9.7	11.3							×		✖		★ (blue)	–
Troy Community, Troy	305	9.8	9.6			–	–	–		–		–	–	–	–
Tyler, Tunkhannock	1,205	11.1	12.2										–		–
Tyrone Hospital, Tyrone	764	12.3	12.8								–		–		–
Union City Memorial, Union City	425	12.9	***17.1***	✖	✖	–	×	✖		–	–	–	–	–	–
Uniontown Hospital, Uniontown	6,076	11.4	12.8	×	×						✖				
United, Grove City	1,725	13.9	***16.3***	✖	✖	✖			✖	×		✖	×	✖	×
UPMC Bedford, Everett	1,375	12.0	***15.3***	✖	✖				✖		–	✖		★ (blue)	–
UPMC Horizon, Greenville[1]	5,258	10.6	11.2	★	★				★ (blue)						★ (blue)
UPMC Lee Regional, Johnstown	4,944	12.3	11.8						✖						
Warren General, Warren	1,673	10.8	12.5												–
Washington Hospital, Washington	7,411	11.7	***13.6***	✖	✖			✖	✖		✖				✖
Wayne, Honesdale	1,991	12.6	11.1			★ (blue)				★ (blue)		×			
Waynesboro Hospital, Waynesboro	1,997	11.1	11.2										★ (blue)		
Westmoreland Regional, Greensburg	6,396	11.8	***12.9***	✖	✖			✖	✖	✖					
Williamsport Hospital, Williamsport	4,078	9.6	12.0												
Windber Medical Center, Windber	1,567	13.6	10.6	★	★		★ (blue)								
WVHCS, Kingston	10,593	11.8	***13.1***	✖	✖		✖	✖							✖
York Hospital, York	10,209	11.3	12.1			★ (blue)	✖					×			×
Puerto Rico															
Ashford Presbyterian, San Juan	2,147	12.2	13.2					★ (blue)	✖		✖	★ (blue)			
Auxilio Mutuo, Hato Rey[1]	7,774	12.2	12.6	×	✖	×					✖				
Bella Vista, Mayaguez	3,914	13.2	12.7			✖							×		✖

Footnotes are on page 350.

Hospital outcomes: better (★) or worse (×) than average — Adjusted Death rates — Surgical cases: All selected surgical cases	Coronary artery bypass surgery	Large bowel surgery	Adjusted Adverse outcome rates — Surgical cases: All selected surgical cases	Coronary artery bypass surgery	Large bowel surgery	Gall bladder removal	Total knee replacement	Total hip replacement	Simple prostatectomy	Carotid endarterectomy	Results of accreditation review on full survey: Accreditation status*	Overall evaluation score (higher is better)	Other facts: Number of beds	Major medical school affiliation?	Number of residents	Computerized drug order system (1 to 5 scale, higher is preferred; see page 23 for details)
2.3	3.8	6.5	7.7	10.3	11.9	7.5	6.7	6.4	5.4	8.2	–	91	161	–	–	–
	–	–	★	–		–	–	–	–	–	4	94	124	No	0	–
		✖	×				✖	✖			–[2]	–[2]	245	No	22	–
★	★			★		✖		×	✖		4	83	531	Yes	112	–
	–	–	★	–		–	–	–	–	–	4	89	66	No	0	–
			★				★		–		4	92	422	No	23	–
✖	–	–		–		–	–	–	–	–	–[2]	–[2]	46	No	0	–
★	–	★		–	★	×					4	95	194	Yes	0	–
×	–	–		–			–	–	–	–	4	92	83	No	0	–
	–	–		–		–	–	–	×	–	4	93	115	No	0	–
	–			–			–	–	–	–	–[2]	–[2]	98	No	0	–
–	–	–		–	–	–	–	–	–	–	–[2]	–[2]	60	No	0	–
–	–	–	–	–	–	–	–	–	–	–	–[2]	–[2]	32	No	0	–
–	–	–		–		–	–	–	–	–	4	91	60	No	0	–
–	–	–		–	–	–	–	–	–	–	4	91	59	No	0	–
–	–	–	–	–	–	–	–	–	–	–	4	89	23	No	0	–
	–		✖	–				✖		✖	4	92	187	No	0	–
	–	–		–		–	–	–	–	–	–[2]	–[2]	84	No	0	–
–	–	–		–		–	–	–	–	–	4	95	27	No	0	–
	–			–			✖	★			4	93	205	No	15	–
	–			–			★			✖	4	94	202	No	0	–
✖	–	✖		–		–		–	–	–	–[2]	–[2]	89	No	0	–
			★	★							4	95	220	No	24	–
	–			–			–	–		–	4	91	78	No	0	–
	–			–		–	–	–	–	–	4	97	62	No	0	–
			✖		✖		✖			✖	4	92	263	No	0	–
			★	★		–	★		–	★	4	97	238	No	21	–
	–	–		–	–	–	–	–	–	–	4	88	67	No	0	–
										×	4	85	183	No	–	–
											5	96	437	No	147	3
✖	–	–		–	✖	★	✖	–	–	–	4	90	187	No	0	–
	–	★	✖	–	★	✖		–	✖	–	4	96	402	No	45	–
	–	–	✖	–		✖	✖	–	★	–	4	85	155	No	12	–

***Accreditation Status:** 5=Accredited with commendation or with full standards compliance; 4=Accredited with requirements for improvement; 3=Conditional accreditation.

Detailed Ratings for All Areas

See more information on "Key Ratings for Metro Areas" table beginning on page 32

Blue is most favorable
Bold Italic is least favorable
Blank means neither better nor worse than average
"–" means insufficient data

	Death rates for all selected case types			Hospital outcomes: better (★) or worse (×) than average — Adjusted Death rates											
					Medical Cases										
	Number of cases	Actual death rate (%)	Adjusted death rate (%) (lower is better)	All selected cases	All selected medical cases	Heart attack	Congestive heart failure	Obstructive pulmonary disease	Pneumonia	Respiratory failure and arrest	Septicemia	Stroke	Gastrointestinal hemorrhage	Fluid, electrolyte, & acid-base disorders	Kidney failure
National Average	–	–	12.1	12.1	14.8	21.2	10.6	6.5	16.9	34.4	25.1	18.4	6.7	11.0	20.9
Puerto Rico *(continued)*															
Castaner General, Castaner	153	5.2	7.8			–	–	–		–	–	–	–	–	–
Centro Cardiovascular de PR y del Caribe, Rio Piedras	1,632	6.3	***14.9***	✖				–	–	–	–	–	–	–	–
Clinica Espanola, Mayaguez	867	14.8	***16.2***	✖	✖				✖		–	✖	–	–	–
Clinica San Agustin, Manati	339	7.4	13.9			–	–	–		–	–	–	–	–	–
Doctors, Santurce	1,140	13.1	***15.6***	✖	✖				✖	–	✖		–		–
Doctors Center, Manati	4,129	11.8	***15.6***	✖	✖	✖			✖	–	✖		✖		×
Dr Alejandro Otero Lopez, Manati	4,716	12.6	***18.1***	✖	✖	✖		✖	✖		✖	✖	×		
Dr I Gonzalez Martinez Oncology, San Juan	214	15.0	14.2			–	–	–	–		–	–	–		–
Dr Ramon E Betances, Mayaguez[1]	901	28.6	***24.4***	✖	✖	✖	✖	–	✖	✖	✖	✖	✖	–	✖
Font Martelo, Humacao	1,794	11.2	11.8					★					✖	–	–
Hospital Damas, Ponce[1]	4,270	11.9	12.6						✖						
Hospital de La Concepcion, San German	4,331	17.0	12.8	×	×					–		✖	✖		
Hospital de La Universidad de Puerto Rico, Carolina	1,854	24.6	***24.8***	✖	✖	✖	✖		✖	✖	✖	✖	✖	×	✖
Hospital del Maestro, San Juan[1]	4,243	11.5	12.6			✖		★			✖	★		★	
Hospital Doctor Gubern, Fajardo	976	12.0	***16.1***	✖	✖			–	✖	–	✖		–	–	–
Hospital Doctor Pila, Ponce	3,369	15.5	***15.3***	✖	✖	✖			✖		✖	✖			
Hospital Dr Cayetano Coll Y Toste, Alares	4,562	17.9	***16.2***	✖	✖	✖			✖	✖	✖				
Hospital Dr Dominguez, Humacao	1,024	11.4	12.7						×					–	–
Hospital Dr Susoni, Arecibo	3,734	11.9	***15.6***	✖	✖		✖		✖	×	✖		✖	✖	–
Hospital Episcopal Cristo Redentor, Guayama	1,410	17.8	***17.8***	✖	✖		✖		✖	×	✖	✖	✖	–	–
Hospital Episcopal San Lucas, Ponce	4,168	11.0	***14.5***	✖	✖	✖					✖				
Hospital Hermanos Melendez, Bayamon[1]	4,272	11.5	12.8	×		×					×		×		✖
Hospital Interamericano Medicina Avanzada, Caguas	8,500	11.0	12.0				★	★	✖		✖				✖
Hospital Matilde Brenes, Bayamon	1,853	15.3	***16.7***	✖	✖	✖			✖	✖	✖				–
Hospital Menonita de Cayey, Cayey	2,710	12.7	12.2							–			★		
Hospital Metropolitan, San Juan	2,653	13.2	12.8			✖							★		–
Hospital Oncologico Andres Grillasca, Ponce	86	16.3	18.7	×	✖	–	–	–	–	–	–	–	–	–	–
Hospital Pavia, Santurce	4,892	12.3	***13.5***	✖					✖			★			
Hospital Perea, Mayaguez	3,034	14.3	12.5							✖	✖				–
Hospital San Cristobal, Coto Laurel	2,191	14.5	***14.6***	✖	✖	✖			×	✖	✖				–
Hospital San Francisco, Rio Piedras[1]	4,517	13.2	***14.4***	✖	✖				✖		✖				✖
Hospital San Pablo, Bayamon	9,575	10.5	***14.4***	✖	✖	✖	✖		✖	✖	✖			✖	
Hospital San Pablo del Este, Fajardo	1,156	15.7	***17.9***	✖	✖	–			✖	✖	✖	✖	–	–	
Hospital Santa Rosa, Guayama	1,207	14.3	***16.7***	✖	✖	×			✖		✖	✖	–	–	–
Hospital Universitario de Adultos, Rio Piedras	649	19.4	***15.2***	✖	✖	–	–	–	✖	–	–		–	–	

Footnotes are on page 350.

Hospital outcomes: better (★) or worse (×) than average											Results of accreditation review on full survey		Other facts			
Adjusted Death rates			Adjusted Adverse outcome rates													
Surgical cases			Surgical cases													
All selected surgical cases	Coronary artery bypass surgery	Large bowel surgery	All selected surgical cases	Coronary artery bypass surgery	Large bowel surgery	Gall bladder removal	Total knee replacement	Total hip replacement	Simple prostatectomy	Carotid endarterectomy	Accreditation status*	Overall evaluation score (higher is better)	Number of beds	Major medical school affiliation?	Number of residents	Computerized drug order system (1 to 5 scale, higher is preferred; see page 23 for details)
2.3	3.8	6.5	7.7	10.3	11.9	7.5	6.7	6.4	5.4	8.2	–	91	161	–	–	–
–	–	–	–	–	–	–	–	–	–	–	–[2]	–[2]	24	No	0	–
✖	✖	–	✖	✖	–	–	–	–	–	✖	–[2]	–[2]	192	No	–	–
–	–	–	–	–	–	–	–	–	–	–	–[2]	–[2]	69	No	0	–
–	–	–	–	–	–	–	–	–	–	–	–[2]	–[2]	12	No	0	–
–	–	–		–	–	–	–	–	–	–	–[2]	–[2]	89	No	0	–
	–	–		–			–	–	✖	–	–[2]	–[2]	150	No	1	–
✖	–	–	✖	–			–	–	✖	–	4	90	178	No	18	–
–	–	–	–	–	–	–	–	–	–	–	–[2]	–[2]	85	**Yes**	0	–
–	–	–	–	–	–	–	–	–	–	–	4	***86***	206	No	14	–
–	–	–		–	–		–	–	–	–	–[2]	–[2]	64	No	0	–
	–			–		★	✖	–	✖	–	4	**98**	267	**Yes**	9	–
	–			–		✖	–	–		–	4	**94**	123	No	4	–
–	–	–	✖	–	–	✖	–	–	–	–	–[2]	–[2]	220	No	5	–
	–		✖	–		✖	–	–		–	4	92	247	**Yes**	0	–
–	–	–		–	–		–	–	–	–	–[2]	–[2]	51	No	0	–
	–	–		–			–	–		–	4	91	177	No	12	–
	–	–	×	–	–		–	–	✖	–	4	90	188	No	10	–
–	–	–		–	–		–	–	–	–	–[2]	–[2]	54	No	0	–
	–	–	✖	–	✖	✖	–	–		–	–[2]	–[2]	138	No	1	–
–	–	–		–	–	–	–	–	–	–	–[2]	–[2]	155	No	6	–
✖	✖	–	✖				–	–		✖	4	90	168	No	9	–
	–	✖	×	–	✖		–	–	✖	–	4	93	211	No	0	–
	–			–			✖	–		–	5	**97**	300	**Yes**	–	–
	–	–	✖	–	–		✖	–	✖	–	–[2]	–[2]	95	No	0	–
	–	–	★	–	–		–	–	★	–	–[2]	–[2]	50	No	0	–
	–	–		–			–	–	–	–	–[2]	–[2]	119	No	3	–
–	–	–	–	–	–	–	–	–	–	–	4	93	50	No	0	–
✖	✖	–	✖	✖		✖		–			4	93	183	No	1	–
✖	–	–	✖	–	✖		–	–	–	–	–[2]	–[2]	82	No	0	–
	–	–		–	–	✖	–	–	–	–	–[2]	–[2]	103	No	–	–
	–		✖	–	✖		–	–	–	–	4	***81***	160	No	0	–
★			✖				✖	–			4	92	364	**Yes**	8	–
–	–	–	✖	–	–	✖	–	–	–	–	3	***79***	180	No	–	–
–	–	–		–	–	–	–	–	–	–	–[2]	–[2]	89	No	0	–
–	–	–		–	–	–	–	–	–	–	4	**94**	297	**Yes**	15	–

***Accreditation Status:** 5=Accredited with commendation or with full standards compliance; 4=Accredited with requirements for improvement; 3=Conditional accreditation.

Detailed Ratings for All Areas

See more information on "Key Ratings for Metro Areas" table beginning on page 32

Blue is most favorable
Bold Italic is least favorable
Blank means neither better nor worse than average
"–" means insufficient data

	Death rates for all selected case types			Hospital outcomes: better (★) or worse (×) than average — Adjusted Death rates	Medical Cases										
	Number of cases	Actual death rate (%)	Adjusted death rate (%) (lower is better)	All selected cases	All selected medical cases	Heart attack	Congestive heart failure	Obstructive pulmonary disease	Pneumonia	Respiratory failure and arrest	Septicemia	Stroke	Gastrointestinal hemorrhage	Fluid, electrolyte, & acid-base disorders	Kidney failure
National Average	–	–	12.1	12.1	14.8	21.2	10.6	6.5	16.9	34.4	25.1	18.4	6.7	11.0	20.9
Puerto Rico *(continued)*															
Hospital Universitario Dr Ruiz Arnau, Bayamon	1,338	24.8	***20.5***	✖	✖	✖	✖		✖	×	✖	✖	✖	–	–
Hospital Wilma N Vazquez, Vega Baja	2,524	12.6	***14.3***	✖	✖				✖			×	–	–	–
Lafayette, Arroyo	1,101	9.4	11.3				★	★	✖	–			–		–
Mennonite General, Aibonito	3,510	10.3	***14.4***	✖	✖				✖		✖				
Hospital San Juan - Dr. Rafel Lopez Nussa, Rio Piedras	777	27.0	***22.7***	✖	✖		✖	–	✖	×	✖	✖	✖	–	–
Nuevo Hospital Episcopal San Lucas, Ponce	1,959	20.6	***19.3***	✖	✖	✖		✖	✖	✖	✖	✖	✖	×	
Ryder, Humacao	2,989	18.1	***16.9***	✖	✖		✖		✖	✖	✖	✖	✖	✖	×
San Carlos General, Santurce	1,472	10.9	***14.4***	✖	✖						✖		✖	–	–
San Gerardo Centro de Rehabilitacion, Rio Piedras	497	20.1	***18.3***	✖	✖	–	✖	–	✖		✖		–	–	–
San Juan Bautista, Caguas	1,696	20.8	***17.4***	✖	✖				✖	✖	✖		✖	–	✖
Southern Medical Center, Yauco	1,573	19.5	***18.3***	✖	✖		✖	✖	✖		✖		–		–
Rhode Island															
Kent County, Warwick	7,310	13.1	11.3	★	★				★						
Landmark, Woonsocket	3,996	12.6	***14.2***	✖	✖	✖	×	★	✖						
Memorial of Rhode Island, Pawtucket	3,934	12.7	10.2	★	★		★		★		★			★	
Miriam, Providence	4,857	9.3	10.3	★	★	★						★		★	
Newport Hospital, Newport	2,425	10.8	11.2												
Rhode Island, Providence	9,483	11.5	10.9	★	★	★	★		★					★	
Roger Williams, Providence	4,393	17.0	***12.9***	✖	✖				✖		×	✖	★		
St Joseph of Rhode Island, Providence	4,928	10.0	9.6	★	★		★	★	★		★	★			
South County, Wakefield	2,614	11.1	11.3								★				
Westerly Hospital, Westerly	2,499	10.6	11.5			×									★
Women and Infants of Rhode Island, Providence	289	2.8	16.5		–	–	–	–	–	–	–	–	–	–	–
South Carolina															
Abbeville County, Abbeville	701	12.1	11.2					–			★				–
Aiken Regional, Aiken	4,314	12.7	***13.2***	✖	✖			✖			✖				
Allen Bennett, Greer	1,738	13.9	***15.2***	✖	✖	×		✖	✖	–		✖			–
Allendale County, Fairfax	180	7.8	9.5			–	–	–		–	–	–	–	–	–
Anderson Area, Anderson	7,361	11.8	11.8					★							
B J Workman, Woodruff	542	9.6	9.3	★	★	–		–		–		–	–		–
Bamberg County, Bamberg[1]	625	12.6	9.6	★	★	–	★	–		–			–	–	–
Barnwell County, Barnwell	460	10.0	14.4			–		–	✖	–	–		–	–	–
Beaufort Memorial, Beaufort	2,238	11.8	***13.9***	✖	✖	✖		✖	✖						
Bon Secours - St Francis Xavier, Charleston	2,268	9.5	10.5	★	★					★					×

Footnotes are on page 350.

Hospital outcomes: better (★) or worse (×) than average											Results of accreditation review on full survey		Other facts			
Adjusted Death rates			Adjusted Adverse outcome rates													
Surgical cases			Surgical cases													
All selected surgical cases	Coronary artery bypass surgery	Large bowel surgery	All selected surgical cases	Coronary artery bypass surgery	Large bowel surgery	Gall bladder removal	Total knee replacement	Total hip replacement	Simple prostatectomy	Carotid endarterectomy	Accreditation status*	Overall evaluation score (higher is better)	Number of beds	Major medical school affiliation?	Number of residents	Computerized drug order system (1 to 5 scale, higher is preferred; see page 23 for details)
2.3	3.8	6.5	7.7	10.3	11.9	7.5	6.7	6.4	5.4	8.2	–	91	161	–	–	–
–	–	–	–	–	–	–	–	–	–	–	3	**83**	341	**Yes**	0	–
✖	–	–		–	–	✖	–	–	–	–	–[2]	–[2]	110	No	0	–
–	–	–	–	–	–	–	–	–	–	–	–[2]	–[2]	41	No	0	–
	–	–	✖	–	–	×		✖	✖	–	–[2]	–[2]	131	No	5	–
–	–	–	–	–	–	–	–	–	–	–	4	**95**	311	**Yes**	53	–
–	–	–		–	–	–	–	–	–	–	–[2]	–[2]	324	**Yes**	71	–
✖	–	–		–	–			–		–	–[2]	–[2]	144	No	0	–
–	–	–		–	–	–	–	–	–	–	–[2]	–[2]	66	No	0	–
–	–	–	–	–	–	–	–	–	–	–	–[2]	–[2]	60	No	–	–
–	–	–		–	–	–	–	–	–	–	4	**95**	256	No	15	–
–	–	–		–	–	–	–	–	–	–	–[2]	–[2]	111	No	4	–
	–		★	–							4	91	339	No	21	–
	–			–				–	★	×	4	93	139	No	0	–
	–			–				–			4	**94**	199	**Yes**	72	–
											4	93	227	**Yes**	0	–
	–			–		–		–	–		5	**96**	116	No	0	–
★											4	92	529	**Yes**	455	–
	–			–		×		–	–	–	4	92	146	**Yes**	88	–
	–		★	–		★	★				4	89	261	**Yes**	0	–
	–			–	★	–		✖	–	–	4	**94**	83	No	0	–
	–			–			★	–	–	–	4	93	125	No	0	–
–	–	–		–	–	–	–	–	–	–	5	**94**	197	**Yes**	27	–
–	–	–		–	–	–	–	–	–	–	4	93	60	No	0	–
			✖					–	–	✖	5	**94**	269	No	0	–
	–	–	★	–		★	–	–	–	–	–[2]	–[2]	58	No	0	–
–	–	–	–	–	–	–	–	–	–	–	–[2]	–[2]	36	No	0	–
	–		✖	–		✖	★			✖	–[2]	–[2]	369	No	27	–
–	–	–	–	–	–	–	–	–	–	–	–[2]	–[2]	43	No	0	–
–	–	–	–	–	–	–	–	–	–	–	4	91	84	No	0	–
–	–	–	–	–	–	–	–	–	–	–	4	90	45	No	0	–
	–	–	×	–					–	–	4	90	135	No	0	–
	–			–				–		–	5	**97**	145	No	0	–

***Accreditation Status:** 5=Accredited with commendation or with full standards compliance; 4=Accredited with requirements for improvement; 3=Conditional accreditation.

Detailed Ratings for All Areas

See more information on "Key Ratings for Metro Areas" table beginning on page 32

Blue is most favorable
Bold Italic is least favorable
Blank means neither better nor worse than average
"–" means insufficient data

	Death rates for all selected case types			Hospital outcomes: better (★) or worse (×) than average — Adjusted Death rates											
					Medical Cases										
	Number of cases	Actual death rate (%)	Adjusted death rate (%) (lower is better)	All selected cases	All selected medical cases	Heart attack	Congestive heart failure	Obstructive pulmonary disease	Pneumonia	Respiratory failure and arrest	Septicemia	Stroke	Gastrointestinal hemorrhage	Fluid, electrolyte, & acid-base disorders	Kidney failure
National Average	–	–	12.1	12.1	14.8	21.2	10.6	6.5	16.9	34.4	25.1	18.4	6.7	11.0	20.9
South Carolina *(continued)*															
Cannon, Pickens	880	14.0	14.0	×	×		✖	–				×	–		–
Carolina Pines Regional, Hartsville	2,139	11.3	12.6												
Carolinas Hospital System, Florence	5,731	12.8	11.6			✖	**★**	×	**★**		★				
Carolinas Hospital System, Kingstree	531	10.7	11.9			–		–		–			–		–
Carolinas Hospital System, Lake City	450	13.6	14.2				×	–		–		✖	–		–
Charleston Memorial, Charleston	138	13.8	9.6			–		–		–	–	–	–	–	–
Chester County, Chester[1]	1,347	10.3	10.0	**★**	**★**				**★**	–		★			
Chesterfield General, Cheraw	798	12.8	9.9	**★**	**★**	×	★	–			★				
Clarendon, Manning	915	16.1	***15.2***	✖	✖				✖	–	✖				–
Colleton, Walterboro	2,371	9.5	8.2	**★**	**★**		**★**	**★**	★	**★**	**★**			★	
Conway Hospital, Conway	3,262	13.1	***15.0***	✖	✖	✖		✖			✖				✖
East Cooper Regional, Mt Pleasant	1,470	11.6	13.5	×	×	×					×				–
Edgefield County, Edgefield	596	11.9	12.1			–		–		–	–		–		–
Fairfield, Winnsboro	527	15.4	***15.9***	✖	✖	–		–	✖	–			–		–
Georgetown Memorial, Georgetown	3,002	11.4	***13.7***	✖	✖	×	×								✖
Grand Strand Regional, Myrtle Beach	6,504	10.4	***13.2***	✖	✖			✖	✖					✖	
Greenville Hospital, Greenville[1]	9,861	11.1	***13.3***	✖	✖							✖			
Hampton Regional, Varnville	414	13.0	12.4			–		–		–	–	–	–		–
Hillcrest, Simpsonville	874	16.2	***19.0***	✖	✖	✖		✖	✖	–	✖	✖	–		–
Hilton Head Medical Center, Hilton Head Island[1]	2,438	10.4	12.9												
Kershaw County, Camden	2,547	10.2	9.7	**★**	**★**		**★**		**★**					★	
Laurens County, Clinton[1]	2,099	16.2	***16.7***	✖	✖	✖			✖	✖	×	✖			
Lexington, West Columbia	5,566	13.7	***15.4***	✖	✖	✖	✖	✖	✖		✖	✖		×	
Loris Community, Loris	1,988	11.0	***13.9***	✖	✖	✖			✖						
Low Country General, Beaufort	284	15.5	13.6			–		–		–	–	–	–		–
Marion County, Marion	2,303	11.5	12.2				**★**			✖					×
Marlboro Park, Bennettsville	1,074	13.9	12.0												
Mary Black, Spartanburg[1]	2,821	11.3	11.7									×		★	
McLeod Health, Florence	7,321	12.4	***13.6***	✖	✖			✖	✖	✖			✖	✖	
Medical University of South Carolina, Charleston	2,817	9.1	13.2	×					×	–	✖				
Newberry County, Newberry	1,226	12.3	13.3												✖
Oconee, Seneca	3,070	10.7	***13.3***	✖	×			✖							
Palmetto Baptist, Columbia	4,223	11.6	***13.2***	✖	✖	✖	✖								
Palmetto Baptist, Easley	1,950	14.8	***15.7***	✖	✖				✖		✖	×			✖
Palmetto Richland, Columbia	5,716	12.1	12.1												

Footnotes are on page 350.

Hospital outcomes: better (★) or worse (×) than average											Results of accreditation review on full survey		Other facts			
Adjusted Death rates			Adjusted Adverse outcome rates													
Surgical cases			Surgical cases													
All selected surgical cases	Coronary artery bypass surgery	Large bowel surgery	All selected surgical cases	Coronary artery bypass surgery	Large bowel surgery	Gall bladder removal	Total knee replacement	Total hip replacement	Simple prostatectomy	Carotid endarterectomy	Accreditation status*	Overall evaluation score (higher is better)	Number of beds	Major medical school affiliation?	Number of residents	Computerized drug order system (1 to 5 scale, higher is preferred; see page 23 for details)
2.3	3.8	6.5	7.7	10.3	11.9	7.5	6.7	6.4	5.4	8.2	–	91	161	–	–	–
–	–	–		–	–	–	–	–	–	–	4	100	42	No	0	–
–	–	–		–	–	–	–	–	–	–	4	98	116	No	0	–
✖	–	✖	✖	–			✖	–	✖		4	95	296	No	0	–
–	–	–	–	–	–	–	–	–	–	–	–[2]	–[2]	47	No	0	–
–	–	–	–	–	–	–	–	–	–	–	5	97	40	No	0	–
–	–	–	–	–	–	–	–	–	–	–	–[2]	–[2]	113	Yes	0	–
–	–	–		–	–	–	–	–	–	–	5	97	54	No	0	–
–	–	–	–	–	–	–	–	–	–	–	4	94	58	No	0	–
–	–	–	–	–	–	–	–	–	–	–	4	86	56	No	0	–
	–	–		–		–	×	–	–	–	4	97	116	No	0	–
	–	–		–	✖			–	★	–	4	97	137	No	0	–
	–		×	–	×	–	–	–	–	–	5	92	112	No	0	–
–	–	–	–	–	–	–	–	–	–	–	4	93	59	No	0	–
–	–	–	–	–	–	–	–	–	–	–	4	91	33	No	0	–
	–			–				–			4	93	141	No	0	–
				★			✖		★		4	94	168	No	0	2
✖	✖		✖		✖		✖				4	83	777	No	135	–
–	–	–	–	–	–	–	–	–	–	–	–[2]	–[2]	36	No	0	–
–	–	–		–	–	–	–	–	–	–	–[2]	–[2]	46	No	0	–
	–			–		✖				–	–[2]	–[2]	79	No	0	–
	–	–		–		–	–	–	–	–	4	93	100	No	0	–
×	–	–		–				–	–	–	4	86	85	No	0	–
	–			–	★						5	96	275	No	0	–
	–	–	★	–				–	–	–	5	97	105	No	0	–
–	–	–	–	–	–	–	–	–	–	–	–[2]	–[2]	31	No	0	–
–	–	–		–	–	–	–	–	–	–	–[2]	–[2]	216	No	0	–
–	–	–		–	–	–	–	–	–	–	4	91	104	No	0	–
	–		★	–			★			–	4	78	212	No	0	–
✖					✖	×					4	91	411	No	16	–
		–			✖	–			–	★	4	97	572	Yes	502	–
	–	–	★	–		–	–	–	–	–	5	96	77	No	0	–
	–			–	×		★	–	–	–	4	88	111	No	1	–
	–		✖	–	✖	✖					4	89	361	No	30	–
★	–			–	★			–		–	4	90	93	No	0	–
									–		4	85	612	Yes	190	–

***Accreditation Status:** 5=Accredited with commendation or with full standards compliance; 4=Accredited with requirements for improvement; 3=Conditional accreditation.

Detailed Ratings for All Areas

See more information on "Key Ratings for Metro Areas" table beginning on page 32

Blue is most favorable
Bold Italic is least favorable
Blank means neither better nor worse than average
"–" means insufficient data

	Death rates for all selected case types				Hospital outcomes: better (★) or worse (×) than average — Adjusted Death rates — Medical Cases											
	Number of cases	Actual death rate (%)	Adjusted death rate (%) (lower is better)	All selected cases	All selected medical cases	Heart attack	Congestive heart failure	Obstructive pulmonary disease	Pneumonia	Respiratory failure and arrest	Septicemia	Stroke	Gastrointestinal hemorrhage	Fluid, electrolyte, & acid-base disorders	Kidney failure
National Average	–	–	12.1	12.1	14.8	21.2	10.6	6.5	16.9	34.4	25.1	18.4	6.7	11.0	20.9
South Carolina *(continued)*															
Piedmont, Rock Hill[1]	5,474	12.4	***14.3***	✖	✖		✖		✖					✖	
Providence, Columbia	6,114	10.9	12.6						×						✖
Regional Medical Center, Orangeburg	4,653	13.5	11.4					×		**★**			×	★	**★**
Roper, Charleston	8,184	10.3	11.4		★	**★**									
Roper North, North Charleston	738	15.6	***14.5***	✖	✖	✖							✖		–
St Eugene, Dillon	1,460	11.4	12.2				**★**			**★**	✖			×	
St Francis, Greenville[1]	6,770	10.8	***13.2***	✖	✖		✖	✖	✖						
Self Regional, Greenwood	4,354	12.1	***15.4***	✖	✖	✖	✖		✖		✖	✖	✖	×	
Spartanburg Regional, Spartanburg[1]	9,215	12.1	***13.2***	✖	✖		✖			✖		✖			
Springs, Lancaster	2,460	13.8	***13.8***	✖	✖	✖			✖	×					
Trident, Charleston[1]	6,791	12.1	11.6												
Tuomey, Sumter[1]	3,980	12.3	***13.4***	✖	✖		×				×			✖	
Upstate Carolina, Gaffney	1,916	13.7	***13.7***	✖	✖	✖				–					×
Wallace Thomson, Union	1,908	12.6	***13.5***	✖	×	✖	×					✖		★	
Wilson, Darlington	644	17.1	***15.2***	✖	✖	–		–	✖	–	–		–		–
South Dakota															
Avera McKennan, Sioux Falls	5,640	8.2	12.6		×	**★**	✖	✖		×					
Avera Queen of Peace, Mitchell	2,425	8.3	8.8	**★**	**★**			**★**	**★**		**★**		**★**		
Avera Sacred Heart, Yankton	2,633	8.7	11.4										★		–
Avera St Benedict, Parkston	377	13.0	14.3			–		–		–	–	–	–	–	–
Avera St Lukes, Aberdeen	3,225	9.3	12.2									✖		**★**	
Avera Weskota, Wessington Springs[1]	310	9.7	10.4			–		–		–	–	–	–	–	–
Brookings Hospital, Brookings	1,080	10.6	11.9					–	✖	–	–				–
Canton - Inwood, Canton	354	14.7	12.2			–		–		–	–		–		–
Coteau Des Prairies, Sisseton	277	14.1	14.8			–		–		–	–	✖	–	–	–
Custer Community, Custer	156	18.6	***20.5***	✖	✖	–	–	–	✖	–	–	–	–	–	–
De Smet Memorial, De Smet	247	8.9	7.4	**★**	**★**	–	★	–	**★**	–	–	–	–	–	–
Dells Area, Dell Rapids	380	13.9	***15.5***	✖	✖	–		–		–	–	–	–	–	–
Gregory Community, Gregory	565	7.8	8.1	**★**	**★**			–	**★**	–		–	–	–	–
Hand County, Miller	400	11.8	13.8			–	✖	–		–	–	–	–	–	–
Holy Infant, Hoven	94	6.4	6.8			–	–	–	–	–	–	–	–	–	–
Huron Regional, Huron	1,181	10.2	13.1					–		–					–
Lookout, Spearfish	854	10.2	12.9					–		–			–		–
Madison Community, Madison	441	13.8	***15.2***	✖		–		–	×	–	–		–		–
Mid-Dakota, Chamberlain	486	7.8	10.0			–				–	–	–	–	–	–

Footnotes are on page 350.

Hospital outcomes: better (★) or worse (×) than average											Results of accreditation review on full survey		Other facts			
Adjusted Death rates			Adjusted Adverse outcome rates													
Surgical cases			Surgical cases													
All selected surgical cases	Coronary artery bypass surgery	Large bowel surgery	All selected surgical cases	Coronary artery bypass surgery	Large bowel surgery	Gall bladder removal	Total knee replacement	Total hip replacement	Simple prostatectomy	Carotid endarterectomy	Accreditation status*	Overall evaluation score (higher is better)	Number of beds	Major medical school affiliation?	Number of residents	Computerized drug order system (1 to 5 scale, higher is preferred; see page 23 for details)
2.3	3.8	6.5	7.7	10.3	11.9	7.5	6.7	6.4	5.4	8.2	–	91	161	–	–	–
✖		✖	✖	✖	✖		★			✖	4	**83**	276	No	0	–
							★	★	–		3	93	228	No	0	–
	–			–	✖		×	–			4	**96**	295	No	0	–
									✖		4	**95**	375	No	0	–
–	–	–	–	–	–	–	–	–	–	–	5	**97**	104	No	0	–
–	–	–		–	–	–	–	–	–	–	4	**99**	96	No	0	–
	–						★				–[2]	–[2]	225	No	0	–
	–		✖	–	×	✖	✖	–			4	89	313	No	27	–
	★		✖			✖	★	✖			4	**96**	408	No	53	–
	–			–			–	–	–	–	4	**86**	194	No	0	–
				×		✖					4	90	280	No	0	3
	–			–				–	–	–	5	**97**	215	No	0	–
	–	–		–		–	–	–	–	–	5	**96**	125	No	0	–
	–	–		–				–	–	–	4	**88**	107	No	0	–
–	–	–	–	–	–	–	–	–	–	–	–[2]	–[2]	49	No	–	–
			★				★	★			4	**95**	325	**Yes**	0	–
	–			–				–		✖	4	90	99	No	0	–
	–			–			×		★	–	4	**83**	144	No	0	–
–	–	–	–	–	–	–	–	–	–	–	–[2]	–[2]	30	No	0	–
	–		★	–		★			★		4	**78**	143	No	0	–
–	–	–	–	–	–	–	–	–	–	–	–[2]	–[2]	28	No	0	–
–	–	–		–		–	–	–	–	–	–[2]	–[2]	61	No	0	–
–	–	–	–	–	–	–	–	–	–	–	–[2]	–[2]	25	No	0	–
–	–	–	–	–	–	–	–	–	–	–	–[2]	–[2]	27	No	0	–
–	–	–	–	–	–	–	–	–	–	–	–[2]	–[2]	11	No	0	–
–	–	–	–	–	–	–	–	–	–	–	–[2]	–[2]	13	No	0	–
–	–	–	–	–	–	–	–	–	–	–	–[2]	–[2]	18	No	0	–
–	–	–	–	–	–	–	–	–	–	–	–[2]	–[2]	26	No	0	–
–	–	–	–	–	–	–	–	–	–	–	–[2]	–[2]	21	No	0	–
–	–	–	–	–	–	–	–	–	–	–	–[2]	–[2]	22	No	0	–
✖	–	✖		–	✖	–	★	–	–	–	–[2]	–[2]	61	No	0	–
	–	–		–		–	–	–	–	–	–[2]	–[2]	32	No	0	–
–	–	–	–	–	–	–	–	–	–	–	–[2]	–[2]	49	No	0	–
–	–	–	–	–	–	–	–	–	–	–	–[2]	–[2]	36	No	0	–

***Accreditation Status:** 5=Accredited with commendation or with full standards compliance; 4=Accredited with requirements for improvement; 3=Conditional accreditation.

Detailed Ratings for All Areas

See more information on "Key Ratings for Metro Areas" table beginning on page 32

Blue is most favorable
Bold Italic is least favorable
Blank means neither better nor worse than average
"–" means insufficient data

	Death rates for all selected case types			Hospital outcomes: better (★) or worse (×) than average — Adjusted Death rates											
				Medical Cases											
	Number of cases	Actual death rate (%)	Adjusted death rate (%) (lower is better)	All selected cases	All selected medical cases	Heart attack	Congestive heart failure	Obstructive pulmonary disease	Pneumonia	Respiratory failure and arrest	Septicemia	Stroke	Gastrointestinal hemorrhage	Fluid, electrolyte, & acid-base disorders	Kidney failure
National Average	–	–	12.1	12.1	14.8	21.2	10.6	6.5	16.9	34.4	25.1	18.4	6.7	11.0	20.9
South Dakota *(continued)*															
Northern Hills General, Deadwood	306	12.1	13.9			**×**	–	–		–	–	–	–	–	–
PHS Indian, Pine Ridge	118	4.2	6.2			–	–	–	–	–	–	–	–	–	–
PHS Indian, Rosebud	81	8.6	14.3			–	–	–	–	–	–	–	–	–	–
PHS Sisseton Indian, Sisseton	51	–	–	–	–	–	–	–	–	–	–	–	–	–	–
Pioneer, Viborg	288	11.8	12.9			–		–		–	–	–	–		–
Prairie Lakes, Watertown	1,879	10.9	***13.7***	**×**	**×**					–			**×**		**×**
Rapid City Regional, Rapid City[1]	5,824	7.8	11.4			★									
St Bernard's Providence, Milbank	358	14.2	***15.9***	**×**	**×**	–	**×**	–		–	–	**×**	–	–	–
St Mary's, Pierre	1,373	9.1	11.7							–	★			–	–
St Michael's, Tyndall	236	9.7	11.9			–	–	–		–	–	–	–	–	–
Sioux San Rapid City Indian Health, Rapid City	102	6.9	10.0			–	–	–	–	–	–	–	–	–	–
Sioux Valley and USD, Sioux Falls	7,914	7.2	10.5	★	★	★						★		★	
Sioux Valley Vermillion, Vermillion[1]	390	10.0	11.2			–		–	★	–	–		–		–
Sturgis Community, Sturgis	600	13.0	14.4	×	×	–		**×**		–	–		–	–	–
US PHS Indian - Cheyenne River, Eagle Butte	96	8.3	11.9			–	–	–	–	–	–	–	–	–	–
Winner Regional, Winner	416	11.5	13.6			–		–		–	–		–	–	–
Tennessee															
Nashville Area															
Baptist, Nashville	10,899	10.7	11.3	★	★				★				★		
Centennial, Nashville	4,593	10.6	11.7				★								
Metropolitan Nashville General, Nashville	677	17.0	***14.8***	**×**	**×**	–		–			**×**	–	–		
St Thomas, Nashville[1]	13,353	8.8	9.8	★	★	★	★	★	★				★	★	
Skyline, Nashville	3,751	13.2	12.1												
Southern Hills, Nashville	2,359	13.5	***13.4***	**×**	**×**			×			×				
Summit, Hermitage	3,327	11.8	11.0	★	★			★	★	★					
Tennessee Christian, Madison	2,000	14.4	11.3								★				★
Vanderbilt University, Nashville[1]	3,766	11.4	10.5	★	★		★		★				★		
Other Areas															
Athens Regional, Athens	1,435	14.6	***15.4***	**×**	**×**		×		**×**	**×**	**×**	**×**			
Baptist, Collierville	200	8.5	10.8			–	–	–	★	–	–	–	–	–	–
Baptist, Huntingdon	1,276	15.3	***15.6***	**×**	**×**		**×**		**×**					×	–
Baptist, Memphis	17,351	11.8	11.8									★			
Baptist, Union City	2,025	15.5	***17.9***	**×**	**×**	**×**	**×**		**×**	★	**×**	**×**	×		
Baptist - Lauderdale, Ripley	870	15.4	***14.3***	**×**	**×**						**×**		**×**		–

Footnotes are on page 350.

Hospital outcomes: better (★) or worse (×) than average											Results of accreditation review on full survey		Other facts			
Adjusted Death rates			Adjusted Adverse outcome rates													
Surgical cases			Surgical cases													
All selected surgical cases	Coronary artery bypass surgery	Large bowel surgery	All selected surgical cases	Coronary artery bypass surgery	Large bowel surgery	Gall bladder removal	Total knee replacement	Total hip replacement	Simple prostatectomy	Carotid endarterectomy	Accreditation status*	Overall evaluation score (higher is better)	Number of beds	Major medical school affiliation?	Number of residents	Computerized drug order system (1 to 5 scale, higher is preferred; see page 23 for details)
2.3	3.8	6.5	7.7	10.3	11.9	7.5	6.7	6.4	5.4	8.2	–	91	161	–	–	–
–	–	–	–	–	–	–	–	–	–	–	–[2]	–[2]	18	No	0	–
–	–	–	–	–	–	–	–	–	–	–	4	95	46	No	0	–
–	–	–	–	–	–	–	–	–	–	–	–[2]	–[2]	35	No	0	–
–	–	–	–	–	–	–	–	–	–	–	4	91	18	No	0	–
–	–	–	–	–	–	–	–	–	–	–	–[2]	–[2]	12	No	0	–
★	–	★	★	–	★				★	–	4	97	68	No	0	–
★			✖							✖	4	93	360	No	18	–
–	–	–	–	–	–	–	–	–	–	–	5	92	35	No	0	–
	–	–		–		–	★	–	–	–	4	91	86	No	0	–
–	–	–	–	–	–	–	–	–	–	–	–[2]	–[2]	25	No	0	–
–	–	–	–	–	–	–	–	–	–	–	–[2]	–[2]	32	No	0	–
★	★	★		★	★			×	✖	×	4	91	496	Yes	0	–
–	–	–	–	–	–	–	–	–	–	–	–[2]	–[2]	29	No	0	–
–	–	–	–	–	–	–	–	–	–	–	–[2]	–[2]	30	No	0	–
–	–	–	–	–	–	–	–	–	–	–	4	87	24	No	0	–
–	–	–	–	–	–	–	–	–	–	–	–[2]	–[2]	35	No	0	–
						✖	★				4	94	534	No	2	1
✖	×			×	✖						4	95	680	No	12	3
–	–	–	–	–	–	–	–	–	–	–	4	96	124	Yes	7	2
★	★						✖			★	4	95	523	No	0	2
	–			–	✖		–	–	–		4	87	285	No	–	4
	–			–				–	–	–	4	95	120	No	0	4
	–			–		×		–	–		4	90	188	No	0	3
–	–	–		–	✖	–	–	–	–	–	4	87	288	No	7	2
						–			–	–	4	89	548	Yes	342	5
–	–	–	★	–	–	–	–	–	–	–	4	88	91	No	0	–
–	–	–	–	–	–	–	–	–	–	–	4	84	60	No	–	–
–	–	–	–	–	–	–	–	–	–	–	4	94	70	No	0	–
			✖	✖			✖				4	82	1,026	No	120	–
	–	–		–		–	–	–	–	–	4	93	133	No	0	–
–	–	–	–	–	–	–	–	–	–	–	4	92	60	Yes	0	–

***Accreditation Status:** 5=Accredited with commendation or with full standards compliance; 4=Accredited with requirements for improvement; 3=Conditional accreditation.

Detailed Ratings for All Areas

See more information on "Key Ratings for Metro Areas" table beginning on page 32

Blue is most favorable
Bold Italic is least favorable
Blank means neither better nor worse than average
"–" means insufficient data

	Death rates for all selected case types			Hospital outcomes: better (★) or worse (×) than average — Adjusted Death rates — Medical Cases											
	Number of cases	Actual death rate (%)	Adjusted death rate (%) (lower is better)	All selected cases	All selected medical cases	Heart attack	Congestive heart failure	Obstructive pulmonary disease	Pneumonia	Respiratory failure and arrest	Septicemia	Stroke	Gastrointestinal hemorrhage	Fluid, electrolyte, & acid-base disorders	Kidney failure
National Average	–	–	12.1	12.1	14.8	21.2	10.6	6.5	16.9	34.4	25.1	18.4	6.7	11.0	20.9
Tennessee *(continued)*															
Other Areas *(continued)*															
Baptist - Tipton, Covington	1,531	16.2	13.1			✖									
Baptist DeKalb, Smithville	1,257	13.5	11.3								–	✖	–		
Baptist of Cocke County, Newport	1,187	16.5	***13.8***	✖	✖				×					–	×
Baptist of East Tennessee, Knoxville	6,859	11.3	11.2	**★**	**★**	★									
Bedford County, Shelbyville	1,314	13.9	***14.8***	✖	✖	×		×	✖				–		
Blount, Maryville	5,581	13.4	11.4		★					**★**				**★**	
Bolivar General, Bolivar	528	19.7	***17.1***	✖	✖	–		–		–	✖	–	–		–
Bradley, Cleveland	3,539	15.8	***13.3***	✖	×					✖				✖	
Bristol Regional, Bristol[1]	5,468	13.4	12.2									✖			
Camden General, Camden	497	22.3	***22.9***	✖	✖	–	✖	–	✖	–	–	✖	–	×	–
Claiborne County, Tazewell[1]	1,792	14.8	12.4												✖
Cleveland Community, Cleveland	828	14.5	***15.1***	✖	✖		✖			×	×		–		–
Coffee, Manchester	599	13.2	10.3					–		–	–		–	–	
Cookville Regional, Cookeville	4,145	12.2	11.6				✖	★	★		★				✖
Copper Basin, Copperhill	695	8.6	8.8	**★**	**★**		★		★			**★**	–	–	
Crockett, Lawrenceburg	2,135	14.6	***15.0***	✖	✖			✖	✖						
Cumberland, Crossville	4,312	10.6	12.4						✖					★	
Cumberland River, Celina	1,194	9.0	6.9	**★**	**★**				**★**	**★**			–	**★**	×
Decatur County General, Parsons	1,079	13.7	13.4			✖			×	–			–		–
Delta, Memphis	889	15.9	***15.4***	✖	✖	✖		✖	×	✖	×		–	★	
Erlanger, Chattanooga[1]	5,404	14.6	***13.9***	✖	✖		×	✖	✖		✖			×	✖
Fentress County General, Jamestown	1,865	7.6	9.0	**★**	**★**		**★**	**★**			**★**		–		
Fort Sanders, Loudon	630	15.7	13.9							✖			–		–
Fort Sanders Parkwest, Knoxville	5,323	11.2	11.4			**★**				**★**		×			★
Fort Sanders Regional, Knoxville	5,785	11.2	12.6						✖						
Fort Sanders Sevier, Sevierville	1,241	17.2	***19.6***	✖	✖		✖	–	✖		–	✖		✖	–
Frank T Rutherford, Carthage	1,309	12.1	12.6			×				–	✖				–
Gateway, Clarksville[1]	3,785	15.2	***15.1***	✖	✖	✖	✖	✖	✖	✖	×	✖	✖		
Gibson General, Trenton	632	17.9	***22.5***	✖	✖	–		✖	✖	–	–	✖	–	✖	–
Grandview, Jasper	1,218	16.5	***14.3***	✖	✖								✖	×	×
Hardin County General, Savannah	999	22.3	***19.9***	✖	✖	✖	✖	✖	✖			✖			✖
HCA River Park, McMinnville	2,521	12.4	12.4			✖				★		×	×		
Hendersonville Medical Center, Hendersonville	1,210	15.5	12.9				✖								
Henry County, Paris	2,185	14.0	***16.4***	✖	✖	✖	✖		✖	–	✖		✖		✖

Footnotes are on page 350.

Hospital outcomes: better (★) or worse (✕) than average											Results of accreditation review on full survey		Other facts			
Adjusted Death rates			Adjusted Adverse outcome rates													
Surgical cases			Surgical cases													
All selected surgical cases	Coronary artery bypass surgery	Large bowel surgery	All selected surgical cases	Coronary artery bypass surgery	Large bowel surgery	Gall bladder removal	Total knee replacement	Total hip replacement	Simple prostatectomy	Carotid endarterectomy	Accreditation status*	Overall evaluation score (higher is better)	Number of beds	Major medical school affiliation?	Number of residents	Computerized drug order system (1 to 5 scale, higher is preferred; see page 23 for details)
2.3	3.8	6.5	7.7	10.3	11.9	7.5	6.7	6.4	5.4	8.2	–	91	161	–	–	–
–	–	–		–	–	–	–	–		–	4	93	70	No	0	–
–	–	–	–	–	–	–	–	–	–	–	4	91	52	No	0	–
–	–	–	–	–	–	–	–	–	–	–	4	98	53	No	2	–
					★				★		4	91	299	No	14	4
–	–	–	–	–	–	–	–	–	–	–	4	92	180	No	4	–
	–			–				–			4	91	123	No	0	4
–	–	–	–	–	–	–	–	–	–	–	4	93	47	No	0	–
✖	–	✖	✖	–	✖			–		✖	4	93	174	No	0	2
✖	✖								–		5	86	318	Yes	30	–
–	–	–	–	–	–	–	–	–	–	–	4	86	24	No	0	–
–	–	–	–	–	–	–	–	–	–	–	3	89	65	No	0	–
–	–	–		–	–	–	–	–	–	–	–[2]	–[2]	70	No	0	2
–	–	–	–	–	–	–	–	–	–	–	–[2]	–[2]	36	No	0	–
	–							–			5	93	168	No	0	–
–	–	–	–	–	–	–	–	–	–	–	4	88	44	No	0	–
–	–	–		–	–	–	–	–	–	–	4	89	98	No	0	–
	–		★	–			★	★	✖	–	3	94	146	No	0	–
–	–	–	–	–	–	–	–	–	–	–	3	82	66	No	0	–
–	–	–	–	–	–	–	–	–	–	–	4	92	40	No	0	–
–	–	–	–	–	–	–	–	–	–	–	4	86	130	No	1	–
			✕		✖	✖	✕				4	79	536	No	181	4
–	–	–	–	–	–	–	–	–	–	–	4	87	73	No	0	–
–	–	–	–	–	–	–	–	–	–	–	4	92	50	No	0	–
											4	89	244	No	9	4
											5	96	398	No	0	4
–	–	–		–	–	–	–	–	–	–	4	93	50	No	0	–
–	–	–	–	–	–	–	–	–	–	–	4	88	50	No	0	–
	–	–	✖	–			✖	–	–	✖	4	87	136	No	0	–
–	–	–	–	–	–	–	–	–	–	–	4	88	42	No	0	–
–	–	–	–	–	–	–	–	–	–	–	4	89	50	No	0	3
–	–	–	–	–	–	–	–	–	–	–	4	89	50	No	0	–
	–	–		–			–	–	–	–	4	89	90	No	0	2
–	–	–		–	–	–	–	–	–	–	4	96	56	No	0	–
✕	–	–		–				–	–	–	4	90	95	No	0	–

***Accreditation Status:** 5=Accredited with commendation or with full standards compliance; 4=Accredited with requirements for improvement; 3=Conditional accreditation.

Detailed Ratings for All Areas

See more information on "Key Ratings for Metro Areas" table beginning on page 32

Blue is most favorable
Bold Italic is least favorable
Blank means neither better nor worse than average
"–" means insufficient data

	Death rates for all selected case types			Hospital outcomes: better (★) or worse (×) than average												
				Adjusted Death rates												
					Medical Cases											
	Number of cases	Actual death rate (%)	Adjusted death rate (%) (lower is better)	All selected cases	All selected medical cases	Heart attack	Congestive heart failure	Obstructive pulmonary disease	Pneumonia	Respiratory failure and arrest	Septicemia	Stroke	Gastrointestinal hemorrhage	Fluid, electrolyte, & acid-base disorders	Kidney failure
National Average	–	–	12.1	12.1	14.8	21.2	10.6	6.5	16.9	34.4	25.1	18.4	6.7	11.0	20.9
Tennessee *(continued)*															
Other Areas *(continued)*															
Hillside, Pulaski	1,514	12.7	**9.9**	★	★				★				★	★	–
Horizon, Dickson	3,216	12.3	12.0				✖			✖					✖
Humboldt General, Humboldt	690	15.5	***15.0***	✖	✖	–		–		–		✖	–		–
Indian Path, Kingsport	2,781	14.1	11.4							★					×
Jackson - Madison County General, Jackson	12,296	12.6	12.2							✖	✖				
Jefferson Memorial, Jefferson City	1,590	17.5	***17.7***	✖	✖	✖		✖	✖	✖	✖		✖	×	–
Jellico Community, Jellico	1,165	14.8	**10.1**	★	★		★						–		
John W Harton Regional, Tullahoma	1,872	13.0	***14.3***	✖	✖		✖					×			
Johnson City Medical Center, Johnson City	8,278	11.4	***13.2***	✖	✖				✖					✖	✖
Lakeway Regional, Morristown	1,206	14.3	***14.5***	✖	✖	✖		✖							★
Laughlin, Greeneville	3,393	11.9	***13.1***	✖	×				×		×	×			
Lincoln, Fayetteville[1]	1,190	15.0	12.5												–
Livingston Regional, Livingston	2,174	14.4	12.9												✖
Macon County General, Lafayette	883	11.4	10.7			✖				–			–		–
Marshall, Lewisburg	1,020	15.7	***15.2***	✖	✖				✖	✖			–		–
Maury Regional, Columbia	5,715	12.3	***13.0***	✖	×	×			✖		✖	★			
Medical Center, Manchester	616	11.0	12.6			–				–	✖	–	–		–
Memorial, Chattanooga	11,982	10.6	12.3						✖	✖			✖		
Methodist, McKenzie[1]	537	18.4	***21.8***	✖	✖		✖	✖	✖	–	–	✖	–	✖	–
Methodist, Oak Ridge	7,320	11.2	11.8			★	✖								
Methodist Healthcare, Brownsville[1]	686	16.0	***14.8***	✖	✖					–	✖	✖	–		
Methodist Healthcare - Dyersburg Hospital, Dyersburg	2,039	19.9	***16.1***	✖	✖	✖			✖		×	✖		✖	
Methodist Healthcare - Fayette Hospital, Somerville	538	14.3	***17.3***	✖	✖	–		–	×	–	✖	–	✖	×	–
Methodist Healthcare - Lexington Hospital, Lexington	774	16.4	***19.2***	✖	✖	–	✖		✖	–	–	×	✖	–	–
Methodist Healthcare - McNairy Hospital, Selmer	845	16.0	***17.9***	✖	✖	–	✖		✖	–	–		–		
Methodist Healthcare - Memphis Hospitals, Memphis	18,866	13.1	***13.4***	✖	✖		✖		✖		✖				
Methodist Healthcare - Volunteer Hospital, Martin	1,868	17.0	12.0					★		★		✖			
Methodist Le Bonheur, Jackson	2,376	9.8	10.7	★	★						×	★		★	
Middle Tennessee, Murfreesboro	4,681	12.6	12.3									×			★
Milan General, Milan	576	14.9	***15.6***	✖	✖	–	×	–		–	–	✖	–	–	–
Morristown - Hamblen, Morristown[1]	2,945	14.0	***14.6***	✖	✖	×	✖		✖				✖	✖	
Northcrest, Springfield	2,051	12.7	**9.9**	★	★		★				★				
Northside, Johnson City	1,467	13.6	***14.2***	✖	✖					✖	✖				–
Parkridge, Chattanooga[1]	5,102	12.5	***13.0***	✖	✖				✖						★

Footnotes are on page 350.

Hospital outcomes: better (★) or worse (×) than average											Results of accreditation review on full survey		Other facts			
Adjusted Death rates			Adjusted Adverse outcome rates													
Surgical cases			Surgical cases													
All selected surgical cases	Coronary artery bypass surgery	Large bowel surgery	All selected surgical cases	Coronary artery bypass surgery	Large bowel surgery	Gall bladder removal	Total knee replacement	Total hip replacement	Simple prostatectomy	Carotid endarterectomy	Accreditation status*	Overall evaluation score (higher is better)	Number of beds	Major medical school affiliation?	Number of residents	Computerized drug order system (1 to 5 scale, higher is preferred; see page 23 for details)
2.3	3.8	6.5	7.7	10.3	11.9	7.5	6.7	6.4	5.4	8.2	–	91	161	–	–	–
–	–	–		–	–	×	–	–	–	–	4	89	86	No	0	–
	–	–	★	–		★	–	–	–	–	5	90	142	No	0	2
–	–	–	–	–	–	–	–	–	–	–	4	92	42	No	0	–
×	–	–	★	–		–	–	–	–	–	4	**87**	166	**Yes**	0	–
								★			4	92	692	No	205	–
–	–	–	–	–	–	–	–	–	–	–	4	89	29	No	0	–
–	–	–	–	–	–	–	–	–	–	–	4	**86**	54	No	0	–
–	–	–		–	–	–	–	–	–	–	4	**87**	137	No	1	–
		✖	✖		✖					✖	4	90	376	**Yes**	0	–
–	–	–	–	–	–	–	–	–	–	–	4	93	135	No	1	–
	–			–			–		–	–	4	**87**	140	No	0	–
–	–	–		–	–	–	–	–	–	–	4	**95**	51	No	0	–
–	–	–	–	–	–	–	–	–	–	–	4	**88**	73	No	0	–
–	–	–	–	–	–	–	–	–	–	–	4	93	43	No	0	–
–	–	–	–	–	–	–	–	–	–	–	4	92	77	No	0	–
✖	–			–							4	**87**	255	No	18	–
–	–	–	–	–	–	–	–	–	–	–	–[2]	–[2]	49	No	0	–
											4	**96**	355	No	43	2
–	–	–	–	–	–	–	–	–	–	–	–[2]	–[2]	29	No	0	–
		✖	★							★	4	**84**	290	No	12	4
–	–	–	–	–	–	–	–	–	–	–	4	**96**	44	No	0	–
	–			–	✖		–	–	–	–	4	**94**	105	No	0	–
–	–	–	–	–	–	–	–	–	–	–	4	**96**	38	No	0	–
–	–	–	–	–	–	–	–	–	–	–	4	93	32	No	0	–
–	–	–	–	–	–	–	–	–	–	–	4	**95**	48	No	0	–
×	✖		✖	✖					✖		4	**95**	1,248	**Yes**	324	–
	–	–		–		–	–	–	–	–	4	93	65	No	0	–
×	–			–		–			–	–	4	**94**	120	No	0	–
	–			–			✖	–		✖	4	**95**	184	No	0	2
–	–	–		–		–	–	–	–	–	4	93	49	No	0	–
✖	–	–		–	–		–	–	–	–	4	**94**	143	No	3	–
	–	–		–		–	–	–	–	–	4	93	100	No	0	–
	–	–		–		–	–	–	–	–	4	91	98	No	0	–
			★				★				4	**88**	517	No	6	2

***Accreditation Status:** 5=Accredited with commendation or with full standards compliance; 4=Accredited with requirements for improvement; 3=Conditional accreditation.

Detailed Ratings for All Areas

See more information on "Key Ratings for Metro Areas" table beginning on page 32

Blue is most favorable
Bold Italic is least favorable
Blank means neither better nor worse than average
"–" means insufficient data

	Death rates for all selected case types				Hospital outcomes: better (★) or worse (×) than average — Adjusted Death rates — Medical Cases										
	Number of cases	Actual death rate (%)	Adjusted death rate (%) (lower is better)	All selected cases	All selected medical cases	Heart attack	Congestive heart failure	Obstructive pulmonary disease	Pneumonia	Respiratory failure and arrest	Septicemia	Stroke	Gastrointestinal hemorrhage	Fluid, electrolyte, & acid-base disorders	Kidney failure
National Average	–	–	12.1	12.1	14.8	21.2	10.6	6.5	16.9	34.4	25.1	18.4	6.7	11.0	20.9
Tennessee *(continued)*															
Other Areas *(continued)*															
Perry, Linden	706	15.7	***14.3***	✖	✖	–		–		–	–		–	✖	
Regional, Memphis	756	18.7	***15.3***	✖	✖	–		–	✖		✖	✖	–	×	
Rhea, Dayton	839	14.3	12.9					–		×				–	–
Roane, Harriman	2,576	13.1	12.6			✖		**★**				×			
St Francis, Memphis	9,457	13.3	***13.9***	✖	✖		✖		✖	✖	✖				
St Mary's Campbell County, La Follette	2,035	13.8	**8.5**	**★**	**★**		**★**	**★**	**★**	**★**		**★**			
St Marys, Knoxville[1]	7,990	12.8	12.0							**★**			✖		
Scott County, Oneida	1,691	11.9	**9.9**	**★**	**★**			**★**		★		✖	**★**		
Smith County, Carthage	836	11.1	**9.8**	**★**	**★**	–			★	–			–		
Southern Tennessee, Winchester	2,660	13.0	12.9				×			×					
Stones River, Woodbury	585	13.3	10.8			–		–		–	**★**	✖	–	–	–
Sumner Regional, Gallatin	2,502	13.5	***14.3***	✖	✖				✖		✖				
Sweetwater Hospital, Sweetwater[1]	1,557	14.8	13.4	×	×			✖	×		×				
Sycamore Shoals, Elizabethton	1,289	16.9	***16.1***	✖	✖	✖	✖	–			✖			✖	
Takoma Adventist, Greeneville	1,524	13.3	11.7												
Trinity, Erin	825	13.8	**9.9**	**★**	**★**	–		–	**★**	✖	**★**		–		✖
Unicoi County, Erwin	821	12.8	***15.0***	✖	✖	–		–	×	–	–		–		–
University, Lebanon	2,789	11.4	11.7			×								★	
University of Tennessee, Knoxville	5,766	10.9	11.5												
University of Tennessee Bowld, Memphis	951	17.0	***15.2***	✖	✖			–	✖	×					
Wayne Medical Center, Waynesboro	954	12.1	13.0			–	×			–	–		–		–
Wellmont Hawkins County, Rogersville[1]	731	11.8	11.3								–		–		
Wellmont Holston Valley, Kingsport[1]	6,541	14.6	***14.2***	✖	✖		✖	✖	✖		×			✖	
White County, Sparta	939	13.4	11.7											✖	–
Williamson, Franklin	2,493	11.2	11.4												
Woods, Etowah[1]	1,387	15.4	***14.4***	✖	✖		✖		✖	–					
Texas															
Austin Area															
Brackenridge, Austin	1,605	11.2	**9.9**	**★**	**★**		**★**				★				
Heart Hospital, Austin	–	–	–	–	–	–	–	–	–	–	–	–	–	–	–
North Austin Medical Center, Austin	3,228	11.7	11.4					✖							
St David's, Austin	5,676	11.9	11.4		★	**★**			**★**						
Seton Medical Center, Austin	7,958	9.7	11.8											**★**	

Footnotes are on page 350.

Hospital outcomes: better (★) or worse (×) than average											Results of accreditation review on full survey		Other facts			
Adjusted Death rates			Adjusted Adverse outcome rates													
Surgical cases			Surgical cases													
All selected surgical cases	Coronary artery bypass surgery	Large bowel surgery	All selected surgical cases	Coronary artery bypass surgery	Large bowel surgery	Gall bladder removal	Total knee replacement	Total hip replacement	Simple prostatectomy	Carotid endarterectomy	Accreditation status*	Overall evaluation score (higher is better)	Number of beds	Major medical school affiliation?	Number of residents	Computerized drug order system (1 to 5 scale, higher is preferred; see page 23 for details)
2.3	3.8	6.5	7.7	10.3	11.9	7.5	6.7	6.4	5.4	8.2	–	91	161	–	–	–
–	–	–	–	–	–	–	–	–	–	–	–[2]	–[2]	53	No	0	–
–	–	–	–	–	–	–	–	–	–	–	4	**86**	335	Yes	0	–
–	–	–	–	–	–	–	–	–	–	–	4	92	42	No	0	–
–	–	–		–			–	–	–	–	4	**87**	85	No	0	–
					×		★				4	**87**	461	No	0	–
–	–	–	–	–	–	–	–	–	–	–	4	95	67	No	0	–
				★				✖			4	**84**	300	No	31	4
–	–	–	–	–	–	–	–	–	–	–	4	91	77	No	0	–
–	–	–	–	–	–	–	–	–	–	–	4	92	40	No	0	–
	–			–			–	–	–	–	4	89	140	No	0	–
–	–	–	–	–	–	–	–	–	–	–	4	92	55	No	0	–
–	–	–		–	–		–	–	–	–	4	93	140	No	0	–
–	–	–		–	–	–	–	–	–	–	4	**83**	59	No	0	–
–	–	–		–		–	–	–	–	–	4	92	93	No	0	–
×	–	–		–	–	–	–		–	–	5	**84**	80	No	0	–
–	–	–	–	–	–	–	–	–	–	–	3	**82**	31	No	0	–
–	–	–		–	–	–	–	–	–	–	4	93	28	No	0	–
	–	–		–		★		–	–	–	5	**88**	225	No	0	–
★		★				✖	★			★	4	**84**	422	Yes	171	4
–	–	–		–	–	–	–	–	–	–	4	**82**	101	Yes	28	–
–	–	–	–	–	–	–	–	–	–	–	4	93	32	No	0	–
–	–	–	–	–	–		–	–	–	–	4	**88**	50	No	0	–
	★			★					–		4	93	336	No	0	–
–	–	–	–	–	–	–	–	–	–	–	4	93	60	No	0	–
	–		✖	–			✖	✖	–	–	4	90	126	No	0	–
–	–	–		–	–	–	–	–	–	–	4	99	160	No	4	–
	–	–	★	–		–	–	–	–	–	4	**83**	312	No	0	–
–	–	–	–	–	–	–	–	–	–	–	4	**85**	58	–	0	–
				★			–	–	–		4	93	128	No	0	–
									✖		4	92	298	No	0	–
			✖				✖	✖			3	**88**	527	No	77	–

***Accreditation Status:** 5=Accredited with commendation or with full standards compliance; 4=Accredited with requirements for improvement; 3=Conditional accreditation.

Detailed Ratings for All Areas

See more information on "Key Ratings for Metro Areas" table beginning on page 32

Blue is most favorable
Bold Italic is least favorable
Blank means neither better nor worse than average
"–" means insufficient data

	Death rates for all selected case types			Hospital outcomes: better (★) or worse (×) than average — Adjusted Death rates — Medical Cases											
	Number of cases	Actual death rate (%)	Adjusted death rate (%) (lower is better)	All selected cases	All selected medical cases	Heart attack	Congestive heart failure	Obstructive pulmonary disease	Pneumonia	Respiratory failure and arrest	Septicemia	Stroke	Gastrointestinal hemorrhage	Fluid, electrolyte, & acid-base disorders	Kidney failure
National Average	–	–	12.1	12.1	14.8	21.2	10.6	6.5	16.9	34.4	25.1	18.4	6.7	11.0	20.9
Texas *(continued)*															
Austin Area *(continued)*															
Seton Northwest, Austin	–	–	–	–	–	–	–	–	–	–	–	–	–	–	–
South Austin Hospital, Austin	3,927	11.9	10.6	★	★	★	★								
Dallas-Ft. Worth Area															
All Saints Episcopal, Fort Worth	5,054	13.3	***14.9***	✖	✖	✖	✖	✖	✖				×		
Arlington Memorial, Arlington	4,843	12.9	***15.8***	✖	✖		✖		✖		✖	✖	✖		×
Baylor, Garland	3,154	12.7	***14.4***	✖	✖		✖		✖		✖				
Baylor, Grapevine	1,261	13.6	***14.1***	✖	✖	✖							✖		–
Baylor, Irving	3,416	13.0	12.4			★	✖			★					
Baylor - Richardson Medical Center, Richardson	1,681	15.2	13.0					✖			★				
Baylor All Saints of Cityview, Fort Worth	–	–	–	–	–	–	–	–	–	–	–	–	–	–	–
Baylor University, Dallas	10,756	9.2	10.6	★	★	★		★	★	★		★		★	
Charlton Methodist, Dallas	3,418	14.3	11.3												
Children's, Dallas	–	–	–	–	–	–	–	–	–	–	–	–	–	–	–
Cook Children's, Fort Worth	–	–	–	–	–	–	–	–	–	–	–	–	–	–	–
Dallas - Fort Worth, Grand Prairie	1,068	18.9	***14.2***	✖	✖	✖		✖							–
Dallas Southwest, Dallas	1,037	12.2	10.3	★	★		★	–			×				
Doctors, Dallas	4,701	12.8	11.9							★					
Harris Methodist Fort Worth, Fort Worth	7,526	10.8	12.0					✖		★					
Harris Methodist H-E-B, Bedford	3,711	14.5	***14.3***	✖	✖		✖	✖	✖	×					
Harris Methodist Northwest, Azle	962	14.7	10.2	★	★				★		★		✖		
Harris Methodist Southwest, Fort Worth	1,651	15.1	***13.8***	✖	✖						×				–
Huguley, Fort Worth[1]	2,765	16.2	***14.1***	✖	✖							✖	✖		
JPS, Fort Worth[1]	1,000	16.1	***16.2***	✖	✖		✖	✖	✖		✖		–	–	
Lake Pointe, Rowlett	2,276	16.1	11.9									★			
Las Colinas, Irving	93	4.3	6.3			–	–	–	–	–	–	–	–	–	–
Leland, Garland	367	18.8	***16.2***	✖	✖	–		–	✖	–		–	–	×	–
Medical Center, Arlington	1,632	11.8	10.4	★	★						★				–
Medical Center, Lancaster	1,319	19.9	11.2				★	–	★						
Medical Center, Mesquite	2,651	14.3	12.4												
Medical City Dallas Hospital, Dallas	4,156	10.7	10.9	★	★						★				
Mesquite Community, Mesquite	1,608	19.3	***14.4***	✖	✖						✖			✖	
Methodist, Dallas	4,510	12.4	11.2	★	★									★	
North Hills, North Richland Hills	2,337	16.0	12.5					✖							

Footnotes are on page 350.

Hospital outcomes: better (★) or worse (×) than average											Results of accreditation review on full survey		Other facts			
Adjusted Death rates			Adjusted Adverse outcome rates													
Surgical cases			Surgical cases													
All selected surgical cases	Coronary artery bypass surgery	Large bowel surgery	All selected surgical cases	Coronary artery bypass surgery	Large bowel surgery	Gall bladder removal	Total knee replacement	Total hip replacement	Simple prostatectomy	Carotid endarterectomy	Accreditation status*	Overall evaluation score (higher is better)	Number of beds	Major medical school affiliation?	Number of residents	Computerized drug order system (1 to 5 scale, higher is preferred; see page 23 for details)
2.3	3.8	6.5	7.7	10.3	11.9	7.5	6.7	6.4	5.4	8.2	–	91	161	–	–	–
–	–	–	–	–	–	–	–	–	–	–	–[2]	–[2]	–	–	–	–
								–	×		4	**94**	200	No	0	–
✖	✖			✖						★	4	93	249	No	0	–
×	✖				✖				–		5	**98**	339	No	0	–
			★						–		4	92	175	No	18	–
	–	–	★	–		–	–	–	–	–	4	**94**	88	No	0	–
×		✖	✖		✖	×	✖		–	×	4	91	217	No	0	–
	–	–		–		★	–	–	–	–	5	90	97	No	0	–
–	–	–	–	–	–	–	–	–	–	–	–[2]	–[2]	–	–	–	–
★										★	4	89	847	No	158	–
	–			–	★			–	–	–	4	***84***	130	No	18	–
–	–	–	–	–	–	–	–	–	–	–	5	**96**	224	–	0	–
–	–	–	–	–	–	–	–	–	–	–	4	91	181	–	0	–
✖	–	–		–		–	–	–	–	–	–[2]	–[2]	136	No	16	–
–	–	–		–	–	–	–	–	–	–	4	92	107	No	16	–
				★	×		✖	–			4	**96**	179	No	0	–
×							★				5	**97**	507	No	0	–
✖	✖	✖				✖			–		–[2]	–[2]	165	No	0	–
–	–	–	–	–	–	–	–	–	–	–	5	**96**	36	No	0	–
	–	–		–		–	–	–	–	–	5	**96**	83	No	0	–
✖	–	–		–		–	★	–	–	✖	4	89	156	No	0	–
–	–	–		–		–	–	–	–	–	4	***88***	278	No	137	–
✖	–	–		–		–	–	–	–	–	4	**97**	87	No	0	–
–	–	–	–	–	–	–	–	–	–	–	4	**94**	77	No	0	2
–	–	–	–	–	–	–	–	–	–	–	4	90	113	No	0	–
	–	–	★	–		–	–	–	–	–	4	**95**	188	No	0	2
–	–	–		–	–	–	–	–	–	–	5	**97**	79	No	0	–
	–	–		★	×	–	–	–	–	–	4	91	166	No	0	–
								×			4	**97**	496	No	0	3
✖	–	–		–	–	–	–	–	–	–	4	92	115	No	0	–
	–							–	–	✖	4	***82***	362	No	41	–
✖	–					–	–	–	–	–	5	**98**	115	No	0	–

***Accreditation Status:** 5=Accredited with commendation or with full standards compliance; 4=Accredited with requirements for improvement; 3=Conditional accreditation.

Detailed Ratings for All Areas

See more information on "Key Ratings for Metro Areas" table beginning on page 32

Blue is most favorable
Bold Italic is least favorable
Blank means neither better nor worse than average
"–" means insufficient data

	Death rates for all selected case types			Hospital outcomes: better (★) or worse (×) than average — Adjusted Death rates — Medical Cases											
	Number of cases	Actual death rate (%)	Adjusted death rate (%) (lower is better)	All selected cases	All selected medical cases	Heart attack	Congestive heart failure	Obstructive pulmonary disease	Pneumonia	Respiratory failure and arrest	Septicemia	Stroke	Gastrointestinal hemorrhage	Fluid, electrolyte, & acid-base disorders	Kidney failure
National Average	–	–	12.1	12.1	14.8	21.2	10.6	6.5	16.9	34.4	25.1	18.4	6.7	11.0	20.9
Texas *(continued)*															
Dallas-Ft. Worth Area *(continued)*															
Osteopathic of Texas, Fort Worth	2,719	17.9	***14.0***	✖	✖				✖	✖				✖	
Parkland, Dallas[1]	1,933	13.2	11.0		★										
Plaza, Fort Worth	4,140	13.4	12.5												
Presbyterian, Dallas	7,629	10.8	12.2												
RHD, Dallas	1,823	15.1	12.5									×			
St Paul University, Dallas	3,500	10.9	12.4												
Texas Scottish Rite for Children, Dallas	–	–	–	–	–	–	–	–	–	–	–	–	–	–	–
Zale Lipshy University, Dallas	1,063	6.1	10.5			–		–		–			–	–	–
Houston Area															
Baycoast, Baytown	839	10.1	10.2				★	–		–			–	–	✖
Bayou City (Belleaire Blvd), Houston	607	14.2	11.3					–					–		
Bayou City (Portsmouth St), Houston	–	–	–	–	–	–	–	–	–	–	–	–	–	–	–
Bayshore, Pasadena	3,908	13.7	12.0						★	★			✖		
Bellaire, Houston	778	14.0	**9.2**	★	★		★	–	★					★	
Ben Taub General, Houston[1]	1,836	15.2	***13.8***	✖	✖	✖					✖				
Christus St John, Nassau Bay	1,186	12.7	***14.2***	✖	×						✖		–	×	–
Christus St Joseph, Houston	3,860	12.4	12.3				×							×	
Clear Lake Regional, Webster	3,493	14.7	12.8				✖		×						
Columbia Spring Branch, Houston	3,632	13.1	11.7							★	✖				
Cypress Fairbanks, Houston	2,010	14.2	11.7												
Doctors - Parkway, Houston	2,174	12.0	**9.5**	★	★		★		★			★			
Doctors - Tidwell, Houston	905	7.7	**6.8**	★	★		★		★	★	★		–		★
East Houston Regional, Houston	1,976	13.5	11.9			×							★		★
Houston Northwest, Houston	4,283	13.4	12.1												✖
Kingwood Medical Center, Kingwood	1,641	10.8	10.7		★			★					–	★	
Lyndon B Johnson General, Houston[1]	–	–	–	–	–	–	–	–	–	–	–	–	–	–	–
Memorial Hermann, Houston	2,454	15.2	***13.4***	✖								✖			
Memorial Hermann Memorial City, Houston	5,095	11.8	12.3			×		×				★			
Memorial Hermann Northwest, Houston	–	–	–	–	–	–	–	–	–	–	–	–	–	–	–
Memorial Hermann Southeast, Houston	–	–	–	–	–	–	–	–	–	–	–	–	–	–	–
Memorial Hermann Southwest, Houston[1]	–	–	–	–	–	–	–	–	–	–	–	–	–	–	–
Methodist, Houston	9,344	7.7	11.6		★				★			★			
Methodist Diagnostic, Houston	2,259	8.9	**9.5**	★	★	★		★		★					

Footnotes are on page 350.

Hospital outcomes: better (★) or worse (×) than average											Results of accreditation review on full survey		Other facts			
Adjusted Death rates			Adjusted Adverse outcome rates													
Surgical cases			Surgical cases													
All selected surgical cases	Coronary artery bypass surgery	Large bowel surgery	All selected surgical cases	Coronary artery bypass surgery	Large bowel surgery	Gall bladder removal	Total knee replacement	Total hip replacement	Simple prostatectomy	Carotid endarterectomy	Accreditation status*	Overall evaluation score (higher is better)	Number of beds	Major medical school affiliation?	Number of residents	Computerized drug order system (1 to 5 scale, higher is preferred; see page 23 for details)
2.3	3.8	6.5	7.7	10.3	11.9	7.5	6.7	6.4	5.4	8.2	–	91	161	–	–	–
×	✖					–	★	–	–		4	93	197	**Yes**	66	–
	–	–		–		–	–	–	–	–	4	**94**	702	**Yes**	678	–
						×					5	**97**	235	No	0	2
✖	✖		×	✖				×			4	**96**	604	No	47	–
	–	–	✖		–	✖	–	–	–		4	**96**	141	No	0	–
		×	×				✖	✖	✖		5	**94**	339	No	39	–
–	–	–	–	–	–	–	–	–	–	–	5	**97**	52	–	0	–
	–	–			–	–		–			5	**98**	145	**Yes**	0	–
–	–	–	–	–	–	–	–	–	–	–	4	***82***	171	No	0	–
–	–	–	–	–	–	–	–	–	–	–	–[2]	–[2]	190	No	–	–
–	–	–	–	–	–	–	–	–	–	–	3	***83***	341	–	0	–
✖	✖			✖			×	–	–		4	92	271	No	0	2
–	–	–	–	–	–	–	–	–	–	–	4	89	194	No	0	–
–	–	–		–		–	–	–	–	–	4	***86***	801	**Yes**	0	–
–	–	–	✖	–	–	–	✖	–	–	–	4	**95**	135	No	0	–
	–							–	–	–	4	93	395	No	73	–
	–			★				–			4	**97**	338	No	0	4
	–			★				–			4	**96**	269	No	0	–
–	–	–		–	–		–	–	–	–	4	***87***	140	No	0	–
–	–	–		–	–	–	–	–	–	–	–[2]	–[2]	134	No	0	–
–	–	–	–	–	–	–	–	–	–	–	4	89	101	No	0	–
–	–	–		–		–	–	–	–	–	4	91	121	No	1	–
	✖							–	–		4	**94**	366	No	0	–
–	–	–		–	–	–	–	–	–		4	**98**	153	No	0	–
–	–	–	–	–	–	–	–	–	–	–	4	***86***	–	–	–	–
✖	✖	✖			✖	–	–	–	–	✖	5	**98**	610	**Yes**	0	–
											5	**96**	300	No	0	–
–	–	–	–	–	–	–	–	–	–	–	5	**98**	–	–	–	–
–	–	–	–	–	–	–	–	–	–	–	–[2]	–[2]	–	–	–	–
–	–	–	–	–	–	–	–	–	–	–	5	**97**	788	–	0	–
	✖			✖					✖		4	**96**	854	**Yes**	0	–
★	–	★	★	–	★		★	–	–	–	4	93	84	No	0	–

***Accreditation Status:** 5=Accredited with commendation or with full standards compliance; 4=Accredited with requirements for improvement; 3=Conditional accreditation.

Detailed Ratings for All Areas

See more information on "Key Ratings for Metro Areas" table beginning on page 32

Blue is most favorable
Bold Italic is least favorable
Blank means neither better nor worse than average
"–" means insufficient data

	Death rates for all selected case types			Hospital outcomes: better (★) or worse (×) than average — Adjusted Death rates — Medical Cases											
	Number of cases	Actual death rate (%)	Adjusted death rate (%) (lower is better)	All selected cases	All selected medical cases	Heart attack	Congestive heart failure	Obstructive pulmonary disease	Pneumonia	Respiratory failure and arrest	Septicemia	Stroke	Gastrointestinal hemorrhage	Fluid, electrolyte, & acid-base disorders	Kidney failure
National Average	–	–	12.1	12.1	14.8	21.2	10.6	6.5	16.9	34.4	25.1	18.4	6.7	11.0	20.9
Texas *(continued)*															
Houston Area *(continued)*															
Northeast, Humble	2,894	10.5	11.4												
Northside General, Houston	261	5.7	**6.8**	**★**	**★**	–	–	–		–	–	–	–	–	–
Park Plaza, Houston	3,309	11.8	**10.9**	**★**	**★**							**★**			
Riverside General, Houston	10	–	–	–	–	–	–	–	–	–	–	–	–	–	–
St Lukes Episcopal, Houston[1]	7,877	8.6	**10.8**	**★**	**★**	★			**★**	**★**		**★**			**★**
San Jacinto Methodist, Baytown	3,462	14.0	***13.1***	**✖**	**✖**		×		×	**✖**		★			
Texas Children's, Houston	–	–	–	–	–	–	–	–	–	–	–	–	–	–	–
Texas Orthopedic, Houston	341	–	–	–	–	–	–	–	–	–	–	–	–	–	–
Tomball Regional, Tomball	2,845	10.6	**10.5**	**★**	**★**				★		**★**				
University of Texas M D Anderson Cancer Ctr, Houston	1,306	15.5	***14.7***	**✖**	**✖**	–	–	**✖**	**✖**	**★**		×	**✖**		
West Houston Medical Center, Houston	1,654	15.5	12.0												**✖**
Woman's of Texas, Houston	96	–	–	–	–	–	–	–	–	–	–	–	–	–	–
San Antonio Area															
Baptist, San Antonio[1]	16,384	12.5	**11.4**	**★**	**★**		**★**		**★**					×	**★**
Christus Santa Rosa (Babcock Rd), San Antonio	–	–	–	–	–	–	–	–	–	–	–	–	–	–	–
Christus Santa Rosa (N Santa Rosa St), San Antonio[1]	5,091	10.4	**9.6**	**★**	**★**		**★**		**★**	**★**	**★**				**★**
Methodist Ambulatory Surgery NW, San Antonio	64	–	–	–	–	–	–	–	–	–	–	–	–	–	–
Methodist Specialty and Transplant, San Antonio[1]	1,841	12.2	13.4	×				×					**✖**		
Metropolitan Methodist, San Antonio	–	–	–	–	–	–	–	–	–	–	–	–	–	–	–
Nix, San Antonio[1]	1,630	8.3	10.7					★						×	
North Central Baptist, San Antonio	–	–	–	–	–	–	–	–	–	–	–	–	–	–	–
Northeast Baptist, San Antonio	–	–	–	–	–	–	–	–	–	–	–	–	–	–	–
Northeast Methodist, San Antonio	1,638	16.4	12.9						**✖**						★
Southeast Baptist, San Antonio	–	–	–	–	–	–	–	–	–	–	–	–	–	–	–
Southwest General, San Antonio	1,952	10.5	**8.5**	**★**	**★**		**★**		**★**			★			
Southwest Texas Methodist, San Antonio[1]	10,083	10.5	11.8												
University, San Antonio	1,080	12.6	12.5					–					–		
Other Areas															
Abilene Regional, Abilene	3,019	11.2	12.3												
Alice Regional, Alice	1,886	13.6	11.7				**★**			**✖**	**✖**			**★**	
Angleton - Danbury, Angleton	963	14.5	***16.7***	**✖**	**✖**			×	**✖**		–		–		
Anson General, Anson	495	9.5	**7.2**	**★**	**★**	–			**★**	**★**	–	–	–		–
Atlanta Memorial, Atlanta	1,422	13.0	12.8			**✖**						**✖**			–

Footnotes are on page 350.

Hospital outcomes: better (★) or worse (✖) than average											Results of accreditation review on full survey		Other facts			
Adjusted Death rates			Adjusted Adverse outcome rates													
Surgical cases			Surgical cases													
All selected surgical cases	Coronary artery bypass surgery	Large bowel surgery	All selected surgical cases	Coronary artery bypass surgery	Large bowel surgery	Gall bladder removal	Total knee replacement	Total hip replacement	Simple prostatectomy	Carotid endarterectomy	Accreditation status*	Overall evaluation score (higher is better)	Number of beds	Major medical school affiliation?	Number of residents	Computerized drug order system (1 to 5 scale, higher is preferred; see page 23 for details)
2.3	3.8	6.5	7.7	10.3	11.9	7.5	6.7	6.4	5.4	8.2	–	91	161	–	–	–
	–	–		–		★	–	–		✖	4	**88**	188	No	0	–
–	–	–	–	–	–	–	–	–	–	–	–[2]	–[2]	39	No	0	–
	–			–				★	–	–	4	92	259	No	0	–
–	–	–	–	–	–	–	–	–	–	–	4	**88**	69	No	0	–
✖	✖		✖	✖	✖						4	**96**	648	**Yes**	7	–
	–		★	–			★	–	–	★	4	89	186	**Yes**	24	–
–	–	–	–	–	–	–	–	–	–	–	5	**96**	378	–	0	–
–	–	–	✖	–	–	–	✖		–	–	4	**96**	40	No	0	–
	–			★				–	–	–	4	**94**	110	No	8	–
	–		×	–		–	–	–	–	–	5	**97**	437	No	228	–
✖	–	–			–	–	–	–	–		5	**97**	151	No	0	–
–	–	–		–	–	–	–	–	–	–	5	**99**	199	No	0	–
		×	✖		×		✖	✖	✖		4	**79**	414	No	3	–
–	–	–	–	–	–	–	–	–	–	–	–[2]	–[2]	–	–	–	–
				★				–	✖	–	4	**88**	531	**Yes**	0	–
–	–	–	–	–	–	–	–	–	–	–	4	**96**	37	No	0	–
		–	★			–		–			4	93	198	No	0	2
–	–	–	–	–	–	–	–	–	–	–	–[2]	–[2]	212	–	0	–
★	–	–				–			–	–	4	**87**	152	No	0	–
–	–	–	–	–	–	–	–	–	–	–	–[2]	–[2]	126	–	0	–
–	–	–	–	–	–	–	–	–	–	–	–[2]	–[2]	234	–	0	–
	–	–	★	–		–	–	–	–	–	5	**98**	89	No	0	2
–	–	–	–	–	–	–	–	–	–	–	–[2]	–[2]	153	–	0	–
–	–	–		–	–		–	–	–	–	4	92	175	No	0	–
						×		★			4	**83**	736	No	0	2
	–	–			–	–	–	–	–	–	4	**79**	547	**Yes**	540	2
		–		★	★			✖	✖	✖	4	**94**	162	No	0	–
★	–	–		–	–		–	–	–	–	5	**97**	90	No	0	–
×	–	–		–		–	–	–	–	–	4	**97**	49	No	0	–
–	–	–	–	–	–	–	–	–	–	–	–[2]	–[2]	22	No	0	–
–	–	–		–	–	–	–	–	–	–	–[2]	–[2]	44	No	0	–

***Accreditation Status:** 5=Accredited with commendation or with full standards compliance; 4=Accredited with requirements for improvement; 3=Conditional accreditation.

Detailed Ratings for All Areas

See more information on "Key Ratings for Metro Areas" table beginning on page 32

Blue is most favorable
Bold Italic is least favorable
Blank means neither better nor worse than average
"–" means insufficient data

	Death rates for all selected case types			Hospital outcomes: better (★) or worse (×) than average											
				Adjusted Death rates											
					Medical Cases										
	Number of cases	Actual death rate (%)	Adjusted death rate (%) (lower is better)	All selected cases	All selected medical cases	Heart attack	Congestive heart failure	Obstructive pulmonary disease	Pneumonia	Respiratory failure and arrest	Septicemia	Stroke	Gastrointestinal hemorrhage	Fluid, electrolyte, & acid-base disorders	Kidney failure
National Average	–	–	12.1	12.1	14.8	21.2	10.6	6.5	16.9	34.4	25.1	18.4	6.7	11.0	20.9
Texas *(continued)*															
Other Areas *(continued)*															
Baptist St Anthony, Amarillo[1]	8,423	8.9	12.8	×	×		×	✖	✖						
Baylor - Ellis County, Waxahachie	2,067	14.8	***15.1***	✖	✖	×			✖						×
Bellville General, Bellville[1]	553	18.8	***17.4***	✖	✖	✖	✖						–		
Big Bend Regional, Alpine	440	11.4	***15.5***	✖	×	–		✖		–		–	–	–	–
Big Bend Regional Home Health, Alpine	104	10.6	15.0			–	–	–	–	–	–	–	–	–	–
Bowie Memorial, Bowie	1,148	15.1	13.5	×	×	✖	✖			–	–				
Brazosport, Lake Jackson	2,313	11.8	12.9									×			
Brownfield Regional, Brownfield	289	18.3	***15.9***	✖	✖			–	✖	–	–		–	–	–
Brownsville Medical Center, Brownsville	4,006	12.3	10.5	★	★				★			★			★
Brownwood Regional, Brownwood	4,033	12.1	11.7											★	
Burleson St Joseph, Caldwell	186	16.7	14.4			–	–	–		–	–	–	–	–	–
Campbell, Weatherford	1,313	14.5	***14.6***	✖	✖	✖	×		×	✖					–
Central Texas, Cameron	532	15.2	14.1					–	✖	–			–		–
Central Texas, San Marcos	2,060	12.5	***13.5***	✖	✖	✖		×							–
Childress Regional, Childress	486	16.0	***19.9***	✖	✖	–	✖			–	–	✖	–	–	–
Chillicothe Hospital, Chillicothe[1]	90	7.8	10.0			–	–	–	–	–	–	–	–	–	–
Christus, Jasper	1,163	15.0	***14.9***	✖	✖	✖				✖					–
Christus St Elizabeth, Beaumont	9,126	11.4	12.7	×	✖		✖	✖							
Christus St Joseph's, Paris	3,987	14.3	***14.9***	✖	✖	✖	✖		✖	✖					
Christus St Mary, Port Arthur	3,547	11.9	10.8	★	★					★					
Christus St Michael, Texarkana[1]	6,422	12.5	***13.0***	✖	✖				✖	★				✖	
Christus Spohn, Alice	311	10.9	13.1			–		–		–	–	–	–	–	–
Christus Spohn, Beeville	1,429	13.4	13.6	×	×					×		✖			–
Christus Spohn, Corpus Christi	4,543	10.6	11.6												
Christus Spohn Kleberg, Kingsville	1,997	10.3	12.2				×								✖
Citizens, Victoria	4,215	8.6	11.7												
Clay County, Henrietta	396	11.6	9.1	★	★			–		–		★	–		
Cleveland Regional, Cleveland	1,605	11.0	9.2	★	★				★	★	★		★	★	
Cochran, Morton	163	15.3	15.2			–	–	–	✖	–	–	–	–	–	–
Coleman County, Coleman	1,059	12.1	10.3	★	★	–			★	★		✖	–		
College Station Medical Center, College Station	1,095	11.3	9.8	★	★				★					★	
Collingsworth General, Wellington	299	19.1	13.9			–	–	–		–		–	–		–
Colorado - Fayette, Weimar	1,095	14.6	10.8					–		–					–
Columbus Community, Columbus	632	12.8	14.6	×	×	–		–	✖	–		–	–	–	–

Footnotes are on page 350.

Hospital outcomes: better (★) or worse (×) than average											Results of accreditation review on full survey		Other facts			
Adjusted Death rates			Adjusted Adverse outcome rates													
Surgical cases			Surgical cases													
All selected surgical cases	Coronary artery bypass surgery	Large bowel surgery	All selected surgical cases	Coronary artery bypass surgery	Large bowel surgery	Gall bladder removal	Total knee replacement	Total hip replacement	Simple prostatectomy	Carotid endarterectomy	Accreditation status*	Overall evaluation score (higher is better)	Number of beds	Major medical school affiliation?	Number of residents	Computerized drug order system (1 to 5 scale, higher is preferred; see page 23 for details)
2.3	3.8	6.5	7.7	10.3	11.9	7.5	6.7	6.4	5.4	8.2	–	91	161	–	–	–
	✖		✖				✖	✖		★	4	**87**	427	No	0	–
	–		★	–	★			–	–	–	4	89	66	No	0	–
–	–	–	–	–	–	–	–	–	–	–	4	**88**	26	No	0	–
–	–	–	–	–	–	–	–	–	–	–	–[2]	–[2]	36	No	0	–
–	–	–	–	–	–	–	–	–	–	–	–[2]	–[2]	40	No	–	–
–	–	–		–	–		–	–	–	–	–[2]	–[2]	44	No	0	–
×	–	–		–	×	–		–	–	–	4	89	156	No	0	2
–	–	–	–	–	–	–	–	–	–	–	–[2]	–[2]	42	No	0	–
×	✖			✖			–	–	–	–	4	91	219	No	0	–
	–			–	★			–		–	4	**94**	143	No	0	–
–	–	–	–	–	–	–	–	–	–	–	–[2]	–[2]	30	No	0	–
–	–	–	★	–	–	–		–	–	–	4	92	67	No	0	–
–	–	–	–	–	–	–	–	–	–	–	–[2]	–[2]	34	No	0	–
	–	–		–				–	–	–	4	**95**	108	No	0	–
–	–	–	–	–	–	–	–	–	–	–	–[2]	–[2]	35	No	0	–
–	–	–	–	–	–	–	–	–	–	–	–[2]	–[2]	12	No	0	–
–	–	–	–	–	–	–	–	–	–	–	–[2]	–[2]	57	No	0	–
			✖		✖		✖		✖		4	**94**	420	No	0	–
			★				★				4	**95**	175	No	0	–
		–			★		✖	–	–		4	93	223	No	0	–
✖							★		✖	✖	4	92	239	No	0	–
–	–	–	–	–	–	–	–	–	–	–	4	90	49	No	0	–
–	–	–		–	–	–	–	–	–	–	4	**88**	67	No	0	–
	✖					★		–			4	92	270	**Yes**	30	–
–	–	–		–	–	–	–	–	–	–	4	**85**	85	No	0	–
	✖					★			✖	×	4	**98**	231	No	0	–
–	–	–	–	–	–	–	–	–	–	–	–[2]	–[2]	25	No	0	–
–	–	–	–	–	–	–	–	–	–	–	3	**79**	104	No	0	–
–	–	–	–	–	–	–	–	–	–	–	–[2]	–[2]	15	No	0	–
–	–	–	–	–	–	–	–	–	–	–	–[2]	–[2]	27	No	0	–
	–	–	★			–	–	–	–	–	4	93	119	No	0	–
–	–	–	–	–	–	–	–	–	–	–	–[2]	–[2]	20	No	0	–
–	–	–		–	–	–	–	–	–	–	4	**94**	24	No	0	–
–	–	–		–	–	–	–	–	–	–	–[2]	–[2]	36	No	0	–

***Accreditation Status:** 5=Accredited with commendation or with full standards compliance; 4=Accredited with requirements for improvement; 3=Conditional accreditation.

Detailed Ratings for All Areas

See more information on "Key Ratings for Metro Areas" table beginning on page 32

Blue is most favorable
Bold Italic is least favorable
Blank means neither better nor worse than average
"–" means insufficient data

	Death rates for all selected case types			Hospital outcomes: better (★) or worse (×) than average — Adjusted Death rates — Medical Cases											
	Number of cases	Actual death rate (%)	Adjusted death rate (%) (lower is better)	All selected cases	All selected medical cases	Heart attack	Congestive heart failure	Obstructive pulmonary disease	Pneumonia	Respiratory failure and arrest	Septicemia	Stroke	Gastrointestinal hemorrhage	Fluid, electrolyte, & acid-base disorders	Kidney failure
National Average	–	–	12.1	12.1	14.8	21.2	10.6	6.5	16.9	34.4	25.1	18.4	6.7	11.0	20.9
Texas *(continued)*															
Other Areas *(continued)*															
Comanche Community, Comanche	465	16.3	13.3			–		★		–		–	–	–	–
Community General, Dilley	404	5.4	7.3	★	★	–		–			–	–	–	–	–
Concho County, Eden	252	15.9	13.0			–		–		–	–	–	–	–	–
Conroe Regional, Conroe	3,468	14.1	***13.6***	✖	✖				✖					✖	
Coon, Dalhart	303	16.8	***16.8***	✖	✖	–		–	✖	–	–	✖	–	–	–
Cornerstone Regional, Edinburg	82	–	–	–	–	–	–	–	–	–	–	–	–	–	–
Corpus Christi - Bay Area, Corpus Christi	3,588	12.3	12.1										★		
Corpus Christi Doctors Regional, Corpus Christi	2,437	11.8	***13.3***	✖				✖							
Coryell, Gatesville	723	13.7	***14.4***	✖	✖			–			–	✖	–	–	–
Covenant, Levelland	763	14.3	13.3			–	✖	–		–			–	–	–
Covenant, Plainview	998	13.3	11.9					–		–					–
Covenant - Lakeside, Lubbock[1]	10,297	10.8	12.5			★			✖				✖		★
Cozby - Germany, Grand Saline	415	14.9	12.3			–		–		✖		–	–	–	–
Crane Memorial, Crane	154	14.9	***20.3***	✖	✖	–	–	–	✖	–	–	–	–	–	–
Crosbyton Clinic, Crosbyton	707	10.7	9.1	★	★	–		–	★	–			–	★	–
Cuero Community, Cuero	1,452	14.3	12.0												
D M Cogdell, Snyder	595	12.8	14.5	×	×	–		✖	✖	–	–		–		–
De Leon Hospital, De Leon	644	15.2	***16.0***	✖	✖	–		–	×	–			–		–
Del Sol, El Paso	5,721	13.7	11.4		★				★						
Denton Community, Denton	2,355	12.7	11.4								★				
Denton Regional, Denton	2,515	13.9	***13.3***	✖	✖					✖		✖			
DeTar - Navarro, Victoria	2,320	11.1	12.8												
DeTar - North, Victoria	1,223	12.1	12.2										–		–
Dimmit County, Carrizo Springs	678	13.4	***15.1***	✖	✖			–		–	–		–		✖
Doctor's, New Boston	110	10.0	12.1			–	–	–	–	–	–	–	–	–	–
Doctors, Groves	1,042	11.1	7.4	★	★		★	★	★			★			
Doctors, Laredo	2,179	11.3	11.2			×			★						
Doctors, Tyler	830	18.2	11.7					–		★					
Dolly Vinsant, San Benito	725	9.1	9.4	★	★	–		–		–			–		
East Texas, Athens	3,648	12.6	12.8			✖					✖			★	✖
East Texas, Carthage	680	14.0	***14.9***	✖	✖			–		–		×	–		–
East Texas, Clarksville	1,371	12.3	10.9										–		–
East Texas, Crockett	1,784	16.4	***14.9***	✖	✖	×	✖		✖		×				
East Texas, Fairfield	404	14.9	15.0	×	×	–		–		–		–	–	–	–

Footnotes are on page 350.

Hospital outcomes: better (★) or worse (×) than average											Results of accreditation review on full survey		Other facts			
Adjusted Death rates — Surgical cases			Adjusted Adverse outcome rates — Surgical cases													
All selected surgical cases	Coronary artery bypass surgery	Large bowel surgery	All selected surgical cases	Coronary artery bypass surgery	Large bowel surgery	Gall bladder removal	Total knee replacement	Total hip replacement	Simple prostatectomy	Carotid endarterectomy	Accreditation status*	Overall evaluation score (higher is better)	Number of beds	Major medical school affiliation?	Number of residents	Computerized drug order system (1 to 5 scale, higher is preferred; see page 23 for details)
2.3	3.8	6.5	7.7	10.3	11.9	7.5	6.7	6.4	5.4	8.2	–	91	161	–	–	–
–	–	–	–	–	–	–	–	–	–	–	–[2]	–[2]	19	No	0	–
–	–	–	–	–	–	–	–	–	–	–	4	**86**	18	No	–	–
–	–	–	–	–	–	–	–	–	–	–	–[2]	–[2]	20	No	0	–
				★		✖	–	–	★		4	91	232	No	0	–
–	–	–	–	–	–	–	–	–	–	–	–[2]	–[2]	23	No	0	–
–	–	–	–	–	–	–	–	–	–	–	4	91	6	No	0	–
✖	✖			✖				–	✖	★	4	90	372	No	20	–
×	✖	–		✖		✖		–			–[2]	–[2]	237	No	7	–
–	–	–	–	–	–	–	–	–	–	–	4	**96**	48	No	0	–
–	–	–	–	–	–	–	–	–	–	–	4	89	49	No	0	–
✖	–	–		–	–	–	–	–	–	–	4	**96**	36	No	0	–
✖	✖		✖	✖				★	✖	×	4	92	410	No	60	–
–	–	–	–	–	–	–	–	–	–	–	–[2]	–[2]	20	No	0	–
–	–	–	–	–	–	–	–	–	–	–	–[2]	–[2]	28	No	0	–
–	–	–	–	–	–	–	–	–	–	–	–[2]	–[2]	30	No	0	–
–	–	–	–	–	–	–	–	–	–	–	5	**96**	60	No	0	–
–	–	–	–	–	–	–	–	–	–	–	5	**86**	39	No	0	–
–	–	–	–	–	–	–	–	–	–	–	–[2]	–[2]	14	No	0	–
							★	–		–	5	**98**	270	No	0	2
	–	–		–		–		–	–	–	4	93	122	No	0	–
		–				–		–	–		4	92	197	No	0	2
✖	–			–				–	×	–	5	**99**	191	No	0	–
–	–	–		–	–	–		–	–	–	–[2]	–[2]	156	No	0	–
–	–	–	–	–	–	–	–	–	–	–	–[2]	–[2]	35	No	0	–
–	–	–	–	–	–	–	–	–	–	–	4	93	63	No	0	–
–	–	–	–	–	–	–	–	–	–	–	–[2]	–[2]	106	No	–	–
★	–	–	★	–			–	–	–	–	4	93	108	No	0	–
–	–	–	–	–	–	–	–	–	–	–	–[2]	–[2]	46	No	0	–
–	–	–	–	–	–	–	–	–	–	–	4	**83**	33	No	0	–
	–			–			–	–		–	4	**95**	108	No	0	–
–	–	–	–	–	–	–	–	–	–	–	4	**87**	30	No	0	–
–	–	–	–	–	–	–	–	–	–	–	4	91	36	No	0	–
–	–	–	★	–	–	–	–	–	–	–	4	**94**	68	No	0	–
–	–	–	–	–	–	–	–	–	–	–	–[2]	–[2]	19	No	0	–

***Accreditation Status:** 5=Accredited with commendation or with full standards compliance; 4=Accredited with requirements for improvement; 3=Conditional accreditation.

Detailed Ratings for All Areas

See more information on "Key Ratings for Metro Areas" table beginning on page 32

Blue is most favorable
Bold Italic is least favorable
Blank means neither better nor worse than average
"–" means insufficient data

	Death rates for all selected case types			Hospital outcomes: better (★) or worse (×) than average — Adjusted Death rates	Medical Cases										
	Number of cases	Actual death rate (%)	Adjusted death rate (%) (lower is better)	All selected cases	All selected medical cases	Heart attack	Congestive heart failure	Obstructive pulmonary disease	Pneumonia	Respiratory failure and arrest	Septicemia	Stroke	Gastrointestinal hemorrhage	Fluid, electrolyte, & acid-base disorders	Kidney failure
National Average	–	–	12.1	12.1	14.8	21.2	10.6	6.5	16.9	34.4	25.1	18.4	6.7	11.0	20.9
Texas (continued)															
Other Areas (continued)															
East Texas, Jacksonville	1,659	16.0	13.1			✖		✖							
East Texas, Mt Vernon	663	11.8	10.6				★	–		–			–	–	–
East Texas, Pittsburg	1,101	13.4	13.2							–			–		✖
East Texas, Quitman	1,064	14.5	***15.5***	✖	✖						✖	×	✖		–
East Texas, Trinity	515	11.3	11.1			–				–	–	–	–		–
East Texas, Tyler	7,725	13.4	***12.7***	✖		★		✖						×	
Eastland Memorial, Eastland	1,006	13.1	***15.7***	✖	✖	–			✖	–	–	✖			–
Edinburg Regional, Edinburg	1,863	10.5	9.8	★	★				★	★					
El Campo Memorial, El Campo	607	17.8	13.6					–		–			–		✖
Electra Memorial, Electra	465	9.5	10.7			–		–		–	–		–	–	–
Faith, Jacksboro	352	11.6	9.4			–	–			–		–	–	–	–
Falls, Marlin	1,168	18.1	11.3			✖		–	★	–	✖				–
Fayette, La Grange	1,160	14.0	12.4							–	✖		★		–
Fort Duncan, Eagle Pass	2,365	9.2	6.7	★	★		★	★	★		★		★	★	★
Frio, Pearsall	471	14.0	***15.4***	✖	✖	–				–	–		–	✖	–
Gainesville Memorial, Gainesville	1,046	17.8	***16.9***	✖	✖		×	–	✖	–	✖				–
Georgetown Hospital, Georgetown[1]	1,370	13.4	***15.4***	✖	✖				✖			✖			✖
Glen Rose Medical Center, Glen Rose	512	14.3	13.2			–		–		–			–	–	–
Golden Plains, Borger	667	11.2	12.7			–	★	✖		–	–		–		–
Good Shepherd, Longview	8,957	11.9	9.7	★	★	★	★		★	★	★	★	★		★
Goodall - Witcher, Clifton	1,057	16.8	***17.9***	✖	✖		✖		✖	–	–	✖	–	–	✖
Graham Regional, Graham	1,006	16.7	***17.4***	✖	✖	×	✖		✖	–			–		–
Guadalupe Valley, Seguin	2,020	11.7	12.9			✖	✖				✖				
Gulf Coast, Wharton	1,498	10.7	9.8	★	★				★			★			
Hall County, Memphis	257	17.1	***15.9***	✖	✖	–	–	–		–	–	–	–		–
Hamilton, Olney	630	12.9	10.8					–			–		–		
Hamilton General, Hamilton	589	14.6	13.4							–	–		–		–
Hamlin Memorial, Hamlin	351	11.7	12.2			–		–		–	–	–	–		–
Hansford, Spearman	140	10.7	11.1			–	–	–		–	–	–	–	–	–
Hardeman County, Quanah	196	14.8	11.6			–		–		–	–	–	–		–
Harris Methodist Erath County, Stephenville	1,987	12.2	12.2										×		
Haskell Memorial, Haskell	286	19.9	***18.4***	✖	✖	–		–		–	–	✖	–	–	–
Heart of Texas, Brady	726	11.4	11.5			–							–		
Hemphill County, Canadian	135	12.6	11.2			–	–	–		–	–	–	–	–	–

Footnotes are on page 350.

Hospital outcomes: better (★) or worse (×) than average											Results of accreditation review on full survey		Other facts			
Adjusted Death rates			Adjusted Adverse outcome rates													
Surgical cases			Surgical cases													
All selected surgical cases	Coronary artery bypass surgery	Large bowel surgery	All selected surgical cases	Coronary artery bypass surgery	Large bowel surgery	Gall bladder removal	Total knee replacement	Total hip replacement	Simple prostatectomy	Carotid endarterectomy	Accreditation status*	Overall evaluation score (higher is better)	Number of beds	Major medical school affiliation?	Number of residents	Computerized drug order system (1 to 5 scale, higher is preferred; see page 23 for details)
2.3	3.8	6.5	7.7	10.3	11.9	7.5	6.7	6.4	5.4	8.2	–	91	161	–	–	–
	–	–		–		–	–	–	–	–	4	91	65	No	0	–
–	–	–	–	–	–	–	–	–	–	–	–[2]	–[2]	30	No	0	–
–	–	–	–	–	–	–	–	–	–	–	4	**97**	42	No	0	–
–	–	–	–	–	–	–	–	–	–	–	4	93	15	No	0	–
–	–	–	–	–	–	–	–	–	–	–	–[2]	–[2]	22	No	0	–
×			★							★	4	91	340	No	0	–
–	–	–	–	–	–	–	–	–	–	–	–[2]	–[2]	40	No	0	–
	–	–		–	–				–	–	4	92	163	No	0	–
–	–	–	–	–	–	–	–	–	–	–	4	**96**	42	No	0	–
–	–	–	–	–	–	–	–	–	–	–	–[2]	–[2]	23	No	0	–
–	–	–	–	–	–	–	–	–	–	–	–[2]	–[2]	17	No	0	–
–	–	–	–	–	–	–	–	–	–	–	–[2]	–[2]	36	No	0	–
–	–	–		–	–		–	–	–	–	4	91	45	No	0	–
–	–	–		–	–		–	–	–	–	3	***84***	69	No	0	–
–	–	–	–	–	–	–	–	–	–	–	–[2]	–[2]	22	No	0	–
–	–	–		–	–	–	–	–	–	–	–[2]	–[2]	44	No	0	–
	–	–		–		–	–	–	–	–	4	**96**	56	No	0	–
–	–	–	–	–	–	–	–	–	–	–	4	92	16	No	0	–
–	–	–	–	–	–	–	–	–	–	–	–[2]	–[2]	48	No	0	–
×	×		×	×		★	×			×	4	92	295	No	0	–
–	–	–	–	–	–	–	–	–	–	–	–[2]	–[2]	40	No	0	–
–	–	–	–	–	–	–	–	–	–	–	–[2]	–[2]	38	No	0	–
	–	★	★	–	★			–		–	4	***86***	105	No	0	–
	–			–			–	–	–	–	4	**94**	141	No	0	–
–	–	–	–	–	–	–	–	–	–	–	–[2]	–[2]	20	No	0	–
–	–	–	–	–	–	–	–	–	–	–	–[2]	–[2]	41	No	0	–
–	–	–	–	–	–	–	–	–	–	–	–[2]	–[2]	22	No	0	–
–	–	–	–	–	–	–	–	–	–	–	–[2]	–[2]	23	No	0	–
–	–	–	–	–	–	–	–	–	–	–	–[2]	–[2]	28	No	0	–
–	–	–	–	–	–	–	–	–	–	–	–[2]	–[2]	23	No	0	–
	–	–		–	×			–	★	–	5	**97**	75	No	0	–
–	–	–	–	–	–	–	–	–	–	–	–[2]	–[2]	30	No	0	–
–	–	–	–	–	–	–	–	–	–	–	–[2]	–[2]	27	No	0	–
–	–	–	–	–	–	–	–	–	–	–	–[2]	–[2]	19	No	0	–

***Accreditation Status:** 5=Accredited with commendation or with full standards compliance; 4=Accredited with requirements for improvement; 3=Conditional accreditation.

Detailed Ratings for All Areas

See more information on "Key Ratings for Metro Areas" table beginning on page 32

Blue is most favorable
Bold Italic is least favorable
Blank means neither better nor worse than average
"–" means insufficient data

	Death rates for all selected case types			Hospital outcomes: better (★) or worse (×) than average — Adjusted Death rates — Medical Cases											
	Number of cases	Actual death rate (%)	Adjusted death rate (%) (lower is better)	All selected cases	All selected medical cases	Heart attack	Congestive heart failure	Obstructive pulmonary disease	Pneumonia	Respiratory failure and arrest	Septicemia	Stroke	Gastrointestinal hemorrhage	Fluid, electrolyte, & acid-base disorders	Kidney failure
National Average	–	–	12.1	12.1	14.8	21.2	10.6	6.5	16.9	34.4	25.1	18.4	6.7	11.0	20.9
Texas *(continued)*															
Other Areas *(continued)*															
Henderson Memorial, Henderson	1,836	11.8	11.6				✖		★						–
Hendrick, Abilene[1]	6,509	11.4	11.6				×				★			★	
Hereford Regional, Hereford	443	14.4	***17.5***	✖	✖	–	✖	–	✖	–	–	–	–	–	–
Hi-Plains, Hale Center	238	13.9	13.6			–	×	–		–	–	–	–	–	–
Highland, Lubbock	538	8.4	8.5	★	★	–		–					–		–
Hill Country, Fredericksburg	2,116	11.7	***14.2***	✖	✖				✖				✖		
Hill Regional, Hillsboro	1,307	14.5	12.0			✖									
Hillcrest, West	374	12.6	***15.9***	✖	✖	–	×	–		–	–	–	–	–	–
Hillcrest Baptist, Waco	4,912	12.6	***14.2***	✖	✖			✖	✖				✖		
Hopkins County, Sulphur Springs	1,914	12.4	***14.0***	✖	✖		✖								
Huntsville Memorial, Huntsville	1,527	13.0	***16.8***	✖	✖		✖	✖	✖	✖		✖			–
Jackson County, Edna	248	20.6	***17.6***	✖	✖	–		–		–	–	–	–	–	–
Johns, Taylor	815	14.8	***16.5***	✖	✖				✖	–	–		–		–
Kell West Regional, Wichita Falls	206	2.4	9.8			–	–	–	–	–	–	–	–	–	–
Kimble, Junction	280	15.7	14.4			–	–	–		–	–	–	–		–
King's Daughters, Temple	1,088	13.1	***15.2***	✖	✖			★	✖				–		–
Knapp, Weslaco	4,097	10.8	11.4			✖			★						
Knox County, Knox City	294	12.9	13.7			–	–	–		–	✖	–	–		–
Lake Granbury Medical Center, Granbury	1,187	17.4	***15.3***	✖	✖	×	×	×	✖						–
Lake Whitney Medical Center, Whitney	395	13.4	11.4					–		–	–		–	–	–
Lamb, Littlefield	581	11.2	13.9			–	✖	–		–	–	–	–	★	–
Lavaca, Hallettsville	678	19.2	***14.5***	✖	✖			–		–			–		✖
Liberty - Dayton, Liberty	560	16.6	14.2	×	×	–	×				×		–	–	–
Lillian M Hudspeth, Sonora	77	6.5	5.6	★	★	–	–	–	–	–	–	–	–	–	–
Limestone, Groesbeck	124	15.3	12.2			–	–	–		–	–	–	–	–	–
Llano Memorial, Llano[1]	1,144	16.0	***17.3***	✖	✖	–	✖		✖	–	✖	×	–	✖	–
Longview Regional, Longview	2,874	15.4	10.2	★	★		★		★		★	★			
Lynn County, Tahoka	186	18.3	***20.6***	✖	✖	–	–	–	✖	–	–	–	–	–	–
Mainland, Texas City	2,581	15.2	***13.3***	✖	✖	✖									
Marshall Regional, Marshall	2,019	15.0	12.1				★								
Martin County, Stanton	82	26.8	***26.0***	✖	✖	–	–	–	✖	–	–	–	–	–	–
Matagorda County, Bay City[1]	1,115	15.2	***16.3***	✖	✖		✖	✖					–		
McAllen Medical Center, McAllen	7,713	11.5	10.5	★	★		★		★	★				★	★
McAllen Medical Heart Hospital, McAllen	2,316	6.8	10.1	★	★	★							–		–

Footnotes are on page 350.

Hospital outcomes: better (★) or worse (×) than average											Results of accreditation review on full survey		Other facts			
Adjusted Death rates			Adjusted Adverse outcome rates													
Surgical cases			Surgical cases													
All selected surgical cases	Coronary artery bypass surgery	Large bowel surgery	All selected surgical cases	Coronary artery bypass surgery	Large bowel surgery	Gall bladder removal	Total knee replacement	Total hip replacement	Simple prostatectomy	Carotid endarterectomy	Accreditation status*	Overall evaluation score (higher is better)	Number of beds	Major medical school affiliation?	Number of residents	Computerized drug order system (1 to 5 scale, higher is preferred; see page 23 for details)
2.3	3.8	6.5	7.7	10.3	11.9	7.5	6.7	6.4	5.4	8.2	–	91	161	–	–	–
–	–	–		–	–	–	–	–	–	–	4	**87**	80	No	0	–
×											4	**97**	369	No	0	–
–	–	–	–	–	–	–	–	–	–	–	4	**86**	40	No	0	–
–	–	–	–	–	–	–	–	–	–	–	–[2]	–[2]	40	No	0	–
–	–	–		–	–	–	–	–	–	–	3	**78**	115	No	0	–
	–	–	✖	–			✖	✖	★	–	4	**83**	59	No	0	–
–	–	–		–	–	–	–	–	–	–	4	93	63	No	0	–
–	–	–	–	–	–	–	–	–	–	–	–[2]	–[2]	19	No	0	–
✖	✖						★				4	**96**	272	No	0	–
	–	–		–	★		–	–	–	–	4	**96**	94	No	0	–
–	–	–		–	–	–		–	–	–	4	**95**	104	No	0	–
–	–	–	–	–	–	–	–	–	–	–	–[2]	–[2]	19	No	0	–
–	–	–	–	–	–	–	–	–	–	–	4	**96**	50	No	0	–
–	–	–		–	–	–	–	–	–	–	4	**86**	27	No	0	–
–	–	–	–	–	–	–	–	–	–	–	–[2]	–[2]	15	No	0	–
–	–	–		–		–	–	–	–	–	4	**97**	108	No	0	–
	–			–						★	4	**99**	233	No	0	–
–	–	–	–	–	–	–	–	–	–	–	–[2]	–[2]	14	No	0	–
	–	–		–		–	–	–	–	–	4	**84**	34	No	0	–
–	–	–	–	–	–	–	–	–	–	–	–[2]	–[2]	30	No	0	–
–	–	–	–	–	–	–	–	–	–	–	–[2]	–[2]	41	No	0	–
–	–	–	–	–	–	–	–	–	–	–	–[2]	–[2]	36	No	0	–
–	–	–	–	–	–	–	–	–	–	–	4	**87**	29	No	0	–
–	–	–	–	–	–	–	–	–	–	–	–[2]	–[2]	13	No	0	–
–	–	–	–	–	–	–	–	–	–	–	–[2]	–[2]	15	No	0	–
–	–	–	★	–		–	–	–	–	–	–[2]	–[2]	30	No	0	–
✖	–			✖				–	–	–	5	**96**	149	No	0	–
–	–	–	–	–	–	–	–	–	–	–	–[2]	–[2]	24	No	0	–
	–	–		–		–	–	–	–	–	4	92	152	No	0	2
	–	–		–				–	–	–	4	92	91	No	0	–
–	–	–	–	–	–	–	–	–	–	–	–[2]	–[2]	21	No	0	–
–	–	–	–	–	–	–	–	–	–	–	4	91	67	No	0	–
			★				★	–			–[2]	–[2]	435	No	0	–
		–		✖	–		–	–	–		4	91	70	No	–	–

***Accreditation Status:** 5=Accredited with commendation or with full standards compliance; 4=Accredited with requirements for improvement; 3=Conditional accreditation.

Detailed Ratings for All Areas

See more information on "Key Ratings for Metro Areas" table beginning on page 32

Blue is most favorable
Bold Italic is least favorable
Blank means neither better nor worse than average
"–" means insufficient data

	Death rates for all selected case types			Hospital outcomes: better (★) or worse (×) than average — Adjusted Death rates — Medical Cases											
	Number of cases	Actual death rate (%)	Adjusted death rate (%) (lower is better)	All selected cases	All selected medical cases	Heart attack	Congestive heart failure	Obstructive pulmonary disease	Pneumonia	Respiratory failure and arrest	Septicemia	Stroke	Gastrointestinal hemorrhage	Fluid, electrolyte, & acid-base disorders	Kidney failure
National Average	–	–	12.1	12.1	14.8	21.2	10.6	6.5	16.9	34.4	25.1	18.4	6.7	11.0	20.9
Texas (continued)															
Other Areas (continued)															
McCuistion Regional, Paris	2,722	11.9	***13.7***	✖	✖	✖			✖						
McKenna, New Braunfels	2,630	11.5	***13.3***	✖	×	✖					✖				
Medical Arts, Lamesa	314	14.6	14.6			–		–		–	–	–	–		–
Medical Center, Lewisville	2,043	12.0	10.2	★	★		★				★				
Medical Center, Odessa	5,746	10.7	11.6				×		★						
Medical Center, Plano	3,284	12.8	12.4			★		✖	✖						
Medical Center, Terrell	1,532	16.7	***13.6***	✖	✖	✖						×	✖		
Medina, Hondo	551	14.2	13.7			–	★	–		–		✖	–		–
Memorial, Gonzales	594	15.2	14.0					–			×		–		–
Memorial, Livingston	1,057	11.0	13.0			–				–			–		–
Memorial, Port Lavaca	860	13.1	***14.6***	✖	✖	✖		✖		–			–		–
Memorial, San Augustine	430	14.0	11.7			–		–		–	–		–	–	–
Memorial, Seminole	281	14.9	***15.9***	✖	✖	–	✖	–		–	–	–	–	–	–
Memorial Hermann Baptist, Beaumont	4,118	13.5	11.1	★	★						★	★			
Memorial Hermann Baptist, Orange	1,765	14.3	12.7												–
Memorial Hermann Fort Bend, Missouri City	569	12.3	10.3			–		–					–	–	–
Memorial Jermann Haty, Katy	1,182	15.3	11.8					–					–		
Memorial of East Texas, Lufkin[1]	4,721	13.0	10.5	★	★		★	★				★			
Mercy, Laredo	5,361	14.1	11.3	★											✖
Methodist Health Center, Sugar Land	79	–	–	–	–	–	–	–	–	–	–	–	–	–	–
Metroplex Adventist, Killeen[1]	2,870	12.7	***13.5***	✖	✖	✖				–	×			★	✖
Mid-Jefferson, Nederland	1,355	15.1	12.9			×	✖			–					–
Midland Memorial, Midland	5,235	12.4	***13.5***	✖	✖	★		✖				✖			
Mission Hospital, Mission	2,273	9.9	9.3	★	★				★						★
Mitchell County, Colorado City	457	16.4	***17.7***	✖	✖	–			✖	–	–	×	–	–	–
Moore County, Dumas[1]	736	12.0	9.6	★	★	–	★	–	★				–	–	
Mother Frances Regional, Tyler[1]	8,470	12.1	12.0				★			✖		★			
Muenster Memorial, Muenster	198	15.7	16.4	×	×	–		–		–	–	–	–	–	–
Muleshoe Area, Muleshoe	309	10.0	11.5			–	–	–		–	–	–	–		–
Nacogdoches Medical Center, Nacogdoches	3,313	11.5	***14.1***	✖	✖			✖							✖
Nacogdoches Memorial, Nacogdoches	2,668	11.3	11.8								✖			★	
Navarro Regional, Corsicana	2,316	16.8	***14.9***	✖	✖	✖	✖	✖		✖					
Nocona General, Nocona	651	15.5	11.6				★						–		–
North Bay, Aransas Pass	1,296	14.7	13.2				✖								–

Footnotes are on page 350.

Hospital outcomes: better (★) or worse (✕) than average											Results of accreditation review on full survey		Other facts			
Adjusted Death rates			Adjusted Adverse outcome rates													
Surgical cases			Surgical cases													
All selected surgical cases	Coronary artery bypass surgery	Large bowel surgery	All selected surgical cases	Coronary artery bypass surgery	Large bowel surgery	Gall bladder removal	Total knee replacement	Total hip replacement	Simple prostatectomy	Carotid endarterectomy	Accreditation status*	Overall evaluation score (higher is better)	Number of beds	Major medical school affiliation?	Number of residents	Computerized drug order system (1 to 5 scale, higher is preferred; see page 23 for details)
2.3	3.8	6.5	7.7	10.3	11.9	7.5	6.7	6.4	5.4	8.2	–	91	161	–	–	–
	–	✕		–				–		–	4	93	152	No	0	–
	–			–		✕		–		★	4	84	114	No	0	–
–	–	–	–	–	–	–	–	–	–	–	–[2]	–[2]	38	No	0	–
	–			–		–	–	–	–	–	5	96	100	No	0	–
										✖	4	94	309	Yes	0	–
		★			★		–	–			5	97	245	No	0	2
–	–	–		–		–	–	–	–	–	4	89	112	No	0	–
–	–	–	–	–	–	–	–	–	–	–	–[2]	–[2]	32	No	0	–
–	–	–	–	–	–	–	–	–	–	–	–[2]	–[2]	34	No	0	–
–	–	–	–	–	–	–	–	–	–	–	4	97	31	No	0	–
–	–	–	–	–	–	–	–	–	–	–	4	100	56	No	0	–
–	–	–	–	–	–	–	–	–	–	–	–[2]	–[2]	16	No	0	–
–	–	–	–	–	–	–	–	–	–	–	–[2]	–[2]	33	No	0	–
	–		✖			✕		–	–	✖	5	92	153	No	0	–
	–	–		–		–	–	–	–	–	4	92	104	No	0	–
–	–	–	–	–	–	–	–	–	–	–	4	96	65	No	0	–
–	–	–	–	–	–	–	–	–	–	–	4	91	80	No	0	–
	–			–	★			–	–	–	4	91	203	No	0	–
			★	★				–	–	–	4	94	273	No	0	–
–	–	–	–	–	–	–	–	–	–	–	4	95	22	No	0	–
	–	–		–		–		–	–	–	4	92	200	No	0	–
–	–	–		–	–	–	–	–	–	–	5	99	120	No	0	–
✖	✖							★		★	4	86	255	No	0	–
	–	✖	✖	–	✖		✖	–	–	–	4	83	138	No	0	–
–	–	–	–	–	–	–	–	–	–	–	–[2]	–[2]	25	No	0	–
–	–	–	–	–	–	–	–	–	–	–	4	94	58	No	0	–
✕											4	92	295	No	0	–
–	–	–	–	–	–	–	–	–	–	–	–[2]	–[2]	18	No	0	–
–	–	–	–	–	–	–	–	–	–	–	–[2]	–[2]	25	No	0	–
✖	✖			✕				–	–	–	4	97	124	No	0	–
	–	–						–	–	–	4	89	140	No	0	–
✖	–	✖		–	✖		–	–	★		4	91	144	No	0	–
–	–	–	–	–	–	–	–	–	–	–	–[2]	–[2]	33	No	0	–
–	–	–		–	–	–	–	–	–	–	4	94	69	No	0	–

***Accreditation Status:** 5=Accredited with commendation or with full standards compliance; 4=Accredited with requirements for improvement; 3=Conditional accreditation.

Detailed Ratings for All Areas

See more information on "Key Ratings for Metro Areas" table beginning on page 32

Blue is most favorable
Bold Italic is least favorable
Blank means neither better nor worse than average
"–" means insufficient data

	Death rates for all selected case types				Hospital outcomes: better (★) or worse (×) than average — Adjusted Death rates — Medical Cases											
	Number of cases	Actual death rate (%)	Adjusted death rate (%) (lower is better)	All selected cases	All selected medical cases	Heart attack	Congestive heart failure	Obstructive pulmonary disease	Pneumonia	Respiratory failure and arrest	Septicemia	Stroke	Gastrointestinal hemorrhage	Fluid, electrolyte, & acid-base disorders	Kidney failure
National Average	–	–	12.1	12.1	14.8	21.2	10.6	6.5	16.9	34.4	25.1	18.4	6.7	11.0	20.9
Texas *(continued)*															
Other Areas *(continued)*															
North Central, McKinney	2,344	15.2	12.6			✖								×	
Northeast, Bonham	1,012	16.4	10.8				★	★		×					–
Northwest Regional, Corpus Christi	1,664	13.2	12.8									×			–
Northwest Texas, Amarillo[1]	3,649	14.0	***14.1***	✖	✖			✖	✖	✖	×				
Ochiltree General, Perryton	418	15.3	***16.4***	✖	✖	–	✖			–	–		–	–	–
Odessa Regional, Odessa	834	7.0	10.7			×					–	–	–	–	–
Otto Kaiser, Kenedy	358	24.9	***27.8***	✖	✖	–	✖	✖	✖	–	–	✖	–	–	–
Palestine Regional, Palestine	1,877	14.1	***17.6***	✖	✖		✖		✖	✖	✖		✖		✖
Palo Pinto General, Mineral Wells[1]	1,480	12.7	***14.2***	✖	✖	✖					✖	×			–
Pampa Regional, Pampa	1,700	9.2	9.6	★	★				★						
Park Place, Port Arthur	2,179	13.2	12.6			★								✖	
Parkview, Wheeler	429	8.2	5.5	★	★	–		–	★	–	★	–	–	★	–
Parkview Regional, Mexia	1,347	14.8	11.9					✖							★
Pecos County, Fort Stockton	372	18.5	***19.9***	✖	✖	–	✖	–		–	–	–	–	✖	–
Permian General, Andrews	393	14.5	***19.1***	✖	✖	✖	–	–	×	–	–	–	–		–
Plains, Dimmitt	214	7.9	8.2	★	★	–	–	–		–	–	–	–	–	–
Polly Ryon, Richmond[1]	1,294	15.7	***13.9***	✖	✖							✖	–	✖	–
Presbyterian, Commerce	405	18.3	13.1			✖		–		–			–	–	–
Presbyterian, Greenville[1]	2,527	14.3	12.7			✖					✖				
Presbyterian, Kaufman	1,449	15.8	***17.3***	✖	✖	✖			✖		✖	✖			✖
Presbyterian, Plano	1,221	4.7	12.5			✖		–		–	–		–	–	–
Presbyterian, Winnsboro	843	12.2	13.1			–		–					–		
Providence, El Paso	5,742	10.9	10.4	★	★				★	★	★				
Providence, Waco	4,859	12.6	***15.3***	✖	✖	×	✖		✖				×	✖	
R E Thomason General, El Paso	943	12.9	11.9					–		✖			–	–	
Reeves County, Pecos	360	13.1	13.7			–				–	–	–	–		–
Refugio County, Refugio[1]	99	10.1	8.4			–	–	–		–	–	–	–	–	–
Richards, Rockdale	359	15.0	11.7			–		–		–			–	–	–
Rio Grande Regional, McAllen	4,963	10.8	11.9			×			★				×		✖
Rolling Plains, Sweetwater	1,197	10.8	11.5			–				–					
Round Rock Medical Center, Round Rock	1,334	10.3	11.0			✖									
Roy H Laird, Kilgore	934	11.7	9.0	★	★			–	★	✖			–	–	
Sabine County, Hemphill	534	11.6	12.9			–				–	–	✖	–	–	–
St Joseph Regional, Bryan	6,271	11.3	12.8	×	×										

Footnotes are on page 350.

Hospital outcomes: better (★) or worse (×) than average											Results of accreditation review on full survey		Other facts			
Adjusted Death rates			Adjusted Adverse outcome rates													
Surgical cases			Surgical cases													
All selected surgical cases	Coronary artery bypass surgery	Large bowel surgery	All selected surgical cases	Coronary artery bypass surgery	Large bowel surgery	Gall bladder removal	Total knee replacement	Total hip replacement	Simple prostatectomy	Carotid endarterectomy	Accreditation status*	Overall evaluation score (higher is better)	Number of beds	Major medical school affiliation?	Number of residents	Computerized drug order system (1 to 5 scale, higher is preferred; see page 23 for details)
2.3	3.8	6.5	7.7	10.3	11.9	7.5	6.7	6.4	5.4	8.2	–	91	161	–	–	–
✖	–	✖		–	✖	–		–	–	–	4	87	159	No	0	2
–	–	–	–	–	–	–	–	–	–	–	4	82	39	No	0	–
	–	–		–	–	–		–	–	–	4	96	73	No	0	–
✖	✖								–	–	4	96	353	Yes	0	–
–	–	–	–	–	–	–	–	–	–	–	–[2]	–[2]	45	No	0	–
–	–	–		–	–	–	–	–	–	–	4	87	100	No	0	–
–	–	–	–	–	–	–	–	–	–	–	–[2]	–[2]	30	No	0	–
✖	–	–		–		–	★	–	–	–	–[2]	–[2]	150	No	1	–
–	–	–	★	–	–	–	–	–	–	–	4	92	44	No	0	–
	–	–	★	–		–	–	–	★	–	4	91	91	No	0	–
		–	★			–	★	–	–		5	87	198	No	0	–
–	–	–	–	–	–	–	–	–	–	–	–[2]	–[2]	25	No	0	–
	–	–		–		–	–	–	–	–	4	93	44	No	0	–
–	–	–	–	–	–	–	–	–	–	–	4	95	31	No	0	–
–	–	–		–	–	–	–	–	–	–	4	85	74	No	0	–
–	–	–	–	–	–	–	–	–	–	–	–[2]	–[2]	36	No	0	–
–	–	–		–	–	–	–	–	–	–	4	97	144	No	0	–
–	–	–	–	–	–	–	–	–	–	–	4	93	30	No	–	–
	–	–		–			–	–	–	–	4	91	124	No	0	–
–	–	–		–	–	–	–	–	–	–	4	96	56	No	0	–
	–	–		–	–	–			–	–	5	98	155	No	0	–
–	–	–		–	–	–	–	–	–	–	4	93	38	No	0	–
				×				–			4	88	328	No	0	–
✖		×					★	–	–		–[2]	–[2]	218	No	0	–
✖	–	–		–	–	–	–	–	–	–	4	90	267	Yes	6	–
–	–	–	–	–	–	–	–	–	–	–	–[2]	–[2]	44	No	0	–
–	–	–	–	–	–	–	–	–	–	–	4	88	20	No	0	–
–	–	–	–	–	–	–	–	–	–	–	–[2]	–[2]	47	No	0	–
			×	✖				–		✖	4	92	230	No	0	–
–	–	–		–	–	–	–	–	–	–	4	97	54	No	0	–
	–		★	–	★	–	–	–		–	4	94	96	No	0	–
–	–	–	–	–	–	–	–	–	–	–	–[2]	–[2]	50	No	0	–
–	–	–	–	–	–	–	–	–	–	–	–[2]	–[2]	36	No	0	–
		✖	★	★			★		✖		4	93	259	No	0	–

***Accreditation Status:** 5=Accredited with commendation or with full standards compliance; 4=Accredited with requirements for improvement; 3=Conditional accreditation.

Detailed Ratings for All Areas

See more information on "Key Ratings for Metro Areas" table beginning on page 32

Blue is most favorable
Bold Italic is least favorable
Blank means neither better nor worse than average
"–" means insufficient data

	Death rates for all selected case types			Hospital outcomes: better (★) or worse (×) than average — Adjusted Death rates — Medical Cases											
	Number of cases	Actual death rate (%)	Adjusted death rate (%) (lower is better)	All selected cases	All selected medical cases	Heart attack	Congestive heart failure	Obstructive pulmonary disease	Pneumonia	Respiratory failure and arrest	Septicemia	Stroke	Gastrointestinal hemorrhage	Fluid, electrolyte, & acid-base disorders	Kidney failure
National Average	–	–	12.1	12.1	14.8	21.2	10.6	6.5	16.9	34.4	25.1	18.4	6.7	11.0	20.9
Texas (continued)															
Other Areas (continued)															
San Angelo Community, San Angelo	2,274	9.8	12.8										✖		–
Scenic Mountain, Big Spring	2,401	13.0	***13.3***	✖					×		×				
Scott and White, Temple	9,569	9.9	**11.2**	**★**	**★**	**★**									
Seton Edgar B Davis, Luling	761	14.6	***17.7***	✖	✖	✖		✖		–	✖	✖	–	–	–
Seton Highland Lakes, Burnet	933	17.0	***16.9***	✖	✖		✖			✖		✖	✖		–
Seymour Hospital, Seymour	582	11.5	13.7			–		–		–	–	✖	–	–	–
Shamrock General, Shamrock	288	10.1	9.6			–		–	★		–	–	–		–
Shannon, San Angelo	6,100	11.3	***13.5***	✖	✖	✖	✖							×	✖
Shelby Regional, Center	835	16.2	13.6			–				✖		✖	–		✖
Sid Peterson, Kerrville	3,680	9.6	12.5			×				–					
Sierra, El Paso	5,845	11.2	**11.0**	**★**	**★**				★						
Smithville Regional, Smithville	858	13.6	12.0				×						–		–
South Texas Regional, Jourdanton	1,186	9.4	10.2	★	★		**★**		★	–	✖		–		
Southwestern General, El Paso	556	7.9	9.5	★	★	–			**★**	–	–	–	–	★	–
Stamford Memorial, Stamford	316	13.6	15.0			–	–	–	×	–	–	–	–	–	–
Starr County, Rio Grande City	472	13.6	***16.0***	✖	✖	–		–		–	–	–	–		–
Stephens, Breckenridge	541	17.0	***18.6***	✖	✖	✖	✖	–	✖	–	–	×	–		–
Swisher, Tulia[1]	149	15.4	15.6			–	–	–		–	–	–	–	–	–
Texoma, Denison[1]	4,525	11.1	12.2					×							
Throckmorton County, Throckmorton	120	10.8	8.1			–	–	–	**★**	–	–	–	–	–	–
Titus Regional, Mt Pleasant	2,211	11.7	11.6						★	–					✖
Trinity, Brenham	1,281	16.3	***18.2***	✖	✖			✖	✖		–		✖	✖	–
Trinity, Carrollton	1,057	14.3	13.1			✖							–		–
Tyler County, Woodville	863	16.9	***14.1***	✖	✖	✖				–			–	–	✖
United Regional, Wichita Falls	6,603	11.9	***13.8***	✖	✖				✖		✖		×	✖	
University, Lubbock	2,121	15.3	***15.9***	✖	✖		✖		✖		✖			✖	
University of Texas, Tyler	2,257	9.5	12.5												
University of Texas Medical Branch, Galveston[1]	4,220	11.6	11.3		★				★		✖				**★**
Uvalde Memorial, Uvalde[1]	1,383	12.3	12.9										–		
Val Verde Regional, Del Rio	1,600	13.4	***14.2***	✖	✖			✖							✖
Valley Baptist, Harlingen	8,591	11.7	12.0					×							**★**
Valley Regional, Brownsville	2,285	9.5	**10.0**	**★**	**★**		**★**		**★**			★			
W J Mangold, Lockney	287	10.8	11.0			–	–	–	**★**	–	–	–	–		–
Wadley Regional, Texarkana	5,690	11.8	**11.0**	**★**	**★**							★			

Footnotes are on page 350.

Hospital outcomes: better (★) or worse (×) than average											Results of accreditation review on full survey		Other facts			
Adjusted Death rates			Adjusted Adverse outcome rates													
Surgical cases			Surgical cases													
All selected surgical cases	Coronary artery bypass surgery	Large bowel surgery	All selected surgical cases	Coronary artery bypass surgery	Large bowel surgery	Gall bladder removal	Total knee replacement	Total hip replacement	Simple prostatectomy	Carotid endarterectomy	Accreditation status*	Overall evaluation score (higher is better)	Number of beds	Major medical school affiliation?	Number of residents	Computerized drug order system (1 to 5 scale, higher is preferred; see page 23 for details)
2.3	3.8	6.5	7.7	10.3	11.9	7.5	6.7	6.4	5.4	8.2	–	91	161	–	–	–
	–		★	★				–	–	–	5	97	136	No	0	–
✖	–	–		–		–	–	–		–	4	92	110	No	0	–
			★	★			★	★		★	4	86	411	Yes	269	–
–	–	–	–	–	–	–	–	–	–	–	4	79	15	No	0	–
–	–	–		–	–	–	–	–	–	–	4	84	26	No	0	–
–	–	–	–	–	–	–	–	–	–	–	–[2]	–[2]	34	No	0	–
–	–	–	–	–	–	–	–	–	–	–	–[2]	–[2]	16	No	0	–
			★				★			★	4	91	224	No	0	–
–	–	–	–	–	–	–	–	–	–	–	4	89	46	No	0	–
	–			–		×			–		4	89	104	No	0	–
									–		4	92	328	No	0	–
–	–	–	–	–	–	–	–	–	–	–	–[2]	–[2]	24	No	0	–
–	–	–	–	–	–	–	–	–	–	–	4	92	30	No	0	–
–	–	–		–	–	–	–	–	–	–	–[2]	–[2]	102	No	0	–
–	–	–	–	–	–	–	–	–	–	–	–[2]	–[2]	26	No	0	–
–	–	–	–	–	–	–	–	–	–	–	–[2]	–[2]	44	No	0	–
–	–	–	–	–	–	–	–	–	–	–	–[2]	–[2]	33	No	0	–
–	–	–	–	–	–	–	–	–	–	–	–[2]	–[2]	26	No	0	–
×		✖	✖			×	✖				4	93	206	No	0	–
–	–	–	–	–	–	–	–	–	–	–	–[2]	–[2]	25	No	0	–
	–		★	–	★		–	–	–	★	4	92	151	No	0	–
	–	–	★	–		–		–		–	4	99	60	No	0	–
–	–	–		–	–	–	–	–	–	–	4	96	125	No	0	–
–	–	–	–	–	–	–	–	–	–	–	–[2]	–[2]	26	No	0	–
×			✖			✖					4	92	385	No	0	–
×	–	–		✖		–	✖	–	–	–	4	94	301	Yes	0	–
	–	–	✖	✖		–	–	–	–	✖	4	93	112	No	23	–
✖		✖	✖	×	✖	–		–	–	✖	4	87	776	Yes	585	5
–	–	–		–	–	–		–	–	–	4	81	54	No	0	–
	–	–		–	–		–	–		–	4	84	81	No	0	–
			★	✖			★	✖		★	–[2]	–[2]	343	No	13	–
	✖	–		✖			–	–		–	4	92	177	No	0	–
–	–	–	–	–	–	–	–	–	–	–	–[2]	–[2]	27	No	0	–
	–							–	✖		4	95	335	No	0	–

***Accreditation Status:** 5=Accredited with commendation or with full standards compliance; 4=Accredited with requirements for improvement; 3=Conditional accreditation.

Detailed Ratings for All Areas

See more information on "Key Ratings for Metro Areas" table beginning on page 32

Blue is most favorable
Bold Italic is least favorable
Blank means neither better nor worse than average
"–" means insufficient data

	Death rates for all selected case types			Hospital outcomes: better (★) or worse (✖) than average — Adjusted Death rates — Medical Cases											
	Number of cases	Actual death rate (%)	Adjusted death rate (%) (lower is better)	All selected cases	All selected medical cases	Heart attack	Congestive heart failure	Obstructive pulmonary disease	Pneumonia	Respiratory failure and arrest	Septicemia	Stroke	Gastrointestinal hemorrhage	Fluid, electrolyte, & acid-base disorders	Kidney failure
National Average	–	–	12.1	12.1	14.8	21.2	10.6	6.5	16.9	34.4	25.1	18.4	6.7	11.0	20.9
Texas *(continued)*															
Other Areas *(continued)*															
Walls Regional, Cleburne	1,994	14.4	13.0												–
Ward, Monahans	394	8.4	11.1			–		–		–	–	–	–	–	–
Westwood, Midland	1,039	7.5	7.1	★	★	–	★	★	★			★	–		
Wilbarger General, Vernon	1,191	11.7	13.3							–		✖	–		–
Wilson, Floresville	541	15.2	11.7					–		–			–		–
Wilson N Jones, Sherman	4,374	12.6	***13.2***	✖	✖			×	✖	✖					
Wilson N Jones - North Campus, Sherman	1,471	12.6	11.8							✖					
Wise Regional, Decatur[1]	1,283	14.9	***14.8***	✖	✖	✖		×			✖		–		
Woodland Heights, Lufkin	2,623	10.4	10.2	★	★			★	★						
Yoakum Community, Yoakum	719	15.2	***16.6***	✖	✖					–	–	✖	✖		–
Utah															
Salt Lake City Area															
Alta View, Sandy	1,214	15.2	13.2					–						✖	–
Cottonwood, Murray	2,586	10.9	10.0	★	★	★			★		★				
Jordan Valley, West Jordan	544	17.8	***18.6***	✖	✖	✖	✖	–		–	✖		–	–	–
LDS, Salt Lake City	5,691	8.4	10.3	★	★	★			★				★		
Pioneer Valley, West Valley	1,260	11.6	12.4											–	
Primary Children's, Salt Lake City	–	–	–	–	–	–	–	–	–	–	–	–	–	–	–
St Mark's, Salt Lake City	5,087	10.5	11.5			★	×		★	★		×	✖		×
Salt Lake Regional, Salt Lake City	1,891	10.9	11.5												
University of Utah, Salt Lake City[1]	2,515	10.4	10.8	★	★	★		×			★				
Other Areas															
Allen, Moab	193	9.8	14.3			–	–	–		–	–	–	–	–	–
American Fork Hospital, American Fork	1,094	11.5	12.2					–		✖					
Ashley Valley, Vernal	458	9.2	9.1	★	★			–	★			–	–	–	–
Bear River Valley, Tremonton	175	21.7	***23.9***	✖	✖	–	–	–	✖	–	–	–	–	–	–
Beaver Valley, Beaver	260	3.1	3.6	★	★	–	★	–	★	–	–	–	–	–	–
Brigham City Community, Brigham City	528	11.7	9.9				–	–		–	★		–		–
Castleview, Price	1,094	13.9	11.7					–							
Central Valley, Nephi	254	13.0	14.4			–	–	–		–	–	–	–	–	–
Davis, Layton	1,586	12.2	***15.1***	✖	✖	★		–	✖			✖	×		
Delta Community, Delta	135	12.6	11.9			–	–	–		–	–	–	–	–	–
Dixie Regional, St George	3,858	10.0	11.9				×								

Footnotes are on page 350.

Hospital outcomes: better (★) or worse (✕) than average											Results of accreditation review on full survey		Other facts			
Adjusted Death rates			Adjusted Adverse outcome rates													
Surgical cases			Surgical cases													
All selected surgical cases	Coronary artery bypass surgery	Large bowel surgery	All selected surgical cases	Coronary artery bypass surgery	Large bowel surgery	Gall bladder removal	Total knee replacement	Total hip replacement	Simple prostatectomy	Carotid endarterectomy	Accreditation status*	Overall evaluation score (higher is better)	Number of beds	Major medical school affiliation?	Number of residents	Computerized drug order system (1 to 5 scale, higher is preferred; see page 23 for details)
2.3	3.8	6.5	7.7	10.3	11.9	7.5	6.7	6.4	5.4	8.2	–	91	161	–	–	–
	–	–	✕	–			✕	–	–	–	5	**97**	126	No	0	–
–	–	–	–	–	–	–	–	–	–	–	–[2]	–[2]	36	No	0	–
–	–	–		–	–	–	–	–	–	–	4	***82***	86	No	0	–
–	–	–		–	–	–	–	–	–	–	4	91	49	No	0	–
–	–	–	–	–	–	–	–	–	–	–	–[2]	–[2]	30	No	0	–
	–				★			–			4	***86***	158	No	0	–
★	–	–	★	–	★	–	–	–	–	–	–[2]	–[2]	105	No	0	–
	–	–	★	–		–	–	–	–	–	4	**99**	59	No	0	–
	★	–		★		✕		–	–		4	91	122	No	0	–
–	–	–	–	–	–	–	–	–	–	–	–[2]	–[2]	28	No	0	–
–	–	–		–	–	–	–	–	–	–	4	**95**	72	No	0	–
✕	–			–						–	4	90	182	No	0	–
–	–	–	–	–	–	–	–	–	–	–	4	91	50	No	0	–
							✕	★	★		4	90	401	No	34	–
–	–	–	✕	–	–	–	✕	–	–	–	4	**96**	127	No	1	–
–	–	–	–	–	–	–	–	–	–	–	4	**94**	191	–	12	–
				★					–		4	92	229	No	0	–
						–	–	–		–	–[2]	–[2]	138	No	0	–
		–			✕	–		★	–		4	***88***	346	**Yes**	403	–
–	–	–	–	–	–	–	–	–	–	–	–[2]	–[2]	38	No	0	–
–	–	–		–	–			–	–	–	4	**96**	72	No	0	–
–	–	–	–	–	–	–	–	–	–	–	4	**94**	29	No	0	–
–	–	–	–	–	–	–	–	–	–	–	–[2]	–[2]	20	No	0	–
–	–	–	–	–	–	–	–	–	–	–	–[2]	–[2]	12	No	0	–
–	–	–		–	–	–	–	–	–	–	5	**97**	49	No	0	–
★	–	★	★	–	★	–		–	–	–	4	93	60	No	0	–
–	–	–	–	–	–	–	–	–	–	–	–[2]	–[2]	20	No	0	–
	–	–		–				–	–	–	4	91	126	No	1	–
–	–	–	–	–	–	–	–	–	–	–	–[2]	–[2]	20	No	0	–
	–			–	★				–		4	90	116	No	4	–

***Accreditation Status:** 5=Accredited with commendation or with full standards compliance; 4=Accredited with requirements for improvement; 3=Conditional accreditation.

Detailed Ratings for All Areas

See more information on "Key Ratings for Metro Areas" table beginning on page 32

Blue is most favorable
Bold Italic is least favorable
Blank means neither better nor worse than average
"–" means insufficient data

	Death rates for all selected case types			Hospital outcomes: better (★) or worse (×) than average — Adjusted Death rates											
					Medical Cases										
	Number of cases	Actual death rate (%)	Adjusted death rate (%) (lower is better)	All selected cases	All selected medical cases	Heart attack	Congestive heart failure	Obstructive pulmonary disease	Pneumonia	Respiratory failure and arrest	Septicemia	Stroke	Gastrointestinal hemorrhage	Fluid, electrolyte, & acid-base disorders	Kidney failure
National Average	–	–	12.1	12.1	14.8	21.2	10.6	6.5	16.9	34.4	25.1	18.4	6.7	11.0	20.9
Utah *(continued)*															
Other Areas *(continued)*															
Fillmore Community, Fillmore	115	10.4	10.9			–	–	–		–	–	–	–	–	–
Garfield, Panguitch[1]	138	13.8	11.4			–	–	–	–	–	–	–	–	–	–
Gunnison Valley, Gunnison	284	10.2	12.2			–	–	–		–	–		–	–	–
HCA Mountain Star - Lake View, Bountiful	1,439	12.1	12.0					–		★				–	–
Heber Valley, Heber City	143	14.7	13.4			–	–	–		–	–	–	–	–	–
Kane County, Kanab	155	7.7	10.5			–	–	–		–	–	–	–	–	–
Logan Regional, Logan	1,858	10.3	12.9							–					
McKay - Dee, Ogden	4,122	8.9	10.9	★	★	★			★	✖		×			
Milford Valley, Milford	179	9.5	14.0			–		–		–	–	–	–	–	–
Mountain Star Mountain View, Payson	1,234	9.7	10.8					–					–		–
Ogden Regional, Ogden	1,836	10.8	10.9			★	✖		★						
San Juan, Monticello	142	14.8	***18.0***	✖	✖	–	–	–		–	–	–	–	–	–
Sanpete Valley, Mt Pleasant	143	7.0	6.2	★	★	–	–	–		–	–		–	–	–
Sevier Valley, Richfield	522	12.3	10.9			–		–		–	–		–	–	–
Timpanogos Regional, Orem	302	13.6	14.8			–		–		–	–		–	–	–
Tooele Valley Regional, Tooele	374	10.7	11.1			–		–		–		–	–	–	–
Uintah Basin, Roosevelt	389	12.6	***18.9***	✖	✖	–	✖	–	✖	–	–	✖	–	–	–
Utah Valley Regional, Provo	4,578	10.2	12.9	×											
Valley View, Cedar City	551	9.8	13.3				✖	–		–	–		–	–	–
Vermont															
Brattleboro Memorial, Brattleboro	1,176	10.9	13.3		×				×			×			✖
Central Vermont, Barre	1,798	14.8	***13.8***	✖	✖		✖			×		✖			
Copley, Morrisville	738	11.9	13.7					–		–	–		–	–	–
Fletcher Allen of Vermont, Burlington	5,554	9.6	***13.0***	✖	✖		×	✖		✖	×				
Grace Cottage, Townshend	213	16.4	***16.5***	✖	✖	–		–		–	–		–	–	–
Mt Ascutney, Windsor	461	18.2	***19.3***	✖	✖		✖	✖	✖		–	×	–	–	–
North Country, Newport[1]	1,164	12.8	12.3				✖								–
Northeastern Vermont Regional, St Johnsbury	868	14.7	***17.2***	✖	✖			✖	✖	–		✖		–	–
Northwestern, St Albans	1,412	12.4	***15.4***	✖	✖		✖					✖	✖	–	✖
Porter, Middlebury[1]	957	8.3	9.1	★	★	★	★	–		–	–		–	–	–
Rutland Regional, Rutland	3,612	11.0	***13.4***	✖	✖				✖	★		✖			
Southwestern Vermont, Bennington	2,745	11.5	11.9												
Springfield Hospital, Springfield	1,319	12.1	13.1									✖		–	–

Footnotes are on page 350.

Hospital outcomes: better (★) or worse (×) than average											Results of accreditation review on full survey		Other facts			
Adjusted Death rates			Adjusted Adverse outcome rates													
Surgical cases			Surgical cases													
All selected surgical cases	Coronary artery bypass surgery	Large bowel surgery	All selected surgical cases	Coronary artery bypass surgery	Large bowel surgery	Gall bladder removal	Total knee replacement	Total hip replacement	Simple prostatectomy	Carotid endarterectomy	Accreditation status*	Overall evaluation score (higher is better)	Number of beds	Major medical school affiliation?	Number of residents	Computerized drug order system (1 to 5 scale, higher is preferred; see page 23 for details)
2.3	3.8	6.5	7.7	10.3	11.9	7.5	6.7	6.4	5.4	8.2	–	91	161	–	–	–
–	–	–	–	–	–	–	–	–	–	–	–[2]	–[2]	20	No	0	–
–	–	–	–	–	–	–	–	–	–	–	–[2]	–[2]	44	No	0	–
–	–	–	–	–	–	–	–	–	–	–	–[2]	–[2]	20	No	0	–
	–	–		–		–		✖	–	–	5	95	118	No	0	–
–	–	–	–	–	–	–	–	–	–	–	–[2]	–[2]	20	No	0	–
–	–	–	–	–	–	–	–	–	–	–	–[2]	–[2]	33	No	0	–
	–			–					–	–	4	87	97	No	0	–
							✖				4	87	293	No	19	–
–	–	–	–	–	–	–	–	–	–	–	–[2]	–[2]	34	No	0	–
	–	–		–		–			–	–	4	95	126	No	0	4
				★		–			–	–	5	95	179	No	0	–
–	–	–	–	–	–	–	–	–	–	–	–[2]	–[2]	26	No	0	–
–	–	–	–	–	–	–	–	–	–	–	–[2]	–[2]	20	No	0	–
–	–	–	–	–	–	–	–	–	–	–	4	94	26	No	0	–
–	–	–	–	–	–	–	–	–	–	–	4	93	51	No	0	4
–	–	–	–	–	–	–	–	–	–	–	–[2]	–[2]	24	No	0	–
–	–	–	–	–	–	–	–	–	–	–	–[2]	–[2]	42	No	0	–
×	×		✖	×			✖	✖		★	4	87	314	No	45	–
–	–	–		–	–	–	★	–	–	–	4	96	36	No	0	–
★	–	–	★	–	–			–	–	–	4	95	61	No	0	–
	–	–		–		–	★	–	–	–	4	94	141	No	0	–
–	–	–		–	–	–	–	–	–	–	4	87	41	No	0	–
			×							✖	–[2]	–[2]	508	Yes	248	–
–	–	–	–	–	–	–	–	–	–	–	–[2]	–[2]	18	No	0	–
–	–	–	–	–	–	–	–	–	–	–	–[2]	–[2]	33	No	0	–
	–	–	★	–		–	–	–	–	–	4	93	27	No	0	–
–	–	–		–		–	–	–	–	–	4	88	49	No	0	–
–	–	–		–		–		–	–	–	4	89	53	No	0	–
–	–	–		–		–	–	–	–	–	4	83	45	No	0	–
	–	×		–						×	4	85	132	No	4	–
	–		★	–		–		★	–	–	–[2]	–[2]	76	No	0	–
	–	–		–		–	–	–	–	–	4	88	69	No	0	–

***Accreditation Status:** 5=Accredited with commendation or with full standards compliance; 4=Accredited with requirements for improvement; 3=Conditional accreditation.

Detailed Ratings for All Areas

See more information on "Key Ratings for Metro Areas" table beginning on page 32

Blue is most favorable
Bold Italic is least favorable
Blank means neither better nor worse than average
"–" means insufficient data

	Death rates for all selected case types			Hospital outcomes: better (★) or worse (×) than average — Adjusted Death rates — Medical Cases											
	Number of cases	Actual death rate (%)	Adjusted death rate (%) (lower is better)	All selected cases	All selected medical cases	Heart attack	Congestive heart failure	Obstructive pulmonary disease	Pneumonia	Respiratory failure and arrest	Septicemia	Stroke	Gastrointestinal hemorrhage	Fluid, electrolyte, & acid-base disorders	Kidney failure
National Average	–	–	12.1	12.1	14.8	21.2	10.6	6.5	16.9	34.4	25.1	18.4	6.7	11.0	20.9
Virgin Islands															
Gov Juan F Luis, St Croix	596	16.6	***18.9***	✖	✖	–		–	✖	✖	✖	✖	–	×	
Roy Lester Schneider, Charlotte Amalie St Thomas	572	15.2	***17.7***	✖	✖	–		–	✖		–		✖		–
Virginia															
Norfolk Area															
Bon Secours DePaul, Norfolk	3,965	15.0	12.4												
Sentara Leigh, Norfolk	5,458	10.5	9.5	★	★		★		★		★	★			
Sentara Norfolk General, Norfolk	5,825	10.3	10.0	★	★	★	★	★	★	★					
Washington, DC, Area															
Inova Alexandria Hospital, Alexandria	4,464	11.5	10.6	★	★		★	★							
Inova Fair Oaks, Fairfax	2,264	10.8	11.1			✖	★	★							★
Inova Fairfax, Falls Church	9,143	10.0	10.3	★	★		★		★			★			★
Inova Mount Vernon, Alexandria	3,757	8.5	9.8	★	★				★		★	★			★
Loudoun, Leesburg	1,893	12.9	12.4			✖				★					
Northern Virginia, Arlington	1,570	17.7	11.9												
Potomac, Woodbridge	1,731	11.3	11.2					×	★						
Prince William, Manassas	2,007	17.2	***17.3***	✖	✖	×	✖	✖	✖			✖		✖	
Reston Hospital, Reston	2,284	10.9	10.9							★	★				
Virginia, Arlington	5,162	12.3	10.2	★	★		★				★				★
Other Areas															
Augusta, Fishersville	6,413	11.6	9.7	★	★	★	★	★		★	★		★	★	
Bon Secours - Stuart Circle, Richmond	1,862	14.2	***13.9***	✖	✖				✖				✖	✖	
Bon Secours Maryview, Portsmouth	6,370	12.5	11.6				★	★				×			
Bon Secours Memorial Regional, Mechanicsville	4,787	11.8	10.7	★	★	★	★	★		★		★		✖	★
Bon Secours Richmond Community, Richmond	939	17.9	13.6	×		×		–			✖		–		
Bon Secours St Mary's, Richmond	7,724	11.0	11.2	★	★		★			★		★			×
Buchanan General, Grundy	2,807	8.3	11.0			✖		★			✖				–
Capitol, Richmond	1,182	13.7	8.4	★	★		★		★		★				★
Carilion, Roanoke	11,291	9.8	10.5	★	★	★	★		★	★			★	★	
Carilion Bedford, Bedford	1,098	15.4	12.1			×		★							–
Carilion Franklin, Rocky Mount	1,433	17.0	***16.2***	✖	✖	✖			×	✖	✖				
Carilion Giles, Pearisburg	1,221	8.8	8.1	★	★		★		★	★				★	–
Carilion New River Valley, Christiansburg	2,467	11.4	11.8									×	★	★	✖
Chesapeake General, Chesapeake	6,138	13.0	11.6				★				✖				
CJW Johnston Willis, Richmond	11,163	12.0	10.3	★	★	★	★		★	★		★	★		★

Footnotes are on page 350.

Hospital outcomes: better (★) or worse (×) than average											Results of accreditation review on full survey		Other facts			
Adjusted Death rates			Adjusted Adverse outcome rates													
Surgical cases			Surgical cases													
All selected surgical cases	Coronary artery bypass surgery	Large bowel surgery	All selected surgical cases	Coronary artery bypass surgery	Large bowel surgery	Gall bladder removal	Total knee replacement	Total hip replacement	Simple prostatectomy	Carotid endarterectomy	Accreditation status*	Overall evaluation score (higher is better)	Number of beds	Major medical school affiliation?	Number of residents	Computerized drug order system (1 to 5 scale, higher is preferred; see page 23 for details)
2.3	3.8	6.5	7.7	10.3	11.9	7.5	6.7	6.4	5.4	8.2	–	91	161	–	–	–
–	–	–	–	–	–	–	–	–	–	–	–[2]	–[2]	160	No	0	–
–	–	–	–	–	–	–	–	–	–	–	–[2]	–[2]	160	No	–	–
	–			–	×		★	–	–		4	91	293	Yes	0	–
	–			–					–		–[2]	–[2]	212	Yes	0	–
							–	–	–		4	94	478	No	0	–
									✖		5	96	311	No	0	–
	–	–		–				–	–	–	4	96	151	No	0	–
★	★					✖					4	93	656	No	27	–
	–	–	✖	–		×	★	✖	–	–	4	94	229	No	0	–
	–	–		–			–	–	–	–	4	97	92	No	0	–
	–	–		–		–	–	–	–		4	83	96	No	0	–
	–	–		–		–	–	–	–	–	4	98	137	No	0	–
	–	–		–		–	–	–	–	–	4	97	135	No	0	–
	–	–		–		–		–	–	–	4	86	121	No	0	–
											4	90	283	No	33	–
★	–	★		–							4	95	205	No	0	–
	–	–		–		–	★	–	–	–	–[2]	–[2]	158	No	3	–
	–	×		–	×	×	★	×			4	81	346	No	0	–
	–	–	★		★				–		4	96	180	No	0	–
–	–	–		–	–	–	–	–	–	–	4	91	102	No	1	–
									–	✖	4	87	348	No	0	–
–	–	–	★	–	–	–	–	–	–	–	4	92	144	No	0	–
–	–	–	–	–	–	–	–	–	–	–	–[2]	–[2]	135	No	0	–
★			×	★				✖	✖		–[2]	–[2]	740	Yes	143	–
	–	–		–	★	–	–	–	–	–	4	96	49	No	0	–
–	–	–		–	–	–	–	–	–	–	5	99	37	No	0	–
–	–	–		–	–	–	–	–	–	–	4	99	31	No	0	–
	–			–				–	–		–[2]	–[2]	175	No	–	–
	–			–					–		4	92	260	No	0	–
	★										–[2]	–[2]	764	No	15	–

***Accreditation Status:** 5=Accredited with commendation or with full standards compliance; 4=Accredited with requirements for improvement; 3=Conditional accreditation.

Detailed Ratings for All Areas

See more information on "Key Ratings for Metro Areas" table beginning on page 32

Blue is most favorable
Bold Italic is least favorable
Blank means neither better nor worse than average
"–" means insufficient data

	Death rates for all selected case types			Hospital outcomes: better (★) or worse (×) than average — Adjusted Death rates — Medical Cases											
	Number of cases	Actual death rate (%)	Adjusted death rate (%) (lower is better)	All selected cases	All selected medical cases	Heart attack	Congestive heart failure	Obstructive pulmonary disease	Pneumonia	Respiratory failure and arrest	Septicemia	Stroke	Gastrointestinal hemorrhage	Fluid, electrolyte, & acid-base disorders	Kidney failure
National Average	–	–	12.1	12.1	14.8	21.2	10.6	6.5	16.9	34.4	25.1	18.4	6.7	11.0	20.9
Virginia *(continued)*															
Other Areas *(continued)*															
Clinch Valley, Richlands	2,983	8.3	8.5	★	★		★	★	★	★			★	★	
Columbia Allegheny Regional, Lowmoor	2,797	13.6	10.7	★	★	★									
Community Memorial, South Hill	2,568	13.3	11.2												
Culpeper Regional, Culpeper[1]	1,744	11.9	12.8												
Danville Regional, Danville	6,167	13.6	***13.8***	✖	✖	✖	×	✖	×	✖				★	
Dickenson County, Clintwood	888	11.9	11.7								×	–	–		–
Fauquier, Warrenton	2,402	11.4	11.9							×				**★**	
Greensville, Emporia	2,064	11.9	10.5	★	★		**★**								
Halifax Regional, South Boston[1]	3,297	14.2	***14.7***	✖	✖	✖		✖	✖	×	×			×	
Healthsouth, Richmond	2,883	11.7	***13.5***	✖	✖		✖	★			✖				
Henrico Doctors', Richmond	6,318	10.7	10.8	★	★			**★**		★					
John Randolph, Hopewell	2,658	15.2	12.2			✖									
Johnston, Abingdon	3,107	15.8	***15.1***	✖	✖	✖	✖	×	✖			×			✖
Lee County, Pennington Gap	1,706	10.7	8.5	★	★		★	**★**	★					★	
Lewis - Gale, Salem	7,125	11.3	11.4										★		
Louise Obici, Suffolk	3,800	13.1	***13.6***	✖	✖					✖	✖		✖		×
Martha Jefferson, Charlottesville	5,591	10.9	11.1	★	**★**			**★**	★						
Mary Immaculate, Newport News[1]	2,091	14.3	***14.9***	✖	✖			✖	✖	✖		✖		✖	★
Mary Washington, Fredericksburg	7,575	11.1	10.8	★	★	★	**★**						★		
Memorial, Martinsville	4,009	14.0	***13.4***	✖	✖			✖							✖
Montgomery Regional, Blacksburg	2,440	13.2	12.2												
Norton Community, Norton	2,117	9.0	9.2	★	★			**★**	★	★			★		
Page, Luray	1,233	11.0	9.6	★	★					★			–		★
Pulaski Community, Pulaski	2,070	11.4	11.0					★						★	
R J Reynolds - Patrick County, Stuart	674	13.1	13.4							–			–		–
Rappahannock General, Kilmarnock	1,679	13.1	12.5							–				✖	
Retreat, Richmond	2,241	11.5	10.6	★	**★**										
Riverside, Tappahannock	1,619	14.1	***13.6***	✖	✖	×	×								★
Riverside Regional, Newport News	7,735	12.2	***12.9***	✖	✖			✖	✖						
Riverside Walter Reed, Gloucester	1,700	15.8	***14.3***	✖	✖		✖	✖					✖		✖
Rockingham, Harrisonburg	6,016	11.5	9.6	★	★		**★**	★	★	★	★		★	★	**★**
Russell County, Lebanon	1,985	12.7	12.2			×									
St Mary's, Norton	1,522	8.7	8.9	★	★			★	★						×
Sentara Bayside, Virginia Beach	2,415	15.8	12.2											×	

Footnotes are on page 350.

Hospital outcomes: better (★) or worse (✕) than average											Results of accreditation review on full survey		Other facts			
Adjusted Death rates			Adjusted Adverse outcome rates													
Surgical cases			Surgical cases													
All selected surgical cases	Coronary artery bypass surgery	Large bowel surgery	All selected surgical cases	Coronary artery bypass surgery	Large bowel surgery	Gall bladder removal	Total knee replacement	Total hip replacement	Simple prostatectomy	Carotid endarterectomy	Accreditation status*	Overall evaluation score (higher is better)	Number of beds	Major medical school affiliation?	Number of residents	Computerized drug order system (1 to 5 scale, higher is preferred; see page 23 for details)
2.3	3.8	6.5	7.7	10.3	11.9	7.5	6.7	6.4	5.4	8.2	–	91	161	–	–	–
–	–	–		–	–		–	–	–	–	4	89	178	No	0	–
	–	✕		–		★		–	–	–	3	***78***	156	No	7	–
	–	–		–			–	–	–	–	4	**95**	123	No	0	–
	–	–	★	–	★			–	–	–	5	**99**	70	No	0	–
	–		★	–			★				4	92	143	No	0	–
–	–	–	–	–	–	–	–	–	–	–	4	***85***	41	No	0	–
	–		★	–		–	★	–	–	–	4	90	83	No	0	–
–	–	–		–	–	–		–	–	–	4	***87***	89	No	0	–
	–	–		–		–	–	–	–	–	4	***88***	138	**Yes**	0	–
	–			–	★	–			–		5	93	147	No	0	–
							★		–		4	92	340	No	0	–
✕	–	✕		–			–	–	–	–	4	90	98	No	0	–
	–	–		–		–		★	–		4	***88***	135	No	0	–
–	–	–	–	–	–	–	–	–	–	–	4	***88***	80	No	0	–
						✕	★	★			4	90	521	No	8	–
✕	–	✕	✕	–				–	–	✕	4	91	160	No	0	–
★	–	★	★	–						–	4	92	156	No	0	–
	–	–		–		–	–	–	–	–	4	***88***	110	No	3	–
				✕							5	**96**	318	No	0	–
✕	–			–					✕	–	4	***83***	152	No	0	–
	–			–			–	–	–	–	4	92	104	No	0	–
–	–	–		–	–	–	–	–	–	–	4	90	55	No	0	–
–	–	–	–	–	–	–	–	–	–	–	4	90	54	No	0	–
–	–	–	★	–	–	–	–	–	–	–	4	***84***	87	No	0	2
–	–	–	–	–	–	–	–	–	–	–	4	**98**	33	No	0	–
	–	–		–		★	–	–	–	–	4	**95**	76	No	0	–
	–		★	–		–	–	–	–		4	91	100	No	0	–
–	–	–		–	–	–	–	–	–	–	5	**98**	67	No	0	–
			✕	★			✕			✕	4	**95**	360	No	62	–
–	–	–		–		–	–	–	–	–	4	93	71	No	0	–
	–			–			✕				4	90	251	No	0	–
✕	–	–	–	–	–	–	–	–	–	–	4	93	78	No	0	–
–	–	–		–	–	–	–	–	–	–	4	93	89	No	0	–
	–		★	–			–	–	–	★	4	***86***	100	No	0	–

***Accreditation Status:** 5=Accredited with commendation or with full standards compliance; 4=Accredited with requirements for improvement; 3=Conditional accreditation.

Detailed Ratings for All Areas

See more information on "Key Ratings for Metro Areas" table beginning on page 32

Blue is most favorable
Bold Italic is least favorable
Blank means neither better nor worse than average
"–" means insufficient data

	Death rates for all selected case types				Hospital outcomes: better (★) or worse (×) than average — Adjusted Death rates — Medical Cases										
	Number of cases	Actual death rate (%)	Adjusted death rate (%) (lower is better)	All selected cases	All selected medical cases	Heart attack	Congestive heart failure	Obstructive pulmonary disease	Pneumonia	Respiratory failure and arrest	Septicemia	Stroke	Gastrointestinal hemorrhage	Fluid, electrolyte, & acid-base disorders	Kidney failure
National Average	–	–	12.1	12.1	14.8	21.2	10.6	6.5	16.9	34.4	25.1	18.4	6.7	11.0	20.9
Virginia *(continued)*															
Other Areas *(continued)*															
Sentara Hampton General, Hampton	4,123	14.8	12.3				★				×		✖		★
Sentara Virginia Beach General, Virginia Beach	5,655	11.6	**10.5**	**★**	**★**	★			**★**		★				
Shenandoah, Woodstock	1,643	11.3	10.7		★				**★**						
Shore, Nassawadox[1]	2,638	14.2	12.2					**★**		★					
Smyth County, Marion	1,805	16.9	***16.0***	✖	✖		✖	✖	✖			✖	★		✖
Southampton, Franklin	1,620	12.7	13.4	×	×				✖	–					
Southside, Farmville	2,228	19.0	***19.2***	✖	✖	✖	✖	✖	✖	✖	✖	✖	✖	✖	✖
Southside Regional, Petersburg	5,139	11.4	11.5			✖	**★**						**★**		
Stonewall Jackson, Lexington	983	11.8	***14.5***	✖	✖		✖	–		–	–			✖	–
Tazewell Community, Tazewell	1,083	15.6	13.7	×	×		✖	**★**		✖	✖		**★**		–
Twin County Regional, Galax	2,288	17.8	***17.9***	✖	✖		✖	×	✖	×		✖		✖	–
University of Virginia, Charlottesville[1]	6,187	10.3	**10.6**	**★**	**★**				**★**				**★**	**★**	
Virginia Baptist, Lynchburg	9,549	11.4	***12.8***	✖	✖		✖		✖		×				
Virginia Commonwealth University, Richmond[1]	4,007	11.8	11.9				**★**							✖	
Warren, Front Royal	1,182	14.7	12.8				×		✖						
Wellmont Lonesome Pine, Big Stone Gap	841	15.7	11.5											–	×
Williamsburg Community, Williamsburg	3,246	10.4	11.4						★					×	
Winchester Medical Center, Winchester	9,187	8.8	**10.9**	**★**	**★**	**★**			**★**						✖
Wythe County, Wytheville	1,773	14.0	12.6									✖			
Washington															
Seattle Area															
Allenmore, Tacoma	–	–	–	–	–	–	–	–	–	–	–	–	–	–	–
Auburn Regional, Auburn	2,146	13.3	12.7				×			✖				**★**	
Cascade Valley, Arlington	552	12.7	12.1			–	×	–			–		–	–	–
Children's, Seattle	–	–	–	–	–	–	–	–	–	–	–	–	–	–	–
Enumclaw Community, Enumclaw	579	13.8	***15.6***	✖	✖			–	✖	–	–		–	–	–
Evergreen, Kirkland	2,756	15.5	***13.9***	✖	✖			×		✖	✖				✖
Good Samaritan, Puyallup	4,185	13.2	***13.8***	✖	✖		✖	✖	×						✖
Harborview, Seattle	1,385	20.3	13.3	×	×							✖			**★**
Harrison, Bremerton	6,203	13.1	12.0							×					
Highline, Burien	2,469	14.4	***13.6***	✖	✖		✖		×	✖					
Northwest, Seattle	5,375	13.4	12.2						✖		**★**	**★**	×	×	
Overlake, Bellevue	4,861	12.3	***13.2***	✖	✖	**★**	✖	✖	✖						

Footnotes are on page 350.

Hospital outcomes: better (★) or worse (×) than average											Results of accreditation review on full survey		Other facts			
Adjusted Death rates			Adjusted Adverse outcome rates													
Surgical cases			Surgical cases													
All selected surgical cases	Coronary artery bypass surgery	Large bowel surgery	All selected surgical cases	Coronary artery bypass surgery	Large bowel surgery	Gall bladder removal	Total knee replacement	Total hip replacement	Simple prostatectomy	Carotid endarterectomy	Accreditation status*	Overall evaluation score (higher is better)	Number of beds	Major medical school affiliation?	Number of residents	Computerized drug order system (1 to 5 scale, higher is preferred; see page 23 for details)
2.3	3.8	6.5	7.7	10.3	11.9	7.5	6.7	6.4	5.4	8.2	–	91	161	–	–	–
✖	–	✖	✖	–	✖	–		–	✖	–	5	97	167	No	0	–
			×					✖			4	94	193	No	0	–
–	–	–		–	–	–	–	–	–	–	4	90	95	No	0	–
	–	–		–		–	–	–	–	–	4	88	143	No	0	–
✖	–	–		–	–	–	–	–	✖	–	4	97	279	No	4	–
	–	–	★	–		–		–	–	–	4	93	72	No	0	–
	–			–			–	–		–	4	91	88	No	0	–
	–			–			–	–	✖	–	4	89	272	No	0	–
–	–	–		–	–	–	–	–	–	–	4	88	80	No	0	–
–	–	–	–	–	–	–	–	–	–	–	4	98	38	No	0	–
	–	–		–			✖	–	✖	–	5	88	76	No	0	–
		★			★				–		4	94	555	Yes	604	–
★	★				★					✖	–[2]	–[2]	323	Yes	0	–
	✖					–		✖	–	–	4	87	714	Yes	420	–
–	–	–		–	–	–	–	–	–	–	4	93	51	No	0	–
–	–	–	–	–	–	–	–	–	–	–	5	95	49	No	0	–
★	–			–				–		★	4	91	139	No	4	–
									–		4	91	387	No	0	–
–	–	–		–	–	–	–	–	–	–	4	97	82	No	0	–
–	–	–	–	–	–	–	–	–	–	–	–[2]	–[2]	–	–	–	–
	–			–				–	–	–	5	88	100	No	1	4
–	–	–	★	–	–	–	–	–	–	–	4	90	48	No	0	–
–	–	–	–	–	–	–	–	–	–	–	4	96	208	–	0	–
–	–	–		–	–	–	–	–	–	–	–[2]	–[2]	27	No	0	–
	–			–		–			–	★	4	87	149	No	0	2
	–			–		✖		★			4	94	211	No	0	4
	–	–		–		–	–	–	–	–	5	96	348	Yes	0	4
	–		★	–						★	4	81	219	No	6	2
	–			–		–			–	–	3	94	203	No	7	2
	–		★		★				–		4	84	187	No	0	4
							✖		–		4	86	218	No	7	3

***Accreditation Status:** 5=Accredited with commendation or with full standards compliance; 4=Accredited with requirements for improvement; 3=Conditional accreditation.

Detailed Ratings for All Areas

See more information on "Key Ratings for Metro Areas" table beginning on page 32

Blue is most favorable
Bold Italic is least favorable
Blank means neither better nor worse than average
"–" means insufficient data

	Death rates for all selected case types			Hospital outcomes: better (★) or worse (×) than average											
				Adjusted Death rates											
					Medical Cases										
	Number of cases	Actual death rate (%)	Adjusted death rate (%) (lower is better)	All selected cases	All selected medical cases	Heart attack	Congestive heart failure	Obstructive pulmonary disease	Pneumonia	Respiratory failure and arrest	Septicemia	Stroke	Gastrointestinal hemorrhage	Fluid, electrolyte, & acid-base disorders	Kidney failure
National Average	–	–	12.1	12.1	14.8	21.2	10.6	6.5	16.9	34.4	25.1	18.4	6.7	11.0	20.9
Washington *(continued)*															
Seattle Area *(continued)*															
Providence, Everett	4,169	13.3	13.0	×	✖			✖	✖		★			✖	
St Clare, Lakewood	1,611	14.4	11.7						★	✖					
St Francis, Federal Way	1,572	16.3	11.5											★	
St Joseph, Tacoma	3,977	14.0	11.8												
Stevens, Edmonds	3,013	14.2	12.9				×								
Swedish, Seattle	8,334	10.6	11.6												
Swedish - Ballard, Seattle	–	–	–	–	–	–	–	–	–	–	–	–	–	–	–
Swedish - Providence Campus, Seattle	4,157	10.0	11.8			★	✖							★	
Tacoma General, Tacoma[1]	5,739	12.6	***13.4***	✖	✖		✖	✖							✖
University of Washington, Seattle	1,706	8.0	11.3								–	★	–		
Valley, Renton	3,925	12.8	12.6								×			×	
Valley General, Monroe	455	14.3	***16.5***	✖	✖	–	×	–	✖	–	–	–	–	–	–
Virginia Mason, Seattle	4,632	7.9	**10.2**	★	★							★	★		
Other Areas															
Affiliated, Mt Vernon	2,784	12.9	12.2												
Capital, Olympia	1,942	12.6	***14.4***	✖	✖		✖					✖			
Central Washington, Wenatchee	3,418	12.0	***13.2***	✖	✖					✖	★	✖			✖
Columbia Basin, Ephrata	120	16.7	16.2			–	–	–	–	–	–	–	–	–	–
Deaconess, Spokane	3,893	8.6	**10.0**	★	★	★	★				★			★	
East Adams Rural, Ritzville	168	9.5	8.2			–	–	–	★	–	–	–	–	–	–
Ferry County, Republic	147	6.1	**4.3**	★	★	–	–	–		★	–	–	–	–	–
Forks Community, Forks	157	9.6	11.1			–	–	–		–	–	–	–	–	–
Grays Harbor, Aberdeen	2,924	12.3	11.4				★	★	×	–	★				
Holy Family, Spokane	3,743	12.4	12.7			×		✖					★		×
Island, Anacortes	1,001	11.9	***14.4***	✖	✖			–		✖		✖		–	
Jefferson General, Port Townsend	964	12.6	13.1								–	×			–
Kadlec, Richland	2,222	9.5	11.3				✖					★	★		
Kennewick General, Kennewick	1,768	12.5	11.9				✖								
Kittitas Valley, Ellensburg	836	15.4	***15.5***	✖	✖		✖	–	✖	✖	–		–	–	–
Klickitat Valley, Goldendale	245	14.7	14.6			–		–		–	–	–	–	–	–
Lake Chelan Community, Chelan	164	13.4	10.7			–	–	–		–	–	–	–	–	–
Lourdes, Pasco[1]	1,415	13.0	***13.9***	✖	✖										
Mason General, Shelton	1,222	10.3	12.0										★		–

Footnotes are on page 350.

Hospital outcomes: better (★) or worse (✖) than average											Results of accreditation review on full survey		Other facts			
Adjusted Death rates			Adjusted Adverse outcome rates													
Surgical cases			Surgical cases													
All selected surgical cases	Coronary artery bypass surgery	Large bowel surgery	All selected surgical cases	Coronary artery bypass surgery	Large bowel surgery	Gall bladder removal	Total knee replacement	Total hip replacement	Simple prostatectomy	Carotid endarterectomy	Accreditation status*	Overall evaluation score (higher is better)	Number of beds	Major medical school affiliation?	Number of residents	Computerized drug order system (1 to 5 scale, higher is preferred; see page 23 for details)
2.3	3.8	6.5	7.7	10.3	11.9	7.5	6.7	6.4	5.4	8.2	–	91	161	–	–	–
						✖			–		4	***87***	283	No	0	3
	–	–	★	–		–	★		–	–	–[2]	–[2]	60	No	0	2
	–	–		–		–	–	–	–	–	–[2]	–[2]	99	No	0	2
						–	★	★			4	***80***	283	No	19	2
	–			–			★		–	–	5	**94**	124	No	0	4
								★			4	**94**	601	**Yes**	41	3
–	–	–	–	–	–	–	–	–	–	–	–[2]	–[2]	–	–	–	–
	✖					–					–[2]	–[2]	245	**Yes**	36	3
				✖							4	***84***	377	No	24	4
		–				–			–	–	4	91	376	**Yes**	237	4
	–		★	–						★	4	92	165	No	24	3
–	–	–	–	–	–	–	–	–	–	–	4	90	69	No	0	–
★	★	★	★	★			★	★		★	4	***83***	282	No	108	4
	–		★	–		–			–	★	4	89	166	No	0	–
	–		★	–		–			–	★	4	90	101	No	0	4
	–		★	–				★	★		4	89	133	No	0	–
–	–	–	–	–	–	–	–	–	–	–	–[2]	–[2]	56	No	0	–
			★					✖	★	★	4	**96**	326	**Yes**	8	–
–	–	–	–	–	–	–	–	–	–	–	–[2]	–[2]	17	No	0	–
–	–	–	–	–	–	–	–	–	–	–	–[2]	–[2]	11	No	0	–
–	–	–	–	–	–	–	–	–	–	–	–[2]	–[2]	17	**Yes**	0	–
	–			–				–		–	4	89	112	No	0	–
	–			–							4	93	190	No	0	–
	–	–	★	–		–	★	–	–	–	–[2]	–[2]	43	No	0	–
–	–	–	★	–	–	–	–	–	–	–	–[2]	–[2]	35	No	0	–
	–			–					–	–	4	89	124	No	0	–
	–	–	★	–		–	–	–	–	–	4	**96**	71	No	0	–
–	–	–		–		–	–	–	–	–	–[2]	–[2]	32	No	0	–
–	–	–	–	–	–	–	–	–	–	–	–[2]	–[2]	15	No	0	–
–	–	–	–	–	–	–	–	–	–	–	–[2]	–[2]	30	No	0	–
–	–	–		–		–	–	–	–	–	4	**88**	32	No	4	–
–	–	–		–		–		–	–	–	4	**88**	51	No	0	–

***Accreditation Status:** 5=Accredited with commendation or with full standards compliance; 4=Accredited with requirements for improvement; 3=Conditional accreditation.

Detailed Ratings for All Areas

See more information on "Key Ratings for Metro Areas" table beginning on page 32

Blue is most favorable
Bold Italic is least favorable
Blank means neither better nor worse than average
"–" means insufficient data

	Death rates for all selected case types			Hospital outcomes: better (★) or worse (×) than average — Adjusted Death rates												
				Medical Cases												
	Number of cases	Actual death rate (%)	Adjusted death rate (%) (lower is better)	All selected cases	All selected medical cases	Heart attack	Congestive heart failure	Obstructive pulmonary disease	Pneumonia	Respiratory failure and arrest	Septicemia	Stroke	Gastrointestinal hemorrhage	Fluid, electrolyte, & acid-base disorders	Kidney failure
National Average	–	–	12.1	12.1	14.8	21.2	10.6	6.5	16.9	34.4	25.1	18.4	6.7	11.0	20.9
Washington *(continued)*															
Other Areas *(continued)*															
Mid-Valley, Omak	511	14.9	***18.9***	✖	✖		✖	–	✖	–	–	×	–	–	–
Morton General, Morton	206	17.0	***16.8***	✖	✖	–	–	–		–	–	–	–	–	–
Mount Carmel, Colville	799	9.9	10.2					–	★			✖	–		–
Newport Community, Newport	352	15.1	***16.6***	✖	✖	–		–	✖	–	–	–	–	–	–
North Valley, Tonasket	175	12.6	13.1			–	–	–		–	–	–	–	–	–
Ocean Beach, Ilwaco	483	15.1	***15.6***	✖	✖	✖		–			–	✖	–	–	–
Okanogan - Douglas, Brewster	423	14.4	13.4			✖	–	–		–	–		–	–	–
Olympic, Port Angeles	3,069	12.9	***13.9***	✖	✖				✖					×	✖
Othello Community, Othello	184	9.8	12.8			–	–	–	–	–	–	–	–	–	–
Peacehealth St John, Longview	3,738	12.9	12.9	×	×	✖	✖	★ (blue)				✖			
Prosser Memorial, Prosser	136	14.0	14.4			–	–	–		–	–	–	–	–	–
Providence, Centralia	2,326	13.0	***14.0***	✖	✖	✖							✖		
Providence, Toppenish	465	11.8	10.5					–		–	–		–	–	–
Providence, Yakima	3,138	12.8	***13.6***	✖	✖	★	✖	✖				×			×
Providence St Peter, Olympia	5,367	11.7	12.2				✖	✖						✖	
Pullman Memorial, Pullman	287	9.1	11.8			–	–	–	–	–	–		–	–	–
Quincy Valley, Quincy	119	8.4	9.3			–	–	–	–	–	–	–	–	–	–
Sacred Heart, Spokane	8,342	11.2	***12.8***	✖	✖		✖						✖		
St Joseph, Bellingham	5,257	10.9	12.9	×	✖	★ (blue)	✖	✖							×
St Joseph's, Chewelah[1]	414	8.2	8.9	★	★	–		–	★		–		–	–	–
St Mary, Walla Walla	1,792	10.1	12.4				×							★ (blue)	–
Samaritan, Moses Lake[1]	971	13.9	***14.7***	✖	✖		✖	×					×	–	–
Skyline, White Salmon	334	11.1	9.9					–		–	–		–	–	–
Southwest Washington, Vancouver	6,488	13.4	***15.2***	✖	✖		✖		✖	×	×	✖	✖	✖	
Sunnyside Community, Sunnyside	880	13.0	12.2					✖							
Tri-State, Clarkston	1,003	9.6	13.8		×	✖				–	✖			–	
Valley, Spokane	2,044	12.3	11.9												–
Walla Walla General, Walla Walla	800	11.6	12.5					–					–	–	–
Whidbey General, Coupeville	1,192	11.6	13.1				✖	✖							–
Whitman, Colfax	631	11.4	13.1			–				–			–	–	–
Yakima Valley, Yakima	3,701	12.4	***13.1***	✖	✖	★			×			✖			
West Virginia															
Beckley Appalachian Regional, Beckley	4,393	10.9	10.0 (blue)	★ (blue)	★ (blue)	✖	★ (blue)		★ (blue)				★		

Footnotes are on page 350.

Hospital outcomes: better (★) or worse (✕) than average											Results of accreditation review on full survey		Other facts			
Adjusted Death rates			Adjusted Adverse outcome rates													
Surgical cases			Surgical cases													
All selected surgical cases	Coronary artery bypass surgery	Large bowel surgery	All selected surgical cases	Coronary artery bypass surgery	Large bowel surgery	Gall bladder removal	Total knee replacement	Total hip replacement	Simple prostatectomy	Carotid endarterectomy	Accreditation status*	Overall evaluation score (higher is better)	Number of beds	Major medical school affiliation?	Number of residents	Computerized drug order system (1 to 5 scale, higher is preferred; see page 23 for details)
2.3	3.8	6.5	7.7	10.3	11.9	7.5	6.7	6.4	5.4	8.2	–	91	161	–	–	–
–	–	–	★	–	–	–	–	–	–	–	–[2]	–[2]	30	No	0	–
–	–	–	–	–	–	–	–	–	–	–	–[2]	–[2]	18	No	0	–
–	–	–		–	–	–	–	–	–	–	4	89	33	No	0	–
–	–	–	–	–	–	–	–	–	–	–	–[2]	–[2]	24	No	0	–
–	–	–	–	–	–	–	–	–	–	–	–[2]	–[2]	92	No	0	–
–	–	–	–	–	–	–	–	–	–	–	–[2]	–[2]	14	No	0	–
–	–	–	–	–	–	–	–	–	–	–	–[2]	–[2]	43	No	0	–
★	–	★	★	–	★				★	–	4	89	78	No	0	–
–	–	–	–	–	–	–	–	–	–	–	–[2]	–[2]	32	No	0	–
	–		★	–					–	★	4	80	178	No	8	–
–	–	–	–	–	–	–	–	–	–	–	–[2]	–[2]	24	No	0	–
	–			–					–	★	4	94	79	No	0	–
–	–	–	–	–	–	–	–	–	–	–	4	91	48	No	0	–
						–	★		–		4	87	197	No	0	–
★			★	★	★		★	★	–	★	4	88	314	No	15	2
–	–	–	–	–	–	–	–	–	–	–	4	88	24	No	0	–
–	–	–	–	–	–	–	–	–	–	–	–[2]	–[2]	38	No	0	–
									★		4	94	607	Yes	0	–
★	★		★			★		★	★		4	88	189	No	0	–
–	–	–	–	–	–	–	–	–	–	–	–[2]	–[2]	65	No	0	–
	–	–	★	–		–	★		★	–	4	94	107	No	0	–
–	–	–		–		–		–	–	–	–[2]	–[2]	50	No	0	–
–	–	–	–	–	–	–	–	–	–	–	–[2]	–[2]	24	No	0	–
			★				★				4	88	279	No	19	–
	–	–		–		–	–	–	–	–	–[2]	–[2]	38	No	0	–
	–	–	★	–		–		–	–	–	4	90	41	No	0	–
★	–	★	★	–		–			–		4	95	117	No	2	–
	–	–	★	–		–	–	–	–	–	4	95	72	No	0	–
	–	–		–		–	–	–	–	–	4	89	51	No	0	–
–	–	–	–	–	–	–	–	–	–	–	–[2]	–[2]	31	No	0	–
	–	–	★	–		–	★				4	91	210	No	0	–
	–			–		★	–	–	–	✕	4	87	173	No	0	–

***Accreditation Status:** 5=Accredited with commendation or with full standards compliance; 4=Accredited with requirements for improvement; 3=Conditional accreditation.

Detailed Ratings for All Areas

See more information on "Key Ratings for Metro Areas" table beginning on page 32

Blue is most favorable
Bold Italic is least favorable
Blank means neither better nor worse than average
"–" means insufficient data

	Death rates for all selected case types				Hospital outcomes: better (★) or worse (×) than average — Adjusted Death rates — Medical Cases											
	Number of cases	Actual death rate (%)	Adjusted death rate (%) (lower is better)	All selected cases	All selected medical cases	Heart attack	Congestive heart failure	Obstructive pulmonary disease	Pneumonia	Respiratory failure and arrest	Septicemia	Stroke	Gastrointestinal hemorrhage	Fluid, electrolyte, & acid-base disorders	Kidney failure
National Average	–	–	12.1	12.1	14.8	21.2	10.6	6.5	16.9	34.4	25.1	18.4	6.7	11.0	20.9
West Virginia *(continued)*															
Bluefield Regional, Bluefield	5,137	11.3	10.1	★	★					★					
Boone, Madison	490	19.2	***19.4***	✖	✖	–				–	✖	✖	–	–	–
Cabell, Huntington[1]	3,636	12.3	***14.0***	✖	✖	✖	×				✖				
Camden - Clark, Parkersburg	6,694	11.6	***13.2***	✖	✖							✖	✖		
Charleston Area, Charleston	13,342	10.7	12.3					✖	×			★		✖	★
City, Martinsburg	2,547	11.1	12.1												
Davis, Elkins	3,576	11.6	***13.9***	✖	✖	✖					✖	×			
Fairmont General, Fairmont	4,147	12.3	12.2										★		
Grant, Petersburg	1,129	12.2	13.2							–					
Greenbrier Valley, Ronceverte	2,690	14.1	***13.5***	✖	✖			×		★		×			×
Hampshire, Romney	382	12.0	12.6			–		–			–	–	–	–	–
Herbert J Thomas, South Charleston	4,939	12.9	***12.9***	✖	×	✖					×		×	×	✖
Jackson General, Ripley	2,156	11.9	12.4			✖	★					✖			–
Jefferson, Ranson	1,113	12.8	***14.7***	✖	✖					–			–	✖	–
Logan General, Logan	3,350	11.4	12.2				★								
Monongalia General, Morgantown	5,059	8.2	10.9	★	★				★				★		
Montgomery General, Montgomery	1,172	12.1	13.2							✖					–
Ohio Valley, Wheeling	2,950	11.9	11.8												★
Plateau, Oak Hill	961	10.7	10.7						★				–	★	–
Pleasant Valley, Point Pleasant	2,564	13.9	***15.7***	✖	✖	✖		✖	✖		–	✖	✖		–
Pocahontas, Marlinton	765	10.6	12.1							–	–		–	★	–
Potomac Valley, Keyser	1,055	12.1	9.3	★	★					★				–	
Preston, Kingwood	589	16.3	***16.3***	✖	✖			–	✖	–	–		–	–	–
Princeton Community, Princeton	4,038	12.2	9.9	★	★		★	★		★	★				★
Putnam General, Hurricane	2,042	14.5	12.6						✖						×
Raleigh General, Beckley	5,091	12.8	10.3	★	★		★		★		★				
Reynolds, Glen Dale	2,250	12.3	***15.4***	✖	✖			✖	✖						✖
St Francis, Charleston	3,474	10.3	9.9	★	★			★	★	★		★			★
St Joseph's, Buckhannon	1,228	14.3	***17.9***	✖	✖		✖	✖	✖	–	–	×			–
St Joseph's, Parkersburg	4,186	10.8	11.2									★	★		
St Luke's, Bluefield	1,322	10.1	10.9				★						–	–	
St Mary's, Huntington	9,461	11.6	***13.1***	✖	✖		✖		✖			✖			
Stonewall Jackson, Weston	2,299	8.5	9.5	★	★		★	★							
Summersville Memorial, Summersville	1,304	12.3	10.1	★	★			★	★						
United, Clarksburg	7,626	10.4	11.1	★	★	✖	★	★	★	★					

Footnotes are on page 350.

Hospital outcomes: better (★) or worse (×) than average											Results of accreditation review on full survey		Other facts			
Adjusted Death rates			Adjusted Adverse outcome rates													
Surgical cases			Surgical cases													
All selected surgical cases	Coronary artery bypass surgery	Large bowel surgery	All selected surgical cases	Coronary artery bypass surgery	Large bowel surgery	Gall bladder removal	Total knee replacement	Total hip replacement	Simple prostatectomy	Carotid endarterectomy	Accreditation status*	Overall evaluation score (higher is better)	Number of beds	Major medical school affiliation?	Number of residents	Computerized drug order system (1 to 5 scale, higher is preferred; see page 23 for details)
2.3	3.8	6.5	7.7	10.3	11.9	7.5	6.7	6.4	5.4	8.2	–	91	161	–	–	–
	–			–					–	–	4	**88**	265	No	0	–
–	–	–	–	–	–	–	–	–	–	–	4	91	38	No	0	–
	–			–				–	–		5	**98**	278	**Yes**	0	–
	–			–						×	4	**88**	214	No	0	–
					✖						4	**87**	765	**Yes**	134	–
	–			–				–	–	–	4	**84**	145	No	0	–
	–	–		–			–	–	✖	–	4	**88**	115	No	0	–
	–	–	★	–			★	–	★		4	**86**	156	No	0	–
–	–	–		–	–	–	–	–	–	–	–[2]	–[2]	51	No	0	–
	–	–		–			–	–	★	–	4	**97**	122	No	6	–
–	–	–	–	–	–	–	–	–	–	–	4	92	17	No	0	–
	–		×	–				–		✖	4	91	212	No	0	–
–	–	–		–		–	–	–	–	–	4	**83**	74	No	0	–
–	–	–		–	–	–	–	–	–	–	4	92	62	No	0	–
	–	–		–		★	–	–		–	4	**82**	132	No	10	–
		★			★		★		✖		4	91	207	No	0	–
–	–	–	–	–	–	–	–	–	–	–	5	**96**	55	No	0	–
	–		★	–		–	–	–	–		4	90	191	No	23	–
–	–	–	–	–	–	–	–	–	–	–	4	91	74	No	0	–
–	–	–		–		–	–	–	–	–	4	93	102	No	0	–
–	–	–	–	–	–	–	–	–	–	–	–[2]	–[2]	27	No	0	–
–	–	–	–	–	–	–	–	–	–	–	4	**88**	42	No	0	–
–	–	–	–	–	–	–	–	–	–	–	4	93	56	No	0	–
	–		★	–				★		–	4	89	188	No	0	–
	–			–			–	–	–	–	4	**87**	64	No	0	–
	–			–	★		✖	–		–	4	90	325	No	8	2
	–	–	✖	–		–	–	–	–	✖	4	92	120	No	0	–
	–		★	–			★		–		4	**96**	121	No	0	–
–	–	–		–	–	–	–	–	–	–	4	**86**	79	No	0	–
	–			–	★			–			4	**84**	259	No	0	–
–	–	–		–	–	–	–	–	–	–	4	**87**	52	No	0	–
	★	✖	✖	★	✖		–			✖	4	91	365	**Yes**	0	–
–	–	–		–	–	–	–	–	–	–	4	**94**	70	No	0	–
–	–	–		–		–	–	–	–	–	–[2]	–[2]	57	No	0	–
	–			–			★		✖		4	93	316	No	22	–

***Accreditation Status:** 5=Accredited with commendation or with full standards compliance; 4=Accredited with requirements for improvement; 3=Conditional accreditation.

Detailed Ratings for All Areas

See more information on "Key Ratings for Metro Areas" table beginning on page 32

Blue is most favorable
Bold Italic is least favorable
Blank means neither better nor worse than average
"–" means insufficient data

	Death rates for all selected case types				Hospital outcomes: better (★) or worse (×) than average — Adjusted Death rates — Medical Cases										
	Number of cases	Actual death rate (%)	Adjusted death rate (%) (lower is better)	All selected cases	All selected medical cases	Heart attack	Congestive heart failure	Obstructive pulmonary disease	Pneumonia	Respiratory failure and arrest	Septicemia	Stroke	Gastrointestinal hemorrhage	Fluid, electrolyte, & acid-base disorders	Kidney failure
National Average	–	–	12.1	12.1	14.8	21.2	10.6	6.5	16.9	34.4	25.1	18.4	6.7	11.0	20.9
West Virginia *(continued)*															
Weirton Medical Center, Weirton	4,461	9.0	11.0	★	★										
Welch Emergency, Welch	720	13.9	14.1	×	×			×			–	×	–		–
West Virginia University, Morgantown	2,393	14.0	***14.8***	✖	✖				✖			×		×	
Wetzel County, New Martinsville	994	15.0	***15.5***	✖	✖				✖	–	–		×	–	–
Wheeling Hospital, Wheeling	6,542	10.9	***13.4***	✖	✖		✖		✖					✖	
Williamson Memorial, Williamson	2,136	8.9	7.6	★	★			★	★	★			–	★	★
Wisconsin															
Milwaukee Area															
Children's of Wisconsin, Wauwatosa	–	–	–	–	–	–	–	–	–	–	–	–	–	–	–
Columbia, Milwaukee	4,766	8.9	11.9												
Froedtert Memorial Lutheran, Milwaukee	3,295	11.7	11.2		★		★							★	
Northwest General, Milwaukee	180	10.6	10.7			–	–	–	–	–	–	–	–	–	–
St Francis, Milwaukee	5,066	9.6	12.1												
St Joseph's, Milwaukee	6,503	12.2	12.6						✖						
St Joseph's Bluemound, Wauwatosa	–	–	–	–	–	–	–	–	–	–	–	–	–	–	–
St Luke's, Milwaukee	17,177	10.4	10.9	★	★	★	★				★			★	★
St Luke's South Shore, Cudahy	–	–	–	–	–	–	–	–	–	–	–	–	–	–	–
St Mary's, Milwaukee	2,394	11.1	12.3												
St Michael, Milwaukee	2,950	13.9	13.0	×									✖	×	✖
Sinai Samaritan, Milwaukee	3,334	11.8	11.1	★	★									★	
West Allis Memorial, West Allis	4,351	12.0	12.8												
Other Areas															
Agnesian, Fond Du Lac[1]	3,155	10.5	12.6												×
All Saints, Racine[1]	5,815	13.4	***16.0***	✖	✖	✖	✖	✖	✖				✖	✖	✖
Appleton Medical Center, Appleton	3,625	10.0	11.9				✖		★	–				★	×
Aurora, Kenosha	265	9.4	16.1			–	–	–		–	–	–	–	–	–
Aurora of Manitowoc County, Two Rivers[1]	750	15.3	***16.3***	✖	✖	✖	×	–		–				–	–
Baldwin Area, Baldwin	482	11.2	12.1			–				–	–	–	–	–	–
Barron Medical Center, Barron	584	13.4	***16.7***	✖	✖			–	✖	–	–		–	✖	–
Bay Area, Marinette	2,545	13.2	12.7			✖		×			★			×	
Beaver Dam Community, Beaver Dam	1,509	11.3	12.7												–
Bellin, Green Bay	4,051	6.3	10.9	★	★				★	★					
Beloit Memorial, Beloit	2,652	12.2	***15.5***	✖	✖	✖	✖		✖	✖	✖	×			
Berlin Memorial, Berlin	1,336	9.7	12.8				✖			–					

Footnotes are on page 350.

Hospital outcomes: better (★) or worse (×) than average											Results of accreditation review on full survey		Other facts			
Adjusted Death rates			Adjusted Adverse outcome rates													
Surgical cases			Surgical cases													
All selected surgical cases	Coronary artery bypass surgery	Large bowel surgery	All selected surgical cases	Coronary artery bypass surgery	Large bowel surgery	Gall bladder removal	Total knee replacement	Total hip replacement	Simple prostatectomy	Carotid endarterectomy	Accreditation status*	Overall evaluation score (higher is better)	Number of beds	Major medical school affiliation?	Number of residents	Computerized drug order system (1 to 5 scale, higher is preferred; see page 23 for details)
2.3	3.8	6.5	7.7	10.3	11.9	7.5	6.7	6.4	5.4	8.2	–	91	161	–	–	–
	–		★	–		★	★	–	–	★	4	90	205	No	0	–
–	–	–	–	–	–	–	–	–	–	–	–[2]	–[2]	49	No	0	–
✖		–	✖			–			–		4	93	381	**Yes**	232	–
–	–	–	–	–	–	–	–	–	–	–	4	**94**	39	No	0	–
											5	**97**	252	No	21	–
–	–	–	–	–	–	–	–	–	–	–	4	93	76	No	0	–
–	–	–	–	–	–	–	–	–	–	–	4	**94**	222	–	5	–
★			★			★	★				4	**86**	328	**Yes**	0	–
						–		–	–		4	**98**	472	**Yes**	0	–
–	–	–	–	–	–	–	–	–	–	–	–[2]	–[2]	98	No	1	–
✖	✖	★	✖	✖	★			✖			4	91	212	No	0	–
											4	90	445	No	19	–
–	–	–	–	–	–	–	–	–	–	–	–[2]	–[2]	72	–	0	–
★		★			★		★				4	93	747	No	63	–
–	–	–	–	–	–	–	–	–	–	–	–[2]	–[2]	–	–	–	–
		★		✖		–			–	–	4	**83**	241	**Yes**	0	–
							–	–	✖	–	4	92	179	**Yes**	0	–
	✖			×	★	–			–	–	4	92	255	No	72	–
	–			–					★		4	**96**	147	No	0	–
★	–	★	★	–	★			–		–	4	**85**	90	No	0	–
						×					4	93	215	No	0	–
										★	–[2]	–[2]	146	No	0	–
–	–	–	–	–	–	–	–	–	–	–	4	**95**	44	No	–	–
–	–	–		–	–	–	–	–	–	–	4	**94**	53	No	0	–
–	–	–	–	–	–	–	–	–	–	–	–[2]	–[2]	27	No	0	2
–	–	–		–	–		–	–	–	–	–[2]	–[2]	92	No	0	–
	–	×		–		★		✖		★	4	92	115	No	0	–
	–		★	–		–	★	–	★	–	–[2]	–[2]	93	No	0	–
									★		4	**86**	179	No	0	–
	–			–			★	–	–	–	4	**82**	124	No	0	–
	–		★	–				–	–		4	91	61	No	0	–

***Accreditation Status:** 5=Accredited with commendation or with full standards compliance; 4=Accredited with requirements for improvement; 3=Conditional accreditation.

Detailed Ratings for All Areas

See more information on "Key Ratings for Metro Areas" table beginning on page 32

Blue is most favorable
Bold Italic is least favorable
Blank means neither better nor worse than average
"–" means insufficient data

	Death rates for all selected case types			Hospital outcomes: better (★) or worse (×) than average											
				Adjusted Death rates											
				Medical Cases											
	Number of cases	Actual death rate (%)	Adjusted death rate (%) (lower is better)	All selected cases	All selected medical cases	Heart attack	Congestive heart failure	Obstructive pulmonary disease	Pneumonia	Respiratory failure and arrest	Septicemia	Stroke	Gastrointestinal hemorrhage	Fluid, electrolyte, & acid-base disorders	Kidney failure
National Average	–	–	12.1	12.1	14.8	21.2	10.6	6.5	16.9	34.4	25.1	18.4	6.7	11.0	20.9
Wisconsin *(continued)*															
Other Areas *(continued)*															
Black River Falls Memorial, Black River Falls	794	8.7	9.6	★	★		★	★		–	–			–	✖
Bloomer Memorial, Bloomer[1]	281	14.6	14.6			–	×	–		–	–	×	–	–	–
Boscobel Area, Boscobel	251	11.2	12.5					–		–	–	–	–	–	–
Burnett, Grantsburg	457	10.1	12.5			–		–		–	–	×	–		–
Calumet, Chilton	573	14.0	***16.6***	✖	✖	✖			✖	–	–		–		–
Columbus Community, Columbus	1,081	9.6	11.1			★		–		–					–
Community, Menomonee Falls	2,919	11.3	***14.3***	✖	✖	×		✖	✖			✖			✖
Community, Oconto Falls	675	11.3	12.4					–		–	–		–		–
Cumberland Memorial, Cumberland[1]	493	7.3	8.5	★	★			–		–	–		–	–	–
Divine Savior, Portage	1,296	12.5	13.0							✖		✖			–
Door County, Sturgeon Bay	1,306	10.0	12.8							–	–			–	–
Elmbrook, Brookfield	2,920	10.9	***13.7***	✖	✖		×		✖		✖				
Flambeau, Park Falls	696	18.4	***17.0***	✖	✖	×	✖		✖		✖		–	–	–
Fort Atkinson Memorial, Fort Atkinson	2,121	12.7	***13.8***	✖	✖	✖	×							✖	–
Franciscan Skemp, La Crosse	2,915	9.9	12.7							✖					
Good Samaritan, Merrill	722	8.4	7.9	★	★		★	★		–	–		–		–
Grant Regional, Lancaster	450	15.3	14.7	×	✖		✖	–	✖	–	–		–		–
Gundersen Lutheran, La Crosse	5,097	10.2	12.3				×					✖	★		
Hartford Memorial, Hartford	963	12.8	12.3					–		–					–
Hayward Area, Hayward[1]	696	12.6	11.9					–			–		★	–	–
Holy Family, Manitowoc	3,188	11.6	***13.5***	✖	✖	✖	×							★	×
Holy Family, New Richmond	464	8.6	12.2			–		–		–	–	✖	–		–
Howard Young, Woodruff	2,369	7.3	9.9	★	★							★			
Hudson Hospital, Hudson	465	11.0	12.8					–		–	–		–	–	–
Indianhead, Shell Lake	448	10.3	13.2			×				–	–	–	–	–	–
Kenosha Hospital, Kenosha	3,636	10.5	12.0												
Lakeland, Elkhorn	1,952	13.9	***14.5***	✖	✖	✖		✖		✖		✖			–
Lakeview, Rice Lake	1,675	10.6	***14.6***	✖	✖			✖		–			✖		–
Langlade, Antigo	1,265	10.1	11.1						★						–
Luther, Eau Claire	4,612	9.8	11.7			★	✖		×		★				×
Memorial, Ashland	1,524	10.8	13.3					✖		–		✖			–
Memorial, Burlington	1,825	12.8	12.7			✖						✖	×		
Memorial, Neillsville	523	16.4	13.7					–		–	–		–		
Memorial Community, Edgerton	561	11.9	13.6				✖	–		–			–	–	–

Footnotes are on page 350.

Hospital outcomes: better (★) or worse (✕) than average											Results of accreditation review on full survey		Other facts			
Adjusted Death rates			Adjusted Adverse outcome rates													
Surgical cases			Surgical cases													
All selected surgical cases	Coronary artery bypass surgery	Large bowel surgery	All selected surgical cases	Coronary artery bypass surgery	Large bowel surgery	Gall bladder removal	Total knee replacement	Total hip replacement	Simple prostatectomy	Carotid endarterectomy	Accreditation status*	Overall evaluation score (higher is better)	Number of beds	Major medical school affiliation?	Number of residents	Computerized drug order system (1 to 5 scale, higher is preferred; see page 23 for details)
2.3	3.8	6.5	7.7	10.3	11.9	7.5	6.7	6.4	5.4	8.2	–	91	161	–	–	–
–	–	–	★	–	–	–	–	–	–	–	4	**88**	38	No	0	–
–	–	–	–	–	–	–	–	–	–	–	4	**94**	32	No	0	–
–	–	–	–	–	–	–	–	–	–	–	–[2]	–[2]	44	No	0	–
–	–	–	–	–	–	–	–	–	–	–	–[2]	–[2]	17	No	0	–
–	–	–		–	–	–	–	–	–	–	4	**87**	26	No	0	–
–	–	–		–	–	–		–	–	–	4	**97**	34	No	0	–
	–		★	–						★	4	**96**	142	No	0	–
–	–	–		–	–	–	–	–	–	–	–[2]	–[2]	27	No	0	–
–	–	–	–	–	–	–	–	–	–	–	4	**94**	40	No	0	–
–	–	–	★	–	–	–	–	–	–	–	4	**99**	42	No	0	–
	–	–		–		–	✕	–	–	–	4	**84**	45	No	0	–
	–			–		★	★				4	**86**	136	No	0	–
–	–	–		–	–	✕	–	–	–	–	4	**85**	42	No	0	–
	–			–				–		–	–[2]	–[2]	74	No	0	–
	–			–			★			–	4	**84**	345	No	–	–
–	–	–		–	–	–	–	–	–	–	4	**87**	63	No	0	–
–	–	–	★	–	–	–	–	–	–	–	4	**96**	28	No	0	–
	✕		★				★			★	4	**87**	277	No	0	–
–	–	–		–	–	–	–	–	–	–	5	**99**	71	No	0	–
–	–	–	–	–	–	–	–	–	–	–	4	**95**	41	No	0	–
	–		★	–							4	**85**	176	No	0	–
–	–	–	★	–	–	–	–	–	–	–	–[2]	–[2]	20	No	0	1
★	–		★	–			★	★			4	**95**	65	No	0	–
–	–	–	–	–	–	–	–	–	–	–	4	**95**	39	No	0	2
–	–	–	–	–	–	–	–	–	–	–	4	**95**	49	No	0	–
			★				★	★			4	89	143	No	0	–
	–	–		–		–		–	–	–	4	**96**	78	No	0	–
	–	–		–		–			–	–	4	93	69	No	0	–
	–	–		–		–	–	–	–	–	4	91	43	No	0	–
								★			4	**87**	179	No	0	–
	–	–		–	–	–	✕	–		–	4	**88**	101	No	0	–
★	–		★	–		–	★	–	–		4	**96**	87	No	0	–
–	–	–	–	–	–	–	–	–	–	–	–[2]	–[2]	29	No	0	–
–	–	–		–	–	–	–	–	–	–	–[2]	–[2]	64	No	0	–

***Accreditation Status:** 5=Accredited with commendation or with full standards compliance; 4=Accredited with requirements for improvement; 3=Conditional accreditation.

Detailed Ratings for All Areas

See more information on "Key Ratings for Metro Areas" table beginning on page 32

Blue is most favorable
Bold Italic is least favorable
Blank means neither better nor worse than average
"–" means insufficient data

	Death rates for all selected case types			Hospital outcomes: better (★) or worse (✕) than average — Adjusted Death rates — Medical Cases											
	Number of cases	Actual death rate (%)	Adjusted death rate (%) (lower is better)	All selected cases	All selected medical cases	Heart attack	Congestive heart failure	Obstructive pulmonary disease	Pneumonia	Respiratory failure and arrest	Septicemia	Stroke	Gastrointestinal hemorrhage	Fluid, electrolyte, & acid-base disorders	Kidney failure
National Average	–	–	12.1	12.1	14.8	21.2	10.6	6.5	16.9	34.4	25.1	18.4	6.7	11.0	20.9
Wisconsin *(continued)*															
Other Areas *(continued)*															
Memorial Health Center, Medford[1]	703	11.1	11.1					–		–	–		–	–	–
Memorial of Iowa County, Dodgeville	800	13.4	12.8							–	–				✖
Memorial of Lafayette County, Darlington	287	14.6	15.1				–	–		–	–	–	–	–	–
Mercy, Janesville[1]	3,452	11.9	13.0	✕	✕							✖			
Mercy, Oshkosh[1]	3,963	9.4	10.4	★	★	★			★		★				
Meriter, Madison	4,936	9.9	11.8											★	
Mile Bluff, Mauston[1]	1,041	9.6	11.8				✕			–	–				–
Monroe Clinic, Monroe	2,166	8.9	11.9			✕									
Myrtle Werth, Menomonie[1]	1,083	12.0	11.6					–							
New London Family, New London	859	12.2	13.0					–		–		✕	–	–	–
Oconomowoc Memorial, Oconomowoc	1,518	10.5	12.7												
Oconto Memorial, Oconto	150	19.3	***18.0***	✖	✖	–	–	–		–	–	–	–	–	–
Osceola Medical Center, Osceola	258	19.8	***21.2***	✖	✖	–	✖	–	✖	–	✖	–	–	–	–
Osseo Area, Osseo[1]	54	11.1	12.6			–	–	–	–	–	–	–	–	–	–
Prairie Du Chien Memorial, Prairie Du Chien	910	13.5	13.6							✖					–
Reedsburg Area, Reedsburg	808	7.8	10.4			–		★	★	–	–		–	–	–
Richland Hospital, Richland Center	965	10.1	11.0							–	–	★			–
Ripon Medical Center, Ripon	771	11.9	12.9							–	–		–	–	–
River Falls Area, River Falls	558	13.4	***15.2***	✖	✖		✕	–	✕	–	–		–	–	–
Riverside, Waupaca	1,038	19.0	***18.4***	✖	✖	✖	✖	–	✖	✖	✖	✖			–
Riverview, Wisconsin Rapids	1,753	10.7	***13.7***	✖	✖				✖						–
Rusk County, Ladysmith[1]	577	11.8	12.1							–		✕	–	★	–
Sacred Heart, Eau Claire	3,020	9.2	11.5												
Sacred Heart, Tomahawk	478	13.8	***15.8***	✖	✖	–		–	✖	–			–	–	–
Sacred Heart - St Mary's, Rhinelander[1]	1,824	9.4	12.5									✖			–
St Catherine's, Kenosha	1,344	16.1	***15.2***	✖	✖			✖	✖			✕			
St Clare, Baraboo	1,293	11.1	11.7												–
St Croix Regional, St Croix Falls	970	8.8	9.3	★	★			–	★	–					
St Elizabeth, Appleton	2,807	10.0	10.8	★	★	★		★							
St Joseph's, Chippewa Falls	1,487	11.9	11.9												
St Joseph's, Marshfield	6,818	9.1	12.1				✕								
St Joseph's, West Bend	2,008	9.4	10.5	★	★						★				
St Mary's, Green Bay	2,683	9.4	13.3	✕	✖				✖			✕		★	
St Mary's, Superior	952	12.7	***15.0***	✖	✖		✕	–	✖		–		–	–	–

Footnotes are on page 350.

Hospital outcomes: better (★) or worse (×) than average											Results of accreditation review on full survey		Other facts			
Adjusted Death rates			Adjusted Adverse outcome rates													
Surgical cases			Surgical cases													
All selected surgical cases	Coronary artery bypass surgery	Large bowel surgery	All selected surgical cases	Coronary artery bypass surgery	Large bowel surgery	Gall bladder removal	Total knee replacement	Total hip replacement	Simple prostatectomy	Carotid endarterectomy	Accreditation status*	Overall evaluation score (higher is better)	Number of beds	Major medical school affiliation?	Number of residents	Computerized drug order system (1 to 5 scale, higher is preferred; see page 23 for details)
2.3	3.8	6.5	7.7	10.3	11.9	7.5	6.7	6.4	5.4	8.2	–	91	161	–	–	–
–	–	–	–	–	–	–	–	–	–	–	4	91	49	No	0	–
	–		★	–	★	–	–	–	–	–	4	97	40	No	0	–
–	–	–	–	–	–	–	–	–	–	–	–[2]	–[2]	28	No	0	–
	–		★					★	–		4	87	192	No	12	–
			✖	✖		✖	×			★	4	86	175	No	0	–
				×					★		4	91	369	Yes	4	–
–	–	–		–	–	–	–	–	–	–	4	93	37	No	0	–
	–			–							4	96	117	No	0	–
–	–	–	★	–	–	–	–	–	–	–	4	91	55	No	0	–
–	–	–	★	–	–	–	–	–	–	–	4	97	39	No	0	–
	–			–	★	×		–	–		4	92	72	No	0	–
–	–	–	–	–	–	–	–	–	–	–	–[2]	–[2]	17	No	0	–
–	–	–	–	–	–	–	–	–	–	–	–[2]	–[2]	19	No	0	–
–	–	–	–	–	–	–	–	–	–	–	–[2]	–[2]	16	No	0	–
–	–	–		–	–	–	–	–	–	–	4	92	43	No	0	–
–	–	–	★	–	–	–	–	–	–	–	4	91	38	No	0	–
–	–	–	–	–	–	–	–	–	–	–	4	92	38	No	0	–
–	–	–	★	–		–	–	–	–	–	4	95	29	No	0	–
–	–	–		–	–	–	–	–	–	–	4	91	31	No	0	2
–	–	–		–	–	–	–	–	–	–	4	87	32	No	0	–
	–			–		✖		–	–	–	4	96	79	No	0	–
–	–	–	–	–	–	–	–	–	–	–	–[2]	–[2]	35	No	0	–
	–		★	–			★	★			4	94	179	No	0	–
–	–	–	–	–	–	–	–	–	–	–	–[2]	–[2]	60	No	–	–
	–	–		–					–	–	4	94	53	No	0	–
	–	–		–		–	–	–	–	–	–[2]	–[2]	114	No	0	–
	–	–		–		–		–	–	–	4	91	82	No	0	–
–	–	–		–	–	–	–	–	–	–	4	95	69	No	0	–
			★		★			★	★		4	87	166	Yes	0	–
	–	–		–		–		–	–	–	4	92	127	No	0	–
						×		✖			4	92	524	Yes	0	–
	–			–		–		–	–	–	4	89	103	No	0	–
	–		★	–			★		–	★	4	83	119	No	0	–
–	–	–	★	–	–	–	–	–	★	–	4	92	42	No	0	1

***Accreditation Status:** 5=Accredited with commendation or with full standards compliance; 4=Accredited with requirements for improvement; 3=Conditional accreditation.

Detailed Ratings for All Areas

See more information on "Key Ratings for Metro Areas" table beginning on page 32

Blue is most favorable
Bold Italic is least favorable
Blank means neither better nor worse than average
"–" means insufficient data

	Death rates for all selected case types			Hospital outcomes: better (★) or worse (×) than average — Adjusted Death rates — Medical Cases											
	Number of cases	Actual death rate (%)	Adjusted death rate (%) (lower is better)	All selected cases	All selected medical cases	Heart attack	Congestive heart failure	Obstructive pulmonary disease	Pneumonia	Respiratory failure and arrest	Septicemia	Stroke	Gastrointestinal hemorrhage	Fluid, electrolyte, & acid-base disorders	Kidney failure
National Average	–	–	12.1	12.1	14.8	21.2	10.6	6.5	16.9	34.4	25.1	18.4	6.7	11.0	20.9
Wisconsin *(continued)*															
Other Areas *(continued)*															
St Mary's Ozaukee, Mequon	2,089	13.1	***14.0***	✖	✖		✖			×					
St Marys, Madison	6,768	9.7	12.5					✖				✖	✖		
St Michaels, Stevens Point	2,163	12.3	***15.0***	✖	✖				✖	✖		×			×
St Nicholas, Sheboygan	2,052	13.4	***15.8***	✖	✖		✖			–		✖			×
St Vincent, Green Bay	4,997	9.9	10.7	★	★				★						
Sauk Prairie, Prairie Du Sac[1]	1,232	7.3	10.7					✖	★	–				–	–
Shawano Medical Center, Shawano	1,416	15.0	***13.9***	✖	✖		×						✖		✖
Sheboygan Memorial, Sheboygan	1,926	13.3	***17.0***	✖	✖		✖	✖	✖	–		✖	×	✖	×
Southwest, Platteville	547	15.9	***18.2***	✖	✖		✖	✖	×	–	–	✖	–	–	–
Spooner Health System, Spooner	540	13.7	***14.8***	✖	×			–		–	–	✖	–		–
Stoughton Hospital, Stoughton[1]	808	13.7	***15.6***	✖	✖		✖			–	–	×	–		–
Theda Clark, Neenah	3,824	7.2	10.8	★	★		★			×	★		★		
Tomah Memorial, Tomah	567	14.5	***14.9***	✖	✖			–	×	–	–		–	–	–
University of Wisconsin, Madison[1]	3,466	8.9	9.4	★	★	★	★		★					★	★
Valley View, Plymouth[1]	636	11.9	13.2					–		–	–		–	–	–
Vernon, Viroqua	1,054	10.5	12.3					–		–		×			
Victory, Stanley	567	10.4	10.8					–		–			–	★	–
Watertown Memorial, Watertown	1,091	12.6	12.8							–					
Waukesha Memorial, Waukesha	5,554	10.6	11.5				★		✖	✖					★
Waupun Memorial, Waupun	686	11.5	13.9			×		–		–	–	✖	–	–	–
Wausau Hospital, Wausau	5,396	8.6	11.2			★	✖								
Wyoming															
Campbell County, Gillette	684	10.7	10.5								–		–		–
Community, Torrington	379	12.9	***15.6***	✖	×	–		✖		–	–	–	–	–	–
Crook County, Sundance[1]	91	12.1	13.8			–	–	–	–	–	–	–	–	–	–
Evanston Regional, Evanston	302	13.9	10.8			–			★	–	–		–	–	–
Hot Springs County, Thermopolis	580	10.3	12.6			–		–		–	–		–		–
Ivinson, Laramie	825	9.5	***14.8***	✖	✖	–		–	✖	–	–		–	–	–
Johnson County, Buffalo	297	9.4	11.2			–	–	–		–	–	–	–	–	–
Lander Valley, Lander	712	12.4	13.9		×	–		–		–	✖		–	★	–
Memorial - Sweetwater County, Rock Springs	881	13.1	***14.5***	✖	✖	×				✖					–
Memorial of Carbon County, Rawlins	596	9.4	11.5			–		–	★	–	–	✖	–	–	–
Memorial of Converse County, Douglas	263	11.8	***17.1***	✖	×	–	–	–	–	–	–	–	–	–	–

Footnotes are on page 350.

Hospital outcomes: better (★) or worse (×) than average											Results of accreditation review on full survey		Other facts			
Adjusted Death rates			Adjusted Adverse outcome rates													
Surgical cases			Surgical cases													
All selected surgical cases	Coronary artery bypass surgery	Large bowel surgery	All selected surgical cases	Coronary artery bypass surgery	Large bowel surgery	Gall bladder removal	Total knee replacement	Total hip replacement	Simple prostatectomy	Carotid endarterectomy	Accreditation status*	Overall evaluation score (higher is better)	Number of beds	Major medical school affiliation?	Number of residents	Computerized drug order system (1 to 5 scale, higher is preferred; see page 23 for details)
2.3	3.8	6.5	7.7	10.3	11.9	7.5	6.7	6.4	5.4	8.2	–	91	161	–	–	–
×	–			–		–	★		–	–	4	**86**	82	No	0	–
		★			★		×			★	4	91	287	**Yes**	0	–
×	–			–		×		★	–	–	4	91	114	No	0	–
×	–			–					–	–	4	**87**	185	No	0	–
★	–		★	–	★	★					4	91	285	No	0	–
★	–	–	★	–	★	–			–	★	4	**95**	36	No	0	–
–	–	–		–		–	–	–	–	–	4	**95**	46	No	0	–
	–		★	–	★	–		★		–	4	90	157	No	0	–
–	–	–		–	–	–	–	–	–	–	4	**96**	33	No	0	–
–	–	–	–	–	–	–	–	–	–	–	4	**94**	46	No	0	–
–	–	–		–		–	–	–	–	–	4	**94**	38	No	0	–
	–		×				×		★		4	90	216	No	0	–
–	–	–	–	–	–	–	–	–	–	–	4	**94**	45	No	0	–
	×		×	×					–		4	92	467	**Yes**	436	–
–	–	–		–	–	–	–	–	–	–	4	91	92	No	0	–
–	–	–		–	–	–		–	–	–	–[2]	–[2]	17	No	0	–
–	–	–	–	–	–	–	–	–	–	–	–[2]	–[2]	41	No	0	–
	–	–				–		–	–	–	4	91	45	No	0	–
								★	×		4	**81**	288	No	0	–
–	–	–		–	–	–	–	–	–	–	4	**94**	30	No	0	–
★		★	★		★					★	5	**94**	218	No	0	–
–	–	–		–	–	–	–	–	–	–	4	92	76	No	0	–
–	–	–	–	–	–	–	–	–	–	–	4	**87**	36	No	0	–
–	–	–	–	–	–	–	–	–	–	–	–[2]	–[2]	16	No	0	–
–	–	–	–	–	–	–	–	–	–	–	4	93	38	No	0	–
–	–	–	–	–	–	–	–	–	–	–	4	92	49	No	0	–
–	–	–		–	–			–	–	–	4	**94**	72	No	0	–
–	–	–	–	–	–	–	–	–	–	–	4	92	15	No	0	–
–	–	–	–	–	–	–	–	–	–	–	4	93	81	No	0	–
–	–	–		–	–	–	–	–	–	–	4	**94**	99	No	0	–
–	–	–	–	–	–	–	–	–	–	–	–[2]	–[2]	35	No	0	–
–	–	–	–	–	–	–	–	–	–	–	–[2]	–[2]	34	No	0	–

***Accreditation Status:** 5=Accredited with commendation or with full standards compliance; 4=Accredited with requirements for improvement; 3=Conditional accreditation.

Detailed Ratings for All Areas

See more information on "Key Ratings for Metro Areas" table beginning on page 32

Blue is most favorable
Bold Italic is least favorable
Blank means neither better nor worse than average
"–" means insufficient data

	Death rates for all selected case types			Hospital outcomes: better (★) or worse (×) than average — Adjusted Death rates — Medical Cases											
	Number of cases	Actual death rate (%)	Adjusted death rate (%) (lower is better)	All selected cases	All selected medical cases	Heart attack	Congestive heart failure	Obstructive pulmonary disease	Pneumonia	Respiratory failure and arrest	Septicemia	Stroke	Gastrointestinal hemorrhage	Fluid, electrolyte, & acid-base disorders	Kidney failure
National Average	–	–	12.1	12.1	14.8	21.2	10.6	6.5	16.9	34.4	25.1	18.4	6.7	11.0	20.9
Wyoming *(continued)*															
Memorial of Sheridan County, Sheridan	1,328	10.7	11.8												–
North Big Horn, Lovell	201	15.4	16.4	×	×	–		–		–	–	–	–	–	–
Platte County, Wheatland[1]	527	13.3	***19.0***	✖	✖	–	✖		✖	–	–	–	✖		–
Powell Hospital, Powell[1]	359	10.6	13.5			×		–		–	–		–	–	–
Riverton Memorial, Riverton	902	10.1	10.5												★
St Johns, Jackson[1]	526	4.9	**8.2**	★	★	–	★	–		–	–		–	–	–
South Lincoln, Kemmerer	81	13.6	19.8	×	×	–	–	–	–	–	–	–	–	–	–
Star Valley, Afton	102	6.9	10.0			–	–	–	–	–	–	–	–	–	–
United, Cheyenne	3,094	12.1	***13.4***	✖	✖				✖						
Washakie, Worland	561	10.7	12.9			✖		–		–	–	★	–		–
West Park, Cody[1]	668	7.5	11.4							–	–		–	–	–
Weston County, Newcastle	164	12.2	12.8			–	–	–		–	–	–	–	–	–
Wyoming, Casper	3,275	10.3	***13.3***	✖	×		×					✖			

Footnotes:

[1] Some data for this hospital may reflect information from a larger entity or multiple hospitals.

[2] Researchers could not determine information for this item from the data sources that were used.

Notes on Naming and Identifying Hospitals

The Metro Areas and All Areas tables in this book are based on several data sources.

The data on mortality and adverse outcomes come from Medicare records of patient discharge information for the years ending September 30, 1997, 1998, and 1999. Mortality and adverse outcomes information is shown for a hospital only for years for which the hospital's Medicare identification number shown on the "Providers of Services" (POS) file Medicare issued in July 2001 is the same as the Medicare hospital identification number shown on the Medicare records of patient discharges. The data on medical school affiliation come from the Medicare POS file. The data on the results of accreditation surveys conducted by the Joint Commission on the Accreditation of Healthcare Organizations (JCAHO) come from information provided by JCAHO in September 2001. The data on bed size and number of residents come from hospital industry data sources that we believe to be reliable or from the Medicare POS file if not available from our other industry sources. The physicians ratings data come from our own physician survey, in which the names we used to identify hospitals were drawn from industry data sources that we believe to be reliable.

Readers need to be aware that hospitals change names, locations, and ownership over time. It is possible that a hospital listed in this book under a given name was operating under a different name and/or ownership and/or at a different location when the data reported here were collected. Even if there have been no changes of this kind, it is likely that the hospitals have changed their level of performance since the data-collection period, and performance changes are probably even more likely if there have been changes in name, location, or ownership.

We had to apply some judgment in dealing with name, location, and possible ownership differences. We had two main objectives: first, to use the most current name we could get for each hospital to help readers identify the hospitals, and, second, to exclude data in cases where changes were significant enough that in our judgment there had ceased to be a relationship between the hospital for which we had data and the hospital name and location that would be listed in the book. Where we found what we judged to be a significant name difference for a hospital among our data sources, we called the hospital to check on current name and location. We also sent letters to hospital administrators noting the data and the identification numbers within those sources that we were missing to match hospital names with the data. We asked the administrators for corrections or updates. This entire process resulted in many updates of names and the elimination of some data.

Even where there may have been no change in name, we sometimes found differences among our data sources in the specific name given to a hospital at a single location. In some cases, one source might have been reporting on a larger or smaller unit than another. For instance, the data from one source might be for a hospital and rehabilitation center while another source might be reporting only on the hospital. So long as each source appeared to be reporting on an entity that included the same acute-care hospital, we reported the data under what appeared to be an acute-care hospital name. But we added a note if there appeared to be differences in the inclusiveness of the facility or facilities referred to by the different data sources.

Hospital outcomes: better (★) or worse (×) than average											Results of accreditation review on full survey		Other facts			
Adjusted Death rates			Adjusted Adverse outcome rates													
Surgical cases			Surgical cases													
All selected surgical cases	Coronary artery bypass surgery	Large bowel surgery	All selected surgical cases	Coronary artery bypass surgery	Large bowel surgery	Gall bladder removal	Total knee replacement	Total hip replacement	Simple prostatectomy	Carotid endarterectomy	Accreditation status*	Overall evaluation score (higher is better)	Number of beds	Major medical school affiliation?	Number of residents	Computerized drug order system (1 to 5 scale, higher is preferred; see page 23 for details)
2.3	3.8	6.5	7.7	10.3	11.9	7.5	6.7	6.4	5.4	8.2	–	91	161	–	–	–
–	–	–	★	–	–	–	–	–	–	–	4	**83**	60	No	0	–
–	–	–	–	–	–	–	–	–	–	–	–[2]	–[2]	13	No	0	–
–	–	–	–	–	–	–	–	–	–	–	4	93	43	No	0	–
–	–	–	–	–	–	–	–	–	–	–	4	93	30	No	0	–
–	–	–	–	–	–	–	–	–	–	–	4	89	59	No	0	–
–	–	–	★	–	–	–	–	–	–	–	4	**87**	42	No	0	–
–	–	–	–	–	–	–	–	–	–	–	–[2]	–[2]	16	No	3	–
–	–	–	–	–	–	–	–	–	–	–	–[2]	–[2]	12	No	0	–
	✖			×					–	–	4	**83**	178	No	0	–
–	–	–	–	–	–	–	–	–	–	–	4	**87**	30	No	0	–
–	–	–	★	–	–	–	★	–	–	–	4	**98**	32	No	0	–
–	–	–	–	–	–	–	–	–	–	–	–[2]	–[2]	23	No	0	–
		×					★		–		4	91	201	No	0	–

***Accreditation Status:** 5=Accredited with commendation or with full standards compliance; 4=Accredited with requirements for improvement; 3=Conditional accreditation.

Appendix A:

A Few Nationally Recognized Centers for Difficult Cases

Our survey or physicians included the following open-ended request of the doctors: "If there are any major kinds of cases in which you would want your loved one to get care at a medical center in some other part of the country, please tell us below the type(s) of cases and the name(s) and location(s) of the facility or facilities you would recommend."

This was a very informal approach, and compiling a list of medical centers for you from the named facilities was a judgmental process for us. Since some types of diseases were mentioned only a few times, we listed some centers with only a few mentions; for frequently mentioned diseases, the threshhold was higher.

For the most part, the following list addresses broad categories of cases. You might want a facility that has expertise in your particular condition, defined much more narrowly. Still, you might find it useful to use one of the listed facilities as a starting point for getting more specific referrals.

There are many types of cases that are not covered. That is simply because we got too few mentions of those types to be useful.

We include this informal list because we think you might find it a useful addition to the much more quantitative information presented elsewhere in this book.

- **Aneurysm, abdominal or thoracic**—Methodist Hospital, Houston, TX (Baylor College of Medicine)
- **Biliary diseases**—Johns Hopkins, Baltimore, MD
- **Bone marrow transplant**—Fred Hutchinson Cancer Research Center (University of Washington Medical Center), Seattle, WA
- **Cancer, pancreas**—Johns Hopkins, Baltimore, MD
- **Cancer, prostate**—Johns Hopkins, Baltimore, MD
- **Cancer, various types**—*Mentioned most often*: Memorial Sloan-Kettering, New York, NY; M. D. Anderson Cancer Center (University of Texas), Houston, TX. *Also mentioned often*: Dana Farber Cancer Institute (Brigham and Women's and Children's hospitals), Boston, MA; Mayo Clinic (Saint Marys and Rochester Methodist hospitals), Rochester, MN; Johns Hopkins, Baltimore, MD
- **Cardiac surgery**—*Mentioned most often*: Cleveland Clinic Foundation, Cleveland, OH. *Also mentioned often*: New York Presbyterian, New York, NY
- **Cardiology/cardiac care**—*Mentioned most often*: Cleveland Clinic Foundation, Cleveland, OH. *Also mentioned often*: New York Presbyterian, New York, NY; Mayo Clinic (Saint Marys and Rochester Methodist hospitals), Rochester, MN; Texas Heart Institute (Saint Luke's Episcopal Hospital), Houston, TX
- **Developmental problems**—NIH National Institute of Child Health and Human Development, Bethesda, MD
- **Difficult diagnostic problems**—Mayo Clinic (Saint Marys and Rochester Methodist hospitals), Rochester, MN
- **Eye care**—Johns Hopkins, Baltimore, MD
- **Neurology**—Mayo Clinic (Saint Marys and Rochester Methodist hospitals), Rochester, MN; Johns Hopkins, Baltimore, MD
- **Neurosurgery**—*Mentioned most often*: Johns Hopkins, Baltimore, MD. *Also mentioned often*: Massachusetts General, Boston, MA; Mayo Clinic (Saint Marys and Rochester Methodist hospitals), Rochester, MN; UCLA Medical Center, Los Angeles, CA
- **Orthopedics**—Harborview, Seattle, WA; Hospital for Special Surgery, New York, NY
- **Pancreatic disease**—Johns Hopkins, Baltimore, MD
- **Pediatrics, cardiac care and surgery**—Children's Hospital Boston, Boston, MA
- **Pediatrics, neurosurgery**—Johns Hopkins, Baltimore, MD
- **Pediatrics, various cases**—Children's Hospital Boston, Boston, MA; Children's Hospital of Philadelphia, Philadelphia, PA; Johns Hopkins, Baltimore, MD; Texas Children's Hospital, Houston, TX; St. Jude, Memphis, TN
- **Pulmonary disease and asthma**—National Jewish, Denver, CO
- **Rare diseases**—Mayo Clinic (Saint Marys and Rochester Methodist hospitals), Rochester, MN; Johns Hopkins, Baltimore, MD
- **Transplants, liver**—UPMC Presbyterian, Pittsburgh, PA
- **Transplants, various types**—*Mentioned most often*: UPMC Presbyterian, Pittsburgh, PA; Stanford Hospital, Stanford, CA; UCLA Medical Center, Los Angeles, CA; Duke University Hospital, Durham, NC
- **Urology cases**—Johns Hopkins, Baltimore, MD; Cleveland Clinic Foundation, Cleveland, OH
- **Vascular surgery**—Cleveland Clinic Foundation, Cleveland, OH; Mayo Clinic (Saint Marys and Rochester Methodist hospitals), Rochester, MN

The following hospitals were mentioned by a large number of doctors for a wide variety of types of cases—Mayo Clinic (Saint Marys and Rochester Methodist hospitals), Rochester, MN; Johns Hopkins, Baltimore, MD; Cleveland Clinic Foundation, Cleveland, OH; Massachusetts General, Boston, MA; UCLA Medical Center, Los Angeles, CA; New York Presbyterian, New York, NY; UCSF Medical Center, San Francisco, CA; Stanford Hospital, Stanford, CA; and Brigham and Women's, Boston, MA.

Appendix B:

Special Considerations for Cancer Cases

The types of cases used in our calculation of risk-adjusted death rates did not include cases in which cancer was the diagnosis listed as the primary reason for hospital admission. Calculating risk-adjusted death rates is not as meaningful for cancer cases as for many other types of cases. Often, what the hospital does can have little or no effect on whether the patient dies within 30 days after hospital admission, which is the period for which the hospital death rates were calculated. The death from cancer may be unavoidable, and the hospital's efforts may be focused on pain reduction or treatment of secondary problems. Some hospitals may have a higher proportion of advanced cancer cases than other hospitals have, depending in part on community customs and resources for treating such cases in nursing homes, hospices, or other settings.

Nonetheless, it is important to choose a top-quality institution for the treatment of cancer, whether inpatient or outpatient. Choice of such an institution might have a big effect on the long-term outcome.

One indication of an institution's competence in the treatment of cancer is designation by the National Cancer Institute (NCI) as a Comprehensive Cancer Center or a Clinical Cancer Center. This designation is given to major academic and research institutions throughout the United States with broad-based, coordinated, interdisciplinary programs in cancer research. These institutions have been selected by the NCI for scientific excellence and capability to integrate a diversity of research approaches to focus on the problem of cancer. In addition to doing research, the institutions also treat patients.

A further indication of an institution's competence in treating cancer is membership in the National Comprehensive Cancer Network (NCCN). NCCN is a not-for-profit alliance of leading cancer centers. It seeks to help member institutions to do excellent research, measure the outcomes of the care they provide, and provide state-of-the-art cancer care to as many patients as possible.

The following is a list of NCI-designated Comprehensive and Clinical Cancer Centers and NCCN network members. All institutions on the list are NCI-designated Centers except where noted. Those that are also NCCN members are identified. Bear in mind that there are many other high-quality institutions that might be more convenient for you, but you or your physician might want to seek advice or referrals from professionals at the listed institutions.

Alabama

University of Alabama at Birmingham Comprehensive Cancer Center, Birmingham, AL (NCCN member hospital)

Arizona

Arizona Cancer Center, Tucson, AZ

California

City of Hope National Medical Center & Beckman Research Institute, Duarte, CA (NCCN member hospital)

University of California at San Diego Cancer Center, La Jolla, CA

Jonsson Comprehensive Cancer Center, Los Angeles, CA

University of Southern California/Norris Comprehensive Cancer Center, Los Angeles, CA

Chao Family Comprehensive Cancer Center, Orange, CA

Stanford Hospitals and Clinics, Stanford, CA (NCCN member hospital but not an NCI-designated Cancer Center)

University of California San Francisco Cancer Center & Cancer Research Institute, San Francisco, CA (NCCN member hospital)

Colorado

Univ. of Colorado Cancer Center, Denver, CO

Connecticut

Yale Cancer Center, New Haven, CT

District of Columbia

Lombardi Cancer Research Center, Washington, DC

Florida

H. Lee Moffitt Cancer Center & Research Institute at the University of South Florida, Tampa, FL (NCCN member hospital)

Hawaii

Cancer Research Center of Hawaii, Honolulu, HI

Illinois

University of Chicago Cancer Research Center, Chicago, IL

Robert H. Lurie Cancer Center, Chicago, IL (NCCN member hospital)

Indiana

Indiana Univ. Cancer Center, Indianapolis, IN

Iowa

Holden Comprehensive Cancer Center at the University of Iowa, Iowa City, IA

Maryland

The Sidney Kimmel Comprehensive Cancer Center at Johns Hopkins, Baltimore, MD (NCCN member hospital)

Massachusetts

Dana-Farber/Harvard Cancer Center, Boston, MA (NCCN member hospital)

Michigan

University of Michigan Comprehensive Cancer Center, Ann Arbor, MI (NCCN member hospital)

Barbara Ann Karmanos Cancer Institute, Detroit, MI

Minnesota

University of Minnesota Cancer Center, Minneapolis, MN

Mayo Clinic Cancer Center, Rochester, MN

Missouri

Siteman Cancer Center, St. Louis, MO

Nebraska

University of Nebraska Medical Center/Eppley Cancer Center, Omaha, NE (NCCN member hospital)

New Hampshire

Norris Cotton Cancer Center/Dartmouth-Hitchcock Medical Center, Lebanon, NH

New Jersey

The Cancer Institute of New Jersey, New Brunswick, NJ

New York

Cancer Research Center/Albert Einstein College of Medicine, Bronx, NY

Roswell Park Cancer Institute, Buffalo, NY (NCCN member hospital)

Kaplan Cancer Center/New York University Medical Center, New York, NY

Memorial Sloan-Kettering Cancer Center, New York, NY (NCCN member hospital)

Herbert Irving Comprehensive Cancer Center, New York, NY

North Carolina

University of North Carolina Lineberger Comprehensive Cancer Ctr, Chapel Hill, NC

Duke Comprehensive Cancer Ctr, Durham, NC (NCCN member hospital)

Comprehensive Cancer Center/Wake Forest Univ., Winston-Salem, NC

Ohio

Ireland Cancer Center, Cleveland, OH

Arthur G. James Cancer Hospital & Richard J. Solove Research Institute, Columbus, OH (NCCN member hospital)

Oregon

Oregon Cancer Center, Portland, OR

Pennsylvania

University of Pennsylvania Cancer Center, Philadelphia, PA

Fox Chase Cancer Center, Philadelphia, PA (NCCN member hospital)

Kimmel Cancer Center, Philadelphia, PA

University of Pittsburgh Cancer Institute, Pittsburgh, PA

Tennessee

St. Jude Children's Research Hospital, Memphis, TN (NCCN member hospital)

Vanderbilt-Ingram Cancer Center, Nashville, TN

Texas

M.D. Anderson Cancer Center, Houston, TX (NCCN member hospital)

San Antonio Cancer Institute, San Antonio, TX

Utah

Huntsman Cancer Institute, Salt Lake City, UT (NCCN member hospital)

Vermont

Vermont Cancer Center, Burlington, VT

Virginia

Cancer Center/University of Virginia, Health Sciences Center, Charlottesville, VA

Massey Cancer Center, Richmond, VA

Washington

Fred Hutchinson Cancer Research Center, Seattle, WA (NCCN member hospital)

Wisconsin

Comprehensive Cancer Center/University of Wisconsin, Madison, WI

Appendix C:

Hospitals Recognized for Excellence in Nursing Services

Another indicator of hospital quality, not shown on the tables in this book, is recognition of a hospital by the Magnet Nursing Services Recognition Program for Excellence in Nursing Services. This recognition is given by the American Nurses Credentialing Center, established by the American Nurses Association. Forty-six acute care hospitals currently have this recognition. They are listed below. We have found that these hospitals also have significantly lower risk-adjusted mortality rates than other hospitals in our "all cases" category, and they were rated much higher than other hospitals by the physicians we surveyed.

Alabama
University of Alabama, Birmingham

California
Cedars - Sinai, Los Angeles
University of California - Davis, Sacramento

Colorado
Poudre Valley, Fort Collins
University of Colorado, Denver

Connecticut
Middlesex, Middletown

Florida
Baptist, Miami
Bayfront, St Petersburg
Mt Sinai, Miami Beach
West Boca, Boca Raton

Georgia
Candler, Savannah
St Joseph's, Savannah
St Joseph's, Atlanta

Idaho
St Luke's Regional, Boise

Illinois
Children's, Chicago

Kentucky
Jewish, Louisville
University of Kentucky, Lexington

Minnesota
Rochester Methodist, Rochester
St Marys, Rochester

New Jersey
Capital - Mercer, Trenton
Hackensack University, Hackensack
Jersey Shore, Neptune
Morristown Memorial, Morristown
Riverview, Red Bank
Robert Wood Johnson Univ., New Brunswick
St Francis, Trenton
St Joseph's Regional, Paterson
St Peter's University, New Brunswick

New York
Long Island Jewish, New Hyde Park
North Shore University, Manhasset

North Carolina
Catawba, Hickory
High Point Regional, High Point
North Carolina Baptist, Winston-Salem

Oregon
Providence St Vincent, Portland

Pennsylvania
Fox Chase Cancer Center, Philadelphia

Rhode Island
Miriam, Providence

South Dakota
Avera McKennan, Sioux Falls

Texas
St Lukes Episcopal, Houston
Univ. of Texas MD Anderson Cancer Ctr, Houston

Virginia
Inova Fairfax, Falls Church

Washington
University of Washington, Seattle

Wisconsin
Hartford Memorial, Hartford
St Luke's, Milwaukee
St Luke's South Shore, Cudahy
Sinai Samaritan, Milwaukee
West Allis Memorial, West Allis

Appendix D:

A Patient's Bill of Rights

A Patient's Bill of Rights was first adopted by the American Hospital Association (AHA) in 1973. This revision was approved by the AHA Board of Trustees on October 21, 1992.

Introduction

Effective health care requires collaboration between patients and physicians and other health care professionals. Open and honest communication, respect for personal and professional values, and sensitivity to differences are integral to optimal patient care. As the setting for the provision of health services, hospitals must provide a foundation for understanding and respecting the rights and responsibilities of patients, their families, physicians, and other caregivers. Hospitals must ensure a health care ethic that respects the role of patients in decision making about treatment choices and other aspects of their care. Hospitals must be sensitive to cultural, racial, linguistic, religious, age, gender, and other differences as well as the needs of persons with disabilities.

The American Hospital Association presents A Patient's Bill of Rights with the expectation that it will contribute to more effective patient care and be supported by the hospital on behalf of the institution, its medical staff, employees, and patients. The American Hospital Association encourages health care institutions to tailor this bill of rights to their patient community by translating and/or simplifying the language of this bill of rights as may be necessary to ensure that patients and their families understand their rights and responsibilities.

Bill of Rights

These rights can be exercised on the patient's behalf by a designated surrogate or proxy decision maker if the patient lacks decision-making capacity, is legally incompetent, or is a minor.

1. The patient has the right to considerate and respectful care.
2. The patient has the right to and is encouraged to obtain from physicians and other direct caregivers relevant, current, and understandable information concerning diagnosis, treatment, and prognosis.

   Except in emergencies when the patient lacks decision-making capacity and the need for treatment is urgent, the patient is entitled to the opportunity to discuss and request information related to the specific procedures and/or treatments, the risks involved, the possible length of recuperation, and the medically reasonable alternatives and their accompanying risks and benefits.

   Patients have the right to know the identity of physicians, nurses, and others involved in their care, as well as when those involved are students, residents, or other trainees. The patient also has the right to know the immediate and long-term financial implications of treatment choices, insofar as they are known.
3. The patient has the right to make decisions about the plan of care prior to and during the course of treatment and to refuse a recommended treatment or plan of care to the extent permitted by law and hospital policy and to be informed of the medical consequences of this action. In case of such refusal, the patient is entitled to other appropriate care and services that the hospital provides or transfer to another hospital. The hospital should notify patients of any policy that might affect patient choice within the institution.
4. The patient has the right to have an advance directive (such as a living will, health care proxy, or durable power of attorney for health care) concerning treatment or designating a surrogate decision maker with the expectation that the hospital will honor the intent of that directive to the extent permitted by law and hospital policy.

   Health care institutions must advise patients of their rights under state law and hospital policy to make informed medical choices, ask if the patient has an advance directive, and include that information in patient records. The patient has the right to timely information about hospital policy that may limit its ability to implement fully a legally valid advance directive.
5. The patient has the right to every consideration of privacy. Case discussion, consultation, examination, and treatment should be conducted so as to protect each patient's privacy.
6. The patient has the right to expect that all communications and records pertaining to his/her care will be treated as confidential by the hospital, except in cases such as suspected abuse and public health hazards when reporting is permitted or required by law. The patient has the right to expect that the hospital will emphasize the confidentiality of this information when it releases it to any other parties entitled to review information in these records.
7. The patient has the right to review the records pertaining to his/her medical care and to have the information explained or interpreted as necessary, except when restricted by law.
8. The patient has the right to expect that, within its capacity and policies, a hospital will make reasonable response to the request of a patient for appropriate and medically indicated care and services. The hospital must provide evaluation, service, and/or referral as indicated by the urgency of the case. When medically appropriate and legally permissible, or when a patient has so requested, a patient may be transferred to another facility. The institution to which the patient is to be transferred must first have accepted the patient for transfer. The patient must also have the benefit of complete information and explanation concerning the need for, risks, benefits, and alternatives to such a transfer.
9. The patient has the right to ask and be informed of the existence of business relationships among the hospital, educational institutions,

other health care providers, or payers that may influence the patient's treatment and care.

10. The patient has the right to consent to or decline to participate in proposed research studies or human experimentation affecting care and treatment or requiring direct patient involvement, and to have those studies fully explained prior to consent. A patient who declines to participate in research or experimentation is entitled to the most effective care that the hospital can otherwise provide.
11. The patient has the right to expect reasonable continuity of care when appropriate and to be informed by physicians and other caregivers of available and realistic patient care options when hospital care is no longer appropriate.
12. The patient has the right to be informed of hospital policies and practices that relate to patient care, treatment, and responsibilities. The patient has the right to be informed of available resources for resolving disputes, grievances, and conflicts, such as ethics committees, patient representatives, or other mechanisms available in the institution. The patient has the right to be informed of the hospital's charges for services and available payment methods.

The collaborative nature of health care requires that patients, or their families/surrogates, participate in their care. The effectiveness of care and patient satisfaction with the course of treatment depend, in part, on the patient fulfilling certain responsibilities. Patients are responsible for providing information about past illnesses, hospitalizations, medications, and other matters related to health status. To participate effectively in decision making, patients must be encouraged to take responsibility for requesting additional information or clarification about their health status or treatment when they do not fully understand information and instructions. Patients are also responsible for ensuring that the health care institution has a copy of their written advance directive if they have one. Patients are responsible for informing their physicians and other caregivers if they anticipate problems in following prescribed treatment.

Patients should also be aware of the hospital's obligation to be reasonably efficient and equitable in providing care to other patients and the community. The hospital's rules and regulations are designed to help the hospital meet this obligation. Patients and their families are responsible for making reasonable accommodations to the needs of the hospital, other patients, medical staff, and hospital employees. Patients are responsible for providing necessary information for insurance claims and for working with the hospital to make payment arrangements, when necessary.

A person's health depends on much more than health care services. Patients are responsible for recognizing the impact of their life-style on their personal health.

Conclusion

Hospitals have many functions to perform, including the enhancement of health status, health promotion, and the prevention and treatment of injury and disease; the immediate and ongoing care and rehabilitation of patients; the education of health professionals, patients, and the community; and research. All these activities must be conducted with an overriding concern for the values and dignity of patients.

Appendix E:

Where to Complain

Alabama
Bureau of Health Provider Standards
Department of Public Health
Complaints Unit, Suite 600
P.O. Box 303017
Montgomery, AL 36130-3017
1-800-356-9596 (in-state) or
334-206-5300

Alaska
State Health Facilities Licensing and Certification
4730 Business Park Boulevard, Suite 18
Anchorage, AK 99503
907-334-2483

Arizona
Assurance & Licensure Services
1647 East Morten Avenue
Phoenix, AZ 85040
602-674-4340

Arkansas
Department of Health Facilities Services
Freeway Medical Building
5800 West 10th Street, Suite 400
Little Rock, AR 72204
501-661-2201

California
Department of Health Services
Licensing and Certification Division
1800 3rd Street, Suite 210
Sacramento, CA 95814
916-445-3054

Colorado
Department of Public Health and Environment
Health Facilities Division
4300 Cherry Creek Drive South
Denver, CO 80246
303-692-2800

Connecticut
Department of Public Health
Division of Health Services Administration
410 Capital Avenue
P.O. Box 340308, M.S. 12HFL
Hartford, CT 06134-0308
860-509-7400

Delaware
Health and Social Services
Health Facilities Licensing and Certification
2055 Limestone Road, Suite 200
Wilmington, DE 19808
800-942-7373

District of Columbia
Department of Public Health
Health Regulation Administration
825 North Capital Street NE, 2nd Floor
Washington, DC 20002
202-442-5888

Florida
Department of Health
Agency for Health Care Administration
2727 Mahan Drive
Tallahassee, FL 32308
888-419-3456

Georgia
Department of Public Health
Office of Regulatory Services
Complaint Unit
2 Peachtree Street NW, 31st Floor
Atlanta, GA 30303
404-657-5726

Hawaii
State Department of Health
Office of Health Assurance
601 Kamokile Boulevard, Suite 395
Kapolei, HI 96797
808-692-7420

Idaho
Department of Health and Welfare
Division of Medicaid Facility Standards
3380 Americana Terrace, Suite 230
Boise, ID 83706
208-334-6626

Illinois
Department of Public Health
Healthcare Facilities and Programs
525 West Jefferson Street, 4th Floor
Springfield, IL 62761
1-800-252-4343 (in-state) or
217-782-7412

Indiana
State Department of Health
Division of Acute Care
2 North Meridian Street
Indianapolis, IN 46204
(317) 233-7474

Iowa
Department of Public Health
Inspection and Appeals
Lucas Office Building, 3rd Floor
321 East 12th Street
Des Moines, IA 50319-0083
1-800-383-4920

Kansas
Deptartment of Health and Environment
Division of Health
Bureau of Health Facilities
1000 SW Jackson, Suite 330
Topeka, KS 66612-1365
1-800-842-0078

Kentucky
Cabinet for Health Services
Office of Inspector General
Division of Community Health Services
908 West Broadway
Louisville, KY 40203
502-595-4079

Louisiana
Department of Public Health and Hospitals
DHH/Health Standards Section
P.O. Box 3767
500 Laurel Street, Suite 100
Baton Rouge, LA 70802
225-342-6429

Maine
Department of Human Services
Bureau of Medical Services
Division of Licensing and Certification
35 Anthony Avenue, Station 11
Augusta, ME 04333
207-624-5443

Maryland
Department of Health and Mental Hygiene
Licensing and Certification Division
Office of Health Care Quality
55 Wade Avenue
Catonsville, MD 21228
410-402-8015

Massachusetts
Department of Public Health
Division of Health Care Quality
Complaint Unit
10 West Street, 5th Floor
Boston, MA 02111
617-753-8000

Michigan
Department of Consumer and Industry Services
Bureau of Health Systems
Division of Licensing and Certification
Complaint Intake Unit
P.O. Box 30664
Lansing, MI 48909
1-800-882-6006

Minnesota
Department of Health
Office of Health Facility Complaints
P.O. Box 64970
St. Paul, MN 55164-0970
1-800-369-7994 or
651-215-8702

Mississippi
State Department of Health
Health Facilities Licensure and Certification
Complaint Dept
P.O. Box 1700
Jackson, MS 39215
1-800-227-7308

Missouri
Health and Senior Services
Bureau of Health Facility Regulation
P.O. Box 570
Jefferson City, MO 65102
573-751-6308

Montana
Department of Health and Human Services
Certification Bureau
2401 Colonial Drive, 2nd Floor
Helena, MT 59601
406-444-2099

Nebraska
Department of HHS Regulation and Licensure
Division of Investigations
Facility Complaints
P.O. Box 94986
Lincoln, NE 68509-4986
(402) 471-1719

Nevada
Health Division
Bureau of Lisensure and Certification
1550 College Parkway, Suite 158
Carson City, NV 89706-7921
775-687-4475

New Hampshire
Department of Health and Human Services
Health Facilities Administration
Licensing Office
129 Pleasant Street
Concord, NH 03301
603-271-4607

New Jersey
Department of Health and Senior Services
Inspection, Compliance, and Complaints
Market and Warren Streets
Trenton, NJ 08625
609-633-7048

New Mexico
Department of Health
Division of Health Improvement
Health Facility Licensing and Certification
2040 South Pacheco Street, 2nd Floor
Sante Fe, NM 87505
1-800-752-8649
505-476-9053

New York
Department of Health
Bureau of Hospitals and Primary Care Services
Hadley Park Place
433 River Street, 6th Floor
Troy, NY 12180
518-402-1003

North Carolina
Division of Public Health
Department of Health and Human Services
Facilities Services Complaints Branch
Broughton Building
805 Biggs Drive, Dix Campus
Raleigh, NC 27603
919-733-7461

North Dakota
Department of Health
Division of Health Facilities
600 East Boulevard Avenue, Department 301
Bismarck, ND 58505-0200
701-328-2352

Ohio
Department of Health
Complaint Unit
246 North High Street
Columbus, OH 43215

Oklahoma
Department of Health
Medical Facilities Division
1000 NE Tenth, Room 1114
Oklahoma City, OK 73117-1299
405-271-6576

Oregon
Public Health Services
Health Care Licensure
800 NE Oregon Street
Portland, OR 97232

Pennsylvania
Department of Health
Bureau of Facility Licensure and Certification
Division of Acute and Ambulatory Care
P.O. Box 90
Harrisburg, PA 17108
1-877-724-2584

Rhode Island
Department of Health
Division of Facilities Regulation
3 Capitol Hill, Room 306
Providence, RI 02908
401-222-2566

South Carolina
Department of Health
Division of Health Licensing
2600 Bull Street
Columbia, SC 29201
803-545-4370

South Dakota
Department of Health
Licensure and Certification Division
615 East 4th Street
Pierre, SD 57501-1700
605-773-3356

Tennessee
Division of Health Care Facilities
Centralized Complaint Intake Unit
425 5th Avenue North
Cordell Hull Building, 1st Floor
Nashville, TN 37247-0508
1-877-287-0010

Texas
Health Facility Licensing and Compliance
Department of Health
1100 West 49th Street
Austin, TX 78756
1-888-973-0022

Utah
Department of Health
Central Office
P.O. Box 142003
288 N 1460 W
Salt Lake City, UT 84114-2003

Vermont
Department of Aging and Disabilities
Division of Licensing and Protection
Ladd Hall
103 South Main Street
Waterbury, VT 055671
1-800564-1612 (in-state) or
802-241-2345

Virginia
Department of Health
Quality Health Care and Consumer Protection
3600 West Broad Street, Suite 216
Richmond, VA 23230-4920
804-367-2133

Washington
Department of Health
Office of Health Care Survey
Facilities and Services Licensing
P.O. Box 47852
Olympia, WA 98504-785
1-800-633-6828 or
360-705-6612

West Virginia
Bureau for Public Health
Health Facility Licensure and Certification
350 Capital Street, Suite 206
Charleston, WV 25301-3718
304-558-0050

Wisconsin
Department of Health and Family Services
Bureau of Quality Assurance
Health Services Section
P.O. Box 2969
Madison, WI 53701-2969
608-266-8084

Wyoming
Department of Health
Office of Health Quality
Healthcare Facilities Complaints
2020 Carey Avenue, 8th Floor
Cheyenne, WY 82002
307-777-7123